Treatment
of Mental Disorders

D0637315

Treatment
of Mental Disorders

edited by

John H. Greist, M.D.
UNIVERSITY OF WISCONSIN MEDICAL SCHOOL

James W. Jefferson, M.D.
UNIVERSITY OF WISCONSIN MEDICAL SCHOOL

Robert L. Spitzer, M.D.
COLUMBIA UNIVERSITY COLLEGE OF PHYSICIANS AND SURGEONS

NEW YORK   OXFORD
Oxford University Press
1982

Copyright © 1982 by Oxford University Press, Inc.

LIBRARY OF CONGRESS CATALOGING IN PUBLICATION DATA
Main entry under title:

Treatment of mental disorders.

  Bibliography: p.
  Includes index.
  1. Psychiatry—Addresses, essays, lectures.
2. Psychotherapy—Addresses, essays, lectures.
I. Greist, John H.   II. Jefferson, James W.
III. Spitzer, Robert L. [DNLM: 1. Mental dis-
orders—Therapy.   WN 400 T7847]
RC458.T73   616.89'1   82-3423
ISBN 0-19-502101-6   AACR2
ISBN 0-19-503107-5 (pbk.)

Printing (last digit): 9 8 7 6 5 4 3 2 1

Printed in the United States of America

To the memory of Adolf Meyer
and those he taught

Preface

The study and treatment of mental disorders have come to a crossroads. Schools of most competing therapies are gradually discarding their reliance on doctrinaire beliefs and beginning to argue from the high scientific ground of study populations relatively homogeneous for important variables, randomization, detailed specification of treatments, ratings by unbiased observers, and suitable follow-up evaluation. Yet the many threads of evidence that make up the fabric of optimal clinical practice are difficult for the individual clinician to find and weave together. The third edition of the *Diagnostic and Statistical Manual of Mental Disorders* (DSM-III) adds another pattern to what may seem an increasingly complex tapestry.

Treatment of Mental Disorders presents the state of the art and science of psychiatric treatments as they are known and practiced today. Its publication provides practitioners in psychiatry, psychiatric nursing, psychology, and social work with a convenient and authoritative source of practical information regarding the treatment of mental disorders in adults. The contributors are experts in their respective areas and they have emphasized treatment methods of proven effectiveness. Critical reviews of the literature, highlighting well-controlled studies, are supplemented with descriptions of current clinical practice when controlled research has not been conducted.

The editors are convinced that although there are logically preferred treatments for specific disorders, patients may not respond logically to standard treatment approaches. Awareness of and willingness to use a range of treatment methods is the hallmark of the compleat clinician. Achieving a balance between and integration of dynamic and behavioral psychotherapies and somatic treatments is a continuing goal for our professions, and it has been our goal in organizing *Treatment of Mental Disorders*. Thus, even in the chapter on organic mental disorders, which some would segregate as requiring organic treatments, the authors also emphasize the psychotherapeutic aspects of caring for patients and their families. Conversely, the chapter on the treatment of personality disorders, long the domain of psychotherapists, highlights the often neglected role of medications. Although few would question the primacy of somatic treatments of schizophrenia, Chapter 5 also emphasizes the important roles and timing of individual and group psychotherapies and community-based supportive therapy. Similarly, affective disorders have come under much better control with the availability of antidepressant and lithium medications, yet Chapter 6 makes clear the demonstrated value of social and psychotherapies as well and specifically addresses issues of relevance to the treatment of women, who make up approximately two-thirds of the population with depression.

Throughout this book, the contributors provide specific guidance for clinicians faced with patients who have particular mental disorders. Where appropriate, they have used a chapter format that proceeds from a description of treatment goals to specific treatment methods to a discussion of treatment controversies and finally a summary. Sharp controversies about treatments still exist in many areas and, to some extent, represent the interface between old and new paradigms of practice. Discussions of these controversies often provide glimmerings of the future.

The essential features of the disorders are extracted from DSM-III and presented with the permission of the American Psychiatric Association. *Treatment of Mental Disorders* thus complements DSM-III by presenting treatments for the adult disorders described therein. Because it follows the DSM-III system of classification, this book can serve as a useful connection between DSM-III diagnostic criteria and current therapeutic practice.

Two chapters not directly related to the DSM-III system have been included because of their clinical importance. Sleep disorders are common and knowledge about them is rapidly advancing. Chapter 18 provides a straightforward classification of sleep disorders and a balanced approach to their management. The issue of compliance or adherence is important across all disorders and to all health care professions. Antidepressants left on the shelf will not relieve depression. Chapter 19 offers a concise summary of the literature on compliance in several psychiatric disorders and specific guidance for helping patients improve compliance.

Learning when and how to use the most appropriate treatments for specific mental disorders and to recognize and manage unwanted treatment effects is an ongoing task for mental health clinicians. The editors are confident that this book will help clinicians select the best treatments available for their patients.

John H. Greist
James W. Jefferson
Robert L. Spitzer

February, 1982

Acknowledgments

The publication of *Treatments for Mental Disorders* required the efforts and good will of many people. Our respective universities, departments, and colleagues have supported this work in ways both hidden and obvious. The contributors have responded in a timely and gracious manner to our repeated requests for revisions and updates.

Jeff House's persistence provided momentum that brought this work to completion. He is truly an editor's editor. Brenda Jones' copy-editing has markedly improved the organization and consistency of presentation, which can be troublesome in multi-authored works.

Georgia Greist has read and remedied deficiencies in the entire manuscript at all stages of preparation. Lynn De Weese, Rosalie Breitenbach, and Jan Montgomery from the Department of Psychiatry at the University of Wisconsin have assisted by typing several chapters. Jean Lechnir's consummate skill with our word processor and unstinting efforts on all chapters of this manuscript throughout their many revisions have brought this book to fruition. She deserves and has our special thanks.

Contents

Contributors xv

Introduction xvii

1. Organic Mental Disorders 3
   CHARLES E. WELLS
   and JOSEPH P. McEVOY

2. Substance Induced and Substance Use Disorders: Alcohol 44
   DONALD W. GOODWIN

3. Substance Induced and Substance Use Disorders: Barbiturates and Similarly Acting Sedative Hypnotics 62
   BARRY LISKOW

4. Substance Induced and Substance Use Disorders (opioids, cocaine, amphetamines and similarly acting sympathomimetics, phencyclidine (PCP), inhalants, hallucinogens and cannabis, tobacco, caffeine) 78
   PHILIP A. BERGER
   and MEREDITH J. DUNN

5. Schizophrenic Disorders 143
   GEORGE M. SIMPSON
   and PHILIP R.A. MAY

6. Affective Disorders 184
   ANDREA JACOBSON
   and WILLIAM T. McKINNEY

7. Anxiety Disorders 234
   ISAAC MARKS

8. Somatoform Disorders 266
   HERBERT OCHITILL,
   ROBERT KELLNER,
   and CARL J. GETTO

9. Dissociative Disorders 309
   GENE COMBS, JR.
   and ARNOLD M. LUDWIG

10. Gender Identity Disorders and Transvestism 320
    RICHARD GREEN

11. Paraphilias and Ego-dystonic Homosexuality 338
    ISAAC MARKS

12. Psychosexual Dysfunctions 365
    HELEN SINGER KAPLAN
    and JAMES LAWRENCE MOODIE

13. Factitious Disorders 387
    JAMES W. JEFFERSON
    and HERBERT OCHITILL

14. Disorders of Impulse Control (not elsewhere classified) 398
ROBERT KELLNER

15. Adjustment Disorders 419
JOHN H. GREIST

16. Personality Disorders 429
ROBERT KELLNER

17. V Codes for Conditions not Attributable to a Mental Disorder that are a Focus of Treatment 455
CARL J. GETTO

18. Diagnosis and Treatment of Sleep Disorders 473
JOYCE D. KALES,
CONSTANTIN R. SOLDATOS,
and ANTHONY KALES

19. Treatment Compliance 501
BARRY BLACKWELL

Subject Index 517

Author Index 540

CONTRIBUTORS

Philip A. Berger, M.D., Department of Psychiatry and Behavioral Sciences, Stanford University, Stanford, California

Barry Blackwell, M.D., Department of Psychiatry, University of Wisconsin-Mt. Sinai, Milwaukee, Wisconsin

Gene Combs, Jr., M.D., Department of Psychiatry, University of Kentucky, Lexington, Kentucky

Meredith J. Dunn, M.A., Dip. Ed., Department of Pediatrics, Stanford University, Stanford, California

Carl J. Getto, M.D., Department of Psychiatry, University of Wisconsin, Madison, Wisconsin

Donald W. Goodwin, M.D., Department of Psychiatry, University of Kansas College of Health Sciences, Kansas City, Kansas

Richard Green, M.D., Department of Psychiatry and Behavioral Sciences, State University of New York at Stony Brook, Stony Brook, New York

John H. Greist, M.D., Department of Psychiatry, University of Wisconsin, Madison, Wisconsin

Andrea Jacobson, M.D., South Bay Psychiatric Clinic, Campbell, California

James W. Jefferson, M.D., Department of Psychiatry, University of Wisconsin, Madison, Wisconsin

Anthony Kales, M.D., Department of Psychiatry, Pennsylvania State University College of Medicine, Hershey, Pennsylvania

Joyce D. Kales, M.D., Department of Psychiatry, Pennsylvania State University College of Medicine, Hershey, Pennsylvania

Helen S. Kaplan, M.D., Ph.D., Payne-Whitney Clinic, Cornell Medical Center, New York, New York

Robert Kellner, M.D., Ph.D., Department of Psychiatry, University of New Mexico, Albuquerque, New Mexico

Gerald L. Klerman, M.D., Harvard Medical School, Massachusetts General Hospital, Boston, Massachusetts

Barry Liskow, M.D., Department of Psychiatry, University of Kansas College of Health Sciences, Kansas City, Kansas

Arnold Ludwig, M.D., Department of Psychiatry, University of Kentucky, Lexington, Kentucky

Isaac Marks, M.D., Institute of Psychiatry, Maudsley and Bethlehem Royal Hospitals, London, England

Philip R.A. May, M.D., Neuropsychiatric Institute, University of California, Los Angeles, California

Joseph P. McEvoy, M.D., Department of Psychiatry, Vanderbilt University School of Medicine, Nashville, Tennessee

William T. McKinney, Jr., M.D., Department of Psychiatry, University of Wisconsin, Madison, Wisconsin

J. Lawrence Moodie, M.D., Department of Psychiatry, Cornell University Medical College, New York, New York

Herbert Ochitill, M.D., Department of Psychiatry, University of California, San Francisco, California

George M. Simpson, M.D., Department of Psychiatry and the Behavioral Sciences, University of Southern California, Los Angeles, California

Constantin R. Soldatos, M.D., Department of Psychiatry, Pennsylvania State University College of Medicine, Hershey, Pennsylvania

Robert L. Spitzer, M.D., New York State Psychiatric Institute, Columbia University College of Physicians and Surgeons, New York, New York

Charles E. Wells, M.D., Department of Psychiatry, Vanderbilt University School of Medicine, Nashville, Tennessee

Introduction

GERALD L. KLERMAN

The editors of this volume and the authors of the individual chapters have provided us with a comprehensive survey of the current "state of the art" of psychiatric treatment. Because the material is so well organized, the reader may not be aware of the significant advances in psychiatric research and therapeutics over the past 25 years which are embodied in this volume.

Three essential features of the book provide a remarkable affirmation of psychiatry as a medical specialty:

1. The chapters are organized around individual mental disorders following the classification in the American Psychiatric Association's *Diagnostic and Statistical Manual*, Third Edition (DSM-III).

2. For each disorder, a range of treatments is discussed, including drug, psychodynamic, behavioral, group, and family therapy.

3. The discussion gives priority to evidence derived from controlled studies over clinical experience or the views of authorities.

That the book incorporates these three features is a testimony to recent progress. A similar volume could not have been written in the early 1950's.

The Principle of Discrete Mental Disorders

The development of DSM-III and the decision to organize this volume around the DSM-III criteria represent a significant reversal of thinking about diagnosis and classification within the mental health professions and elsewhere. The concept of discrete disorders or illnesses was proven valid in the nineteenth century when clinical syndromes initially based on temporal covariation of signs and symptoms were related to two types of biological correlates: anatomical and histopathologic findings at autopsy and bacteria and other microorganisms identified in the laboratory. These advances in basic laboratory biology placed medicine on a scientific basis, and were rapidly applied to psychiatry, particularly in France, Germany, and Austria. In the latter half of the nineteenth century, attempts were made to correlate various psychiatric syndromes with autopsy and bacteriological findings. This, however, left a large residual group of psychotic states unaccounted for. Kraepelin divided these so-called "functional psychoses" into two large groups, which he called "manic depressive insanity" and "dementia praecox." This division of the psychotic disorders became the foundation for subsequent classifications.

There were notable successes in early biological research on "psychiatric" conditions. By 1895, clinical and epidemiological studies had shown that central nervous system syphilis was associated with the syndrome of general paresis, and these associations were confirmed by the development of the Wassermann Test in 1905 and the isolation of the spirochete in brains by Noguchi in 1911. After World War I, Goldberger and his associates in the U.S. Public Health Service discovered the relationship between pellagra and nutritional vitamin B deficiency. In addition to elucidating the biological basis of the disorder, this paved the way for effective treatment and, ultimately, prevention.

From the 1920's through the 1950's, progress in discovering biological correlates of psychiatric disorders seemed to come to a halt. However, this was not the case with mental retardation. Discoveries of chromosomal anomalies led to an understanding of Down's and other syndromes, and discoveries of multiple aminoacidurias further clarified the varied pathogenesis of mental retardation.

Nevertheless, the concept of discrete disorders and the medical model applied to psychiatry came under considerable criticism within the profession and from without. Four lines of criticism were voiced and debated during the 1960's and 70's:

1. The most fundamental was the challenge to the "medical model" made by Szasz (1974). Following his lead, the anti-psychiatrists and the labeling theorists in sociology and psychology rejected the basic premise of psychiatry that mental disorders, such as

psychoses, neuroses, and personality disorders, are true medical illnesses. They argued that in the absence of neurologic or physiologic evidence of biological abnormality, the application of the concept of illness to behavior, and to emotional and cognitive states represented social control of deviance rather than medical practice.

2. A second objection focused on the low reliability of psychiatric diagnoses made by clinicians and researchers. The absence of agreement on diagnoses among clinicians in dramatic court cases undermined the credibility of the mental health professions.

3. A third criticism pointed to the adverse social and psychological consequences of psychiatric diagnosis. This view was expressed forcefully by Karl Menninger in his influential book, *The Vital Balance* (1963). This volume drew attention to the dehumanizing and depersonalizing effects that psychiatric diagnoses often had. This point was taken up by the labeling theorists, particularly Scheff and Lemere, who saw diagnostic practices as indicative of the social control function of psychiatry. Many labeling theorists went further to deny the existence of any intrinsic differences between those individuals who later came to be "labeled" mentally ill and those displaying other forms of deviance. The most dramatic effort to document this phenomenon was described by Rosenhan in his widely quoted article, "On Being Sane in Insane Places" (1973).

4. The fourth line of criticism developed within the research community, mainly from the work of psychologists and statisticians experienced in multivariate statistical techniques. These critics did not challenge the existence of psychiatric illness or the appropriateness of research in psychopathology. Rather, they questioned the categorical or typological nature of the diagnostic systems. Advocating the use of dimensional approaches, they pointed out that sharp boundaries between normal and abnormal do not exist and that many of the phenomena involved in the diagnosis of psychopathology are extensions of normal behavior and emo-

tions such as anxiety and depression. Lorr, Overall, and Eysenck in psychology and Strauss and others in psychiatry are among the researchers who have expanded this view.

Confronted by these challenges, the psychiatric research community responded vigorously. By the early 1960's, there was a growing awareness among clinicians as well as researchers that the absence of an objective and reliable system for the description of psychopathology and for psychiatric diagnosis was limiting progress. In 1965, the National Institute of Mental Health Psychopharmacology Research Branch sponsored a conference on classification in psychiatry that noted the problems created by inadequate diagnosis and classification. In the decade and a half since that conference, there have been major achievements in three areas: understanding sources of cross-national differences in diagnostic practices, improving the precision and reliability of these practices, and developing methods for their validation.

Cross-National Differences in Diagnosis. Two major studies clarified diagnostic practices and helped develop comparable data on mental disorders in different countries. The first, the United States–United Kingdom study organized by Kramer (1969) and Zubin (1969), sought to determine whether reported U.S.–U.K. differences in the rates of depression and schizophrenia among patients admitted to mental hospitals in the two countries were real or artifacts due to different diagnostic practices. It was found that American psychiatrists tended to diagnose as schizophrenic patients who would be considered depressed or manic by British psychiatrists. About the same time the World Health Organization undertook a study to determine whether forms of schizophrenia could be identified in nations with different political and social characteristics (Wing et al., 1974). The results of both studies demonstrated that criteria and methods could be developed for the collection of reliable, uniform, and comparable diagnoses under varying conditions.

Reliability of Diagnosis. Through considerable research in psychopathology, sources of variance were found that contributed to unreliability of diagnosis. Five were identified by Spitzer et al. (1975): (1) subject—the patient actually has different conditions at different times, (2) occasion—the patient is in a different stage of the same condition at different times,

(3) information—the clinicians have different sources of information, (4) observation—clinicians presented with the same stimuli differ in what they observe, and (5) criteria—the formal inclusion and exclusion criteria that clinicians use to summarize patient data into psychiatric diagnosis differ.

Methods to reduce these sources of variance are now available. Structured clinical interviews were developed to elicit the patient's signs and symptoms in a systematic fashion and to reduce that portion of variance due to different interviewing styles and coverage. Operational definitions, with specific inclusion and exclusion criteria for a variety of nosological groups, have reduced the criterion variance that proved to be the largest source of error (Feighner et al., 1972; Robins and Guze, 1972).

The Research Diagnostic Criteria (RDC) evolved from a decade of research on diagnosis, particularly by the group at Washington University, St. Louis. The conditions included in the RDC were chosen because their validity was supported by the most evidence in terms of clinical descriptions, consistency over time, and increased familial incidence.

Spitzer and Endicott, Wing, and others have shown convincingly that these methods increase the reliability of psychiatric diagnosis. While the Research Diagnostic Criteria have received much attention in the United States, parallel work in Great Britain, Scandinavia, and continental Europe, particularly by Wing's group, had led to similar efforts to improve reliability. These efforts have demonstrated that reasonable concordance in psychiatric diagnosis among clinicians and researchers can be achieved.

VALIDITY

Whereas the validity of a classification is limited by its reliability, reliability *per se* does not establish validity. To ascertain that nosological classes in psychiatry are valid, one must correlate clinical phenomena with other kinds of variables, such as long-term outcome, responses to treatment, and familial association.

The traditional approach to validity in psychiatry has been to base diagnostic classification on the best clinical judgment of experienced psychiatrists. Methods for establishing diagnostic validity in psychiatry on a scientific basis were put forth by Robins and Guze (1970). These included careful clinical description, demarcation from other disorders, laboratory studies, follow-up studies, family and genetic studies, response to treatment, and correlation with independent psychological or social variables.

Despite the social and political acrimony surrounding the whole issue of psychiatric diagnosis, the development of operational criteria by the Washington University-St. Louis group codified in the 1972 paper by Feighner et al., opened the way for improved reliability and more empirical tests of validity. Cohen developed the kappa technique for quantifying diagnostic reliability and categorical judgments, and this technique was applied by Spitzer, Fleiss and associates to a wide range of data. Using the clinical experience of the NIMH-CRB Psychobiology Collaborative Project (Katz and Klerman, 1979), the SADS Schedule for Affective Disorders for Schizophrenia and the Research Diagnostic Criteria (RDC) (Spitzer, Endicott, and Robins, 1975) were created. In rapid succession, numerous studies demonstrated that the standardized interview technique originally developed by Burdock and associates and applied to psychiatric diagnosis in the SADS-RDC could provide reliable estimates in clinical settings and in community surveys (Weissman and Myers, 1978). These operational criteria and associated measures of reliability were incorporated in the third edition of the *Diagnostic and Statistical Manual* (DSM-III) (APA, 1980).

Research in genetics provided additional evidence of biological factors in the causation of mental illness. The studies of Heston (1966), and those conducted in Scandinavia by Mednick et al. (1974) and by Kety et al. (1968), using the cross-rearing adoptive technique showed that genetic factors probably were involved in schizophrenia. By dividing patients into unipolar and bipolar groups depending on a history of manic episode, independent studies of the primary affective disorders in the United States, Europe, and Scandinavia in the 1960's demonstrated a strong familial association, thus indicating a genetic transmission of the primary affective disorders, especially bipolar forms.

Evidence for biological factors in psychiatric disorders also came from studies of mental retardation in which the traditional medical strategy led to the discovery of new nosological subclasses. Through the use of laboratory methods, the general category of mental retardation was subdivided according to origin, particularly into aminoacidurias and chromosomal abnormalities.

Together with advances in understanding from basic studies in psychopharmacology, these developments have radically changed psychiatry since World War II. Today there are increasingly sophisticated methods for diagnosis; for personality assessment; and for the assessment of change due to biological and social development, to the natural course of illness, and to specific treatment interventions.

ADVANCES IN PSYCHIATRIC TREATMENT

The introduction of psychotropic drugs in the mid-1950's led to changes in both the scientific investigation and the treatment of psychiatric disorders. The initial contribution of modern psychopharmacology was to stimulate the development of methods for the systematic assessment of patients' symptoms, social function, and diagnosis. Case reports and clinical experience could no longer be relied upon to evaluate the many new agents that followed the introduction of chlorpromazine. The need to determine their efficacy led to controlled clinical trials. Randomized designs, double-blind techniques, and placebo controls became the standards for therapeutic evaluation. These studies demonstrated that the new drugs had varying neuropharmacologic modes of action and different patterns of clinical efficacy, explained partially by diagnostic category. Schizophrenic patients responded to phenothiazines, depressed patients responded to tricyclic antidepressants, and the bipolar subtype of affected patients tended to improve with lithium carbonate. These findings supported the concept that psychiatric disorders were discrete and heterogeneous and prompted the reevaluation of diagnosis.

Although the most dramatic advances during the 1960's and 1970's were in drug therapy, new forms of psychosocial treatment also appeared. Prominent among these were the techniques derived from behavior therapy, such as desensitization, flooding, implosion, and exposure *in vivo* and *in vitro*. These methods have proven effective for the treatment of anxiety disorders, phobias in general, agoraphobia in particular, and obsessive compulsive states. Similarly, new forms of psychodynamically oriented group, family, and brief therapy have diversified the range of treatments available for the mentally ill and have underlined the need for systematic efforts to assess the relative efficacy of the methods and to determine the specific characteristics of patients likely to benefit from one treatment or another. Although advances in the evaluation of psychotherapy have not gained as much attention as those in psychopharmacology, over 400 controlled trials using quantitative methods for the assessment of outcome were recently reviewed by Glass, Smith, and Miller (1980).

If there were only one form of treatment, psychotherapy, and it was applicable to all forms of mental illness, then differential diagnosis would not be a major research or clinical task. This unitary view was dominant within psychiatry in the late 1940's and early 1950's. However, it is no longer tenable. Confronted with multiple forms of drug therapy and a variety of psychotherapies, clinicians need guidance in their selection of the appropriate treatment for individual patients. The renewal of psychiatric diagnosis and classification embodied in DSM-III has provided clinicians with reliable and valid criteria to help decide which patients will benefit from which kinds of therapy.

RESEARCH METHODOLOGY IN THERAPEUTICS

As mentioned above, this book gives priority to evidence derived from controlled studies in making judgments about the appropriateness, safety, and efficacy of various treatments for specific mental disorders. It is widely, if not universally, accepted that the strongest evidence for the efficacy of treatment derives from controlled studies, particularly randomized clinical trials. Prominent medical journals such as the *JAMA*, *New England Journal of Medicine*, and *Lancet* regularly report results from randomized trials of new drugs, surgical procedures, radiation, and even psychotherapy. It is important to recognize that this is a relatively recent innovation. Although the principles of experimentation in scientific research have been known for centuries, they were not applied to therapeutics until the twentieth century. The first randomized trial reported in the United States was conducted by Gold and associates at New York Hospital-Cornell Medical Center in the mid-1930's; they used placebos, a double-blind design, and random assignment to study angina treatments. The major impetus to apply clinical trials more widely came from the 1962 amendments to the U.S. Federal Food and Drug Act introduced by Senators Kefauver and Harris. Before that, evidence of efficacy was not required for the marketing of a new drug, only of purity and safety. To demonstrate the efficacy as well as the safety of drugs required careful attention to the selection of patients and quantitative measures of the intensity of their symptoms and of changes in their behavior that could be used at the time of entrance into the study and repeated during and after the course of drug treatment.

Thus the regulations and guidelines of the Food and Drug Administration in the United States not only have contributed greatly to the acceptance of the randomized controlled trial as the standard method for the evaluation of treatment, but were also an important stimulus to the development of psychosocial assessment methods.

Randomized controlled trials in psychiatry have rapidly generated information of high scientific quality and clinical relevance. They have made it possible to specify clinical conditions for which a particular therapy is effective and also to identify those for which we do not have adequate evidence, either positive or negative, as is the case with many forms of personality disorders represented in DSM-III on Axis II. This volume systematically reviews the available evidence from clinical trials and other studies and places the current state of clinical practice on a firmer basis than has heretofore been possible.

The Resolution of Disputes Within Psychiatry

Contemporary psychiatry has been marked by rivalry among numerous competing schools that have proposed different theories as to the nature and origin of mental illnesses and have advocated different methods of treatment, whether biological, social, interpersonal, psychodynamic, or behavioral. Many observers have noted that these divisions are especially prominent in American psychiatry (Havens, 1973 and Klerman, unpublished). So intense are the loyalties and emotions manifested by the adherents of these various schools that psychiatry sometimes seems like an arena for conflicting ideological sects rather than a scientific discipline based on commonly shared methodological approaches and advances in empirical knowledge.

For many years it appeared that there was no way out of this situation. There were no means by which the claims of various schools as to the causation of mental illness and the efficacy of their form of therapy could be established as valid or dismissed as unsubstantiated by empirical evidence.

This scene has changed dramatically, particularly in the United States and Canada, Great Britain, Western Europe, Scandinavia, Japan, Australia, New Zealand, and other parts of Asia. Within psychiatric research, there has been a rapid diffusion of methods for quantitative assessment of symptoms, social adjustment, life events, and other variables relevant to the diagnosis and classification of psychopathology. Moreover, systematic investigations have been undertaken to test theory, that is, the views of various schools of thought in psychiatry are being translated into hypotheses capable of being tested empirically. It is to be hoped that this process, rather than reliance on polemic, appeals to authority, and the formation of ideological loyalties, will serve to resolve current disputes in psychiatry.

Against this backdrop, the current volume does not promote a particular approach to psychiatric treatment, be it biological, psychodynamic, behavioral, or social psychiatric. Rather the authors provide a balanced and scholarly assessment of the available evidence for a variety of psychiatric treatments. The comprehensive nature of the discussion attests to the progress made in psychiatry and to the increasing acceptance of scientific standards for evaluating treatment.

REFERENCES

American Psychiatric Association, Diagnostic and Statistical Manual of Mental Disorder, (DSM-III) 3rd ed., Washington, D.C., American Psychiatric Association, 1980.

Feighner JD, Robins E, Guze SB et al., Diagnostic criteria for use in psychiatric research. Arch Gen Psychiat. 26: 57–63, 1972.

Glass GV, Smith ML, Miller TI, The Benefits of Psychotherapy, Baltimore, Johns Hopkins Press, 1980.

Havens LB, Approaches to the Mind, Boston, Little, Brown, 1973.

Heston LL, Psychiatric disorders in foster home reared children of schizophrenic mothers. Br. J. Psychiat. 112: 819–825, 1966.

Katz M and Klerman GL, Introduction: Overview of the Clinical Studies Program. Am. J. Psychiat. 136: 49–51, 1979.

Kety SS, Rosenthal D, Wender PH et al., The types and prevalence of mental illness in the biological and adaptive families of adopted schizophrenics. *In* The Transmission of Schizophrenia, Rosenthal, D, and Kety, SS (eds), Oxford, Pergamon Press, 1968, 345–362.

Klerman GL, Diagnosis and Classification of Alcoholism, Drug Abuse and Mental Disorders: The Contemporary American Scene. Paper commissioned as part of the WHO-ADAMHA Joint Program on Diagnosis and Classification of Psychiatric Disorders. (unpublished).

Kramer M, Cross-national study of diagnosis of the mental disorders: origin of the problem. Am. J. Psychiat. 125: 1–11, 1969.

Mednick SA, Schulsenger F, Higgins J et al. (eds). Genetics, Environment and Psychopathology, New York, North Holland, 1974.

Menninger K, Mayman M, Pruyser P, The Vital Balance, New York, Viking, 1963.

Robin E and Guze SB, Classification of affective disorders: The primary secondary, the endogenous reactive, and the neurotic-psychotic concepts. *In* Recent Advances in the Psychobiology of the Depressive Illness, Williams TA, Katz, MM and Sheild, JA (eds). Washington, D.C., U.S. Government Printing Office, 1972, 283–293.

Robins E and Guze SB, Establishment of diagnostic validity in psychiatric illness: its application to schizophrenia. Am. J. Psychiat. 126: 107, 1970.

Rosenhan DA, On being sane in insane places. Science. 179: 250–258, 1973.

Spitzer RL, Endicott J, Robins E, Research Diagnostic Criteria, New York: New York State Department of Mental Hygiene, Biometrics Branch, 1975.

Szasz T, The Myth of Mental Illness, New York, Harper and Row, 1974.

Weissman MM and Myers JK, Affective disorders in a US urban community. Arch Gen Psychiat. 38: 1304–1311, 1978.

Zubin J, Cross-national study of diagnosis of the mental disorders: methodology and planning. Am. J. Psychiat. 125(suppl) 12, 1969.

Treatment
of Mental Disorders

1 | Organic Mental Disorders

CHARLES E. WELLS and JOSEPH P. McEVOY

The diagnosis and treatment of the organic mental disorders have traditionally not received a high priority in the training and practice of most psychiatrists. This relative neglect is surprising in light of the observation that the "organic disorders . . . are the only mental syndromes for which in some cases a probable cause can be found and a specific, rather than empiric, treatment applied" (Detre and Jarecki, 1971). Three factors have probably contributed to this neglect. First, exact diagnosis has not always been highly valued by psychiatrists. As Hunter (1973) acerbically observed: "It is curious that patients [with behavioral and cognitive aberrations] are sent to physicians for diagnosis but to psychiatrists for treatment." Second, the diagnostic nomenclature approved in DSM-II tended to foster inexactness rather than specificity in the diagnosis of organic conditions. Indeed, not until the article by Seltzer and Sherwin appeared (1978) was there a clear demonstration that more precise diagnosis is possible for almost every patient initially given the diagnosis of chronic brain syndrome. Nor can this general lack of interest in organic conditions be attributed to the pervasive, if inaccurate, belief that treatment for the organic disorders is usually ineffective. For, third, once a specific treatment has been developed for an organic brain disorder, it appears that the psychiatrist often defers to other specialists for his patient's treatment. Thus, after specific therapies for syphilis were developed, general physicians assumed most responsibility for its treatment; and after anticonvulsants became available, neurologists began to treat most epileptics. There are signs that these attitudes are shifting and that psychiatrists are once again willing to address themselves to the difficult problems posed by the diagnosis and treatment of the organic disorders.

Treatment for the seven syndromes of organic dysfunction described in DSM-III cannot be considered apart from problems of making an etiologic diagnosis. Thus once a psychiatric syndrome is recognized and appropriately attributed to organic factors, the next and necessary step in patient management is a search for its etiology. These syndromes stand apart from other psychiatric disorders: they are the only ones for which an etiologic diagnosis is possible and, therefore, they require this two-step diagnostic process before appropriate treatment can commence. Therefore, in the discussion that follows we will emphasize for each syndrome the necessary steps in the investigation of etiology which must precede either specific or symptomatic treatment.

DELIRIUM (293.00)

ESSENTIAL FEATURES

The essential feature of *delirium* is a clouded state of consciousness, that is, a reduction in the clarity of awareness of the environment. This is shown by difficulty in sustaining attention to both external and internal stimuli, sensory misperception (for example, illusions and hallucinations), and inability to maintain a coherent stream of thought. The sleep-wakefulness cycle is almost invariably disturbed, frequently involving a depression in the level of consciousness that can range from simple drowsiness through increasing stages of torpor to stupor or semicoma. More rarely there may be hypervigilance and difficulty falling asleep. Psychomotor activity is also disturbed, which may involve restlessness and hyperactivity or decreased psychomotor activity with sluggishness.

TREATMENT

Delirium is the organic mental disorder most likely to be encountered by psychiatrists in consultative, outpatient, or inpatient settings. Unfortunately, the recognition and diagnosis of delirium on the basis of its clinical presentation gives no hint as to etiology. In the individual patient, delirium due to widely differing causes may present with identical clinical manifestations; therefore, the first step in the management of the delirious patient is the search for its cause or causes (more often the

TABLE 1-1.
CAUSES OF DELIRIUM

I. PRIMARY BRAIN DYSFUNCTION
  1. *Epilepsy and postictal states*
  2. *Trauma (especially concussion)*
  3. *Infections*
  4. *Subarachnoid hemorrhage*

II. SECONDARY BRAIN DYSFUNCTION
  1. *Drugs (ingestion and withdrawal) and poisons*
     a. sedatives (including alcohol)
     b. tranquilizers
     c. other drugs
     d. poisons

  2. *Endocrine Dysfunction (hypofunction or hyperfunction)*
     a. pituitary
     b. thyroid
     c. parathyroid
     d. pancreas
     e. adrenal

  3. *Diseases of Nonendocrine Organs*
     a. liver (hepatic encephalopathy)
     b. kidney and urinary tract
     c. lung
     d. cardiovascular system
     e. deficiency diseases
     f. miscellaneous disease states
        (fever, sepsis, electrolyte imbalance of whatever cause, postoperative states)

latter). If these can be identified, treatment is usually directed toward the primary disease process(es). If no etiology can be discovered, or if the patient's behavior is so disordered that treatment is needed on an emergency basis before an etiology can be established, then treatment to counteract specific symptoms rather than specific disease processes may be instituted.

In seeking the cause(s) of delirium, the direction of the search is often determined by the setting in which it occurs. Delirium presenting in a psychiatric inpatient points one in a different direction than it does in the postoperative patient in surgical intensive care. Likewise, delirium in the patient with diagnosed pulmonary insufficiency calls for a different response than it does in the identified alcoholic. The most common causes of delirium are listed in Table 1-1 (modified from Wells and Duncan, 1980).

In the best of circumstances, the history or physical examination pro-

TABLE 1-2

SUGGESTED LABORATORY STUDIES FOR DELIRIOUS PATIENTS

Blood
  glucose
  urea nitrogen
  electrolytes
  liver function measures
  sedative and tranquilizer levels
  arterial PO_2 and PCO_2
Urine
  glucose
  acetone
  cells
Electrocardiogram

---

vides etiologic clues. When these are not helpful and the cause remains obscure, the physician should turn to the laboratory for assistance. We suggest that the procedures listed in Table 1-2 be carried out in delirious patients in whom the etiology cannot be established on clinical grounds alone.

Not infrequently, when the patient's condition is obviously serious and potentially life threatening, treatment must be started in the absence of an etiologic diagnosis to forestall the possibility of irreparable brain damage. In such situations, before looking to other possible causes, the physician takes steps to prevent death or irreversible brain damage from hypoglycemia, hypoxia or anoxia, hyperthermia, or thiamine deficiency.

Hypoglycemia is usually the first diagnostic consideration when a known diabetic under treatment with insulin becomes delirious, but hypoglycemia occurs in other conditions as well, especially in alcoholics with liver failure. Because prolonged hypoglycemia may result in permanent brain damage, every patient with delirium of unknown etiology should be treated to correct any possible hypoglycemia. After blood has been drawn for diagnostic studies (and urine checked if possible for glucose and acetone), the patient should immediately be given 50 ml of 50% dextrose solution intravenously. If the patient has been hypoglycemic for some time, this may not immediately restore the patient's normal sensorium, but it should prevent any further brain damage due to hypoglycemia while a complete diagnostic evaluation is in progress.

Hypoxia and anoxia pose a threat equal to that of hypoglycemia. Cerebral hypoxia results: (1) when there is impaired perfusion of the brain by blood that is adequately oxygenated; (2) when there is normal perfusion by blood whose oxygen content is inadequate to meet the brain's metabolic requirements; or (3) when there is a combination of impaired perfusion and lowered oxygen content of blood. The first most often results from hypotension, myocardial infarction (in the elderly, myocardial infarction presents as delirium in 13% of patients, Pathy, 1967), and cardiac arrhythmias or arrest; the second from pulmonary disease, ventilatory impairment, carbon monoxide poisoning, and profound anemia. With these possibilities in mind, a differential diagnosis can be accomplished quickly and appropriate remedial steps identified. The latter include such diverse therapeutic measures as ventilatory assistance, supplemental oxygen in respired air, pressor agents, blood transfusions, and drugs to normalize cardiac rhythms.

Two other emergency situations deserve mention. Severe hyperthermia (above 105°) of whatever cause may result in delirium or even death. Its occurrence calls for immediate use of rapid cooling methods (alcohol sponges, ice packs, and fans) to reduce body temperature as quickly as possible. Thiamine deficiency is another cause of delirium, which if not promptly corrected may result in permanent brain damage. The Wernicke syndrome is diagnosed specifically by the presence of delirium in combination with impaired extraocular movements (especially nystagmus, either horizontal or vertical), weakness or paralysis of the lateral rectus muscles, and weakness or paralysis of conjugate gaze. When the Wernicke syndrome is suspected, the patient should immediately be given 100 mg of thiamine intravenously and then 50 mg intramuscularly daily for the next week or until oral intake is adequate.

Fortunately most deliria do not call for emergency treatment, and there is usually adequate time for considered diagnostic evaluation. Treatment of the primary disorder should resolve the delirium in most instances; but this does not always suffice, either because remission of the delirium may lag behind cure of the primary disease or because the primary disease cannot be cured by therapeutic measures available at present. In either case, the patient's suffering or behavior may be such that symptomatic treatment is required. In other instances, the cause or causes for the delirium may never be identified (a common situation), and the physician may have nothing to offer except nonspecific measures.

Nonspecific treatment of delirium has three aspects: (1) environmental management; (2) general medical support; (3) medications for relief of specific symptoms.

Environmental Management

The delirious patient is most comfortable and functions best in a quiet, simple, orderly, and unhurried setting. Too many sensory stimuli, especially if they are competing, are likely to aggravate cerebral disorganization, as does sensory deprivation at the other end of the spectrum. A quiet bedroom at home is possibly the best place to nurse a delirious patient; an intensive care unit, probably the worst. Usually a private, simply furnished, softly lighted hospital room which is quiet but not totally silent is the best that can be achieved. The room should be kept softly but adequately lighted at all times, because darkness increases the patient's difficulties with visual perception and sometimes triggers visual hallucinations.

The patient requires attendants around the clock whenever the delirium is severe. The attendants' function is to protect the patient from injury, to orient the patient to reality, and to reassure the patient as to his safety. The fewer the number of different attendants, the better. Two or three trusted relatives or friends are ideal if available. They should be instructed thoroughly about their role and responsibilities and the nature of the problems they may encounter. If close associates are not available, the number of different professionals involved should be as few as possible. Medical and nursing personnel should be clearly identified, by uniform if possible, and they should repeatedly introduce themselves to the patient, state their role, and explain what they are doing. They should orient the patient again and again as to time, place, and situation and reassure the patient of his safety. Each diagnostic and therapeutic procedure should be explained thoroughly to lessen the patient's apprehension and to obtain the best cooperation possible. Telling the patient not to be afraid because the procedure won't hurt is not enough. Above all, attendants must protect the patient from self-injury, deliberate or unwitting. Physical restraints should be used sparingly, but at times their use is clearly required and just as clearly therapeutic.

Medical Support

General medical support is often important, although it may not be aimed at the primary cause of the delirium. Agitation and hyperactivity are often prominent, with resulting mental and physical exhaustion. Insomnia may persist, and dreams and nightmares may recur. Fever often occurs, and at times temperature rises to dangerous levels. Constant movement and fever result in fluid and electrolyte loss, usually augmented by poor alimentation. Severe electrolyte imbalance, dehydration, and even vascular collapse may ensue. Some of the psychiatrist's most severe and complex problems in medical management are encountered in delirious patients, and patients' survival often depends not on identification and treatment of the etiology of the delirium but on sophisticated treatment of its medical complications.

Medications

Drugs may be useful, often for symptom relief, less often for prophylaxis. It should be emphasized that not every delirious patient need be given medication. In those patients whose delirium is manifested primarily by a reduced level of arousal, confusion, and bewilderment, the medications most often used may be contraindicated. Since most of the medications used for symptomatic treatment of delirium are also capable of causing delirium, their use always carries with it the possibility of worsening or prolonging delirium rather than helping. Thus whenever a delirium worsens with treatment, the possibility that the treatment itself is responsible for the negative effect should be considered.

In the past, little attention was paid to the possibility that delirium might be a preventable disorder. Yet delirium occurs with such predictability in certain situations that consideration of its possible prophylaxis should be undertaken. Delirium tremens, for example, occurs in chronic alcoholics only in the period following a reduction or cessation of alcohol ingestion, and although its incidence is low, it is life threatening. Its symptoms are usually improved significantly by benzodiazepines or neuroleptics. It seems likely that if benzodiazepines were administered routinely to all chronic alcoholics undergoing detoxification, delirium tremens might be prevented entirely or at least its severity greatly lessened.

Other preventive measures have recently been suggested. The psychoses (more often affective, less often delirious) that occur so often in patients receiving steroids may sometimes be prevented by concomitant use of lithium (Falk et al., 1979). Another recent study indicated that the commonly observed delirium following cataract surgery is actually an anticholinergic delirium and thus potentially avoidable if drugs possessing anticholinergic properties are used in the smallest amounts possible in the immediate postoperative period (Summers and Reich, 1979). It has also been suggested that alcoholic beverages be fortified with thiamine, a procedure that should prevent development of the Wernicke-Korsakoff syndrome (Centerwall and Criqui, 1978). Studies dealing with the prophylaxis of delirium are still minimal, but this is an area in which progress may soon be made.

For the most part, medications are used in delirium to reduce distressing symptoms (fear, anxiety, irritability, anger, hallucinations, delusions) or to reduce distressing behavior (restlessness, hyperactivity, insomnia, assaultiveness). They do little specifically to improve disorientation, memory impairment, or other cognitive dysfunction, although these may be alleviated as fear and agitation are reduced. For many years, hypnotics were the accepted agents for symptomatic treatment of delirium. They were useful even though the sedation that usually resulted often made evaluation and management more difficult. The use of hypnotics has largely been abandoned in favor of the tranquilizers, either anxiolytics or antipsychotics. Both anxiolytic agents and antipsychotics are effective in treating fear, anxiety, restlessness, hyperactivity, and insomnia, and there is little solid evidence that one group is more effective than the other in providing symptomatic relief. Thus, the choice of one group over the other more often is based on which side effects should be avoided in a particular patient rather than their comparative effectiveness.

The benzodiazepines, especially chlordiazepoxide and diazepam, have been subjected to extensive clinical trials and have been proven safe and effective. Their action on the cardiovascular and respiratory systems is minimal, and both are effective anticonvulsants, which is often an important consideration when delirium results from withdrawal of alcohol or other drugs. Although they are less sedating than the standard hypnotics, their sedative effect may nevertheless be significant, especially in the quantities often required to control other more distressing symptoms. For this reason, antipsychotic agents such as haloperidol, which are thought to depress consciousness less than the other antipsychotics, have been advocated. On the other hand, antipsychotics are said to lower the seizure threshold, sometimes result in undesirable cardiovascular effects, and often produce extrapyramidal symptoms and signs.

For moderate anxiety and restlessness in the young or middle-aged adult, oral doses of 25–50 mg chlordiazepoxide, 5–10 mg diazepam, or 15–30 mg oxazepam can be used initially. For more severe anxiety and agitation, initial doses of 50–100 mg chlordiazepoxide, 10–20 mg diazepam, or 30–60 mg oxazepam might be employed. When the patient is extremely agitated, uncooperative, assaultive, or panicky, parenteral administration of the chosen medication may be required (although more rapid, higher, and more sustained blood levels of chlordiazepoxide and diazepam have been reported after oral dosage as compared to intramuscular administration). When immediate symptom control is necessary, slow, intravenous dosage of 50 mg chlordiazepoxide or 10 mg diazepam may be given (oxazepam is not available for parenteral administration). Repeated doses of the chosen medication (in increasing or decreasing amounts as determined by clinical response) are usually given every one to two hours until control of the clinical symptoms is achieved. For elderly patients and for patients with known cerebral damage, an initial oral dose of 10 mg chlordiazepoxide, 2 mg diazepam, or 10 mg oxazepam might be chosen. Some pharmacokinetic studies suggest that oxazepam may be the preferred benzodiazepine for elderly patients (Shull et al., 1976); it has a short half-life and is not conjugated into other pharmacologically active agents. Both chlordiazepoxide and diazepam have relatively long half-lives; thus the physician must be aware of the danger of accumulation of the drug and its active metabolites with repeated administration.

When the physician decides to treat delirium with an antipsychotic, haloperidol is the drug usually chosen, because it produces little sedation and relatively few cardiovascular side effects. Unfortunately, with haloperidol the incidence of extrapyramidal side effects is significant. The usual initial oral dose is 5 mg, once or twice daily. In emergencies (or if oral administration is not possible) 2 to 5 mg administered intramuscularly each hour until control is achieved has been suggested (Moore, 1977).

In treating most deliria, the problem is not so much the choice of drug as it is the amount to use. As Greenblatt and Shader (1975) stated: "When therapy is inadequate, symptoms rage on, while overdosage produces obtundation, coma, and respiratory depression." The physician must try to titrate the quantities prescribed to reach and maintain a position between these two extremes.

Lipowski (1967) listed four possible outcomes of delirium: (1) full return to premorbid state; (2) transition to dementia or another organic mental disorder; (3) transition to a nonorganic mental disorder; (4) death, due either to brain dysfunction or to primary extracranial disease. Although the first outcome is undoubtedly most frequent, delirium does not uniformly resolve without residua even when it does not lead to another disorder. The longer the delirium goes unrecognized and untreated, or the longer it persists despite treatment, the greater the likelihood of permanent cerebral damage. Transition to a nonorganic mental disorder is rare and should suggest that the functional disorder was present but had not been recognized before the delirium.

DEMENTIA (294.10)

ESSENTIAL FEATURES

The essential feature of *dementia* is the loss of intellectual abilities of sufficient severity to interfere with social or occupational functioning. The disturbance involves memory, judgment, abstract thought, and a variety of other higher cortical functions. Changes in personality and behavior also occur. In mild dementia, memory impairment may be limited to forgetfulness in daily life. In more severe memory impairment, the individual may forget names, telephone numbers, directions, conversations, and events of the day. Impairment of abstract thinking may involve difficulty in coping with novel tasks, especially if pressed for time. Impaired judgment and impulse control may lead to a disregard for the conventional rules of social conduct. Disturbances in higher cortical functioning may be shown by disturbance in language, agnosias, or apraxias. Personality changes may involve either an alteration or an accentuation of premorbid traits.

TREATMENT

Treatment of the demented patient must also be preceded by two-step diagnostic process—first, the diagnosis of dementia and second, the identification of its etiology. Once this diagnosis has been made, the psychiatrist must proceed to establish an etiologic diagnosis. As Seltzer and Sherwin (1978) demonstrated, this is possible in almost every patient.

Wells (1979) has recently tabulated the outcome of diagnostic investigation of six groups of patients with presumed dementia who were hospitalized and thoroughly investigated neurologically for the etiology of their clinical dysfunction (see Table 1-3). Two points should be made about the findings.

TABLE 1-3.

SUMMARY OF DIAGNOSIS IN SIX SERIES COMPRISING 417 PATIENTS FULLY
EVALUATED FOR DEMENTIA

DIAGNOSIS	NUMBER		PERCENT
Dementia of unknown causes	199		47.7
Alcoholic dementia-Korsakoff syndrome	42	b	10.0
Multiinfarct dementia	39		9.4
Normal-pressure hydrocephalus	25		6.0
Intracranial masses	20		4.8
Huntington's disease	12		2.9
Drug toxicity	10		2.4
Posttraumatic	7		1.7
Other identified dementing diseases*	28		6.7
Pseudodementias	28		6.7
Depression 16			
Schizophrenia 5			
Not demented (no diagnosis given) 4			
Mania 2			
Hysteria 1			
Dementia uncertain	7		1.7

*Other diagnoses, each seen in 1% or less of the 417 patients, were as follows: epilepsy, Creutzfeldt-Jakob disease, postsubarachnoid hemorrhage, encephalitis, amyotrophic lateral sclerosis, Parkinson's disease, pernicious anemia, hypothyroidism, hyperthyroidism, syphilis, liver disease, Kuff disease, progressive cerebellar degeneration, cerebral anoxic episode.

First, dementia of unknown cause (or cerebral atrophy of unknown cause) made up the largest diagnostic category, accounting for roughly half of all the cases evaluated. In the DSM-III classification, these cases would be labeled almost entirely as presenile dementia or senile dementia. It is now clear that the vast majority of these patients would be diagnosed by pathological investigation as having Alzheimer's disease (of either presenile or senile onset). Some also show evidence of cerebral infarction, of varying extent and of varying significance, which contributes to the symptoms of dementia. Multi-infarct dementia plays a less important role than does Alzheimer's disease in the etiology of dementia, and it should be the prevalent diagnosis only when clinical features point specifically to cerebral infarction (Wells, 1978). Most commonly, etiologic diagnoses for dementia (presenile and senile dementia of the Alzheimer type) are (at our present level of knowledge) made by exclusion, that is, evidence points to certain causes *only* after others have been ruled out.

TABLE 1-4.
DEMENTING DISORDERS CALLING FOR SPECIFIC THERAPEUTIC
INTERVENTIONS

Chronic alcoholism
Chronic drug toxicity
Endocrine disorders
Chronic cardiovascular, pulmonary, hepatic, or renal disease
Normal-pressure hydrocephalus
Intracranial masses
Epilepsy
Infections (encephalitis, cryptococcal meningitis, syphilis)
Parkinson's disease
Deficiency disorders
Wilson's disease
Pseudodementias

Second, although Alzheimer's disease is the most frequent single cause of dementia, many other diseases, some of which call for specific treatment, result in dementia. Table 1-4 lists a number of dementing disorders whose recognition leads to specific therapeutic interventions. In addition, in virtually every series of patients admitted for diagnostic evaluation because of presumed dementia, several patients turn out, on further evaluation (or by virtue of the passage of time), not to be demented at all but to have functional psychiatric disorders, many of which are responsive to treatment. All in all, thorough diagnostic evaluation uncovers causes for dementia that are potentially reversible in 10–15% of the cases. In an additional 25–30%, such evaluation reveals disorders that call for specific treatment measures, even if restitution to the patient's premorbid status cannot be anticipated (Wells, 1979). In many of these patients, prompt identification of the etiology and prompt treatment may lead to some clinical improvement or to a halt in the progression of dysfunction.

The first responsibility of the psychiatrist then, beyond the diagnosis of dementia per se, is to identify the specific disorder responsible. In most instances, diagnosis can be established with reasonable certainty on the basis of history, general physical examination, and neurologic examination, supplemented by a limited number of ancillary diagnostic procedures chosen to follow up leads obtained from these sources. Unfortunately, in these patients specific diagnostic leads are usually rare, even after detailed histories and examinations have been accomplished. When

TABLE 1-5.
SUGGESTED ANCILLARY DIAGNOSTIC PROCEDURES FOR PATIENTS
WITH DEMENTIA

Blood tests
   complete blood count
   serologic test for syphilis
   Sequential Multiple Analyzer with Computer (SMAC) (or other standard metabolic
     screening test)
   FT4 or TSH
   B-12 and folate
Computed cranial tomography
Chest X-ray
Urinalysis

---

no clue points to a specific etiology, how far should the physician pursue the diagnosis with ancillary diagnostic procedures?

Wells (1979) has suggested routine use of a basic core diagnostic battery (see Table 1-5) for those patients in whom no specific disease diagnosis has been suggested by history or examination. This list of suggested procedures is by no means inclusive; indeed, certain useful tests (such as psychological testing, electroencephalography, and cerebrospinal fluid examination) have not been recommended for every patient. The suggested battery should, however, uncover virtually all of the dementing disorders that call for specific therapeutic measures, and other diagnostic instruments might better be reserved for use when they are likely to be of specific diagnostic assistance. Taking into account the diagnoses recorded in Table 1-3, it would be difficult at this time to justify a more extensive routine diagnostic battery than that set forth. The suggested procedures can all be performed on an outpatient basis, an advantage in that the expense of hospitalization is avoided. Even so, the cost is significant, and it must be admitted that the cost–benefit ratio for the individual procedures has not yet been determined.

Treatment for the varied dementing disorders, such as Parkinson's disease, hypothyroidism, hepatic failure, is outside the scope of this chapter, and the reader is referred elsewhere (Wells, 1977). The discussion of therapy given below deals with symptomatic treatment for the demented patient, that is, treatment to combat the signs and symptoms of dementia and not the primary dementing process. Such symptomatic treatment will be needed even for many of those patients in whom an underlying disease process that is treatable has been identified; it will be needed for all those patients suffering progressive dementing disorders for which no specific therapy is available.

At the outset of this discussion, it is important to emphasize that dementia is *never* a normal phase of a person's life cycle, *never* a normal or inevitable concomitant of aging. When no specific, treatable form of dementia can be identified, too many physicians (other specialists perhaps more often than psychiatrists) still infer and tell the family that the patient suffers only from old age. These same physicians often also fail to recognize that such patients need treatment, even if it is nonspecific, or to accept responsibility for providing such treatment. Yet physicians do not often neglect the medical needs of patients with nondementing medical disorders when no specific remedies are at hand. We insist that dementia must be regarded as a syndrome as worthy of medical and psychiatric attention and care as any other.

Once physicians accept the responsibility for treating demented patients, however, there is little question that providing for their care demands modifications of the physician's usual role. First of all, the social problems faced by demented patients are often equal to or even more severe than the medical problems. The physician who is unwilling to grapple with these social problems will usually be of little use to the demented patient. This does not mean that the physician must *personally* solve these problems, but he must usually take the responsibility for bringing together the various caregivers—nurse, family, social service agencies—and melding them into a team working in concert to provide for the patient's care.

Another modification in the physician's usual role follows because most patients whose dementia is moderately to severely advanced appear to be unaware of and unconcerned about their plight. In fact, most demented patients have reached this point before they are brought for medical evaluation. It is always difficult and usually impossible for the physician to establish anything approximating the usual physician–patient relationship with the patient who is oblivious of his condition and of any need for medical attention. Thus the physician's primary relationship often must be with the family or other caretaker, on whom he relies to serve as his surrogate in the patient's treatment. Furthermore, families and other caretakers often serve as the physician's primary or only source of information about the patient's difficulties. The demented patient often appears at his best in the morning or early afternoon when visiting the physician's office or being visited by the physician. Thus the patient's demeanor may belie the facts of nocturnal wandering, incontinence, or aggressiveness recounted by the patient's attendants. Unless mutual good faith can be established between the physician and the primary caregivers, patient care will suffer.

The physician also should neither neglect nor underestimate the importance of his function as educator. Most lay persons are largely ignorant of the nature of dementia. They are understandably fearful of that disorder which so erodes the personality and the intellect, and family members are usually concerned as well about the genetic implications of the diagnosis. An added hurdle is that family members are often almost as adept as patients at denying the severity of cognitive losses. Thus a husband explains the total disorientation of his wife by saying that "she never did pay much attention to dates anyway." More harmful yet is the denial whereby a family attributes a patient's dysfunction to willful perversity. Thus a husband blames his wife's failure to keep house on her laziness and lack of interest or even on her loss of love for him, while completely ignoring her cognitive incapacity. The physician must penetrate this barrier of denial and educate the family about the extent of cognitive loss, the probable nature of the underlying pathology, prognosis, and probable course. At the same time the physician must assume some responsibility for the well being of the family or other caretakers who are often themselves elderly and frail, taking care that the burdens of looking after the severely demented patient do not stress them beyond their capacities. In these situations, the physician often must step in and insist on outside nursing assistance or even institutionalization, steps which at the same time may require the physician to help assuage the caregiver's sense of failure or guilt.

This is not to suggest that the physician should avoid direct contact with the patient, only that it is likely to be different from the usual physician–patient relationship. The physician is very important to the demented patient as a doctor, but not so important as a person. Identified perhaps only by a white jacket or stethoscope, the physician may calm and sustain the demented person even when his name cannot be learned and face cannot be remembered. In such situations it is not surprising that tone of voice or facial expression may be more important than words, that touch may be more therapeutic than speech, or that simply listening or sitting in silence with the patient may quiet apprehensions better than drugs. As one woman wrote of her demented father: "He . . . recognized the doctor for what he was, and the visit sobered him a little. Even that much relief was something to be thankful for . . ."

A treatment plan for the demented patient can be conceptualized quite easily—the difficulty lies in its execution. The treatment plan for the demented patient is based on: (1) a complete evaluation of the patient's physical condition; (2) a thorough assessment of psychological liabilities (lost functions) and assets (retained functions); (3) a knowledge of pre-morbid personality characteristics; and (4) an understanding of the probable neuropathologic substratum and likely course of the disease. On this basis the physician constructs a plan of treatment which is aimed at: (1) preservation of retained functions and restitution of those lost functions which can be restored; (2) reduction of needs for those functions that are permanently lost; and (3) maximal utilization of those capacities that are retained.

Restitution of Lost Functions

Many demented patients function far below their cerebral capacity because of neglect—medical, nutritional, physical, social. Restitution of lost functions is concerned largely with combatting the consequences of neglect and with promoting the best physical health possible to sustain the failing brain. This treatment aim should have first priority, for unless these needs are attended to, other measures are unlikely to prove useful.

The diseased brain functions best in a body which is healthy and in an environment which is not stressful. Almost every medical disorder has the potential for augmenting co-existing impairment in brain function. The vulnerability of the diseased brain to fever, pain, infection, impaired renal function, cardiac failure, and endocrine dysfunction and to virtually all the drugs used to treat these various ailments is well known but often overlooked. Closer attention to medical disorders is required to maintain the demented than the nondemented patient, yet sadly the converse is often the case. Demented patients with visual or auditory impairments suffer the consequences of these losses more than other persons, but fewer efforts are made to correct them. The demented patient's brain is more vulnerable to the toxic effects of medications than the normal brain, yet it is easy to attribute these effects mistakenly to worsening brain disease rather than to increasing doses and numbers of drugs. In sum, the demented patient needs the best possible general medical care.

The nutritional needs of demented persons, especially the elderly, are often neglected, with resulting vitamin deficiencies and inanition. Demented persons often fail to eat through simple neglect or forgetfulness, even when adequate food is available. The refrigerator may be full, and the patient may confabulate a recent meal, yet the examiner will find no evidence that anything has recently been eaten. Unless the dementia is far advanced, most patients will eat when meals are prepared and served, especially if there is company at the table. Public service agencies, such as "Meals on Wheels," may also be of help.

Many patients regress to wheelchair or bed through neglect of their needs for regular exercise and ambulation. Since the physical, psychiatric, and social problems of the demented patient confined to bed or wheelchair are much more serious than those faced by the ambulatory patient, every effort should be made to preserve and promote ambulation.

Reduction of Need for Lost Functions

Most demented patients have experienced a permanent loss of certain important functions—memory, language, orientation, etc. An accurate assessment of those lost functions is important so that caretakers, with the help of the physician, can organize the patient's environment to minimize the need for these lost functions. Whereas stress may enhance function up to a point in the normal person, it usually has the opposite effect in the person with impaired brain function. Indeed, in the brain-damaged person, too much stress can result in a catastrophic reaction with profound regression and disintegration of the remaining ego. Everything that can help the person avoid confronting inadequacies is to the good. For the person who is disoriented for time, large clocks and placards announcing the day and date may help; for the person disoriented to place, signs labeling rooms may likewise be of use. For the institutionalized subject, color-coded doors and furniture may help. For the person who cannot recall names, introductions at every encounter and explanations of role are in order ("I'm your doctor, Dr. Jones."). For the patient who can't keep up with a daily schedule, a description of each activity is appropriate. For the patient who can't remember to take medicines, a daily telephone call may assure compliance; the patient can be asked to take the medication while keeping the phone connection open. Regular telephone prompting from family members may help assure regular eating, bathing, and other daily habits as well.

Change is stressful even for the healthy; for the brain-damaged person, it is doubly so. Patients do best when they can remain in familiar surroundings with adequate but familiar diversions. If the patient must be institutionalized or hospitalized, the sense of disruption may be lessened if some familiar cherished object(s) can be carried along into the new environment. The darkness and silence of night may increase both agitation and disorientation; a soft light constantly illuminating the bedroom helps prevent this.

The physician must often protect the patient from the well-meaning but ill-directed efforts of those who perceive change and stimulation as panaceas for life's ills, including dementia. New faces, new activities, and new experiences are not therapeutic in most cases of dementia, and they should be discouraged. Encouraging the patient to continue as long as possible to move through life's wellworn furrows is more beneficial.

Utilization of Residual Functions

In this aspect of treatment, the physician must use psychotherapeutic and psychopharmacologic skills to promote the patient's well being.

Psychotherapy in its usual sense is of course impossible with most demented patients. If we define psychotherapy, however, as the use of the physician's interpersonal skills to communicate to the patient a sense of concern, support, and acceptance, then we cannot doubt that the demented patient needs psychotherapy. For the patient whose dementia is mild to moderate, the physician may encourage the patient to continue previous interests, keep seeing old friends, participate in group activities, maintain physical activities, and keep active in productive habits as long as possible. The physician should allow the patient to ventilate feelings of anger, hurt, and rejection, accepting these feelings, in most instances, as reasonable and understandable given the circumstances. The therapist should also assume a more directive stance than might be appropriate in other therapeutic relationships, seeking especially to channel the patient's energy and activity into pathways where they will not inevitably encounter stress, frustration, and failure.

Drug therapy is an important aspect of treatment but most pharmacotherapeutic measures are aimed at helping the demented patient, not at lessening the dementia per se. In the demented patient, therefore, medications are chosen to combat the following symptoms: (1) anxiety; (2) depression or mania; (3) psychotic manifestations such as delusions, hallucinations, or paranoid ideation; (4) distressing behavior such as hyperactivity or assaultiveness; and (5) insomnia. All of these symptoms may further reduce the function of a brain which is already compromised; thus their relief may promote well being even though the primary dementing process is unaffected. These symptoms do not usually respond to psychotropic medications as well as they do in functional disorders, but at times drugs may be remarkably effective. In most instances they are certainly worth a trial.

The same two psychopharmacologic caveats must be given for patients with dementia or other neurological disease that are usually given for the use of the psychotropic agents in the elderly: (1) hypnotics are poorly tolerated in the presence of structural brain disease and should be avoided; (2) the damaged central nervous system is often exquisitely sensitive to psychotropic agents; therefore, treatment should be started with doses quite small in comparison to those that are common in functional disorders. Because so many demented patients are elderly as well, pharmacokinetic differences in the elderly must also be taken into account. In addition, many demented subjects have other medical disorders for which they also take medicines, and the probability of confusing drug–drug interactions is high.

For relief of nonpsychotic anxiety, chlordiazepoxide 5 mg twice daily or diazepam 2 mg twice daily may be useful. The dosage may be raised to achieve better symptom relief, but this should be done slowly, cautiously, and under close supervision. Both these drugs, and indeed most of the anxiolytic agents, appear to lose much of their effectiveness with chronic administration, a significant limitation when using them to control anxiety in a disorder as chronic as dementia. In addition, both chlordiazepoxide and diazepam have a relatively long half-life and thus tend to accumulate in tissues. In elderly subjects, the half-life is markedly increased, and plasma clearance of the active metabolites increases as well (Klotz et al., 1975; Roberts et al., 1978; Shader and Greenblatt, 1979). Among the benzodiazepines, pharmacokinetic studies suggest that oxazepam may be the anxiolytic agents of choice in the elderly (Shull et al., 1976). Its half-life is between 8 and 15 hours, the shortest among the benzodiazepines, and this does not increase with advancing age. In the body the drug is changed directly into an inactive metabolite which is then excreted by the kidneys. Much the same can be said about lorazepam, although it has not been studied as extensively. When these agents are used to control anxiety in dementia, 10 mg of oxazepam or 0.5 mg of lorazepam two or three times daily are probably appropriate beginning doses.

For depression, amitriptyline, nortriptyline, imipramine, or doxepin may be used. In general, the choice of a specific tricyclic antidepressant depends not so much on its antidepressant effectiveness as on which side effects might be desired and which should be avoided. For example, in the depressed and demented patient with insomnia, amitriptyline or doxepin might be chosen for their sedating effect and the entire daily dose given before bedtime. Doxepin is said to result in fewer cardiovascular side effects than some other tricyclics and thus might be the drug of choice when these are especially to be avoided. In patients with dementia plus depression, a starting dose of 30–40 mg daily is probably judicious; the dose can then be raised slowly under supervision, depending on the effectiveness of the medication and the development of side effects.

Pharmacokinetic studies have revealed significant changes with increasing age in the way the body deals with most of the tricyclic antidepressants (Risch et al., in press). For amitriptyline, mean plasma levels are significantly increased in patients over age 65. For imipramine, the plasma half-life of both imipramine and its active metabolite desipramine are increased with increasing age, as are the steady-state plasma levels of both. For desipramine both half-life and steady-state plasma levels are higher in elderly than in young subjects. Among the many tricyclic antidepressants available, pharmacokinetic studies suggest certain advantages for nortriptyline. There are no increases in its plasma levels with advancing age (Ziegler and Biggs, 1977); it has fewer sedating and anticholinergic effects than amitriptyline; and its metabolic breakdown products are probably less active pharmacologically than those of most other tricyclics.

Because 25% of all demented patients have significant depression, because depressive psychosis (especially in the elderly) often mimics dementia (pseudodementia), and because dementia is not infrequently misdiagnosed, it has been suggested that perhaps all patients who appear to be demented should be given a trial period of treatment with antidepressants. To us, this seems overly inclusive, but a trial period of antidepressants would appear appropriate in all patients who have a diagnosis of dementia and also have clinical evidence of depression.

Hypomania and mania secondary to structural brain disease are much rarer than depression (Jamieson and Wells, 1979). Should they occur and require treatment, both lithium and antipsychotic agents are effective. For the elderly, the half-life of lithium carbonate is significantly increased, and evidence of cerebral toxicity may appear at serum levels significantly below those at which toxicity occurs in younger patients. The same is probably also the case in patients with structural brain disease.

For paranoid symptoms, distressing delusions and hallucinations, marked hyperactivity, and intolerable levels of aggressiveness or assaultiveness, the antipsychotic agents are usually suggested. Chlorpromazine or thioridazine, 75–100 mg daily in divided doses, or 1–2 mg haloperidol daily in divided doses may be given initially and the dosage then adjusted upward or downward depending on clinical response. As with the antidepressants, choice of a specific medication usually depends more on wanted or unwanted side effects than on specific antipsychotic effectiveness. For example, both chlorpromazine and thioridazine have more sedating effects than does haloperidol, but haloperidol is more likely to precipitate an acute dystonic reaction.

Because they may result in tardive dyskinesia, the antipsychotic agents must always be employed with caution, especially when they are likely to be needed over a long period of time. This is perhaps a less serious consideration when they are used in progressive diseases such as most of the dementias. Balancing this, however, is the suggestion that the damaged brain may be especially vulnerable to the development of tardive dyskinesia and the evidence that the elderly are more prone to develop tardive dyskinesia than the young. Unfortunately, even though one would prefer to avoid their use, the antipsychotic drugs are often the only medications that have any significant effect on these most distressing symptoms, and without them the patient's suffering would be much greater.

For insomnia in demented patients it is ideal to use agents that promote restful sleep but have minimal hypnotic effects. Promethazine hydrochloride 25–50 mg at bedtime or oxazepam 10–20 mg may be effective. When patients who are being given antidepressants or antipsychotics also have insomnia this can often be overcome by administering most or all of these medications before bedtime. Regrettably, it is not unusual for none of these measures to work, and, even though they would rather avoid them, most physicians at times find themselves pushed to try something with more sedating properties. In these circumstances, chloral hydrate 250–500 mg probably stands the best chance of helping without harming.

What of those many agents that are purported to be effective in treating the primary symptoms and signs of dementia per se? Hydergine, papaverine, other vasodilators, Gerovital-H3, pentylenetetrazol, amphetamines and amphetamine-like drugs, nootropics, choline, lecithin, and doubtless many other agents are suggested as being of value in helping to reverse the ravages of dementing disease. Whenever these agents are brought under serious scientific scrutiny, however, the evidence for their effectiveness becomes evanescent at best (Cole and Branconnier, 1977). There is at least some suggestion that hydergine 1 mg three times daily, sublingually or pentylenetetrazol 200 mg orally three or four times a day, if continued over many weeks may be of some benefit to patients with senile dementia which has not progressed too far. The evidence for this is so equivocal, however, that we hesitate to recommend the use of these drugs. Perhaps the most apt observation is that if a patient with purported dementia should improve strikingly with the use of any of the agents listed above, the diagnosis of dementia was probably an error.

OTHER ORGANIC MENTAL SYNDROMES

The other organic mental syndromes listed in DSM-III may be thought of as falling into two broad groups: (1) those occurring in the presence of clear-cut evidence of cognitive impairment, for example, most instances of the frontal lobe syndrome; (2) those occurring in the absence of clear-cut evidence of cognitive impairment, for example, most instances of reserpine-induced depression. The first group is far more common than the second.

From a practical clinical standpoint, it is important for the psychiatrist to be wary of diagnosing these other syndromes when impaired cognition cannot be demonstrated. Unless the evidence for an organic etiology is compelling, these diagnostic categories should be avoided. This warning takes on added importance because: (1) in the elderly, psychologic distress has commonly been attributed on inadequate grounds to organic factors, and thus functional disorders have gone untreated; and (2) in patients with recognized organic brain disease, all new psychiatric symptoms may be attributed incorrectly to the preexisting disease, and thus a superimposed functional disorder may go unrecognized. In general, the recognition of these other organic mental syndromes requires more psychiatric sophistication than do delirium and dementia, and the uncovering of their etiologies is often equally difficult.

In the section that follows, we will deal primarily with some of the most common causes for the various specific syndromes. Symptomatic treatment is similar to that of dementia and will not be repeated.

AMNESTIC SYNDROME (294.00)

Essential Features

The essential feature of *amnestic syndrome* is impairment in short- and long-term memory occurring in a normal state of consciousness (i.e., not clouded). The disturbance is attributed to a specific organic factor. Amnestic syndrome is not diagnosed if memory impairment exists in the context of clouded consciousness (*delirium*) or in association with a more general loss of intellectual abilities (*dementia*). The individual with an amnestic syndrome has both an ongoing inability to learn new material (short-term memory deficit; anterograde amnesia) and an inability to re-call material that was known in the past (long-term memory deficit; retrograde amnesia).

Precipitating Factors

The most common cause of an amnestic syndrome is *head trauma* (Benson, 1978). The length of time after the trauma for which memory is lost (anterograde amnesia) is proportional to the severity of the injury. Acetylcholine, a neurotransmitter believed to be involved in memory functions, appears in the cerebrospinal fluid in increased amounts after head trauma, and the persistence of this excess is proportional to the degree and duration of altered consciousness. Residual memory defects correlate well with overall outcome, and significant permanent memory impairment is common in the severely disabled.

Thiamine deficiency, especially in individuals with a constitutional deficiency of the enzyme transketolase (for which thiamine is a co-factor), may cause bilateral hemorrhage and sclerosis of the mamillary bodies and a severe impairment in memory. Chronic alcoholics, the isolated elderly, and others with vitamin-deficient diets are at risk. The usual presentation is the Wernicke encephalopathy. If recognized and treated promptly, permanent damage may be avoided. If recognition comes too late or if treatment is inadequate, then permanent damage occurs, and the patient may be left with a severe amnestic (Korsakoff) syndrome. The treatment of Korsakoff amnesia should include abstinence from alcohol, good nutrition, and continued oral thiamine supplementation (after initial parenteral administration). The use of extremely high dosage of thiamine analogs has shown equivocal success; certainly, structural damage cannot be completely overcome by chemical replacement. It has been argued that prevention of the Wernicke-Korsakoff syndrome by supplementing all alcoholic beverages with thiamine would be less expensive financially than the cost of medical care for victims of this illness (Centerwall and Criqui, 1978).

Patients with localized *seizure foci* in the limbic system may behave in a fairly organized fashion during periods of ictal dysrhythmia for which they will have no memory. These episodes are usually brief, but in rare cases may persist for hours. Even subclinical, interictal temporal lobe dysrhythmias may impair learning, as in patients with unilateral foci. Patients with left-sided foci have difficulty learning patterns of verbal stimuli, whereas those with right-sided foci have difficulty learning patterns of nonverbal stimuli (faces, music, drawings). Maximal control of temporal lobe dysrhythmia without lowering consciousness would seem to be the goal of treatment.

An amnestic syndrome usually follows *electroconvulsive treatments*. This can be minimized by applying current unilaterally to the nondominant hemisphere, and using the d'Elia electrode placement (secondary electrode lateral to the vertex).

Bilateral posterior cerebral arterial occlusions with infarction of the medial aspects of both temporal lobes will cause an amnestic syndrome accompanied by cortical blindness (Wells and Duncan, 1980). Left posterior cerebral artery occlusion alone, destroying the left medial temporal and thalamic regions, may occasionally result in an amnestic syndrome and a right hemianopsia.

Surgical excision of both temporal lobes causes persistent amnesia. Unilateral dominant hemisphere temporal lobectomy will occasionally produce an amnestic syndrome, usually when damage to the nondominant temporal lobe was not appreciated before surgery. Complete preoperative evaluation of both temporal lobes is mandatory. Clipping of both fornices will produce an irreversible amnestic syndrome.

An amnestic syndrome may follow *encephalitis*, particularly when the infective agent is Herpes simplex, which has a predilection for medial temporal structures. The new antiviral agent, adenosine arabinoside, has decreased mortality in this illness, but major sequelae are still very common.

Little in the way of specific treatment can be offered for amnestic syndromes resulting from destruction or excision of the structures subserving memory, except to secure custodial care for the patient.

The boundaries between the organic delusional, hallucinatory, and affective syndromes are not clear. We will focus on the area of psychopathology that dominates the clinical picture at the time of examination and categorize the syndromes thereby. Mixed syndromes are frequent, and the predominant area of psychopathology may alter within the same individual during the course of illness.

ORGANIC DELUSIONAL SYNDROME (293.81)

Prolonged use of *amphetamines* is probably the most common cause of an isolated organic delusional syndrome. Amphetamines may produce a paranoid psychosis with agitation, delusional mood, or formed delusions. Disorientation and clouding of consciousness are not part of this toxic reaction, and their presence should suggest other drug abuse or withdrawal. Most patients who suffer an amphetamine psychosis vividly remember the episode after their recovery.

ESSENTIAL FEATURES

The essential feature of *organic delusional syndrome* is the presence of delusions that occur in a normal state of consciousness and that are due to a specific organic factor. The diagnosis is not made if delusions occur in a clouded state of consciousness as in delirium, if there is a significant loss of intellectual abilities as in dementia, or if prominent hallucinations are present as in organic hallucinosis. Persecutory delusions are the most common type.

TREATMENT

Patients with amphetamine psychosis should be allowed to rest. Agitation usually clears within 24–48 hours, and the patient may then spend most of the next few days sleeping, often with long periods of dreaming. Paranoid delusions gradually abate over 7–10 days. Rarely, agitation may require treatment with haloperidol or other neuroleptic. Postwithdrawal depressions may occur, and brief treatment with tricyclic antidepressants may be needed.

In contrast to the majority of patients who have an uncomplicated recovery from amphetamine psychosis, some are subject to recurrent "flashback" experiences of paranoid, delusional beliefs. Flashbacks may be triggered by another single use of small amounts of amphetamine, suggesting that lasting vulnerability has been created. Treatment of flashbacks is similar to that of the acute episode.

Rarely, patients with no personal or family history of mental illness develop acute paranoid psychoses after initial exposure to low dosages of amphetamines. Sometimes these persist for weeks or months. Temporal lobe EEG abnormalities may be present during the phase of acute psychosis. Whether these are basically schizophreniform or epileptiform (or other) psychoses is not clear, nor is the best mode of treatment.

A small percentage of patients who have *temporal lobe epilepsy* will, a decade or more after the onset of seizures, develop psychotic paranoid and/or religious delusions accompanied in some cases by hallucinations (Blumer, 1975; Blumer, 1977). The psychosis is sometimes phasic and may have an inverse relationship to seizure frequency. In fact, effective control of seizures by medication may precipitate a psychotic episode in some patients. These patients usually maintain a good range of affect and interest in others; they do not become schizoid; and they do not deteriorate into a socially regressed state.

In those whose psychosis is inversely related to seizure frequency, treatment may include decreasing the dosage of anticonvulsant medications, thereby allowing an increase in seizure frequency. Obviously the rationale for this must be explained carefully to the patient and family. Rarely, regular electroconvulsive treatments may be given to induce controlled and safe seizures. Neuroleptic drugs usually offer minimal benefit, but on rare occasions the results may be dramatic. Surgery does not benefit the psychotic symptoms.

Epileptic psychosis, left untreated, may progress to generalized brain dysfunction (dementia), while the psychotic symptoms become less prominent.

The most common early psychiatric changes associated with *vitamin B-12 deficiency* are diminution of drive and energy, narrowing of affect, and increased irritability. A disturbance in short-term memory is demonstrable in most patients. Occasionally, a psychosis develops, with paranoid or depressive preoccupations, more often the latter (Smith, 1960). If the disease is not properly diagnosed and treated, delirium leads to progressive dementia.

The presence of a megaloblastic anemia, symptoms or signs of long-tract spinal disease (paresthesias, disturbances in deep sensitivity, pyramidal tract signs ranging from mild weakness to spastic paraparesis), or a history of malabsorption or gastric or ileal resection should alert the clinician to the possibility of vitamin B-12 deficiency. Rarely, psychiatric changes occur alone (Strachan and Henderson, 1965).

Neuropsychiatric symptoms correlate with the degree of vitamin B-12 deficiency, not with the hematologic abnormalities. Indeed, neuropsychiatric dysfunction may appear in the absence of hematologic changes (Smith, 1960). Since the illness often follows a relapsing-remitting course in its early stages, diagnosis may be difficult, especially in those without anemia.

It must be stressed that hematologic abnormalities respond very rapidly to replacement of vitamin B-12 in doses below those needed to correct the primary nervous system defects. High doses of cyanocobalamin (1 mg every two to three days for two weeks, followed by 1 mg each week for two weeks, followed by 1000 gamma monthly) must be given parenterally to arrest nervous tissue damage. The longer the duration of neuropsychiatric symptoms before proper diagnosis and treatment, the longer the time required for remission, and the less likely is complete recovery. However, almost all treated patients will improve, even if slowly and incompletely.

Serum folate levels are generally lower in groups of chronic psychiatric patients than in the general population. Yet documented cases of neuropsychiatric illness related to *folate deficiency* are rare indeed (Thornton and Thornton, 1978). A healthy male physician who placed himself on a low-folate diet became sleepless, forgetful, and irritable after four to five months; these changes disappeared two days after oral folate therapy was begun. Chronic use of anticonvulsant drugs can cause folate deficiency; repletion of folate improves alertness and drive, ability to concentrate, and mood in certain epileptic patients. There have been case reports of megaloblastic anemia associated with dementia, both of which responded to folate.

Serum folate levels vary greatly during the day in response to changes in absorption or utilization. Numerous drugs appear to be capable of altering folate levels. Laboratory measurement of the vitamin is also tricky, although the newly developed radioisotope competitive binding methodology is felt to be more accurate than older microbiological methods. Thus, the details of all case reports must be read critically.

It should be recalled that a megaloblastic anemia due to vitamin B-12 deficiency may show a favorable clinical response to folate therapy, without affecting the progressive deterioration in the nervous system. Therefore, folate should never be given to an anemic patient until the status of his B-12 stores is checked.

Most of the psychoses associated with *Huntington's chorea* are affective. Occasional patients develop paranoid delusional psychoses, often with jealous concerns about the imputed sexual misbehavior of others. Such syndromes should be treated with neuroleptic drugs. How much a diminished ability to critically monitor perception and thought, caused by early dementia, contributes to the development of paranoid delusions must be judged in each case.

As brain-injured patients, boxers, alcoholics, and others who have suffered diffuse damage to the brain enter mid- to late life, they have an increased incidence of paranoid psychoses. They may react to their diminishing sexual potential with jealous concerns regarding their spouse's every absence. Violent outbursts may ensue. Neuroleptic drugs offer some control of agitation but rarely provide complete control of the delusions.

ORGANIC HALLUCINOSIS (293.82)

Essential Features

The essential feature of *organic hallucinosis* is the presence of persistent or recurrent hallucinations that occur in a normal state of consciousness and that are attributable to a specific organic factor.

PRECIPITATING FACTORS

Following the chronic use of hallucinogenic drugs, spontaneous episodic recurrences of portions of prior hallucinogen-induced experiences may occur. These flashbacks are most commonly visual (alterations of colors, geometric designs) but may include primitive somatic or affective experiences (numbness or pain, depersonalization, panic, or sadness). Flashbacks usually do not occur until after many exposures to hallucinogens.

After prolonged and heavy hallucinogen use, a few patients develop persistent hallucinatory psychoses, with many or all of the Schneiderian symptoms and with gross formal thought disorder. Unlike schizophrenic patients who tend to be evasive and secretive regarding the content of their hallucinations, these patients often are eager to describe the vivid, intense, and continuous nature of their hallucinatory experiences. These patients find their hallucinations distressing and will often shout or swing their fists at the air where the hallucinations are perceived. Unformed visual hallucinations ("laser beams," "colors," "knives flashing") are prominent. Affective range and desire for human interaction is usually well preserved in these patients; they do not become "schizoid." These chronic hallucinatory psychoses are extremely resistent to treatment with neuroleptics.

Paroxysmal spike discharges can be recorded from deep temporal lobe and limbic striatal structures of patients who have just ingested hallucinogenic drugs. Neurons subjected to such repeated electrical stimulation develop persistent changes in their electrophysiological properties and even in their anatomical structure over time (kindling) (Ifabumuyi and Jeffries, 1976). Limbic system structures have low seizure thresholds and are easily kindled. Ultimately, spontaneous paroxysmal discharges between episodes of exogenous stimulation occur in kindled structures. This may explain flashbacks.

Up to a point, induced neuronal changes are slowly reversible if stimulation is discontinued. The patient must be cautioned against taking any hallucinogenic substance, including marijuana, as this may restart kindling and cause the return of flashbacks. Ultimately, permanent changes may result from prolonged hallucinogen abuse, resulting in continuous irritability and spontaneous episodic discharges in kindled areas accompanied by the persistent psychopathology of the hallucinatory psychoses.

Antiepileptic drugs have been reported to control flashbacks and the chronic hallucinatory psychoses following hallucinogen use (Ifabumuyi and Jeffries, 1976). Because of the difficulties in distinguishing these patients from schizophrenic patients who incidentally used hallucinogens, a trial of neuroleptic drugs should be instituted as first treatment. However, those who fail to improve with neuroleptic drugs should be given at least a 30-day trial of anticonvulsants at therapeutic plasma levels.

Irritative lesions of any type (tumor, stroke, vascular malformation) in sensory or sensory association structures may cause *ictal hallucinations*. This may be the entire extent of a localized seizure, or merely the aura of a seizure which later spreads. Hallucinations may occur in any sensory modality, and in any degree of complexity, depending on the location of the primary lesion. Treatment is aimed first at the primary lesion, and then at control of the epileptic activity with anticonvulsant drugs.

Destruction of primary sensory pathways may result in continuous, spontaneous activity in the sensory association areas that the primary pathways previously supplied and modulated (Brust, 1977). These release "hallucinations" tend to be continuous rather than paroxysmal, although they may be stimulated by input into a sensory association area from other connections (e.g. a woman developed visual hallucinations in a hemianopic field while watching television). Release hallucinations often are replays of past experiences, like persistent afterimages. They may be projected onto objects actually present.

There is no specific treatment for sensory hallucinations. The patient may be cautioned to avoid those stimuli which seem to precipitate the hallucinations. The course is usually one of slow disappearance of the hallucinations over months.

Sensory deprivation removes input to sensory association structures and results in release hallucinations, most commonly visual. The hallucinations are at first simple amorphous forms—rows of dots, geometric patterns, etc. Later, scenes and people may appear. EEG monitors show no epileptic activity, only a slowing of the basic frequencies. Sensory-deprived individuals, when returned to a normal environment, report illusory movements of objects, distortion of shapes and colors, and accentuation of after-images; this seems compatible with overactivity of sensory association structures.

Loss of hearing or vision are common forms of partial sensory deprivation in the elderly (cataracts, otosclerosis) which may lead to hallucinatory experiences. The individual with some degree of cognitive impairment and diminished ability to critically appraise his or her perceptions is most at risk. If possible, treatment is aimed at correcting the defect in the primary sensory pathway (hearing aids, cataract surgery, etc.), or finding other means to enrich general sensory stimulation.

The major problem in dealing with the topic of *alcohol hallucinosis* is that the syndrome has been defined in widely differing ways by various authors. Some describe the occurrence of vivid, multisensory hallucinations, often at night, in chronic alcoholics despite continued drinking. Sleep studies have shown increased pressure for REM-sleep in these individuals, and it has been hypothesized that the hallucinations are dreams invading the waking state. The patient is usually somewhat out of contact during these hallucinatory episodes but may be roused by vigorous stimuli. It seems reasonable to consider such cases to be alcohol-induced deliria (see above).

The more classical definition of alcoholic hallucinosis refers to a syndrome of persistent auditory hallucinations occurring in long-term alcoholics despite a clear sensorium and continued alcohol use. The voices usually occur at night and say malicious, reproachful things, often accusing males of homosexuality and females of promiscuity. The voices may threaten the patient, who responds with fear and apprehension. Ideas of reference and even delusions of persecution may be present. Patients often must be protected from injuring themselves or others in response to their hallucinations.

TREATMENT

Treatment of alcoholic auditory hallucinosis should begin with withdrawal from alcohol, rest, nutritional supplementation, and vitamins. In 75% of patients the voices will gradually disappear over 14 days with no other treatment; the patient remembers the voices but knows they were imaginary. In the remainder, a chronic auditory hallucinosis persists, sometimes for as long as six months. The voices are less vivid and persistent than during the acute phase, and the patient is less agitated, even though paranoid delusions may continue. Neuroleptic drugs can be helpful in these patients. It has been suggested that persistent hallucinosis tends to occur in "constricted, passive" individuals who represent the inadequate personalities of the schizophrenia spectrum; if this is so, the hallucinosis represents a temporary uncovering of a latent susceptibility.

ORGANIC AFFECTIVE SYNDROME (293.83)

Essential Features

The essential feature of *organic affective syndrome* is a disturbance in mood resembling either a *manic episode* or *major depressive episode* that is due to a specific organic factor. The diagnosis is not made if the disturbance in mood occurs in a clouded state of consciousness as in delirium, if it is accompanied by a significant loss of intellectual abilities as in dementia, or if there are persistent or recurrent hallucinations, as in organic hallucinosis; or if delusions predominate, as in organic delusional syndrome.

Precipitating Factors and Treatment

Approximately 20% of patients treated with reserpine develop psychomotor slowing and subdued affect, but only a quarter of these (5% of the total) suffer a true melancholic mood change with depressive preoccupations, *Med Letter* (1976). A history of prior affective illness is the single most reliable variable for predicting who will develop a true depressive syndrome while on reserpine. Such a history should contraindicate use of reserpine for control of hypertension. Discontinuation of reserpine will terminate the depression in some cases, but more commonly standard treatment (antidepressants or ECT) is required even after reserpine is stopped. *Alphamethyldopa* and, more rarely, *propranolol*, also have been reported to induce depression. The management is the same as that for reserpine.

The most common affective change in patients with *Huntington's chorea* is depression; this may reach psychotic proportions with delusions of sinfulness, blameworthiness, or poverty. The combination of a depressed mood, impulsivity due to early dementing changes, and the awful factual situation of having Huntington's chorea may lead to suicide attempts. These depressive episodes generally respond well to tricyclic antidepressants or to ECT.

Excited episodes with manic features also may occur. These are controllable with neuroleptic drugs and tend to resolve spontaneously after several weeks. Information is inadequate regarding the use of lithium carbonate in such patients.

The incidence of major mental disturbances in spontaneous *Cushing's syndrome* is 35 to 40%, and another 40% will show milder alterations of mental function (Cohen, 1980). The mental changes usually appear early in the course of the illness and may antedate the physical stigmata. The occurrence and severity of mental changes have not been shown to bear any relationship to the clinical severity of the Cushing's syndrome. Depression is the most frequently encountered affective change and may occur with retardation or with irritability and paranoia. There is variability in the clinical psychopathology from patient to patient and within the same patient during the course of the disease. Suicide attempts occur in 10% of cases.

Generally, mental symptoms improve following adrenalectomy, but they persist in some patients. Restlessness and anxiety often disappear rapidly, whereas depressive symptoms may require months to a year to resolve. There is no relationship between the clinical severity and the duration of the Cushing's syndrome and the improvement of mental symptoms following adrenalectomy. However, those patients whose illness is caused by a primary CNS defect in the control of ACTH secretion may form a distinct group who are more likely to have a mood disturbance than those patients with a primary adrenal tumor or an ectopic ACTH-producing tumor (Krieger, 1978). Such patients spend decreased amounts of time in the deeper stages of sleep and do not have normal circadian periodicity in the levels of prolactin, growth hormone, or ACTH; and, unlike patients with other causes of Cushing's syndrome, their alterations in brain function persist after treatment of the syndrome (bilateral adrenalectomy or pituitary irradiation) and clinical remission. This suggests that the neuroendocrine changes and the depression may both be caused by the same CNS defect.

Elevated plasma cortisol levels in a depressed patient do not imply the presence of Cushing's syndrome. Patients with primary major depression with melancholia have more frequent secretory cortisol spikes, higher absolute plasma levels of cortisol, and increased 24-hour secretion of cortisol. They may exhibit early escape from dexamethasone suppression and this test is being evaluated as a possible biologic marker of severe depression (melancholia) (Brown et al., 1980; Carroll et al., 1981). The normal circadian periodicity of cortisol secretion is lost. This is probably not a simple reaction to stress since acutely agitated schizophrenic patients show none of these abnormalities.

The incidence of major mental disturbances in patients receiving long-term treatment with either adrenocortical steroids or ACTH is 1–3% when the dose of prednisone is less than 40 mg/day, 4–6 percent when the dose is between 40 and 80 mg/day, and 18% when the dose is over 80 mg/day (Sachar, 1976). Perhaps a fourth of these are psychotic episodes.

By far the most common mild change with steroid or ACTH treatment is euphoria. In more severe cases, mania or depression with irritability, paranoia, or delirium may occur. Marked variability in clinical psychopathology is present from patient to patient, and within the same patient during the course of illness. There may be sudden exacerbations in the severity of mental symptoms without apparent exciting cause. In some patients premonitory symptoms such as paresthesias, insomnia, restlessness, or agitation warn of impending deterioration of the psychiatric condition.

Recovery often follows a decrease in the dose or discontinuation of ACTH or adrenocortical steroids, although this may be gradual. In patients who require continued treatment with ACTH or adrenocortical steroids because of a life-threatening illness, induced mania can be well controlled with lithium carbonate; and induced depressions can be palliated with neuroleptic drugs in low dosages. Tricyclic antidepressants often provoke delirium in such patients, perhaps because effective blood levels of the tricyclics are increased by steroid therapy. A recent study suggests that lithium carbonate may be an effective prophylaxis for the steroid-induced psychoses (Falk et al., 1979).

In the past, up to 50% of patients with *myxedema* showed at least one psychotic manifestation. At present, only about 10% of patients become psychotic before proper diagnosis and the institution of adequate treatment. In all patients with myxedema, emotional reactivity appears to be low; usually these patients are pleasant, good natured, and have a characteristic dry humor.

No established relationship has been noted between the level of thyroid hormone or the severity of myxedema and the presence of psychosis. Psychosis may occur very early in the course of myxedema. Many of the psychoses are deliria, but in occasional patients, depressions or paranoid syndromes with suspiciousness and irritability occur, with few if any of the stigmata of the underlying myxedema. Such symptoms frequently persist and require separate treatment even after adequate treatment of the myxedema, suggesting that they represent constitutionally determined illnesses precipitated by the myxedema.

Patients with myxedema also may suffer severe cardiovascalar as well as CNS complications if improperly diagnosed and treated with narcotic, tranquilizing, or sedative drugs.

Elderly individuals with *hyperthyroidism* may present an "apathetic," placid, or depressed appearance which develops slowly, often with marked weight loss; there are no eye signs in these elderly patients and thyromegaly, though usually present, is not prominent (Brenner, 1978). Cardiovascular signs such as atrial fibrillation or a high-output form of congestive heart failure often offer a clue to correct diagnosis.

Mania has been reported to occur in individuals with no prior history of affective disorder after various drugs (isoniazid, corticosteroids, procarbazine, levodopa), metabolic disturbances (hemodialysis, postoperative), viral infections, and brain tumors (Krauthammer and Klerman, 1978). It is comforting that in almost every case in which it has been tried, lithium has been successful in controlling such secondary manias.

Epilepsy has been reported to cause mania, and perhaps 25% of patients with bipolar affective illness have abnormal EEGs. Carbamazepine has been shown to be an effective treatment in 70% of cases of unselected bipolar patients, including some who do not respond to lithium carbonate. Any manic patient who is nonresponsive to lithium should have an EEG and be considered for a therapeutic trial of carbamazepine.

ORGANIC PERSONALITY SYNDROME (310.10)

ESSENTIAL FEATURES

The essential feature of an *organic personality syndrome* is a marked change in personality that is due to a specific organic factor but not any of the other organic brain syndromes (discussed above). A common pattern is characterized by emotional lability and impairment of impulse control or social judgment. Another pattern is characterized by marked apathy and indifference. Still another pattern seen in some individuals with temporal lobe epilepsy is a marked tendency to humorless verbosity in both writing and speech, religiosity, and occasionally exaggerated aggressiveness. The major personality change may be the development of suspiciousness or paranoid ideation.

When an individual with no prior history of behavioral disorder undergoes a change in personality, especially if the change is sudden or if the individual is over 40, a search should begin for a specific organic etiologic factor.

PRECIPITATING FACTORS AND TREATMENT

Outside of wartime, blunt, closed-head *brain injuries* are the most common explanation; these usually cause greater and more prolonged disorders of consciousness initially and more serious ultimate mental disability than do penetrating focal (missile) injuries. The age of the brain-injured patient is the most dependable variable in estimating the chances for recovery, which are much better in the young. The duration of the post-traumatic anterograde amnesia provides the most reliable index of the severity of the injury.

In 75% of cases of mild brain injury a "post-concussion syndrome" of headache, irritability, dizziness, fatigue, anxiety, and impaired concentration will last for days, weeks, or even months. Various indications of regional brain dysfunction, generalized abnormalities of cerebral blood flow, faulty processing of information on psychometric testing, and abnormalities of vestibular and labyrinthine function have been found in these patients. Propranolol, in doses up to 320 mg daily, has been reported to control the destructive outbursts of rage sometimes seen in these patients.

After severe closed-head injury, the degree of persistent alteration in intellectual and emotional function tends to correspond to the degree of overall disability. Severely disabled patients and some moderately disabled patients show persistent intellectual and emotional deficits which lead to major problems in personal and social adjustment. The outcome of brain injury represents a continuous interplay between the neuropsychiatric deficits, the patients' life-long pattern of coping mechanisms, and the supports and demands of the social situation (Leigh, 1979). Motivation seems to be an important factor in that certain professional groups (e.g. pilots injured in wartime) have generally good outcomes, in contrast to those who suffer industrial injuries for which they may be paid compensation. Improvement in function occurs gradually, leveling out in most cases after two years, but sometimes continuing for five years.

The brain-injured person loses some or all of his ability to reflect upon a situation in an abstract fashion. Rather, he is "stimulus bound" and tends to respond to familiar situations in routine and predictable ways. Newness or the necessity to shift or change is stressful to him, and his life develops a stereotyped character.

Pressuring the brain-injured person to change or to perform tasks beyond his capabilities will cause rapid fatigue manifested by distractability or perseveration. Continued pressure may result in a "catastrophic reaction": an acute, cognitive disorganization with crying, rage, and complete collapse of all performance abilities.

Higher brain functions which are lost in the brain-injured person cannot be regained by retraining. The brain-injured person must be allowed to do things in the tedious or eccentric way he prefers if they work for him. Misguided attempts to force brain-injured patients into "normality" or to afford them "flexibility" will result in a deterioration of function, not improvement.

Major personality changes most commonly occur after bilateral trauma to the *frontal lobes;* frontal lobe tumors are rare, and cerebrovascular occlusions involving the anterior cerebral arteries are very rare. If the lesions are localized to the orbital aspects of the frontal lobes, a "pseudo-psychopathic" change characterized by a lack of adult tact and restraint will occur, whereas localized lesions of the convexities of the frontal lobes produce a "pseudodepressed" change characterized by decreased initiative, slowness, indifference, and apathy (Blumer and Benson, 1975). Most frontal lobe lesions are not neatly localized and produce a mixed syndrome termed an "irritable, euphoric apathy." The patient has no interests, tends to sit around, and does not get much done. He appears euphoric only to those who do not have to be around him much. He is easily irritated but this, like all his emotions, is fleeting and rarely results in harm to others.

Families must be helped to understand that their brain-injured relatives may never be the same functional individuals they were before. They may require advice on how to deal with disruptive behaviors (indiscretions, sexual changes, violence). Families must be supported in caring for their own needs as well as for those of the patient (Lezak, 1978). Violent or unmanageable patients sometimes must be removed from the home. Medications often help symptomatically (see above).

Those lesions of the temporal lobe which produce personality changes tend to be irritative and may be unilateral (Bear and Fedeo, 1977). Personality changes develop gradually but may be the earliest sign of *temporal lobe epilepsy*. The emotions deepen. Everything is laden with meaning, nothing is trivial. The patients tend to be gloomy and discouraged, sober, with a sense of personal destiny. They pay close intellectual attention to everything and often maintain a voluminous, detailed diary stressing moral and philosophical issues. The obsessive and circumstantial aspects of their attempts to interact with others have led to the use of the term "viscosity" in describing their interpersonal style. Once these changes occur, they remain fixed; they are not related to seizure frequency or success of anticonvulsant treatment.

Episodic irritability which increases during the preictal period, then disappears after a seizure, occurs in some patients. Patients must be handled very carefully during such periods or extremely violent and dangerous outbursts may ensue. Carbamazepine has shown promise in obviating this build-up of irritability (Troupin, 1978). Blumer (1977) has also stressed the value of psychotherapy in some patients with personality disorders secondary to temporal lobe epilepsy.

Most men with temporal lobe epilepsy experience a decreased interest in sex, both in action and in fantasy. This may improve with successful anticonvulsant treatment or with unilateral anterior temporal lobectomy. In fact, hypersexuality may follow lobectomy and require treatment with antiandrogens. Some persons with temporal lobe epilepsy become hypersexual; some also develop homosexuality, fetishism, transvestitism, or other unusual forms of sexual expression.

Personality disturbances such as aggressiveness, loss of sexual inhibitions, or childish behavior, are not uncommon in *Wilson's disease*. Storage of copper in the brain is the etiology, and this will ultimately lead to intellectual deterioration if untreated. Evidence of liver damage, Kayser-Fleisher corneal rings, neurological signs and symptoms, and the family history will lead to proper diagnosis and treatment.

Hypercalcemia, often due to hyperparathyroidism, may reduce initiative and spontaneity and cause depressed mood. The illness may progress slowly over years or even decades and thus suggest a personality disorder (Peterson, 1968). The degree of psychic disorder seems related to the calcium level. Once the calcium level reaches 16 mg% or higher, memory loss and reduced ability to concentrate usually occur, and an acute delirium ultimately supervenes. Increased thirst and polyuria are helpful diagnostic clues. The personality changes are wholly and rapidly reversible with correction of the hypercalcemia, irrespective of the duration of the illness, severity of psychic change, or the patient's age.

Idiopathic *hypoparathyroidism* is a relatively uncommon entity which often presents with neuropsychiatric symptoms (Denko and Kaelbing, 1962). Cataracts, epilepsy, paraesthesias, spasms, electrocardiographic changes of hypocalcemia, or dermatitis should provide diagnostic clues. Post surgical hypoparathyroidism should be the second thought a clinician has after noting a thyroidectomy scar. Nonspecific "hysterical, anxious, neurotic" symptoms appear, usually associated with some dampening of intellectual capabilities in a previously well-functioning individual.

REFERENCES

Medical Letter Drugs Therapeutics. 18:19, 1976.

Bear DM, Fedeo P: Quantitative analysis of interictal behavior in temporal lobe epilepsy. Arch Neurol. 34:454, 1977.

Benson DF: Amnesia. South Med J. 71:1221, 1978.

Blumer D: Temporal lobe epilepsy and its psychiatric significance. In: Psychiatric Aspects of Neurologic Disease, Benson, DF and Blumer, D (eds). Grune and Stratton, New York, 1975.

Blumer D: Treatment of patients with seizure disorders referred because of psychiatric complications. McLean Hosp J. June:53, 1977.

Blumer D, Benson DF: Personality changes with frontal and temporal lobe lesions. In: Psychiatric Aspects of Neurologic Disease, Benson, DF and Blumer, D (eds.). Grune and Stratton, New York. 1975.

Brenner I: Apathetic hyperthroidism. J Clin Psychiat. 39:479, 1978.

Brust JCM: "Release hallucinosis" as the major symptom of posterior cerebral artery occlusion: a report of two cases. Ann Neuro. 2:432, 1977.

Brown WA, Shuey I: Response to dexamethasone and subtype of depression. Arch Gen Psychiat 37:747–751, 1980.

Carroll BJ, Feinberg M, Greden JF, Tarika J, Albala AA, Haskett RF: A specific laboratory test for the diagnosis of melancholia. Arch Gen Psychiat. 38: 15–22, 1981.

Centerwall BS, Criqui JH: Prevention of the Wernick-Korsakoff syndrome: A cost-benefit analysis. NEJM. 299:285, 1978.

Cohen SI: Cushing's syndrome: a psychiatric study of 29 patients. Brit J Psychiat. 136:120, 1980.

Cole JO, Branconnier R: Drugs and senile dementia. McLean Hosp J. 2:210, 1977.

Denko JD, Kaelbing R: The psychiatric aspects of hypoparathyroidism. Acta Psychiat Scand. 38:1, 1962.

Detre TP, Jarecki HG: Modern Psychiatric Treatment. Lippincott, Philadelphia. 1971.

Falk WE, Mahnke MW, Poskanzer DC: Lithium prophylaxis of corticotropin-induced psychosis. JAMA. 241:1011, 1979.

Greenblatt DJ, Shader RI: Treatment of the alcohol withdrawal syndrome. In: Manual of Psychiatric Therapeutics, Shader, RI (ed). Little, Brown, Boston. 1975.

Hunter R: Psychosyndrome or brain disease. Proc Royal Soc Med. 66:359, 1973.

Ifabumuyi OI, Jeffries JJ: Treatment of drug-induced psychosis with diphenylhydantoin. Can Psychiat Assoc J. 21:565, 1976.

Jamieson RC, Wells CE: Case studies in neuropsychiatry: I. Manic psychosis in a patient with multiple metastatic brain tumors. J Clin Psychiat. 40:280, 1979.

Klotz U, Avant GR, Hoyumpa A, Schenker S, Wilkinson GR: The effects of age and liver disease on the disposition and elimination of diazepam in adult man. J Clin Invest. 55:347, 1975.

Krauthammer C, Klerman GL: Secondary mania. Manic syndromes associated with antecedent physical illness or drugs. Arch Gen Psychiat. 35:1333, 1978.

Krieger DT: The central nervous system and Cushing's disease. Med Clin North Am. 62:261, 1978.

Leigh D: Psychiatric aspects of head injury. Psychiatry Digest. 40:21, 1979.

Lezak MD: Living with the characterologically altered brain injured patient. J Clin Psychiat. 39:592, 1978.

Lipowski ZJ: Delirium, clouding of consciousness and confusion. J Nerv Ment Dis. 145:227, 1967.

Moore DP: Rapid treatment of delirium in critically ill patients. Am J Psychiat. 134:1431, 1977.

Pathy MS: Clinical presentation of myocardial infarction in the elderly. Brit Heart J. 29:190, 1967.

Peterson P: Psychiatric disorders in primary hyperparathyroidism. J Clin Endocr. 28:1491, 1968.

Risch SC, Huey LY, Janowsky DS: Plasma levels of tricyclic antidepressants and clinical efficacy: review of the literature. J Clin Psychiat. pp. 40:4, 58, 1979.

Roberts RK, Wilkinson GR, Branch RA, Schenker S: Effect of age and parenchymal liver disease on the disposition and elimination of chlordiazepoxide (Librium). Gastroenterology. 75:479, 1978.

Sachar EJ (ed): Hormones, Behavior and Psychopathology. Raven, New York. 1976.

Seltzer B, Sherwin I: Organic brain syndromes: an empirical study and critical review. Am J Psychiat. 135:13, 1978.

Shader RI, Greenblatt DJ: Pharmacokinetics and clinical drug effects in the elderly. Psychopharmacol Bull. 15:8, 1979.

Shull HJ, Wilkinson GR, Johnson R, Schenker S: Normal disposition of oxazepam in acute viral hepatitis and cirrhosis. Ann Int Med. 84:420, 1976.

Smith ADM: Megalobastic madness. Brit Med J. 2:1840, 1960.

Strachan RW, Henderson JG: Psychiatric syndromes due to avitaminosis B-12 with normal blood and bone marrow. Quart J Med. 34:303, 1965.

Summers WK, Reich TC: Delirium after cataract surgery: review and two cases. Am J Psychiat. 136:386, 1979.

Thornton WE, Thornton BP: Folic acid, mental function, and dietary habits. J Clin Psychiat. 39:315, 1978.

Troupin AS: Carbamazepine in epilepsy. In: Clinical Neuropharmacology, Vol. 3, Klawans, HL (ed). Raven New York. 1978.

Wells CE: Diagnostic evaluation and treatment in dementia. In: Dementia, 2nd ed, Wells, CE (ed). F. A. Davis, Philadephia. 1977.

Wells CE: Role of stroke in dementia. Stroke. 9:1, 1978.

Wells CE: Diagnosis of dementia. Psychosomatics. 20:517, 1979.

Wells CE, Duncan GW: Neurology for Psychiatrists. F. A. Davis, Philadelphia. 1980.

Ziegler VE, Biggs JT: Tricyclic plasma levels. Effects of age, race, sex, and smoking. JAMA. 238:2167, 1977.

2 | Substance Induced and Substance Use Disorders: Alcohol

DONALD W. GOODWIN

Although most people who use alcohol do so in a socially acceptable, nonabusive fashion, there are millions of teenagers and adults in this country who are problem drinkers. DSM-III has two major categories of alcohol-related disorders. The first is a group of organic mental disorders induced by the direct effect of alcohol on the nervous system. These include: *intoxication* (303.00), *idiosyncratic intoxication* (291.40), *withdrawal* (291.80), *withdrawal delirium* (291.00), *hallucinosis* (291.30), *amnestic disorder* (Korsakoff's disease) (291.10), and *dementia* (291.2). The second category, *substance use disorder*, refers to the behaviors associated with the use of alcohol and includes *alcohol abuse* and *alcohol dependence*.

This chapter discusses the treatment of the various types of alcohol-induced organic mental disorder and the treatment of alcoholism (which includes both alcohol abuse and alcohol dependence).

ALCOHOL INTOXICATION (303.00)

ESSENTIAL FEATURES

The essential feature of *alcohol intoxication* is maladaptive behavior due to the recent ingestion of alcohol. This may include aggressiveness, impaired judgment, and other manifestations of impaired social or occupational functioning. Characteristic physiological signs include flushed face, slurred speech, unsteady gait, nystagmus, and incoordination. Characteristic psychological signs include loquacity, impaired attention, irritability, euphoria, depression, and emotional lability.

The amount of alcohol required to produce unconsciousness and the lethal amount differ only slightly, explaining why alcohol was used for anesthesia only until better and safer drugs became available. In order to drink enough alcohol to completely depress the respiratory center and produce death, one must drink strong beverages rapidly. Suicide is uncommon from acute alcohol ingestion because most of those who attempt it lose consciousness before they die. Occasionally death will occur when two drinkers engage in a race to see which one can finish, for example, a fifth of bourbon before the other.

There is little or no evidence that repeated use of alcohol leads to an increase in the amount required to produce death. The lethal level apparently varies somewhat with individuals, with ranges reported between 450 mg-% and 800 mg-%. Some of this variation may be due to the unsuspected presence of other drugs at the time a blood specimen is obtained. Postmortem pooling of alcohol may occur in the stomach or cardiac ventricles, resulting in a falsely high reading.

TREATMENT

Management of intoxicated persons centers primarily on controlling their behavior to prevent harm to themselves or to others. Occasionally, individuals commit suicide while intoxicated, and this possibility, while remote, should be considered (Goodwin, 1973). Also, of course, intoxicated individuals can be combative. Physical restraint may be necessary in the latter case, although police officers, nurses, and others who routinely work with intoxicated people often feel that a patient, reassuring approach to the potentially aggressive intoxicated person is superior to the premature use of physical restraint. It is commonly observed that the intoxicated person becomes more combative as those around him take physical action.

Chemical restraint of the intoxicated patient may be dangerous in that most of the sedative and tranquilizer drugs have additive or potentiating effects with alcohol and, together, may result in respiratory depression and death. It is not clear to what extent benzodiazepines react with alcohol to produce additive effects. In the case of chlorodiazepoxide (Librium) there is evidence from the animal literature that little potentiation with alcohol occurs (Miller et al., 1963). Clinically, chlorodiazepoxide has often been given in fairly high parenteral doses (100 mg. or more) with decided calming effects on the patient but no depression of respiration. Benzodiazepines are absorbed more smoothly when given orally but even the erratic absorption that occurs with IM injection still leads rapidly to a relatively high blood level and can be administrated to an aggressive patient when oral administration is not possible.

Death from alcohol intoxication may occur not only from respiratory depression but also from vomiting and aspiration. Death also occurs, of course, from falls, automobile and other accidents, and fires caused by intoxicated individuals smoking cigarettes. Prevention is the only "treatment" in these deaths.

In a medical setting, aside from controlling aggressive behavior, observation should consist of monitoring vital signs and preventing aspiration of vomit. It is rarely necessary to reduce the blood level of alcohol by medical means such as renal or peritoneal dialysis. Fructose in large intravenous dosage will reduce the blood level significantly, but again this is rarely necessary. Alcohol is eliminated from the body at the rate of about one ounce of beverage alcohol per hour. Therefore, within a short time, it is obvious whether the intoxicated individual is going to recover spontaneously from the intoxication.

Although alcohol intoxication alone rarely causes death, the combination of alcohol and sedative and tranquilizer drugs can be lethal indeed, and the clinician treating the intoxicated patient should be alert to the possibility that other drugs may also be involved. If blood specimens indicate this or there is a history of recent drug use, gastric lavage and/or purging of the lower bowel may be warranted.

Other physical conditions which may either mimic alcohol intoxication or increase the adverse effects should be evaluated. Diabetic acidosis or hypoglycemia, particularly, should be ruled out. This can be done by laboratory means or, in the case of suspected hypoglycemia, by administration of glucose in the form of candy, orange juice, or intravenous injection. Where hypoglycemia is present, such administration will produce rapid improvement and can be considered diagnostic.

The possibility of an alcohol disulfiram reaction should also be considered. Disulfiram (Antabuse) reactions are manifested by a flushed skin, rapid heart rate, and fall of blood pressure. The patient should be treated for shock by the usual means, and ascorbic acid and antihistamines have been recommended for counteracting the symptoms.

Alcohol idiosyncratic intoxication (291.40), which is also known as *pathological intoxication*, is a poorly studied condition in which a person becomes severely intoxicated on what is presumed to be a subintoxicating amount of alcohol. Usually one must rely on history alone to know that only a small amount was consumed; therefore, if facilities for measuring blood levels are available, it is well to see what the actual level is. If, indeed, it is low and the person is still very intoxicated or perhaps comatose, it is important to look for other medical explanations, such as hypoglycemia, hepatic decompensation, or subdural hematoma. Psychological factors are believed by some to contribute to pathological intoxication, but the scanty literature on the subject provides little assistance in managing the patient at time of intoxication.

ALCOHOL WITHDRAWAL (291.80)

Essential Features

The essential features of *alcohol withdrawal* are certain characteristic symptoms such as a coarse tremor of the hand, tongue, and eyelids, nausea and vomiting, malaise or weakness, autonomic hyperactivity (such as tachycardia, sweating, and elevated blood pressure), anxiety, depressed mood or irritability, and orthostatic hypotension, that follow within several hours cessation of or reduction in alcohol ingestion by an individual who has been drinking alcohol for several days or longer. The diagnosis is not made if the disturbance is *alcohol withdrawal delirium.*

Withdrawal from alcohol is usually a transient, benign, self-limited experience (Victor and Adams, 1953). Severity of withdrawal is roughly correlated with amount and frequency of prior alcohol consumption. The alcohol hangover is considered by many to be a mild form of withdrawal. Hangover symptoms vary from time to time and from individual to individual but usually last for no more than a day and require no more than symptomatic treatment (e.g. aspirin for a headache). Symptoms include headache, nausea, vomiting, diarrhea, lethargy, anxiety, depression, and sometimes tremor. These symptoms may also occur in medically more serious forms of withdrawal, together with classical withdrawal symptoms.

Studies in the 1950's and 60's left no doubt that symptoms of alcohol withdrawal were directly attributable to excessive consumption of alcohol followed by cessation of use (Isbell et al., 1955). Medically healthy, well nourished subjects, given large amounts of alcohol over a long period, developed classical withdrawal symptoms in carefully conducted experimental studies.

Of the classical withdrawal symptoms, tremor is the mildest and earliest to appear after drinking stops. A gross tremor of the hands is apparent within a few hours, often accompanied by a feeling of "inward" trembling and tremor of the eyelids and tongue. The tremor usually lasts no more than a day or two. Sedative or antianxiety agents will usually relieve the tremor, as well as resumed drinking (the "hair of the dog that bit you" cure).

In the first day or two after drinking stops, acute hallucinations may occur (Victor and Adams, 1953). These may be visual, auditory, or tactile. Often the individual has insight, recognizing the hallucinations for what they are. They may be very mild and more properly be called illusions or be formed hallucinations with no insight. It is not known whether either minor or major tranquilizers relieve the hallucinations. The major tranquilizers (antipsychotics) presumably would reduce the extent and severity of hallucinations, but probably should not be given to patients in alcohol withdrawal because they may lower blood pressure and the seizure threshold. If the hallucinations are mild, accompanied by insight, and not a source of distress for the person or others, a benzodiazepine tranquilizer is all that is indicated, if that.

Alcohol withdrawal hallucinations almost always pass in a few hours to a few days. If not part of a delirium, they do not pose a danger to the patient or others. Very rarely, the hallucinations persist well past the disappearance of other withdrawal symptoms (Victor and Hope, 1958). They may last for weeks, months, and even years. This is called *alcohol hallucinosis* (291.30).

The cause of this rare phenomenon is not understood. There are two schools of thought. One holds that chronic alcohol hallucinosis is really schizophrenia or some other psychotic disorder occurring in a person with a history of heavy drinking. Others maintain that heavy drinking in rare instances will produce a chronic psychosis de novo. Since the condition is so rare, it has been little studied. Whether antipsychotics are helpful has not been reported, but on empirical grounds they can be tried.

Alcohol withdrawal also includes occasional convulsions of the grand mal type. Typically these occur two or three days after the person has stopped drinking. There is little evidence that phenytoin (Dilantin) prevents withdrawal seizures, although many clinicians give phenytoin to patients with a history of withdrawal seizures. It is likely that benzodiazepines and sedative-hypnotics given during withdrawal reduce the possibility of seizure. Again, controlled evidence for this approach is lacking. Epileptics are more likely to have withdrawal seizures than nonepileptics. However, individuals who have alcohol withdrawal seizures do not usually have seizures in other circumstances (Victor, 1968). There is no reason to maintain them on antiseizure medication. During the period of risk for seizures (one to four days after drinking), patients should be watched carefully because of possible harmful effects from a seizure.

The term *alcohol withdrawal delirium* (291.00) should be reserved for those relatively rare occasions when other withdrawal symptoms are accompanied by gross memory impairment, including disorientation. Perhaps only 5% or fewer alcoholics experiencing withdrawal become delirious. Also known as delirium tremens, the condition typically occurs on about the second to fourth day of withdrawal (Victor and Adams, 1953). Its appearance is ominous. Many times it means that the patient is not experiencing simple withdrawal from alcohol but has a serious intercurrent medical illness, such as a fracture, hepatic decompensation, pancreatitis, pneumonia, or subdural hematoma.

When delirium occurs during alcohol withdrawal, the clinician should be particularly alert to a complicating medical illness. Often the physical examination should be repeated and perhaps consultation requested. Death is uncommon, occurring either from the intercurrent medical illness or, more rarely, cannot be explained.

Also, delirious patients, whatever the cause, are dangerous to themselves and others. Unlike schizophrenics, patients with deliria often take their hallucinations seriously and physically attack the hallucinated and delusional object. Delirious patients should be watched very carefully. Delirium often is worse at night. Having lights or television on around the clock and a constant observer (helpfully a member of the family) is indicated.

It is not known whether any medication is specific for delirium. The gross memory disturbance is usually accompanied by vivid visual, auditory, and tactile hallucinations, tremor, persecutory or grandiose delusions, excitement, hyperactivity, and insomnia. It is a mistake, however, to view hyperexcitability as a required feature of delirium tremens. Some patients will have a "quiet delirium," lying peacefully in bed while hallucinating. Their quietness may be misleading; for no apparent reason they may become violent.

In the absence of complicating medical illnesses, delirium tremens usually lasts no longer than one to five days. Uncomplicated withdrawal almost always disappears within a week after drinking stops, except for sleep disturbances, irritability, and sometimes anxiety or depressive symptoms which may or may not be attributable to alcohol withdrawal per se.

Treatment for alcohol withdrawal includes the following:

1. An antianxiety agent during the acute withdrawal period which is then tapered off during the postwithdrawal period if there are no other indications for its continuation. As a rule, 25 mg of chlorodiazepoxide, four times daily with 100 mg given intramuscularly by injection every four hours as needed, suffices to calm the withdrawing patient, ward off seizures to some extent, and still be relatively safe given the frequent uncertainty about the patient's physical status.

2. Vitamins are obligatory. The Wernicke-Korsakoff syndrome almost certainly is caused by thiamine deficiency and the peripheral neuropathy associated with alcohol apparently results from a deficiency of B vitamins in general (Victor et al., 1971).

Thiamine should be administered parenterally for the first three to five days of withdrawal (100 mg intramuscularly twice daily), with a therapeutic capsule containing the B vitamins and vitamin C administered for the first two weeks and once daily for the indefinite future.

Even if the patient seems well nourished, vitamins should be given. This is one of the rare instances where a devastating chronic brain disorder (*alcohol amnestic disorder*, 291.10, in DSM-III, also known as *Korsakoff's syndrome*) can be prevented. Alcoholics almost always have a malabsorption syndrome involving anatomical changes of the mucosa of the small intestine as well as biochemical alterations, which is why thiamine should be given parenterally for the first few days. It also explains why apparently well-nourished individuals who give a history of three substantial meals a day may still have nutritional deficiencies and require supplemental vitamins.

Some clinicians favor giving patients magnesium sulfate during withdrawal. There is some evidence that hypomagnesemia occurs during withdrawal and this may increase the possibility of seizures (Mendelson, 1970). However, there is no direct evidence that seizures are thereby prevented, and most clinicians forego this treatment.

There is a widespread opinion that heavy use of alcohol produces dehydration. In the absence of vomiting, diarrhea, or objective signs of dehydration, such as an elevated hematocrit, one may assume that the patient is, if anything, *overhydrated* (Ogata et al., 1968). Withdrawal thus is not a universal indication for intravenous fluids. It is not only easier but also wiser to encourage the patient to drink water and orange juice unless there is concern about vomiting and subsequent aspiration.

Other symptoms associated with withdrawal, such as nausea, vomiting, and diarrhea, can be treated symptomatically.

Most alcoholics do not experience hypoglycemia, but occasionally this occurs, and sometimes dramatic improvement can be achieved by giving glucose (Freinkel and Arky, 1966).

TREATMENT OF ALCOHOLISM

Chronic excessive use of alcohol produces a wide range of psychiatric symptoms which, in various combinations, can mimic other psychiatric disorders.* Therefore, while a person is drinking heavily and during the withdrawal period, it is difficult to determine whether he suffers from a psychiatric condition other than alcoholism. First, then, a few observations on differential diagnosis:

The diagnosis of alcoholism itself is relatively easy. However, many alcoholics also use other drugs, and it may be difficult to determine which symptoms are produced by alcohol and which by barbiturates, amphet-

*The "Treatment of Alcoholism" section was adapted from *Psychiatric Diagnosis* by D. W. Goodwin and S. B. Guze, 2nd ed. Oxford University Press, New York, 1979.

amines, and so on. If a patient has been drinking heavily and not eating, he may become hypoglycemic, and this condition may produce symptoms resembling those seen in withdrawal.

The two psychiatric conditions most commonly associated with alcoholism are primary affective disorder and sociopathy. Female alcoholics apparently suffer more often from primary affective disorder than do male alcoholics (Schuckit et al., 1969). The diagnosis of primary affective disorder usually can be made by past history or by observing the patient during long periods of abstinence. According to one study, about one-third of patients with manic depressive illness drink more while depressed and another third drink less (Cassidy et al., 1957). Studies indicate that small amounts of alcohol administered to a depressed patient relieve depressive symptoms, but large amounts worsen depression (Mayfield, 1968).

Many sociopaths drink to excess, although how many would be considered "alcoholic" is uncertain. A follow-up study of convicted felons, about half of whom had alcohol problems, indicates that sociopathic drinkers have a higher "spontaneous" remission rate than do nonsociopathic alcoholics (Goodwin et al., 1971; Guze, 1976). When sociopaths reduce their drinking, their criminal activities are correspondingly reduced.

Various personality disorders have been associated with alcoholism, particularly those in which "dependency" is a feature. The consensus at present is that alcoholism is not connected with a particular constellation of personality traits. Longitudinal studies help little in predicting what types of individuals are particularly susceptible to alcoholism (Jones, 1968; McCord and McCord, 1969).

The treatment of alcoholism should not begin until withdrawal symptoms subside. Treatment has three goals: (1) sobriety when possible, (2) reduction in the social, physical, occupational, and legal consequences of alcoholism, and (3) amelioration of psychiatric conditions associated with alcoholism.

A small minority of alcoholics are eventually able to drink in moderation, but for several months after heavy drinking, total abstinence is desirable for two reasons. First, the physician must follow the patient, sober, for a considerable period to diagnose any coexistent psychiatric problems. Second, it is important for the patient to learn that he can cope with ordinary life problems without alcohol. Most relapses occur within six months of discharge from the hospital; they become less and less frequent after that (Glatt, 1959).

For many patients, disulfiram (Antabuse) is helpful in maintaining abstinence. By inhibiting aldehyde dehydrogenase, the drug leads to an accumulation of acetaldehyde if alcohol is consumed. Acetaldehyde is highly toxic and produces nausea and hypotension. The latter condition, in turn, produces shock and may be fatal. In recent years, however, Antabuse has been prescribed in a lower dosage than was employed previously, and no deaths from its use have been reported for a number of years.

Discontinuation of Antabuse after administration for several days or weeks still deters drinking for a three- to five-day period, since the drug requires that long to be excreted. Thus, it may be useful to give patients Antabuse during office visits at three- to four-day intervals early in the treatment program.

Until recent years, it was recommended that patients be given Antabuse for several days and challenged with alcohol to demonstrate the unpleasant effects that follow. This procedure was not always satisfactory because some patients showed no adverse effects after considerable amounts of alcohol were consumed and other patients became very ill after drinking small amounts of alcohol. At present, the alcohol challenge test is considered optional. The principal disadvantage of Antabuse is not that patients drink while taking the drug but that they stop taking the drug after a brief period. This, again, is a good reason to give the drug on frequent office visits during the early crucial period of treatment.

In recent years, a wide variety of procedures, both psychological and somatic, have been tried in the treatment of alcoholism. None has proven definitely superior to others (Blum and Blum, 1969). There is no evidence that intensive psychotherapy helps most alcoholics, nor are tranquilizers or antidepressants usually effective in maintaining abstinence or controlled drinking (Ditman, 1967). Aversive conditioning techniques have been tried, with such agents as apomorphine and emetine to produce vomiting (Voegtlin, 1940), succinylcholine to produce apnea (Clancy et al., 1967), and electrical stimulation to produce pain (Hsu, 1965). None has been shown to be effective in groups of alcoholics; controlled studies have not been carried out. Lysergic acid diethylamide (LSD) has also been tried, but controlled studies indicate that it is ineffective (Blum and Blum, 1969).

While we do not know how many alcoholics benefit from participating in Alcoholics Anonymous, most clinicians agree that alcoholics should be encouraged to attend AA meetings on a trial basis.

Alcoholics Anonymous has many attractive features: the assurance of a regular sympathetic hearing, the feeling that somebody is taking one's condition seriously, the discovery that others are in the same predicament. Unlike most talking therapies, AA expends little effort in trying to explain *why* anyone is alcoholic. The term "allergy" is sometimes used, but usually properly bracketed in quotation marks (alcoholism does not, of course, resemble the conventional allergies at all).

There is an old idea that alcoholics must become religious in order to stop drinking, and it is true that Alcoholics Anonymous has certain similarities to a religion and that some of its members have been "converted" to AA in the same way they would be to other religions. Its "twelve steps," for example, have a definite religious flavor, emphasizing a reliance on God, the need for forgiveness, and caring for others. Nevertheless, to the extent that it is a religion, AA is one of the least doctrinaire and authoritarian religions imaginable. There is no formal doctrine and atheists can belong to AA as comfortably as believers.

In two double-blind studies, lithium carbonate was found superior to placebo in reducing drinking in depressed alcoholics (Kline et al., 1974; Merry et al., 1976). There was a high dropout rate in both studies and the results can only be considered preliminary.

In conclusion, it should be emphasized that relapses are characteristic of alcoholism and that physicians treating alcoholics should avoid anger or excessive pessimism when such relapses occur. Alcoholics probably see nonpsychiatric physicians more often than they see psychiatrists, and there is evidence that general practitioners and internists are sometimes more helpful (Gerard and Saenger, 1966). This may be particularly true when the therapeutic approach is warm but authoritarian, with little stress on "insight" or "understanding." Since the cause of alcoholism is unknown, "understanding" in fact means acceptance of a particular theory. That may provide temporary comfort but probably rarely any lasting benefit.

There is a non theoretical approach to treating alcoholism that is assured to work, given one stipulation: the patient must do what the doctor says. In this case he must do only one thing: come to the office every three or four days.

Doctors cannot help patients, as a rule, who refuse to do what they say, so there is nothing unusual about the stipulation. Why every three or four days? Because, as noted, the effects of Antabuse last up to five days after a person takes it. If the patient takes Antabuse in the office, in the presence of the doctor, they both know he will not drink for up to five days. They have bought time, a precious thing in the treatment of alcoholism.

This approach involves other things besides Antabuse, but Antabuse makes the other things possible. First it gives hope, and hope by the time the alcoholic sees a doctor is often in short supply. He feels his case is hopeless, his family feels it is hopeless, and often the doctor feels it is hopeless. With this approach the doctor can say, "I can help you with your drinking problem" and mean it. He doesn't mean he can help him forever (forever is a long time) and it doesn't mean the patient won't still be unhappy or that he will become a new man. It merely means he will probably not drink as long as he comes to the office every three or four days and takes the Antabuse.

On the first visit the doctor can say something like this: "Your problem, or at least your immediate problem, is that you have trouble controlling your drinking. Let me take charge; let me control your drinking for a time. This will be my responsibility. Come in, take the pill, and then we can deal with other things.

"I want you to stop drinking for a month. [At this point the doctor makes a note in his desk calendar to remind himself when the patient will have taken Antabuse for a month.] After that we can discuss whether you want to continue taking the pill. It will be your decision.

"You need to stop for a month for two reasons. First, I need to know whether there is anything wrong with you besides drinking too much. You may have another problem that I can treat, such as a depression, but I won't be able to find out until you stop drinking for at least several weeks. Alcohol itself makes people depressed and anxious, and mimics all kinds of psychiatric illnesses.

"Second, I want you to stop drinking for a month to have a chance to see that life is bearable—sometimes just barely bearable—without alcohol. Millions of people don't drink and manage. You can manage too, but you haven't had a chance recently to discover this."

F. Scott Fitzgerald complained that he could never get sober long enough to tolerate sobriety, and at least this much can be achieved with the present approach.

It is important for the patient to see the doctor—or whatever professional is responsible for his care—whenever he comes for the pill. Patients as a rule want to please their doctors; this is probably why they are more punctual in keeping office appointments than doctors are in seeing them. In the beginning the patient may be coming, in part, as a kind of favor to the doctor.

The visits can be as brief or as long as time permits. The essential thing is that rapport be established, that the patient believe something is being done to help him, and that he stay on the wagon (he has no choice if he lives up to his part of the doctor–patient contract). Brief, frequent visits can accomplish these things.

The emphasis during the visits should be not on Antabuse but on problems most alcoholics face when they stop drinking. The major problem is finding out what to do with all the time that has suddenly become available now that drinking can no longer fill it. Boredom is the curse of the nondrinking drinking man. For years, most of the pleasurable things in his life have been associated with drinking: food, sex, companionship, fishing, Sunday-afternoon football. Without alcohol these things lose some of their attraction. Who can enjoy French cooking without wine, tacos without beer, or business luncheons without martinis? The alcoholic is sure he cannot. He tends to withdraw, brood, feel sorry for himself.

The therapist may help him find substitute pleasures—hobbies, social activities not revolving around alcohol, anything that kills time and may give some satisfaction, if not anything as satisfying as a boozy glow. In time he may find these things for himself, but meanwhile life can tend to be monotonous.

Also the patient can bring up problems of living that tend to accumulate when a person has drunk a lot. People usually feel better when they talk about problems, particularly when the listener is warm and friendly. The therapist can help by listening even if he cannot solve the problems.

If he is a psychiatrist, he can also do a thorough psychiatric examination, looking for something other than drinking to diagnose and treat. Occasionally—not often—alcoholics turn out to have a depressive illness, anxiety disorder, or other psychiatric condition.

One thing the therapist can do is help the patient accept his alcoholism. This is sometimes difficult. Alcoholics have spent most of their drinking careers persuading themselves and others that they do not have a drinking problem. The habit of self-deception, set and hardened over so many years, is hard to break. William James describes this habit with his usual verve and concludes that the alcoholic's salvation begins with breaking it:

> How many excuses does the drunkard find when each new temptation comes! Others are drinking and it would be churlishness to refuse; or it is but to enable him to sleep, or just to get through this job of work; or it isn't drinking, it is because he feels so cold; or it is Christmas-day; or it is a means of stimulating him to make a more powerful resolution in favor of abstinence than any he has hitherto made; or it is just this once, and once doesn't count . . . it is, in fact, anything you like except being a drunkard. But if . . . through thick and thin he holds to it that he is a drunkard and nothing else, he is not likely to remain one long. The effort by which he succeeds in keeping the right name unwaveringly present to his mind proves to be his saving moral act. (James, 1890)

After a month of taking Antabuse and talking about problems, what happens then? The patient and doctor negotiate. Almost invariably, in my experience, the patient decides to take Antabuse for another month. The doctor says okay, and this is the first step in a process that must occur if the patient is going to recover: acceptance of personal responsibility for control of his drinking.

Proceeding on a month-to-month basis is a variation on the AA principle that an alcoholic should take each day as it comes. For years, alcohol has been the most important thing in the alcoholic's life, or close to it. To be told he can never drink again is about as depressing as anything he can hear. It may not even be true. Studies indicate that a small percentage of alcoholics return to "normal" drinking for long periods (Pattison, 1966). "Controlled" drinking is probably a better term than "normal" drinking, since alcoholics continue to invest alcohol with a significance that would never occur to the truly normal drinker.

Many people, especially among AA members, reject the notion that alcoholics can ever drink normally. If alcoholism is defined as a permanent inability to drink normally, then obviously any person able to drink normally for a long period was never an alcoholic in the first place. The issue is really a definitional one, and those few alcoholics who reported sustained periods of controlled drinking in the studies were at any rate considered alcoholic when they weren't drinking normally. Most clinicians would agree that it is a mistake to encourage an alcoholic to believe he can ever again drink normally, but on the other hand telling him he can never drink again seems unnecessary and may not be true in every case.

When does treatment end? The minimum period is one month because that is the basis for the doctor–patient contract agreed upon in advance. Ideally, however, the treatment should continue for at least six months, with the patient himself making the decision to continue taking Antabuse on a month-to-month basis. Why six months? Because there is evidence that most alcoholics who begin drinking again do so within the first six months following abstention (Skoloda et al., 1975).

Three objections have been raised concerning the above approach to treating alcoholism. The treatment is said to be based on fear, namely, the fear of getting sick, and fear is held to be one of the least desirable forms of motivation. This is debatable. Fear may be the only reason some alcoholics stop drinking. As mentioned earlier, there is evidence that internists have somewhat better success in treating alcoholics than psychiatrists do, and the reason may be that they are in a better position to frighten the patient (Gerard and Saenger, 1966). They have merely to examine his liver and tell him he may be dead in a year if he keeps on drinking. Innumerable alcoholics have stopped drinking because they were told something like this. Others have stopped because they were afraid of losing their wives or jobs. It is probably no coincidence that the hardest alcoholics to treat are those who have little to lose: those who have already lost their wives, jobs, and health. They have no hope of regaining these. All they have left to lose is their life, and by now living has little appeal. Probably the most effective alcoholism treatment programs are run by industries, where the patient is an employee and his job depends on staying sober (Trice and Roman, 1972).

The second objection to the approach outlined here is that the patient becomes too dependent on a personal relationship with an authority figure, the physician, which must end at some point. In the treatment of alcoholism, the goal is not so much a lifetime cure—although sometimes this happens—as it is to bring about improvement. If the patient stays sober for longer periods after treatment than he did before, the treatment has achieved at least limited success. The physician, in any case, should discourage a dependent relationship. He can insist that the patient must take Antabuse and stay dry for a month (realizing that a month is an arbitrary unit of time and any fixed interval will do), but after that the patient has to realize that he himself has the ultimate responsibility for the control of his drinking.

Finally, the complaint is heard that this approach does not get at the root of the problem; it does not explain how the patient became an alcoholic. This is true but, in my opinion, no one can explain how a person becomes alcoholic because no one knows the cause of alcoholism.

Doctors sometimes blame the patient's upbringing and patients often blame everyday stresses. There is no way to validate either explanation. There is probably no harm in telling the patient that his condition remains a medical mystery. And despite some recent studies indicating a possible genetic predisposition to alcoholism (Goodwin, 1981), it is still premature to say that he inherited his disease.

However, if it is ever shown conclusively that some forms of alcoholism are influenced by heredity, this would not make the prognosis less favorable or the treatment less helpful. Sometimes, when evidence for a genetic factor is presented, you hear the following: "But if it is genetic, then you can't do anything about it." It should be noted that diabetes is almost certainly a genetic disorder and there are excellent treatments for diabetes.

REFERENCES

Blum EM, Blum RH: Alcoholism. Jossey-Bass, San Francisco. 1969.

Cassidy WL, Flanagan NB, Spellman M, Cohen ME: Clinical observations in manic-depressive disease. JAMA. 164:1535–1546, 1957.

Clancy J, Vanderhoof E, Campbell P: Evaluation of an aversive technique as a treatment for alcoholism. Quart J Stud Alcohol. 28:476–485, 1967.

Ditman KS: Review and evaluation of current drug therapies in alcoholism. Int J Psychol. 3:248–258, 1967.

Freinkel N, Arky RA: Effects of alcohol on carbohydrate metabolism in man. Psychosom Med. 28:551–563, 1966.

Gerard DL, Saenger G: Outpatient Treatment of Alcoholism. University of Toronto Press, Toronto. 1966.

Glatt MM: An alcholic unit in a mental hospital. Lancet. 2:397–398, 1959.

Goodwin DW: Alcohol in suicides and homicides. Quart J Stud Alcohol. 34:144–156, 1973.

Goodwin DW: Alcoholism: The Facts. Oxford University Press, London and New York. 1981.

Goodwin DW, Crane JB, Guze SB: Felons who drink. Quart J Stud Alcohol. 32:136–147, 1971.

Guze SB: Criminality and Psychiatric Disorders. Oxford University Press, New York. 1976.

Hsu JJ: Electroconditioning therapy of alcoholics. Quart J Stud Alcohol. 26:449–459, 1965.

Isbell H, Fraser H, Wikler A, Belleville R, Eisenman A: An experimental study of the etiology of rum fits and delirium tremens. Quart J Stud Alcohol. 12:1–33, 1955.

James W: Principles of Psychology. Holt, New York. 1890.

Jones MC: Personality correlates and antecedents of drinking patterns in adult males. J Consul and Clin Psychol. 32:2–12, 1968.

Kline NS, Wren JC, Cooper TB, Varga E, Canal O: Evaluation of lithium therapy in chronic and periodic alcoholism. Am J Med Sci. 268:15–22, 1974.

Mayfield DG: Psychopharmacology of alcohol. I. Affective change with intoxication, drinking behavior and affective state. J Nerv Ment Dis. 146:314–321, 1968.

McCord W, McCord J: Origins of Alcoholism. Stanford, California, Stanford University Press, 1960.

Mendelson JH: Biologic concomitants of alcoholism. NEJM. 283:24–32, 1970.

Merry J, Reynolds CM, Bailey J, Coppen A: Prophylactic treatment of alcoholism by lithium carbonate. Lancet. 2:481–482, 1976.

Miller AI, D'Agostino A, Minsky R: Effects of combined chlordiazepoxide and alcohol in man. Quart J Stud Alcohol. 1:9–13, 1963.

Ogata M, Mendelson J, Mello N: Electrolytes and osmolality in alcoholics during experimental intoxication. Psychosom Med. 30:463–488, 1968.

Pattison EM: A critique of alcoholism treatment concepts; with special reference to abstinence. Quart J Stud Alcohol. 27:49–71, 1966.

Schuckit M, Pitts FN, Reich T, King LJ, Winokur G: Alcoholism. Arch Environ Health. 18:301–306, 1969.

Skoloda TE, Alterman AI, Cornelison FS, Gottheil E: Treatment outcome in a drinking decisions program. *The Journal of Studies on Alcohol* 36:365–379, 1975.

Trice HM, Roman PM: Spirits and Demons at Work. Publications Division, New York State School of Industrial and Labor Relations, Cornell University, Ithaca. 1972.

Victor M: The Pathophysiology of Alcoholic Epilepsy. Association for Research in Nervous and Mental Disease, vol. XLVI, Baltimore, The Williams & Wilkins Co, 1968

Victor M, Adams RD: The effect of alcohol on the nervous system. In: Proceedings of the Association for Research in Nervous and Mental Disease. Williams and Wilkins, Baltimore. 1953.

Victor M, Adams RD, Collins GH: The Wernicke-Korsakoff Syndrome. F. A. Davis, Philadelphia. 1971.

Victor M, Hope JM: The phenomenon of auditory hallucinations in chronic alcoholism. J Nerv Ment Dis. 126:451, 1958.

Voegtlin WL: The treatment of alcoholism by establishing a conditioned reflex. Am J Med Sci. 199:802–809, 1940.

3 | Substance Induced and Substance Use Disorders: Barbiturates and Similarly Acting Sedative Hypnotics

BARRY LISKOW

Sedative hypnotics are general CNS depressants. Clinically, these substances produce sedation in small doses and sleep with larger doses. They do not reliably produce analgesia, although intoxicated individuals may ignore pain. There are several distinct features of the depressant effect of sedative hypnotics that separate them from the opiates. First, all sedative hypnotics require, for physical dependence to develop, that the dose per day exceed a threshold value and be continued for a variable period of time that is specific for each drug. Secondly, only a limited degree of tolerance to the effects of the sedative hypnotics develops and essentially no tolerance develops to the lethal dose of the drug. Thirdly, the withdrawal syndrome associated with sedative hypnotics is medically very serious and can have a fatal outcome.

All sedative hypnotics are synthetic chemicals of fairly recent discovery. The first such chemical, chloral hydrate, was synthesized in 1832 and used clinically as a hypnotic in 1869 (Harvey, 1975a). The barbiturates, the most diverse group of sedative hypnotics, were introduced into clinical medicine in 1903 when barbital was marketed. Phenobarbital was introduced in 1912. Since that time more than 2500 barbiturates have been synthesized, approximately 50 marketed, and 12 or so are in widespread use today (Harvey, 1975b).

Pharmacologically, the barbiturates are categorized as long acting (e.g. phenobarbital) or short acting (e.g. secobarbital, pentobarbital, and amobarbital) according to their serum half-lives. The abuse potential of the long-acting barbiturates appears to be minimal but that of the short-acting ones is significant. This is due, at least in part, to the more rapid and intense psychic effects accompanying the short-acting barbiturates.

In the 1950's and 1960's, a large number of nonbarbiturate sedative hypnotics were introduced into clinical medicine. These drugs differ chemically from the barbiturates, but their pharmacological profile and abuse potential are almost identical to the short-acting barbiturates (Hofmann, 1975). Drugs in this group include glutethimide, methyprylon, ethchlorvynol, meprobamate, ethinamate, and methaqualone.

The most extensively used chemical group of nonbarbiturate sedative hypnotics to be introduced since the 1960's has been the benzodiazepines. In terms of their serum half-lives and hence their pharmacological effects, some of the drugs in this group resemble short-acting barbiturates (e.g. lorazepam and oxazepam), some long-acting barbiturates (e.g. chlordiazepoxide), and some a mixture of long-acting and short-acting barbiturates (e.g. diazepam). The one feature of the benzodiazepines that distinguishes them clinically and pharmacologically from the barbiturates is their high therapeutic index (the wide margin between their therapeutic and lethal effects). It is this advantage which had led the benzodiazepines to become more popular clinically than barbiturates in the treatment of anxiety and insomnia (Greenblatt and Shader, 1974). Also, unfortunately, they are becoming increasingly prevalent as drugs of abuse.

PATTERNS OF ABUSE

ESSENTIAL FEATURES

According to DSM-III, the essential feature of *barbiturate or similarly acting sedative or hypnotic abuse* (305.4) is a pattern of pathological use that causes impairment in social or occupational functioning. *Barbiturate or similarly acting sedative or hypnotic dependence* (304.1) is defined by the presence of tolerance or withdrawal.

There appear to be two distinct groups of sedative hypnotic abusers (Shader et al., 1975). One group is composed of adolescents and young adults, mostly male and often antisocial, who use sedative hypnotics to modify mood and consciousness. The drugs may be used orally or intravenously and are frequently mixed with other drugs, such that each drug intensifies the experience of the other. At times, sedative hypnotics will be used when the preferred drug is not available (e.g. barbiturates for heroin or alcohol) or to modify the unpleasant side effects of another drug (e.g. barbiturates to modify the central and peripheral actions of amphetamines). The most widely abused drugs in this group are secobarbital, pentobarbital, methaqualone, glutethimide, and to a lesser extent diazepam (Shader et al., 1975).

The other group of individuals who abuse sedative hypnotics are middle-aged, often middle-class, individuals who initially receive sedatives or hypnotics for ill-defined anxiety or sleep disorders and who then continue to use the drugs daily for these purposes, slowly increasing the dose as tolerance develops until a physically addicting dose is reached. Such individuals often do not realize they are physically addicted until they attempt to decrease or stop their consumption of the sedative hypnotic. They then begin to experience signs of sedative hypnotic withdrawal, which often leads to the resumption of sedative hypnotic use and abuse.

Most patients seeking treatment in rehabilitation centers are from the young adolescent and young adult group of abusers. Limited data are available on the prevalence of abuse in either group, but it is a reasonable assumption that the larger group is composed of middle-aged iatrogenically addicted individuals (Parry et al., 1973).

A third group, much smaller in relation to the other two, but worthy of special note, is composed of health professionals, especially physicians and nurses. Such individuals are at very high risk for developing sedative hypnotic dependence because of the easy availability of the drugs and the tendency to self-treat symptoms of anxiety and insomnia. Such abuse is often undetected except in those health professionals who come to medical attention for treatment of alcoholism and/or opiate abuse.

SEDATIVE HYPNOTIC INTOXICATION

ESSENTIAL FEATURES

Acute and chronic intoxication with the synthetic sedative hypnotics closely resembles intoxication with alcohol. The essential features of *bar-*

biturate or similarly acting sedative or hypnotic intoxication (305.40) are virtually identical to those of *alcohol intoxication* (see p. 29) except that there is no syndrome of *idiosyncratic intoxication*.

All sedative hypnotics are rapidly absorbed from the GI tract and symptoms and signs may appear within 20 min to one hour after the ingestion or within 30 sec to one min after the intravenous injection of an intoxicating dose. Mild symptoms may appear after a therapeutic sedative dose (e.g. amobarbital 30 mg, diazepam 5 mg) and almost invariably after a therapeutic hypnotic dose in a nontolerant individual. Symptoms and signs increase quantitatively and qualitatively with increasing dose. The lethal dose, in both naive and addicted users, is approximately 15 to 20 times the therapeutic hypnotic dose for all sedative hypnotics except the benzodiazepines in which the margin of safety is much higher (the lethal dose being 500 to 1000 times higher than the therapeutic hypnotic dose) (Greenblatt and Shader, 1974). Small doses of nonbenzodiazepine hypnotics or alcohol added to large doses of benzodiazepines may be as dangerous, however, as large doses of sedative hypnotics (Hofmann, 1975).

The signs and symptoms of sedative hypnotic intoxication include sluggishness, slowness of speech, difficulty thinking and concentrating, decreased attention span, poor judgment, emotional lability, irritability, and hostility. Neurological signs and symptoms include nystagmus, diplopia, dysarthria, vertigo, ataxic gait, positive Romberg sign, dysmetria, and decreased superficial reflexes. Generally, pupils and deep tendon reflexes as well as sensory functions remain unaffected.

The sedative hypnotic abuser often has multiple bruises from frequent falls or collisions. Abscesses and sclerosed veins may be noted in those who take sedative hypnotics intravenously. This is due in part to the very alkaline solution resulting from dissolving barbiturate salts (Harvey, 1975b).

Unlike the alcohol abuser, the sedative hypnotic abuser's nutritional status generally remains good. This is because sedative hypnotics, unlike alcohol, have no caloric value and, unlike other drugs, such as amphetamines, have no pharmacological effect on appetite. Hence, sedative hypnotic abusers generally have a normal appetite and do not show signs and symptoms of nutritional deficit (Hofmann, 1975).

In potentially lethal intoxications, an individual may be very drowsy, stuporous, or comatose depending on the amount of the overdose and the time since ingestion. The lethality of overdoses with sedative hypnotics is due to the depression of respiration and/or the development of shock which result from the depressant effects on CNS control of the respiratory and cardiovascular systems. It must be remembered that these signs and symptoms resemble those of stroke and other types of overdoses and poisonings. The management of patients with suspected sedative hypnotic overdose is discussed below.

TREATMENT OF SEDATIVE HYPNOTIC INTOXICATION AND OVERDOSE

In cases of mild or moderate sedative hypnotic intoxication in which the individual is conscious and ambulatory, the primary concern, after assuring that the vital signs are normal, is the prevention of potentially harmful activities (for example, driving, walking, becoming aggressive). This can usually be accomplished by placing the patient in a quiet room with few sensory stimuli so that sleep can occur. Occasionally, if the patient is very agitated, light restraints may be necessary for a short time. Because the moderately intoxicated individual may have taken a large quantity of sedative hypnotics shortly before being seen, it is essential to monitor vital signs and level of consciousness frequently while the patient is resting quietly. If the patient becomes stuporous and/or vital signs begin to deteriorate, further measures, as noted below, must be initiated.

If a patient is stuporous or comatose when initially seen and/or has a history of just having ingested a large amount of sedative hypnotics, then the first concerns are to prevent further absorption of the drug from the GI tract and to be prepared to support respirations and blood pressure. If the patient is conscious when initially seen, 15 to 30 cc of syrup of Ipecac may be given to induce vomiting. If the patient is stuporous, endotracheal intubation followed by gastric lavage should be done followed by introduction of activated charcoal into the stomach to absorb any remaining drug. Some physicians advise, in addition, instillation of 30 cc of sorbitol or other cathartic to induce diarrhea, and hence hasten the clearing of the drug from the GI tract. However, there are as yet not enough data attesting to the value of the latter procedure to recommend it routinely (Davis and Benvenuto, 1975).

When a comatose patient with depressed respirations is initially evaluated, he or she should be given 0.4 mg of naloxone (Narcan) intraveneously. Naloxone is a pure narcotic antagonist and is given to reverse any possible opiate overdose that may have been taken with or without sedative hypnotics. In addition, 50 cc of 50% glucose to treat possible hypoglycemic coma should also be given at this time. Naloxone and glucose are safe to give regardless of the etiology of the coma and should be given to all comatose patients in whom the etiology of coma is in doubt. If respirations remain at fewer than 10 per min after the above procedures, ventilatory assistance is necessary. Adequacy of treatment should be monitored with regular arterial blood gases. The use of respiratory or cerebral stimulants is of little or no value and may serve only to increase the agitation of an intoxicated patient, making management much more difficult (Franz, 1975). If hypotension develops, it should be treated conservatively with fluid replacement. Rarely are vasopressor medications, colloids, or whole blood required.

The urinary excretion of some barbiturates, such as phenobarbital, can be increased by alkalinizing the urine with sodium bicarbonate. Such a procedure, however, will not hasten the excretion of short-acting barbiturates or most other sedative hypnotics. Forced diuresis with intravenous 20% mannitol at the rate of 50 cc per hour greatly increases the excretion of meprobamate but is of little value in hastening the excretion of barbiturates and other sedative hypnotics.

Quantitative and qualitative blood levels may be monitored both to follow the course of treatment and to rule out simultaneous overdoses with other drugs such as tricyclic antidepressants, aspirin, acetaminophen, etc.

Aqueous or lipid hemodialysis rapidly removes most sedative hypnotics from the blood. However, whether hemodialysis produces a lower morbidity or mortality than vigorous conservative measures is unclear from data currently available. Hemodialysis is of little value in removing glutethimide from the blood due to that drug's protein binding and storage in body fat (Davis and Benvenuto, 1975).

In summary, sedative hypnotic intoxication and overdose is treated by providing a safe, quiet environment in which the level of consciousness and vital signs can be regularly monitored, by removing excess drug from the GI tract, and when necessary by providing for support of vital functions. After the patient is past any danger, a thorough psychiatric evaluation is conducted and arrangements for additional treatment initiated.

SEDATIVE HYPNOTIC WITHDRAWAL SYNDROME

ESSENTIAL FEATURES

The essential features of *barbiturate or similarly acting sedative or hypnotic withdrawal* (292.00) are virtually identical to those of *alcohol withdrawal* (see p. 47). The only exception is that a coarse tremor is not invariably present.

Although the barbiturate withdrawal syndrome was first described in the German literature in 1914 (Isbell, 1950), most American and British physicians did not accept the existence of such a syndrome. This reluctance may have been due to the fact that sedative hypnotics, unlike opiates, require that a threshold dose of the drug be taken for a threshold time period to cause physical dependence and the consequent abstinence syndrome to develop. It was not until 1950 that the existence of physical dependence induced by barbiturates was demonstrated experimentally by Isbell. He administered 1500 to 3000 mg of short-acting barbiturate, which provoked a withdrawal syndrome that appeared to be identical to withdrawal from alcohol in all subjects.

In 1954, the threshold value for inducing physical dependence with pentobarbital was established (Fraser et al., 1954). This group found that 400 mg of pentobarbital given daily for four months to subjects and suddenly withdrawn produced paroxysmal EEGs in 30% of the subjects. Six hundred milligrams of pentobarbital given daily for one to two months and withdrawn suddenly produced minor withdrawal symptoms (insomnia, anorexia, and tremor) in 50% of subjects and seizures in 10%. Finally, 900 to 2200 mg of pentobarbital given daily for one to two months and suddenly withdrawn produced seizures in 75% of subjects, delirium in 65%, and minor withdrawal symptoms in 100%.

Similar but less detailed studies have been done to determine the daily threshold dose and time periods necessary for development of physical dependence for each of the sedative hypnotics. These thesholds are given in Table 3-1. Doses below the threshold dose will not produce abstinence syndrome when suddenly withdrawn, no matter how long they are taken.

TABLE 3-1.
THRESHOLD DOSES AND TIME PERIODS OF SEDATIVE HYPNOTIC USE
NECESSARY FOR DEVELOPMENT OF PHYSICAL DEPENDENCE

Drug	Threshold Dose (mg per day)	Duration of Daily Use (days)
Pentobarbital (Nembutal)	400	30–90
Secobarbital (Seconal)	400	30–90
Ethchlorvynol (Placidyl)	2000	30
Ethinamate (Valmid)	13000	30
Glutethimide (Doriden)	2500	30
Methyprylon (Noludar)	2400	30
Chlordiazepoxide (Librium)	45–300	30–90
Diazepam (Valium)	25–100	30–90
Meprobamate (Miltown, Equinal)	3200–6400	40
Phenobarbital (Luminal)	120–200	90–300

From: Hofmann, 1975; Covi et al., 1973; Winokur et al., 1980; Epstein, 1980; Fraser et al., 1958; Haizlip and Ewing, 1958; Hollister et al., 1963; Hollister et al., 1966; Essig, 1964; Essig, 1966.

PRECIPITATING FACTORS

Signs and symptoms of the withdrawal syndrome begin within 12–48 hours after sudden cessation of the short-acting sedative hypnotics (such as secobarbital) (Fraser et al., 1958), but may be delayed up to 7–10 days after cessation of long-acting sedative hypnotics (such as chlordiazepoxide and diazepam) (Hollister et al., 1963; Hollister et al., 1966). The patient may appear improved in the first 12–16 hours after stopping the sedative hypnotic as signs of intoxication clear and the patient becomes more lucid and alert. The severity of the subsequent withdrawal syndrome is directly related to the dose and duration of use of the sedative hypnotic. The syndrome often begins with increasing restlessness and agitation. Gross body tremors may develop along with diaphoresis, hyperpyrexia, orthostatic hypotension, and tachycardia. Nausea, vomiting, and weakness are common. Perceptual distortions (e.g. walls appearing to bend) may occur. Hyperreflexia and increased startle response have been noted. Visual and auditory hallucinations in a clear sensorium may occur. In more severe cases, seizures, usually one or two in number but occasionally leading to status epilepticus, may ensue. Delirium may follow seizures but can also occur in their absence. The delirium is characterized by extreme psychomotor agitation, profound disorientation, auditory and visual hallucinations, and poorly formed delusional thought patterns. The time course of the sedative hypnotic withdrawal syndrome differs for different sedative hypnotics and is in the range of two to five days. The delirium, if it occurs, lasts and adds two to six days to the withdrawal syndrome period (Hofmann, 1975).

TREATMENT

The treatment of sedative hypnotic withdrawal syndrome entails mildly intoxicating the patient with sedative hypnotics and then withdrawing them slowly at the rate of approximately 10% per day. This method should prevent the withdrawal syndrome (Wikler, 1968). The withdrawal should be carried out in an in-patient hospital setting both to keep the patient from returning to sedative hypnotics during withdrawal and because of the possible need for frequent daily adjustments in the withdrawal schedule.

If it is known that the drug being abused is a short-acting barbiturate (e.g. pentobarbital, secobarbital, or amobarbital), then the barbiturate challenge test can be used to determine a rational withdrawal schedule. This test has a number of variations, but its purpose remains the same, to determine the amount of short-acting barbiturates needed in a 24-hour period to keep a physically dependent individual mildly intoxicated (Wikler, 1968). The following is one method for determining whether a patient is physically dependent on a short-acting barbiturate and, if so, the dosage required for safe withdrawal.

THE BARBITURATE CHALLENGE TEST

If the patient is admitted to the hospital in the middle of the day, or at night, it is often convenient to give the challenge test the following morning. If, at admission, the patient is lucid with no signs of withdrawal or intoxication, then 200 mg of secobarbital or pentobarbital should be given at bedtime and the challenge test started the following morning. If the patient shows signs of withdrawal when initially evaluated, 200 mg of secobarbital or pentobarbital should be given every two hours until the patient is asleep; then no additional medication should be given until 12 hours later or 8:00 AM the following morning (whichever is later), at which time the challenge test should begin. If the patient shows signs of intoxication such as lateral gaze nystagmus, ataxia, slurred speech, and/or positive Romberg sign when first evaluated, then no medication is necessary until the first test dose is given the following morning. While being tested, the patient should ingest nothing except fruit juices. The challenge test and its interpretation are as follows:

8:00 AM	200 mg secobarbital or pentobarbital by mouth.
10:00 AM	If the patient exhibits ataxia or slurred speech, or is asleep, physical dependence on short-acting barbiturates is ruled out and no further medication is necessary. If the patient is not mildly intoxicated an additional 200 mg of pentobarbital or secobarbital is given.
12:00 noon	The patient is checked for signs of intoxication once again and if none are present and the patient is awake, then an additional 200 mg of pentobarbital or secobarbital is given. This procedure continues every two hours until the patient exhibits ataxia, dysarthia, or is asleep. If 400 mg or less is needed to produce this mild intoxication, no further treatment is necessary. If 600 mg or more is needed, the patient is considered physically dependent on short-acting barbiturates. The amount to which he or she is physically dependent is the total dosage necessary to produce signs of intoxication. Once the patient exhibits these signs, no additional barbiturates should be given for the rest of the day. Beginning at 12:00 midnight, divided doses of the barbiturates should be given. For example, if 800 mg of pentobarbital is needed before intoxication is achieved, then the orders for the next day should be written "200 mg pentobarbital every six hours beginning at 12:00 midnight." The dose of pentobarbital is then decreased at the rate of 100 mg per day with the understanding that if signs of withdrawal occur while the dosage is being reduced, the patient will be given an extra 100 mg of secobarbital or pentobarbital.

Phenobarbital may be substituted for secobarbital or pentobarbital once the dosage needs of these short-acting barbiturates have been established. Thirty mg of phenobarbital is equivalent to 100 mg of pentobarbital or secobarbital and is administered orally in divided doses (Smith and Wesson, 1970).

If a short-acting, nonbarbiturate sedative hypnotic is the suspected drug of abuse, then the same schedule as noted above can be utilized. That is, the nonbarbiturate sedative hypnotic is administered at the usual hypnotic dose (e.g. methaqualone 300 mg ethchlorvynol 500 mg, methyprylon 300 mg) in place of secobarbital or pentobarbital at mg (Essig, 1964; Khantziam and McKenna, 1979).

With benzodiazepine, long-acting sedative hypnotic, or mixed sedative hypnotic dependence, a barbiturate challenge test will often be negative or otherwise misleading. In addition, the benzodiazepine withdrawal syndrome may not become apparent for 5 to 10 days after the sudden cessation of medication (Hollister et al., 1966). If such dependence is strongly suspected, the patient can safely be started on 25–30 mg bid of diazepam, 100–150 mg bid of chlordiazepoxide, or 60–120 bid of phenobarbarbital and the dosage reduced by 5 mg of diazepam, 25 mg of chlordiazepoxide, or 30 mg of phenobarbital per day (Khantziam and McKenna, 1979; 1976). It should be emphasized that these are guidelines gained from clinical practice and are yet to be verified by experimental evidence.

An alternative method for withdrawal has recently been described by Martin et al. (1979). In this method, phenobarbital is given to a patient in clinical withdrawal as a slow, continuous IV infusion at the rate of .04 mg per kg per min or in equivalent hourly oral doses of 2.4 mg per kg until the patient exhibits marked nystagmus and at least two other signs of intoxication (asleep but arousable, dysarthic, ataxic, or emotional changes). According to the authors, additional medication is seldom needed beyond this initial dose of phenobarbital. One drawback of this method is the necessity of monitoring the phenobarbital serum concentration to identify the occasional patient who requires supplementation of the initial phenobarbital dose in order to suppress the abstinence syndrome induced by the too rapid elimination of the phenobarbital. The authors state that this rapid elimination occurs only rarely. Another drawback is that the study included only seven patients and awaits confirmation. However, if it is confirmed by others, it would be a valuable way of treating sedative hypnotic abuse because medication would be necessary for less than one day in most patients.

TREATMENT OF WITHDRAWAL DELIRIUM

All sedative hypnotics, including alcohol, can lead to withdrawal delirium upon sudden cessation of a threshold dose that has been taken for a sufficient period of time. The delirium, when it occurs, may or may not be ushered in by a seizure, but seizures seldom occur after delirium manifests itself (Fraser et al., 1958). When withdrawal delirium from alcohol or short-acting sedative hypnotics occurs, it generally starts 36 to 120 hours after sudden cessation or abrupt decrease in the drug intake. Long-acting sedative hypnotics such as chlordiazepoxide and diazepam may not result in withdrawal delirium until 5 to 15 days after sudden cessation or abrupt decrease of the drug (Shader and Greenblatt, 1977).

Withdrawal delirium is treated by administering large doses of sedative hypnotics to control the extreme psychomotor agitation of the patient and to lightly intoxicate him/her (Wulff, 1959). These goals can usually be achieved by administering 500 mg of amobarbital IV or 10 mg of diazepam IV, followed by 30 mg of diazepam by mouth twice a day, 150 mg of chlordiazepoxide by mouth twice a day, or 120 mg of phenobarbital by mouth twice a day, with the understanding that the patient's vital signs will be checked before the next oral dose of medication is given. If the patient is asleep, the medication should be held until the next scheduled administration. In this manner, accidental overdosing can be avoided. The medication is then reduced by 5 mg diazepam, 25 mg chlordiazepoxide, or 30 mg phenobarbital per day with the understanding that the reduction will be slowed or additional medication given if signs of withdrawal occur.

In both withdrawal and withdrawal delirium, medication should be given orally (intravenously for the initial dose for delirium) and not intramuscularly. The barbiturates are painful when injected intramuscularly and are absorbed well from the gastrointestinal tract (Harvey, 1975b). Diazepam and chlordiazepoxide achieve higher blood levels faster when given orally than intramuscularly (Shader and Greenblatt, 1977; Greenblatt et al., 1975).

LONG-TERM TREATMENT AND REHABILITATION OF SEDATIVE HYPNOTIC ABUSERS

There are few studies focused on the rehabilitation and long-term treatment of sedative hypnotic abusers, especially when compared with the studies of opiate and alcohol abusers. No doubt, this reflects the real lack of treatment and rehabilitation options available for the sedative hypnotic abuser. Those studies that have been done have not been very encouraging. For example, Tennant (1979) described 46 patients who voluntarily sought outpatient treatment for prescription drug abuse of various kinds. The most commonly abused drugs were diazepam and barbiturates, accounting for more than 50% of the abuse. The patients were equally divided between men and women and their average age was 27 years. Patients were encouraged to attend sessions with experienced drug abuse counselors after they had withdrawn from their medication. Fewer than 30% of patients reported abstinence 90 days after entering treatment. Even more discouraging were the results of Anderson et al. (1972) who reported on the outpatient treatment of amphetamine, barbiturate, and hallucinogenic drug abusers and found that only 8 of 83 patients even returned for a second visit after initial evaluation. These studies probably indicate that methods for relating to the sedative hypnotic outpatient abuser have not been sufficiently developed to engage them in treatment, much less cure their disorder. Despite these and other discouraging results, there are some general principles to guide the physician confronted with a sedative hypnotic abuser. The first step is to determine whether intoxication or physiological dependence is present; if so, it must be treated (see above).

Together with treatment of the direct toxic effects of the sedative hypnotic, a thorough medical and psychiatric evaluation should be conducted. Such an evaluation may reveal that the abuse is related to self-medication for an underlying psychiatric illness (such as depression) or an underlying medical illness (such as thyrotoxicosis). Treatment of such an underlying illness may lead to remission of the substance use disorder.

Whether or not a concomitant illness is present, the next step is to educate the patient about the hazards of acute and chronic sedative hypnotic abuse. This may be especially beneficial to patients who are iatrogenically dependent on sedative hypnotics. However, it should be pointed out that there are as yet no studies clearly indicating that such education is beneficial and this recommendation, like most others relating to the treatment of sedative hypnotic abusers, is based on clinical impressions.

Some patients may benefit from nonpharmacological therapy. Hypnosis, biofeedback, progressive relaxation, and exposure therapy may all help patients who abuse sedative hypnotics in an attempt to relieve anxiety, phobias, obsessions, compulsions, and/or insomnia.

Group therapy and self-help groups for sedative hypnotic abusers on the AA model would seem to be helpful but at present such groups are so few in number that not enough data has accumulated to make a judgment. The dearth of such groups may be due to lack of public recognition of this disorder, and the relative isolation of those suffering from sedative hypnotic dependence.

The substitution of a sedative hypnotic with lower abuse potential than the sedative hypnotic being abused is a controversial treatment; the evidence for or against such treatment is scanty. Even the positive studies, however, do not take into account the fact that such substitution would ordinarily be done more haphazardly than occurs in a research setting. The ease of taking a pill might tend to discourage alternative treatments and encourage widespread, indiscriminate use of such a form of therapy.

Psychotherapy of sedative hypnotic abusers is often recommended but its value has yet to be proven. Those who advocate individual psychotherapy often view drug dependence as an indication of an underlying personality disorder, usually identified as passive dependent. This view has been criticized by citing the unreliability of personality disorder diagnoses and the tendency of some therapists to neglect the substance abuse problem while treating the putative underlying personality disorder.

Therefore, although data are currently skimpy regarding long-term treatment and rehabilitation of sedative hypnotic abusers, the following steps, based on clinical impressions and common sense would appear to be appropriate:

1. Detoxification and treatment of withdrawal if necessary.
2. Thorough medical and psychiatric examination followed by appropriate treatment of any disorders uncovered.
3. Education of the patient regarding the harmful consequences of acute and chronic sedative hypnotic abuse.
4. Treatment of certain symptoms such as anxiety, phobias, and insomnia with nonpharmacological therapies.
5. Caution in prescribing sedative hypnotics to any patients.

It is hoped that in the future more attention will be given to the recognition and identification of the syndrome of sedative hypnotic abuse. Such increased recognition should lead to an increased interest in exploring the most effective methods for the long-term treatment and rehabilitation of the sedative hypnotic abuser.

REFERENCES

National Polydrug Collaborative Project: Treatment Manual I: Medical Treatment for Complications of Polydrug Abuse. National Institute on Drug Abuse, Rockville, Md. 1976.

Anderson W, O'Malley JE, Lazare A: Failure of outpatient treatment of drug abuse: amphetamines, barbiturates, hallucinogens. Am J Psychiat. 128:122–125, 1972.

Davis JM, Benvenuto JA: Acute Reactions from Drug Abuse Problems. In: Emergency Psychiatric Care, Resnick, HLP and Ruben, HL (eds). Charles Press, Bowie, Md. pp. 81–101, 1975.

Essig CF: Addiction to nonbarbiturate sedative tranquilizing drugs. Clin Pharmacol Therapy. 5:334–343, 1964.

Franz DN: Central Nervous System Stimulants. In: The Pharmacological Basis of Therapeutics. Goodman, LS and Gilman, A (eds). Macmillan, New York. pp. 359–366, 1975.

Fraser HF, Isbell H, Eisenman AJ, Wikler A, Pescor FT: Chronic barbiturate intoxication: further studies. Arch Int Med. 94:34–41, 1954.

Fraser HF, Wikler A, Essig C, Isbell M: Degree of physical dependence induced by secobarbital or pentobarbital. JAMA. 166:126–129, 1958.

Greenblatt DJ, Shader RI: Benzodiazepines in Clinical Practice. Raven, New York. 1974.

Greenblatt DJ, Shader RI, Koch-Wester J: Slow absorption of intramuscular chlordiazepoxide. N Eng J Med 291:1116–1118, 1974.

Harvey SC: Hypnotic and Sedatives. Miscellaneous Agents. In: The Pharmacological Basis of Therapeutics, Goodman, LS and Gilman, A. (eds). Macmillan, New York. pp. 124–136, 1975a.

Harvey SC: Hypnotics and Sedatives. The Barbiturates. In: The Pharmacological Basis of Therapeutics, Goodman, LS and Gilman, A (eds). Macmillan, New York, pp. 102–123, 1975b.

Hofmann FG: A Handbook on Drug and Alcohol Abuse: The Biomedical Aspects. Oxford University Press, New York. pp. 116–128, 1975.

Hollister LE, Bennett JL, Kimbell I: Diazepam in newly admitted schizophrenics. Dis Nerv Syst. 24:746–750, 1963.

Hollister LE, Montzenbecker FP, Degans RO: Withdrawal reactions from chlordiazepoxide. Psychopharmacologia. 2:63–68, 1966.

Isbell H: Addiction to barbiturates and the barbiturate abstinence syndrome. Arch Int Med. 33:108, 1950.

Khantziam EJ, McKenna GJ: Acute toxic and withdrawal reaction associated with drug use and abuse. Annals Int Med. 90:361–372, 1979.

Martin PR, Kapur BM, Whiteside EA, Sellers EM: Intravenous phenobarbital therapy in barbiturate and other hyposedative withdrawal reactions: a kinetic approach. Clin Pharmacol Therapy. 2:256–264, 1979.

Parry HJ, Balter MD, Mellinger GD: National patterns of psychotherapeutic drug use. Arch Gen Psychiat. 28:769–783, 1973.

Shader RI, Caine ED, Meyer RE: Treatment of Dependence on Barbiturates and Sedative Hypnotics. In: Manual of Psychiatric Therapeutics. Practical Psychopharmacology and Psychiatry, Shader, RI (ed). Little, Brown & Company, Boston. pp. 195–202, 1975.

Shader RI, Greenblatt DJ: Clinical implications of benzodiazepine pharmacokinetics. Am J Psychiat. 134:652–655, 1977.

Smith DL, Wesson DR: A new method for treatment of barbiturate dependence. JAMA. 2:294–295, 1970.

Tennant FS: Outpatient treatment and outcome of prescription drug abuse. Arch Int Med. 139:154–156, 1979.

Wikler A: Diagnosis and treatment of drug dependence of the barbiturate type. Am J Psychiat. 125:758–765, 1968.

Wulff MH: The barbiturate withdrawal syndrome: a clinical and electroencephalographic study. Electroenceph Clin Neurophysical Suppl. 14:1–173, 1959.

4 | Substance Induced and Substance Use Disorders

(opioids, cocaine, amphetamines and similarly acting sympathomimetics, phencyclidine (PCP), inhalants, hallucinogens and cannabis, tobacco, caffeine)

PHILIP A. BERGER and
MEREDITH J. DUNN

Throughout history, almost every culture has sought ways to alter consciousness by ingesting substances. Alcohol has always been mankind's most widely used psychoactive (mind-altering) substance. Until recently, drugs such as hashish, opium, and naturally occurring hallucinogens were used in limited ways by certain cultures, but were not a major health problem. Modern technology in chemistry and psychopharmacology has increased the types, quality, and availability of psychoactive substances. These substances are currently used by most cultures. The production, distribution, and consumption of psychoactive substances involves a significant part of the time and energy of humankind. The use of drugs of all types is so widespread that in 1894, William Osler suggested, somewhat seriously, that man has an inborn craving for medicine. More recently, Andrew Weil argued that the widespread use of psychoactive drugs in most societies may suggest that the drive and desire for altered states of consciousness is intrinsic to humankind (Weil, 1972).

Supported by the Medical Research Service of the Veterans Administration and the National Institute of Mental Health Specialized Research Center Grant MH 30854. The authors thank Barbara Graham, Constance Gutt, and Bethany Hampton for help in preparing this chapter.

The popularity of psychoactive substances has given rise to many philosophical, social, and ethical controversies. For example: Has the heavy reliance of busy physicians on prescription medications created a "drug-dependent society?" In a free society, should individuals be able to ingest whatever substances they choose, as long as this drug use does not affect others? Are strict legal controls of psychoactive drugs needed to prevent an epidemic of drug use which could seriously threaten social order? Is it not inconsistent to advertise and allow easy access to such dangerous substances as alcohol and tobacco while severely restricting the use of what may be less dangerous psychoactive substances such as marijuana and cocaine? Has the fragmentation of our society and the decreasing importance of the extended family and traditional religions left a gap that only psychoactive drugs can fill? Can the altered states of consciousness produced by some psychoactive substances give an individual better insight into his own psychological makeup or perhaps even lead to insights or perspectives which might benefit society? Why has research on the risks and benefits of psychoactive substance abuse been given such a low priority when substance abuse is considered to be a threat to both individuals and to society? These questions suggest that the use of psychoactive substances is as much a social and ethical problem as it is a medical problem (Berger and Tinklenberg, 1979).

This chapter will focus primarily on the medical aspects of psychoactive substance use. It is divided into sections, following the major pharmacological classes of substances of abuse, excluding alcohol and sedative hypnotics which are discussed in Chapters 2 and 3, respectively. Each section contains a brief history of the substance, a description of its pattern of use, the reasons for its use, and a description of the medical management of both the acute and chronic adverse reactions to each category of psychoactive substance. The chapter begins with a discussion of the management of the acute toxicity of the polydrug abuser to acquaint the reader with the general principles of managing acute adverse reactions to all psychoactive substances.

Psychoactive substances of abuse can be conveniently classified into ten pharmacological categories. This chapter will discuss eight of these: opioids, psychostimulants, phencyclidine (PCP), inhalants, classical hallucinogens and cannabis, tobacco, and caffeine. These categories will be related to two classes of DSM-III disorders: *substance-induced organic mental disorders* and *substance use disorders*. According to DSM-III, the former refers to the direct acute or chronic effects of these substances on the

TABLE 4-1.

PHARMACOLOGICAL CLASSIFICATION OF ABUSED SUBSTANCES

SUBSTANCE CLASSES	REPRESENTATIVE SUBSTANCES	PROBLEMS REQUIRING TREATMENT
Alcohol (ethanol)	See Chap. 2	See Chap. 2
Barbiturate or similarly acting sedatives or hypnotics	See Chap. 3	See Chap. 3
Opioids (narcotic analgesics)	Heroin (diacetylmorphine), morphine, pepthidine (meperidine), methadone, opium, codeine, propoxyphene, oxycodone, levorphanol, and others.	*Organic Mental Disorders* intoxication withdrawal *Substance abuse Substance dependency*
Cocaine, amphetamine and similarly acting sympathomimetics	Cocaine, amphetamine, dextroamphetamine, methamphetamine, methylphenidate, phenmetrazine, diethylproprion, fenfluramine, phentermine, chlorphentermine, and others.	*Organic Mental Disorders* intoxication delirium delusional syndrome
Phenycyclidine (PCP) and related arylcyclohexylamines	Phencyclidine (PCP) Ketamine	*Organic Mental Disorders* intoxication delirium mixed organic mental disorder *Substance abuse*
Inhalants	Glues, cleaning solutions, solvents, lighter fluids, paint and paint thinners, aerosols and other petroleum products containing toluene, acetates, hexane, benzene, xylene, acetone, gasoline, chloroform, naphtha, nitrous oxide, ether, isoamyl and isobutyl, nitrite, and others.	*Organic Mental Disorders* intoxication delirium delusional syndrome hallucinosis amnestic syndrome mixed organic brain syndrome *Substance abuse*

Substance Classes	Representative Substances	Problems Requiring Treatment
Anticholinergics	Many nonprescription substances for insomnia and anxiety (scopolamine and methapyrilene); colds, hayfever, asthma, motion sickness, and acid-peptic disease. Tricyclic antidepressants, neuroleptics antiparkinsonian agents. *Datura stramonium* (jimson weed), Ditran (JB-329)	*Organic Mental Disorders* intoxication delirium delusional syndrome hallucinosis amnestic syndrome mixed organic brain syndrome
Hallucinogens	Lysergic acid diethylamide (LSD-25), psilocybin dimethyltryptamine (DMT), diethyltryptamine (DET), mescaline, 2,5-dimethoxy-4-methylamphetamine (DOM or STP), methylenedioxyamphetamine (MDA), trimethoxyamphetamine (TMA), muscimol, and others.	*Organic Mental Disorders* hallucinosis delusional syndrome affective syndrome *Substance abuse*
Cannabis	Marijuana, hashish, tetrahydrocannabinol (THC)	*Organic Mental Disorders* intoxication delusional syndrome *Substance abuse*
Tobacco	Cigarette, cigar, pipe, or chewing tobacco.	*Organic Mental Disorders* withdrawal *Substance use*
Caffeine	Coffee, tea, cola drinks, caffeine containing pills [No-Doz^R, Vivarin^R, Zoom (guarana)], and others.	*Organic Mental Disorders* caffeinism

central nervous system and the latter to the maladaptive behavior associated with the more or less regular use of the substances. Examples of each pharmacological category, as well as the adverse reactions to each are listed in Table 4–1.

POLYDRUG ABUSE

Most substance abusers use more than one psychoactive agent for nonmedical or recreational purposes. This polydrug abuse is probably increasing (Cohen, 1978). Many polydrug abusers generally have a regular pattern of substance abuse; for example, psychostimulants in the morning, antianxiety agents during the day, and sedative-hypnotics or alcohol in the evening. Other polydrug abusers generally take whatever psychoactive agents are available or least expensive when their preferred substance of abuse is not available. The general principles for the management of severe toxicity or overdose in the polydrug abuser are the same as those for abusers of specific psychoactive substances.

Treament

In the management of acute, toxic drug reactions, four basic medical procedures are major priorities: to secure the safety of the patient and treatment staff, to establish a tentative working diagnosis, to reduce toxic physiological effects, and to manage acute concomitant behavioral disturbances and problems (Berger and Tinklenberg, 1979; Tinklenberg and Berger, 1977).

Ensuring the safety of the patient and those caring for him or her is the first priority for the physician. The patient should not be left unattended while awaiting medical attention or during diagnostic procedures. Combative, severely disoriented, or extremely agitated patients, who show signs of self-destructive behavior, should be placed in gentle physical restraints. Vital signs (blood pressure, pulse, temperature, and electrocardiogram (EKG)) should be taken immediately so that rapid intervention can begin for patients with fever or with cardiovascular or EKG abnormalities. Vital signs should also be monitored in order to follow the course of intoxication over time (Berger and Tinklenberg, 1979; Tinklenberg and Berger, 1977).

A tentative working diagnosis should be established when initial safety is ensured and vital signs are stabilized. Information about the possible combination of drugs involved in the toxic reaction is best obtained from as many sources as possible. Friends who accompany the intoxicated patient can often give information on the substance or substances that were used and sometimes on the reactions of others who took the same drug. Comparing the patient's reactions with those of other users can yield inferences about doses and possible idiosyncratic reactions. Friends may also be able to help determine the approximate doses, the method of administration, the time the drug was taken, and whether any other drugs were used by the patient.

The patient may have taken or been given another drug in an attempt to treat the adverse reaction to the drugs taken initially. Of course, accompanying friends sometimes give misleading information either because they also are intoxicated or are fearful of legal reprisals. Many emergency wards now maintain a list of drugs currently used in the community which have been identified by a chemical analysis service. These lists often specify the alleged content and the actual content of the drug, and include a description of the substances locally available and in vogue. This information is very helpful, but must be up to date, since drug availability and "street" drug names change rapidly (Berger and Tinklenberg, 1979; Tinklenberg and Berger, 1977).

The results of a physical examination should be integrated with historical information when a working diagnosis is established. Because of polydrug abuse and drug adulteration or contamination, specific physical diagnostic criteria should be sought. The common clinical findings associated with each of the major classes of substances of abuse are described in this chapter.

Treatment of disturbed cardiopulmonary function has the highest priority and cardiopulmonary resuscitation is the first treatment for a comatose patient with depressed respirations or cardiac function. Arrhythmias also require immediate treatment. Every comatose patient should be injected with the opioid antagonist naloxone 0.4 mg intravenously (IV), which can be given three times, once every 2 min. This will reverse respiratory and CNS depression due to opioids and is harmless if opioids are not involved. In addition, 50 ml of a 50% glucose solution should be infused in case hypoglycemia has contributed to the coma. More detailed information on the action and administration of naloxone can be found in the section on management of opioid toxicity.

An attempt should be made to prevent further gastric absorption of ingested drugs. Induction of emesis, gastric lavage, activated charcoal, and a carthartic should be used for this purpose. Emesis should be induced (with ipecac syrup or apomorphine intravenous injection) only if the patient is fully conscious and cooperative. Gastric lavage (after placement of a cuffed endotrachial tube to prevent aspiration) is not as efficient as induced emesis, but is the only safe procedure if the patient is not fully conscious. After the gastric contents have been evacuated, a normal saline solution should be infused and withdrawn until the fluid is clear. Gastric lavage is most effective within 4 hours of ingestion except for alcohol, heroin, or LSD, which are rapidly absorbed. However, lavage should be attempted in every patient since anticholinergic adulterants may retard absorption of any substance of abuse. Following gastric lavage, 30 g of activated charcoal is administered via the gastric tube. A purgative such as sodium sulfate (30 g) or sorbitol (70% solution, 30–50 ml) can be given at the same time. The purgative should be repeated until diarrhea develops (Berger and Tinklenberg, 1979; Tinklenberg and Berger, 1977; Berger and Tinklenberg, 1977; Greenblatt and Shader, 1975a).

As the patient recovers from the acute toxicity, withdrawal syndromes may develop. Management of these syndromes is given below under each specific drug category. When a patient is withdrawing from the combination of alcohol or one of the sedative hypnotics as well as an opioid, the initial focus should be on managing the alcohol/sedative hypnotic withdrawal while the patient is maintained on a stable regimen of methadone. The use of anticonvulsant medications in the treatment of polydrug withdrawal is controversial. If an argument can be made for the prophylactic use of phenytoin, a loading dose of 750–1000 mg at a rate of 50 mg/min will rapidly establish a therapeutic blood level of 20 μg/ml. A maintenance dose of 300–400 mg/day will maintain this plasma level (Berger and Tinklenberg, 1979; Berger and Tinklenberg, 1977).

OPIOIDS

History

Opium use predates written history. The earliest written record is Sumerian and may date from 4000 BC. The Assyrians detailed the method of collecting opium which is still used today. The unripe seed boll of the opium poppy (*Papaver somniferum*) is cut, and after the sap has oozed and dried, it is scraped from the incisions. Greek physicians used opium, as did Galen who combined it with alcohol (laudnum) for medicinal purposes. Opium reached China through the Arabs, probably in the ninth century. In 1803, Serturner, a German pharmacist, isolated the pure alkaloid base from opium, later named morphine after Morpheus, the Greek god of dreams in sleep. In 1874, Wright produced diacetylmorphine or heroin, which was first suggested as a cure for morphine addiction.

In the United States and Europe, the use of opium preparations was widespread during the nineteenth century. Opium preparations were sold in grocery and general stores and could be obtained through mail order catalogs. They were advertised as "pain killers," "cough mixtures," "women's friends," and "consumption cures;" factory workers also used laudnum to quiet crying babies while they worked. A popular drink, called "Godfrey's cordial" contained opium along with molasses and sassafras flavoring. Morphine, and later heroin, preparations became popular after the Civil War for the same purposes. The hypodermic syringe was first widely used during the Civil War, often to administer morphine to wounded soldiers.

While opium was legal in the nineteenth century, it was considered by many to be disreputable, if not immoral. Crusades against opium first led to laws banning "opium dens" and then to increased tariffs on opium imports. The shipping by the British of opium from India to China resulted in two "opium wars" fought between Britain and China. This led to international efforts to regulate the opium trade, and ultimately to the regulation of opium in the United States. The Pure Food and Drug Act of 1906 required that medicines which contained drugs such as opiates state their contents on the label. The Harrison Narcotic Act of 1914 restricted legal distribution of opiates to physicians (Brecher, 1972; Akil, 1977).

Since the relief of pain is a primary task of all physicians, opiates and synthetic narcotic analgesics remain one of the most important drug categories in medicine. The development of specific narcotic antagonists, the identification of the opiate receptors, and the discovery of endogenous substances with opiatelike activity (endorphins) characterize the recent history of this important pharmacological category (Akil, 1977).

PATTERNS OF USE

Before World War II, a significant percentage of opiate users were Caucasians from Southern states, and female users were common. Since then, an increasing proportion of opiate users have been urban blacks, Puerto Ricans, and Chicanos, who primarily use intravenous heroin. These groups probably account for about half of the opiate users today. The number of individuals who regularly use heroin has stabilized during the last few years to about 500,000. There was a tenfold increase in regular heroin use between 1960 and 1969, from about 60,000 to more than 600,000, followed by a slight decline and then leveling off during the late 1970s to 500,000. Urban users typically belong to a drug subculture and obtain daily supplies of illegally synthesized and imported heroin from a "pusher" or "connection." Many enter the heroin subculture with intermittent parenteral heroin injection called "chipping" which gradually escalates to daily injections. Other users illegally obtain prescription medications such as morphine, levorphanol, and propoxyphene. Recently, heroin users have begun using a combination of pentazocine (Talwin) and pyribenzamine. Pentazocine is a mixed opioid agonist-antagonist, while pyribenzamine is an antihistamine. The combination is known on the street as " 'T's and blues," and users report a euphoric rush similar to that from heroin; however, the claim is anecdotal. The pharmacological properties including the toxicity of this unusual combination have not yet been investigated. Opiate users within the medical profession also use preparations manufactured by drug companies, such as morphine, methadone, pethidine (meperidine), oxycodone, and codeine (Berger and Tinklenberg, 1977).

Opiate users, like all users of psychoactive substances, claim they use the substance to produce euphoria (Martin et al., 1978). The euphoria produced by intravenous heroin immediately after injection is described as an intense orgasmic sensation known as the "rush," followed by a peaceful withdrawal from one's physical and psychological environment into a state of quiet bliss "like floating on a cloud." Martin suggests that much drug abuse is an attempt to reverse hypophoria, a state characterized by a poor self-image, that is, feeling unpopular, inept, not respected or appreciated, and a failure (Martin et al., 1978). The peaceful oblivious euphoria of intravenous opiates is one method of reversing hypophoria.

OPIOID INTOXICATION
ESSENTIAL FEATURES

The essential features of *opioid intoxication* (305.50) are specific neurological and psychological signs and maladaptive behavioral effects due to the recent use of an opioid. Psychological signs commonly present include euphoria or dysphoria, apathy, and psychomotor retardation. Pupillary constriction is always present (or dilation due to anoxia from a severe overdose). Other neurological signs commonly observed are drowsiness, slurred speech, and impairment in attention and memory. The maladaptive behavioral effects may include impaired judgment, interference with social or occupational functioning, and failure to meet responsibilities.

The mortality rate for heroin addicts is higher than that of their age-matched peers, 16 per 1000 per year for addicts under 30, 30 per 1000 per year in older addicts. Part of this increased mortality rate is due to acute toxicity reactions to heroin or adulterants. The heroin addict is usually unaware of the purity and hence of the dose of heroin injected, and users vary considerably in their level of tolerance to opioids at any time. After withdrawal, a user who had a high degree of tolerance might experience an acute toxic reaction with the prewithdrawal dose. Children of users on methadone maintenance may unknowingly swallow a toxic amount of methadone dissolved in fruit juice or flavored syrup and stored in the refrigerator for weekend use (Berger and Tinklenberg, 1979; Berger and Tinklenberg, 1977).

For an adult, 60 mg of morphine or the equivalent dose of another opioid may be dangerous; 240 mg can be fatal. Sixty milligrams of morphine, however, was fatal in one reported case, while with careful medical management, recovery from a dose of 760 mg of morphine has also been reported. Children, the elderly, and patients with hypothyroidism or respiratory disease have increased sensitivity to opioid toxicity. The syndrome of acute opioid toxicity includes respiratory distress that often presents as apnea with cyanosis, areflexia, and pupillary miosis, unless anoxia has caused pupillary dilation. Patients are often unresponsive, but the coma is characteristically light relative to the degree of respiratory depression. Evaluation of cardiopulmonary function often reveals hypotension, tachycardia, and at times pulmonary edema. Seizures do occur, but are rare. Acute heroin toxicity probably often represents the combination of opioid toxicity and an allergic or hypersensitivity reaction to the adulterants used to dilute the heroin. The opiate toxicity syndrome is fairly uniform among natural and synthetic opioids, however, pethidine (meperidine) may cause dilated pupils and muscular tremors while both pethidine and dex- tropropoxyphene more frequently cause seizures (Berger and Tinklenberg, 1979; Berger and Tinklenberg, 1977).

These characteristic clinical symptoms are usually sufficiently obvious to make the diagnosis of acute opioid toxicity. Sometimes the individuals accompanying the patient to the emergency room can specify the time of administration of heroin, and for a child with opioid toxicity from methadone, the dose can often be determined. In addition, many users of illegal opioids have scarred veins called "tracks" which result from repeated drug injection in nonmedical settings.

Management of Opioid Toxicity

Cardiorespiratory resuscitation is the initial task in the management of the patient with acute opioid toxicity. Mouth-to-mouth or mouth-to-oral airway resuscitation should be given to the patient who is apneic or cyanotic after the upper respiratory passages have been cleared of obstructions. If the patient has no pulse, external cardiac massage should be given simultaneously. To prevent aspiration, intubation with a cuffed endotracheal tube may be necessary if the patient remains apneic or is vomiting. To monitor the efficacy of the resuscitation efforts, arterial blood oxygen, carbon dioxide, and pH should be determined. A large intravenous line is needed and may require a "venous cutdown" because of scarred surface veins. To correct for the possibility that hypoglycemia has exacerbated the coma, 50 ml of 50% glucose should be given through the intravenous line (Berger and Tinklenberg, 1979; Berger and Tinklenberg, 1977; Greenblatt and Shader, 1975a; Greene and Dupont, 1974).

The correct drug for the management of acute opioid toxicity is the narcotic antagonist naloxone since it causes no respiratory suppression. Naloxone 0.4 mg (1 ml or 1 ampoule of the standard preparation, Narcan) should be given to both adults and children. This dose can be repeated three or four times within the first 10 min if no response is seen. Intravenous naloxone is so safe that it should be used routinely as a diagnostic test in a comatose patient who might have ingested an opioid. Naloxone can be given through the femoral vein in adults, or the external jugular vein in children before the intravenous line is established. Loose physical restraints are often placed on the patient before naloxone is administered. This is advisable, for when naloxone is effective, patients often wake up disoriented, agitated, angry, assaultive, and with severe withdrawal symptoms. Naloxone usually reverses symptoms of opioid toxicity within minutes, and dilation of the pupils is often the first sign of a positive response (Berger and Tinklenberg, 1979; Berger and Tinklenberg, 1977; Greenblatt and Shader, 1975a; Greene and Dupont, 1974).

Unfortunately, naloxone has a short duration of pharmacological activity, and opioid-induced respiratory depression can return within 2 to 4 hours. Thus, patients require continued monitoring of respiratory status. Following a heroin overdose, one or two doses of naloxone are usually sufficient. However, the child who has taken an overdose of methadone will probably require repeateed injections of naloxone and constant observation over the next 12 to 24 hours (Berger and Tinklenberg, 1979; Berger and Tinklenberg, 1977; Greenblatt and Shader, 1975a; Greene and Dupont, 1974).

Since opioid toxicity often results from illegal opioid use, attempts to revive the patient "on the street" may complicate the medical treatment of the opioid abuser. Friends often try to revive heroin addicts with facial slaps, or by squeezing or applying ice to nipples or testicles. Street myths at various times have suggested that intravenous amphetamine, milk, or saline can reverse heroin overdoses. Regrettably, amphetamine can precipitate seizures in patients with hypoxia, milk can cause lipoid pneumonia, and saline, probably the safest of three, may disturb the electrolyte balance (Berger and Tinklenberg, 1979).

OPIOID WITHDRAWAL (292.00)

Opioid withdrawal produces a clinical syndrome which is less serious and easier to manage than the withdrawal syndromes of alcohol or sedative-hypnotics. Eight to twelve hours after the last dose of morphine or heroin, the syndrome begins with restlessness, anxiety, and the urge to sleep, which if successful, results in disturbed and brief sleep. Tearing, nasal discharge, sweating, yawning, and deep sighing respirations appear as agitation increases. By 24 to 36 hours, the patient usually has insomnia, anorexia, severe anxiety, waves of "goose-flesh," and alternating periods of chills and warmth often accompanied by fevers of 38 to 39°C. Muscle and joint pains appear, abdominal cramps, vomiting, and diarrhea are common, and tachycardia and hypertension may be found on physical examination. Severe symptoms usually begin to subside after 72 hours, while weakness, anxiety, and disturbed sleep may persist for weeks or even months. The withdrawal syndrome from other opioids is similar, differing only in intensity and time course. Codeine and pethidine produce mild withdrawal syndromes; the symptoms of codeine withdrawal are slow to appear, while those from pethidine withdrawal appear early. Methadone withdrawal lasts about two weeks, is mild, but can include deep muscle pain (Berger and Tinklenberg, 1979; Berger and Tinklenberg, 1977).

Management of Opioid Withdrawal

There are really two parts to the opioid withdrawal syndrome. The first part is the physiological syndrome described above. The second part is the elaboration or exaggeration of symptoms that opioid addicts frequently use in their attempts to obtain more opioids. It is often hard to distinguish between these two, and heroin users are experts in such behaviors as stealing, forging prescriptions, and conning other patients and staff. For this reason, treatment of the opioid detoxification syndrome requires an inpatient or outpatient unit with adequate security, and an experienced, skeptical, and hypervigilant staff.

Patients withdrawing from opioids require a complete medical and drug abuse medical history, a careful physical examination, and a routine clinical blood evaluation including screening tests for common substances of abuse. A standard method of detoxification begins with oral methadone 20 mg. If this dose causes gross intoxication, the patient will probably not require opioid withdrawal. If the patient develops withdrawal symptoms within the next 12 to 24 hours, a second oral dose of 20 mg of methadone should be given. For most opioid addicts, two oral doses of 20 mg of methadone, that is, 40 mg on the first day, will prevent severe withdrawal symptoms. Only drug dealers who may be heavy users of opiates or patients withdrawing from methadone maintenance may require higher doses on the first day of abstinence. After two or three days at a stable dose, methadone can be reduced by 5 or 10 mg each day, leading to complete detoxification in four to ten days. Diazepam can be given if anxiety is severe, flurazepam can be used for insomnia, and massage and jacuzzi baths can be useful for muscle pain (Berger and Tinklenberg, 1979; Berger and Tinklenberg, 1977).

Mothers addicted to opioids can give birth to children who develop a syndrome that probably represents opioid withdrawal. Within 48 hours after delivery, such infants may become extremely irritable and hyperactive. The hyperactivity can cause extreme irritation of the skin on the side of the face, the elbows, and knees. The infants may also develop fever, coarse tremors, anorexia, and vomiting. Respiratory disturbances such as tachypnea, a shrill, high-pitched "cat-like" cry, and seizures may be seen. The treatment of these infants is more urgent than the treatment of the adult withdrawal syndrome. Infants with seizures and respiratory distress will require immediate treatment. Maintaining fluid and electrolyte balance may require intravenous feedings, and a careful diagnostic evaluation should be carried out. The pharmacological treatment for this syndrome is paregoric camphorated tincture of opium three to ten drops every four hours, it should be titrated to decrease hyperactivity, irritability, and other symptoms without causing oversedation. The dose of paregoric should be gradually tapered over four to five days (Mahender, 1974).

MEDICAL DISORDERS COMPLICATING OPIOID ABUSE

Opioid abusers have an increased incidence of medical disorders, some of which are directly related to the method of opioid abuse, and others which are more a function of the lifestyle of such users. Unsterile conditions lead to an increased incidence of hepatitis, thrombophlebitis, subcutaneous abscesses, infective endocarditis which may involve the right, left, or both sides of the heart, lung abscesses, septic pulmonary emboli, and osteomyelitis. The use of contaminated syringes, needles, and the substance of abuse itself can also transmit tetanus, and rarely, malaria. Pulmonary fibrosis, acute and chronic polyneuropathy, glomerulonephritis, nephrotic syndrome, and transverse myelitis have all been reported in illegal opioid abusers. In addition, pneumonia, tuberculosis, urinary tract infections, and veneral diseases are more common among opioid abusers than the general population. Finally, some opioid abusers have unrelated injuries or illnesses such as tooth or organ abscesses, appendicitis, or an injury whose pain has been masked by the analgesic effect of the opioid (Berger and Tinklenberg, 1979).

Pulmonary edema sometimes occurs as part of the overdose syndrome described above. However, pulmonary edema also occurs at lower doses of opioids, particularly illegal heroin. This may represent a hypersensitivity or allergic phenomenon. The opioid abuser with pulmonary edema needs a chest X-ray, and arterial blood gas determinations. If the patient is hypoxic, the situation is life-threatening and may require sitting the patient up and administering such emergency treatments as oxygen, diuretics, digitalis, and aminophylline (Berger and Tinklenberg, 1979).

COCAINE, AMPHETAMINES, AND SIMILARLY ACTING SYMPATHOMIMETICS

HISTORY

When the Spanish conquered the Inca Empire, they discovered that the Andes Indians of South America chewed coca leaves (*Erythroxylon coca*). Chewing these leaves produced mild euphoria, alertness, a feeling of increased energy, and decreased appetite. Although the chewing of coca leaves was relatively uncommon in Europe or America, small amounts of coca extract were added to various "medicinal" drinks such as the American drink introduced in 1886 by J. S. Pemberton of Atlanta. Pemberton combined the extract of the kola nut, which contains caffeine, and coca leaves, labeling the product *Coca-Cola*. However, by the early 1900's, Coca-Cola was being made from coca leaves from which the cocaine had been removed (Brecher, 1972).

The principal active agent in coca leaves, cocaine, was first isolated in the mid-nineteenth century. Pure cocaine from Merck Laboratories was given to Bavarian soldiers by Aschenbrandt in 1884, who reported that it decreased fatigue. Freud, then a young and ambitious neurologist in Vienna, read this report and began experimenting with cocaine. He described his personal euphoric experience with the drug in 1884. Freud sent cocaine to his fiancée and his colleague, von Fleischl-Marxow, who was addicted to morphine because of painful neuromata. Fleischl began his treatment with small doses of cocaine and gradually increased the dosage. Within a year, he was taking a gram a day, more than 20 times the dose that Freud occasionally used for his depressions. Fleischl developed cocaine delusional disorder, a syndrome that resembles acute paranoid schizophrenia. Because of this incident, Freud abandoned his use of cocaine and his research in psychopharmacology (Brecher, 1972).

One of the best descriptions of the discovery of amphetamines was given by Chauncey Leake (Ayd and Blackwell, 1970). K. K. Chen, who worked with Chauncey Leake at the University of Wisconsin in the 1920's, went to China to begin a systematic investigation of the ancient Chinese drug classification. The desert plant Ma Huang (*Ephedra vulgaris*) was repeatedly recommended for asthma. Chen and Schmidt in 1925 rediscovered the active alkaloid, ephedrine, which is still used as a treatment for asthma (Ayd and Blackwell, 1970).

Gordon Alles, in his attempt to find a synthetic substitute for ephedrine, collaborated with Leake in testing several related phenylethylamines for biological activity. The most active compound of their first series was d,l-phenylisopropylamine (amphetamine or Benzedrine). The dextro rotated isomer, dextroamphetamine, or Dexedrine was clinically tested in 1930. Increased alertness, improved physical and mental performance, euphoria, and decreased appetite were observed and reported (Ayd and Blackwell, 1970).

Both the allied and axis forces made extensive use of amphetamines in World War II. Postwar Japan placed large supplies of amphetamines on the open market, which led to an epidemic of amphetamine abuse and numerous cases of amphetamine delusional disorder. Epidemics of amphetamine abuse also occurred in Sweden and the United States. One of the ironies of the history of psychopharmacology is that the amphetamine epidemic in the Haight-Ashbury District of San Francisco took place six blocks from the University of California Medical Center in San Francisco where Alles and Leake had first synthesized amphetamine 40 years earlier.

PATTERNS OF USE

Cocaine has become an extremely highly valued psychoactive substance. However, although cocaine use continues to increase, most users take the drug sporadically. This is probably due to the high cost and unpredictable availability of cocaine. The 90–100% purity of cocaine, which was typical of the drug available on the illicit market several years ago, has dropped to the approximately 30% purity available today. Of the substances of abuse used at present, cocaine currently holds the highest status among groups of middle and upper-class young people, who consider it the most desirable of the psychoactive substances. Cocaine use is popular among those in the arts and the entertainment industries: musicians, artists, and the "jet set."

Cocaine hydrochloride is usually inhaled as a dry powder through a thin tube inserted into the nostril to the nasal mucosa. It can also be dissolved in water and injected intravenously. The cocaine "free base," extracted as described in the following paragraph, can be smoked.

"Free-basing" is a recent trend in cocaine use. Cocaine hydrochloride, the common preparation, is readily soluble in water (1 g will dissolve in 0.4 ml) (thereby becoming suitable for injection or dissolving on the nasal mucosa). If cocaine hydrochloride is dissolved in water, the pH changed to alkaline, and the solution extracted with ether, which is then evaporated, the result is cocaine "free base." This preparation is volatile (has a low melting point), making it more suitable for smoking. The "free base" is not very water soluble (1 g will dissolve in 600 ml) and therefore cannot be used intranasally or intravenously. In addition to making cocaine more suitable for smoking, the procedure of "free basing" can, if done properly, remove impurities.

Intravenous and nasal administration of cocaine salt as well as cocaine "free base" smoking produce a clinical syndrome of short duration; frequent readministration is required to sustain the effects of the drug. Cocaine users claim they experience a euphoria that is different from that caused by opiates or hallucinogens. Cocaine euphoria is reported to be exhilarating, sometimes enabling the user to feel creative, energetic, articulate, talkative, attractive, excited, motivated, and capable of performing difficult and often grandiose tasks. A subjective sense of improved mental and physical abilities and decreased appetite are also reported. Negative effects are described as restlessness, agitation, anxiety, hyperexcitability, irritability, and hostility (Petersen and Stillman, 1977).

There are several common patterns of use of amphetamine and amphetaminelike substances. These substances accounted for almost 17 million prescriptions in 1977 (Cohen, 1978). Oral amphetamine users include people who feel they require its stimulant qualities to prevent sleep or fatigue for periods of sustained activity, those desiring to lose weight, and those who desire improved athletic or mental performance. Long-distance truck drivers, people holding two jobs, students preparing for or taking examinations, and athletes in almost every sport are among those who use amphetamines or amphetaminelike substances. The syndrome produced by oral amphetamine use is similar to that described for cocaine, but is generally of longer duration and can be milder if lower doses of amphetamine are used. A second pattern of amphetamine use involves the intravenous administration of amphetamine in rapidly increasing doses over a period of days in what is called a "speed-run;" this intravenous use usually stops after four to six sleepless days when the user falls asleep or "crashes" (Berger and Tinklenberg, 1979; Tinklenberg and Berger, 1977; Ellinwood, 1979).

Thus the clinical syndromes produced by cocaine and amphetamine are remarkably similar. For example, the chronic use of both amphetamine and cocaine can produce symptoms that are virtually indistinguishable from those of acute paranoid schizophrenia (Ellinwood, 1979; Snyder, 1972). However, amphetamine and amphetaminelike substances generally have a longer duration of activity than cocaine and amphetamine rapidly produces tolerance. True tolerance to the chronic use of cocaine has not been demonstrated (Ellinwood, 1979).

THE PSYCHOSTIMULANT INTOXICATION SYNDROME—COCAINE (305.60) AND AMPHETAMINE (305.70)

There are two major adverse reactions to psychostimulants. These are the organic delusional syndrome that results from chronic psychostimulant use, and the acute and potentially fatal reaction that results from an overdose. The organic delusional syndrome generally occurs when high concentrations of amphetamines and amphetaminelike drugs are used (Ellinwood, 1979; Snyder, 1972). As tolerance to amphetamines develops with repetitive use, the dosage is increased. Alternatively, high blood concentrations may result from repeated intravenous injections of large doses of amphetamines. These high plasma concentrations or a sudden increase in plasma concentrations can induce paranoid psychosis. This syndrome is characterized by suspiciousness, hostility, persecutory delusions, and visual and auditory misperceptions or hallucinations. The psychosis may also include hyperactivity, repetitive compulsive behavior that is reminiscent of animal stereotypy, and tactile hallucinations of small insects crawling on or just under the skin (parasitosis, formication) (Ellinwood, 1979; Snyder, 1972). Unfortunately, the patient experiencing an amphetamine-induced paranoid state has the potential for assaultiveness and violent behavior because of his suspiciousness and delusions of persecution.

Clinically, case reports have described a cocaine psychosis syndrome that is nearly identical with, and in fact may be indistinguishable from, amphetamine psychosis, although less research has been done on this syndrome (Berger and Tinklenberg, 1979).

Extremely high doses of either amphetamine or cocaine can cause death by suppressing cardiac function or, more commonly, by causing respiratory depression. Hyperpyrexia and seizures are also seen with psychostimulant overdose. In addition, hypertension can complicate the clinical presentation of amphetamine or cocaine overdose (Berger and Tinklenberg, 1979; Petersen and Stillman, 1977, Ellinwood, 1979).

Management of Psychostimulant Toxicity

The general principles for treating psychostimulant toxicity are the same as those for treating toxicity of other psychoactive substances. The first priority is to secure the safety of the patient and the treatment staff. This may mean arranging for someone to stay with the patient and the use of gentle physical restraints to control combative or self-destructive behaviors.

After securing the safety of the patient, a tentative diagnosis should be established. This can often be made by direct questioning of the patient or friends about the use of psychostimulants. The suspected drugs should be discussed, not only by their generic trade names, but also by their common street names; e.g. speed, diet pills, uppers, whites, bennys, crystal, crank, hearts, double crosses, and others for amphetamines, and coke, snow, and others for cocaine. Physical examinations reveal a variety of symptoms which characterize adverse reactions to psychostimulants. A complete physical examination should be performed because of the numerous illnesses associated with psychostimulant use, such as elevated blood pressure and excessive sweating. Chronic psychostimulant users lose weight and may look emaciated because of the appetite suppression activity of amphetamines. Some patients will have cutaneous excoriations from skin picking. Urinary tests can be useful, but it must be remembered that not all amphetaminelike stimulants are detected in standard toxic screening tests (Ellinwood, 1979).

When a tentative diagnosis has been established, the patient's surroundings should be arranged to decrease superfluous or threatening stimuli. Staff members should not be unnecessarily close to or behind the patient. The paranoid patient may feel both overwhelmed by too many nurses and confined by limited space. It must be remembered that a paranoid psychostimulant abuser is capable of unprovoked assault. The psychostimulant user will often improve with supportive nonpharmacological methods, although some patients will need more active intervention (Berger and Tinklenberg, 1979; Ellinwood, 1979).

If paranoid behavior is extreme, or if the blood pressure, pulse rate, or temperature is rising, and it is reasonably certain that psychostimulants were the only drugs taken, the patient should be given an antipsychotic agent such as chlorpromazine or haloperidol. These drugs block dopamine receptors and therefore antagonize some of the effects of psychostimulants. The initial dose of chlorpromazine in adults ranges from 100 to 150 mg orally (PO), or 25 to 50 mg intramuscularly (IM). Haloperidol 2–5 mg can be given either PO or IM. Subsequent doses are determined by the patient's overall response as seen from both behavioral improvement and vital signs. The dosage schedule is determined by the time course of peak drug effects. To avoid cardiopulmonary depression and excessive sedation, repeat doses should not be given until the maximal effect of each dose has been observed. Monitoring body temperatures may be useful in determining subsequent doses; rising temperatures may indicate that the toxicity is dangerous and that larger doses of antipsychotic medications are necessary. Hyperpyrexia can be treated with standard techniques such as cooling blankets, fans, and sponge baths. Aspirin and/or acetaminophen may also be useful. Hydration and acidification of the urine to a pH below 5 can accelerate the excretion of amphetamines. The urine can be acidified by giving ammonium chloride 500 mg to 1 g every 3 to 5 hours orally or through a nasogastric tube until the urine pH is below 5 (Berger and Tinklenberg, 1979).

Psychostimulant toxicity can, on rare occasions, produce severe hypertension. Immediate treatment is required when the systolic blood pressure is above 200 mm Hg or there are indications of an impending cerebral vascular accident such as visual disturbances or other transient neurological signs. An intravenous infusion should be initiated and 1–5 mg of phentolamine should be given over 5 to 10 min while the blood pressure is monitored. The systolic blood pressure should be carefully reduced to 160–170 mm Hg without precipitating hypotension (Berger and Tinklenberg, 1979).

When the psychostimulant toxicity is less severe or when the diagnosis is in doubt, the use of potent antipsychotic drugs is questionable. There is a narrow margin between effective behavioral sedation and excessive cardiovascular depression. The possible interaction of the anticholinergic activity of the antipsychotic agent with the anticholinergic activity in the psychoactive substance renders treatment for psychostimulant toxicity with antipsychotic drugs less than ideal. Thus, if the intoxication is not life-threatening and blood pressure, pulse, and temperature are not rising, reassurance may sufficiently calm the patient. If minor agitation and behavioral disturbances persist, benzodiazepines such as diazepam 10–30 mg PO are useful and safe.

Psychostimulant abusers require hospitalization if paranoid psychosis and/or elevated vital signs continue despite vigorous treatment. Since suicidal ideation sometimes follows the discontinuation of psychostimulants, admission to a high-security facility is recommended. Hospitalization is also necessary if markedly impaired perceptions or cognitive functions persist or if any of the numerous medical problems that can be associated with drug abuse are present. If hospitalization is unnecessary, the patient can be discharged to a responsible relative or friend who should observe him or her closely over the next several days. Irritability, weakness, lethargy, and depression are often seen when psychostimulants are discontinued and these symptoms should be predicted in advance (Berger and Tinklenberg, 1979; Ellinwood, 1979). If these symptoms develop into severe depression, treatment with tricyclic antidepressants may be necessary. Finally, since psychostimulant abuse is associated with increased morbidity and mortality, the physician should offer or arrange for long-term treatment (Ellinwood, 1979).

PHENCYCLIDINE

HISTORY

The history of phencyclidine (PCP) is as strange as the clinical effects of the drug itself. Four distinct phases emerge from the 25-year history of this substance. In the 1950's, Parke-Davis initiated animal studies on PCP, one of a group of arylcyclohexylamines. These studies found PCP to be a highly potent, but relatively nontoxic animal anesthetic even when administered intravenously. The second phase of studies, conducted on medical patients and human volunteers, showed that PCP would not be a useful human anesthetic agent. Even in low doses, it was a uniquely potent psychotomimetic, causing disorientation, delirium, and hallucinations as its anesthetic effect dissipated. PCP was withdrawn as a human anesthetic agent in 1965. In the third phase, between 1965 and 1973, PCP was used as a substitute or an adulterant for LSD, mescaline, DMT, THC, and other drugs. Users accustomed to other psychoactive substances were so negative about the effects of PCP that they had to be tricked into using it. In the fourth phase of its history, which continues today, PCP is used for its inherent properties described below, a phenomenon quite unexpected considering the numerous negative reports of its intoxication syndrome (Pittel and Oppedahl, 1979; Petersen and Stillman, 1978).

PATTERNS OF USE

The emergence of PCP as a drug of choice is difficult to explain. Its intoxication state is both variable and unique. The ratio of euphoria to dysphoria is probably lower for PCP than for any other substance of abuse. Even confirmed and repeated users admit that disturbing and negative experiences with the drug are common. Several patterns of PCP use have emerged over the past several years. Many users smoke cigarettes containing PCP, which is placed on parsley, tobacco, or other leafy mixtures in powdered form. This may enable the user to better titrate the dose. PCP can also be inhaled through the nostrils. Street names for PCP include: angel-dust, dust, crystal, elephant or horse tranquilizer, hog, super or weed killer weed, mist, and KJ or KW (Pittel and Oppedahl, 1979; Petersen and Stillman, 1978).

Approximately half the number of current users of PCP average at least one dose per week. The mean age of those who begin to use PCP continuously is approximately 15 years. PCP is used in a social setting, frequently along with other drugs. In fact, in several surveys, every user of PCP was found to abuse other drugs as well. The user of PCP, as opposed to those who consume other illicit drugs, is more likely to be intoxicated with alcohol, to have more arrests for offenses related to substance abuse, and to have more overdose episodes. Several sources of evidence indicate that PCP use is increasing. For example, more PCP has been confiscated by police departments, more patients intoxicated with PCP are being seen in emergency rooms, and there is an increasing number of referrals by family members, friends, and the criminal justice system for the treatment of PCP users (Cohen, 1978; Pittel and Oppedahl, 1979; Petersen and Stillman, 1978).

Users of PCP say that the drug produces a syndrome which is different from that of other psychoactive substances. Users experience "a dream world" or a "perfect escape." The drug is described as having a pronounced effect on thinking, time perception, sense of reality, and mood. Thinking is perceived as "speeded," the mind going faster while time is slowed down with "no more reality." Experiences assume new perspectives in a fantasy world where things seem more dramatic, where "your wishes are fulfilled," and where everything appears more complete and more beautiful. A sense of "oneness" with others and with animals is reported, and religious and philosophical thoughts and experiences are described (Pittel and Oppedahl, 1979; Petersen and Stillman, 1978).

Intense and euphoric mood states occur, although almost every user has also experienced severe depression and therefore describes the drug as bringing one to either "the heights or the depths." Feelings of "endurance," "power," "energy," and "floating" are reported. Visual hallucinations are rare. These effects are said to "come on" within 1 to 5 min after smoking and peak after 5 to 30 min. Users report staying "loaded or high" for 4 to 6 hours, followed by a "come-down" which lasts from 6 to 24 hours. Nasal insufflation (snorting) leads to a more rapid onset of 30 sec to 1 min, but otherwise the clinical syndrome has a similar duration.

THE PCP INTOXICATION SYNDROME (305.90)

PCP and other arylcyclohexylamines such as ketamine are difficult to classify pharmacologically. The clinical syndrome they produce includes properties which are shared with psychostimulants, hallucinogens, sedative-hypnotics, alcohol, analgesics, and anesthetics. PCP also has sympathomimetic properties that cause increased heart rate and elevated blood pressure (Petersen and Stillman, 1978).

The negative aspects of the PCP syndrome include disorientation, mental confusion, anxiety, irritability, paranoia, and violent or assaultive behavior. In addition, chronic users are reported to have flattened affect, depression, and sometimes agitation. Hostility and belligerence remain long after one would expect the pharmacological effects from the drug to have dissipated. Chronic users may develop a persistent schizophrenic-like syndrome which may last for some months after abstinence. This syndrome resembles chronic schizophrenia more closely than any other syndrome presumed to be drug-induced (Pittel and Oppedahl, 1979; Petersen and Stillman, 1978; Hollister, 1968).

Deaths due to PCP can result from both its pharamacological and behavioral effects. Because PCP users exhibit bizarre, unpredictable, and aggressive behavior, and are often severely agitated and confused, dangerous or life-threatening situations are possible. In California, drowning is a major cause of death related to PCP intoxication. Automobile accidents, falls, fires, and other accidents have been reported in PCP-related fatalities (Cohen, 1978; Petersen and Stillman, 1978).

The pharmacological overdose of PCP can also be fatal due to cardiopulmonary depression. Less severe overdoses present with variable signs that can include severe psychosis, ataxia, assaultiveness, vertical and horizontal nystagmus, catatonic staring, analgesia or anesthesia, increased heart rate and blood pressure, and sometimes seizures. PCP psychosis can last from several days to several weeks and can include paranoia, violent behavior, depression, and suicidal ideation.

Management of PCP Intoxication Syndrome

Patients with PCP overdose who present in coma and with cardiopulmonary depression require cardiopulmonary resuscitation, treatment for seizures, and the general treatment of the overdose syndrome described in the previous section on polydrug abuse. In addition, acidification of the urine may hasten the excretion of PCP. The urine can be acidified by giving 500 mg to 1 g ammonium chloride every 3 to 5 hours orally or through a nasogastric tube until the urine pH is below 5.

As the PCP coma lightens, it is important to remember that the patient may be delirious, disoriented, paranoid, and possibly assaultive. Patients who are less intoxicated may initially present with this psychotic state. The patient with PCP psychosis will usually require physical restraints. There are no specific antagonists for the toxic effects of PCP. However, some experience has been gained in symptomatic treatment of the hypertension and psychosis. Some clinicians prefer haloperidol 5 mg IM given hourly if needed, to control both the psychosis and the assaultive behavior. Other physicians use diazepam 10 to 30 mg orally or intramuscularly to decrease violent behavior. Phenothiazine neuroleptics should probably be avoided because of the possibility of potentiating PCP anticholinergic effects. Both diazoxide and hydralazine have been suggested to treat the hypertensive crisis which can be associated with PCP intoxication. The hypertension usually responds quite rapidly, while

PCP psychosis has a characteristically slow response, sometimes lasting for weeks. Even as the psychosis resolves, unpredictable recrudescence of psychotic symptoms or the appearance of suicidal ideation, depression, anxiety, hostility, and belligerence may complicate the recovery (Pittel and Oppedahl, 1979; Petersen and Stillman, 1978).

INHALANTS

HISTORY

The efficiency of absorption of gases, smoke, and volatile liquids has been recognized and utilized by humankind for centuries. The surface area of the pulmonary epithelium is vast and absorption is rapid. A further advantage of inhalation is that the inhaled substance reaches the brain directly without first passing through the liver with its complex system of detoxifying enzymes. In the past, smoked substances have included opium, cannabis, DMT (N,N-dimethyltriptamine), and cocaine. More recently, ether, chloroform, and nitrous oxide were inhaled recreationally before they were discovered to be useful as general anesthetics. Sporadic use of nitrous oxide, primarily by medical, pharmacy, and dental students continues today. Nitrous oxide causes a transient, giddy, dissociated euphoria. It is only dangerous when inhaled without sufficient oxygen (Sharp and Brehm, 1977, Cohen, 1979a).

The inhalants discussed in this section are different from the psychoactive substances mentioned above in that they are readily available to consumers and are inexpensive. 'Glue sniffing" probably began in California in the early 1950's where it was discovered accidentally by adolescents working on plastic model airplanes. Eventually, large numbers of volatile substances were found to possess intoxicating ingredients and subsequently used as inhalants. These include cements, glues, adhesives, paints, lacquers, and their thinners, dry cleaning fluids, spot removers, liquid waxes and shoe polishes, lighter fluids, degreasers, refrigerants, transmission and brake fluids, gasoline, and many others. Most recently, aerosal sprays from supermarkets were found to be intoxicating and thus became popular. They contain conventional solvents as well as Freons (chlorinated, fluorinated-substituted methane or ethane derivatives) which are also intoxicating. Aerosol "whipped cream" often contains nitrous oxide. Aerosols used for intoxication include glass chillers, non-stick frying pan sprays, cold weather car starters, air sanitizers, window cleaners, insecticides, deodorants, hair sprays, and spray paints, especially gold and bronze. The psychoactive ingredients in inhalants include a wide variety of solvents from several chemical classes including aliphatic and aromatic hydrocarbons, halogenated hydrocarbons, Freons, ketones, esters, alcohols, and glycols (Sharp and Brehm, 1977; Cohen, 1979a).

PATTERNS OF USE

Inhalant use is faddish. Within a given community, one specific inhalant will be used by the young for a specific period of time, then it will lose popularity and be replaced by another substance. In general, inhalant use is a phenomenon of young, poor, white or Chicano males. It is more prevalent among underprivileged Chicanos and native Americans than among blacks or whites. Inhalants are the only psychoactive substance more commonly used in grade or junior high school than high school or college. It is difficult to determine the exact extent of use, but data from a national survey suggest that approximately 8% of all youths, but 25% of Chicano youths in Los Angeles, have experimented with inhalants; about 1% of all youths and 13% of Chicano youths in Los Angeles are currently using inhalants (Sharp and Brehm, 1977; Cohen, 1979a).

Inhalant use is an activity in peer-oriented and peer-perpetuated social settings. Young inhalant users choose these substances because they are cheaper than any other psychoactive intoxicants, and easily available in a convenient and legal package. For example, for $1.00, a small can of varnish remover can be legally carried in the pocket of a 12-year-old and can intoxicate more individuals than a gallon of cheap wine (Sharp and Brehm, 1977; Cohen, 1979a).

The syndrome produced by solvent inhalation is described as resembling alcohol intoxication, but is of shorter duration and produces only a minor "hangover." Users describe the state as a "floating euphoria" that eradicates the unpleasant aspects of life. The intoxication enables these youths to escape temporarily from their chaotic, depressing, and often hopeless home environment, to escape from performance pressure at school, and temporarily to correct their personal sense of inadequacy. Unfortunately, as is the case with alcohol, inhalant intoxication can also release aggressive impulses (Sharp and Brehm, 1977; Cohen, 1979a).

An intoxication syndrome distinct from that described above results from inhalation of the volatile nitrites. Amyl nitrite is used medically to dilate the coronary arteries during an episode of angina pectoris. Isobutyl nitrite is a nonprescription substance with similar pharmacological activity. When either of these substances is used prior to orgasm, a subjective sense of time prolongation and enhanced sensitivity is reported. The popularity of these substances in enhancing sexual activity probably occurred first among homosexuals and subsequently spread to heterosexual adults.

Furthermore, the volatile nitrites are being used to produce a brief "altered state of consciousness" which is probably secondary to the dilation of cerebral blood vessels. The volatile nitrites, known as "poppers" or "snappers," are frequently legally sold in pornography shops under such brand names as Locker Room, Jac Aroma, Rush, Kick, Bullet, Toilet Water, and Vaporole. These preparations contain isobutyl nitrite, isobutyl alcohol, and isopentyl nitrite. The clinical syndrome they produce is clearly different from that of the solvent inhalants. They are used by a different population and almost nothing is known of the adverse effects of chronic use. A recent survey found that 19% of regular cocaine users also reported the use of volatile nitrites (Cohen, 1978; Sigell et al., 1978).

Management of the Inhalant Intoxication Syndrome
The typical user of solvent inhalants is not seen by medical personnel because the acute state ends rapidly either with complete recovery or very rarely with death. Sudden death during inhalant use has at least two causes. The first is asphyxiation due to the method of self-administration of solvent inhalants. These substances are placed on a rag, sponge, article of clothing, or in a paper or plastic bag, which the user places against the nose and/or mouth and breathes deeply. Of these methods, the use of a plastic bag is most dangerous since the user may lose consciousness and suffocate. The second cause of sudden death during inhalant use is cardiac arrest, probably due to cardiac arrhythmias which are induced either directly by the inhaled solvent or by a combination of the toxic effects of the solvent and hypoxia (Sharp and Brehm, 1977, Cohen, 1979a).

For the occasional inhalant user who presents in the emergency room acutely intoxicated, some of the treatments described for abusers of hallucinogens or psychostimulants are appropriate. If the patient is agitated and assaultive, gentle physical restraint may be necessary. If the patient is primarily anxious and confused, a benzodiazepine such as diazepam 10–30 mg administered orally can be helpful.

The chronic effects of solvent inhalation are more likely to be seen by the medical profession. In a recent preliminary study of 37 chronic solvent abusers (average number of inhalations in excess of 7000) using the Halstead Reitan Neuropsychological Battery, investigators found that 40% of the inhalant subjects scored in the brain-damaged range on impairment indices as compared with none of the control subjects (Sharp and Brehm, 1977). These results must be interpreted cautiously, since it is possible that some of the inhalant abusers were impaired prior to solvent abuse. It is also uncertain whether solvent use itself or other factors, such as hypoxic episodes or other drugs, contributed to the deficit seen. In addition, further study is necessary to determine the natural course and long-term reversibility of these impairments.

Careful studies are needed to determine the chronic toxicity syndrome of the various solvents of abuse and whether they cause chronic organic brain syndrome. Toluene, perhaps the most common solvent abused, is relatively safe. However, chronic use has the potential of causing kidney and bone marrow disorders. Chronic use of other solvents has the potential of producing peripheral neuropathy, kidney damage, liver disease, and bone marrow disorders. Unfortunately, much of our information on these potential defects is based on single case reports or on attempts to extrapolate from chronic industrial exposure to the same solvents. The true extent of the toxic consequences of repeated self-administration of solvent inhalants requires reliable and careful epidemiologic study (Sharp and Brehm, 1977; Cohen, 1979a).

ANTICHOLINERGICS

History

Descriptions of toxic anticholinergic plants have been specifically mentioned in many early historical documents. *Datura stramonium* (locoweed, jimsonweed, thorn apple, devil's apple, devil's trumpet, stink weed, apple of Peru) is described as a poison in *The Odyssey*. Cleopatra allegedly used *Datura stramonium* to facilitate her seduction of Caesar. In 38 AD, the troops of Mark Antony partook of the same plant during their retreat from Parthia and suffered the dire consequences of stupor, confusion, and death (Goldfrank and Meliek, 1979).

The name "jimsonweed" has its origin in an incident at Jamestown during Bacon's Rebellion in 1676. British troops, sent to halt the rebellion, prepared a meal of *Datura stramonium*. Many soldiers consequently developed the anticholinergic intoxication syndrome. An excerpt from *Beverly's History of Virginia* describes how "some ate plentifully of it, the effect of which was a very pleasant comedy, for they turned natural fools upon it for several days: One would blow up a feather in the air, another would dart straws at it with much fury, and another, stark naked, was sitting in a corner like a monkey." The plant thus became known as "Jamestown weed" and over the past years the term has been condensed to "jimsonweed." The use of jimsonweed was also reported by Omar Khayyam, Henry Thoreau, and others (Goldfrank and Meliek, 1979).

Patterns of Use

Despite their obvious psychological and physiological toxicity, anticholinergic agents are used as psychoactive substances. In many cases, the use is unintentional. Anticholinergic agents are commonly used as adulterants in other psychoactive substances, such as hallucinogens. Thus, the buyer of what is alleged to be LSD may, in fact, purchase and ingest the combination of LSD and scopolamine, or perhaps atropine or scopolamine alone. In addition to this unintentional use, some substance abusers knowingly use anticholinergic substances. For example, the anticholinergic stramonium, found in the anti-asthma preparation Asthmador, had a brief period of popularity as an intoxicating agent. It is alleged to produce euphoria and altered states of consciousness which allow the user to withdraw from the stresses and boredom of everyday reality into a dreamlike state. Prisoners in areas of the country where jimsonweed is indigenous may bring it back to the prison after working outside the prison walls fighting fires or on road-maintenance crews. A tea is brewed from the jimsonweed and ingested to produce the same altered state of consciousness sought by the users of Asthmador. Since many prisoners and psychiatric patients are given neuroleptics and anticholinergics such as Artane they have discovered that Artane and other anticholinergic antiparkinsonian agents can also produce this syndrome.

In addition, Artane in particular, if the dose is carefully titrated, has been described by some users to produce a feeling of comfort and well-being without the accompanying severe altered state of consciousness. Thus Artane abuse has become a problem for some psychiatric patients and prisoners. Unfortunately, the incidence, prevalence, and consequences of intentional and unintentional anticholinergic abuse are largely unknown because these substances have not been placed in a separate category among the substances of abuse (Berger and Tinklenberg, 1979; Goldfrank and Meliek, 1979; Granacher et al., 1976).

The Anticholinergic Intoxication Syndrome

The intoxication syndrome produced by anticholinergic agents can be caused by drugs used for a variety of purposes. Drugs used to treat the common cold, allergies, asthma, motion sickness, peptic ulcer disease, insomnia, depression, schizophrenia, menstrual symptoms, and Parkinson's disease often have anticholinergic activity. In addition, medications used by ophthalmologists, certain toxic plants, and hallucinogens with anticholinergic activity can also produce the anticholinergic intoxication syndrome. A more comprehensive list of substances with anticholinergic activity is found in Table 4-2.

The anticholinergic intoxication syndrome has both physiological and psychological components. The physiological symptoms can include widely dilated and unreactive pupils, blurred vision, flushed face, warm and dry skin, dry mouth and throat, difficulty in swallowing, foul breath, diminished or absent bowel sounds, urinary retention, tachycardia, hypertension, increased respiratory rate, and fever. The psychological symptoms can include disorientation, incoherence, hallucinations, delusions, bizarre motor behavior, fluctuating levels of awareness, and, at times, profound delirium. Severe impairment of recent memory is a prominent symptom of the anticholinergic intoxication syndrome. A patient who has not been unconscious, but who is unable to recall events in the immediately preceding half-hour or who is unable to remember where or who he is, should be strongly suspected of anticholinergic intoxication.

Occasionally, a massive overdose of an anticholinergic substance can produce coma. Comatose patients with the anticholinergic syndrome often exhibit the peripheral physiological symptoms described above, may have

TABLE 4-2.

SUBSTANCES WITH ANTICHOLINERGIC ACTIVITY

Antipsychotic Neuroleptic Medications
  neuroleptics, especially chlorpromazine (Thorazine), and thioridazine (Mellaril).

Tricyclic Antidepressant Medications
  amitriptyline (Elavil)   doxepin (Sinequan)
  imipramine (Tofranil)   nortriptyline (Aventyl)
  protriptyline (Vivactil)   desipramine (Norpramin)
  trimipramine (Surmontil)

Antispasmodics for the Gastrointestinal Tract
  clidinium (Quarzan and in Librax)   methantheline (Banthine)
  propantheline (Pro-Banthine)   adiphenine (Trasentine)
  dicyclomine (Bentyl)   methscopolamine (Pamine)
  hyoscyamine, atropine, and hyoscine (in   homatropine (Matropinal)
    Donnatal)   oxyphenonium (Antrenyl)
  glycopyrrolate (Robinul)   tridihexethyl (in Milpath with meproba-
  mepenzolate (Cantil)   mate)
  belladonna alkaloids (Belladenal and oth-   isopropamide (Darbid)
    ers)   oxyphencyclimine (Daricon and Enarax)
  diphemanil (Prantal)   hexocyclium (Tral)
  methixene (Trest)   anisotropine (Valpin)

Antihistamines with Anticholinergic Activity
  dimenhydrinate (Dramamine)   diphenhydramine (Benadryl)
  orphenadrine (Disipal)   cyclizine (Marezine)
  methapyrilene (Histadyl)   phrilamine (Histalon)
  tripelennamine (Pyribenzamine)   promethazine (Phenergan a phenothiazine
  chlorpheniramine   (Teldrin,   Chlor-   antihistaminic)
    Trimeton, and Ornade)   plus many others

Antiparkinsonian Medications
  benztropine (Cogentin)   biperiden (Akineton)
  ethopropaine (Parsidol HCl)   procyclidine (Kemadrin)
  trihexyphenidyl (Artane)

Other Over-the-Counter Medications
  Cold remedies: Allerest, Coricidin, Flavihist, Romilar, Sine-Off, Contac, Sinutabs, and
    many others.
  Analgesics with anticholinergic activity: Excedrin PM, Cope, and others.
  Menstrual products: Codurex and others.
  Asthma medications: Asthmador and others.

Ophthalmic Preparations
  atropine 1% ophthalmic solution   cyclopentolate (Cyclogyl)
  tropicamide (Mydriacyl)   eucatropine (Euphthalmine)

Over-the-Counter Tranquilizers and Hypnotics
  Alva Tranquil   Asper-Sleep
  Compoz   CVS Sleep Capsules
  Devarex   Dormin
  Dormirex   Dormutol
  Dozar   Ex Tension
  Masons Timed Sleeping Capsules   McKesson Sleep Tablets
  Neo Nyte   Nite Rest

Nytol	Osco Sleep Tablets
Paradorm	Quietabs
Quiet World	Rexall Sleep Capsules
Rexall Sleep Tablets	Sedacaps
Seda Tabs	Seedate
Sleep-Aid	Sleep Eze
Sleeping Pill-Professional	Sleeprin
Slumba-Plus Time Capsules	Slumba-Tabs
Somets	Sominex Capsules
Somnicaps	Sta-Kalm

There are many other similar preparations which also contain anticholinergics. These medications contain either methapyrilene or scopolamine or both.

Plants with Anticholinergic Activity
   Datura stramonium (Jimson weed and many other names)
   Hyoscyamus niger (Henbane)
   Atropa belladonna (deadly nightshade and belladonna)
   Lycium halimifolium (matrimony vine)
   Cestrum nocturnum (Night blooming jessamine)
   Solanum dulcamara (woody nightshade, bittersweet and other names)
   Solanum nigrum (common nightshade and other names)
   Solanum tuberosum (common potato)
   Solanum pseudocapsicum (Jerusalem cherry and silver leaf nightshade and many other names)
   Lycoperisicon esculentum (Tomato)
   Solandra species (Trumpet flower, chalice vine)
   Physalis heterophylla (Ground cherry)

Sources: Goldfrank L. and Meliek M. Locoweed and other anticholinergics. *Hospital Physician* 8:18–39, 1979.

Berger PA and Tinklenberg JR. Medical management of the drug abuser. *In: Psychiatry for the Primary Care Physician*, A. Freeman, R. Sack, and P. Berger (eds). Williams & Wilkins, Baltimore, 1979, pp 359–380.

Shader R.I. (ed). *Manual of Psychiatric Therapeutics*. Little, Brown, Boston, 1975.

clonic movements, upgoing plantar reflexes (a positive Babinski's sign), and hyperreflexia (Berger and Tinklenberg, 1979; Goldfrank and Meliek, 1979; Granacher et al., 1976).

The cardiac complications of the anticholinergic intoxication syndrome can be complex. In addition to tachycardia, there may be a direct suppression of the myocardium (Goldfrank and Meliek, 1979). EKG abnormalities, similar to those produced by quinidine toxicity, result from enhanced re-entrant excitation secondary to reduced conduction velocity. Widening of the QRS complex, prolonged QT interval, and ST segment depression are seen (Goldfrank and Meliek, 1979; Granacher et al., 1976).

Management of Anticholinergic Toxicity
A careful physical examination, EKG, laboratory evaluation, and psychological assessment are basic preliminary procedures in the treatment

of the anticholinergic intoxication syndrome. The patient who is severely agitated and assaultive may require gentle physical restraints. The patient may be unable to cooperate or give a history of the ingested substance, but family members or friends may be of help in determining what drug or substance was ingested. The first priority of treatment is to support vital functions. The anticholinergic syndrome may very occasionally include respiratory or cardiac arrest. In such cases, cardiopulmonary resuscitation is obviously immediately required. When vital functions are stable, but the diagnosis of anticholinergic toxicity is questionable, diazepam (Valium) can be given for sedation. The patient should not be treated with phenothiazine neuroleptics, even in the presence of obvious psychosis. Thioridazine and chlorpromazine, in particular, can exacerbate the anticholinergic toxicity because of their anticholinergic activity (Berger and Tinklenberg, 1979; Goldfrank and Meliek, 1979; Granacher et al., 1976).

A patient with the classical symptoms of the anticholinergic toxicity syndrome, who also has a fever, is profoundly delirious, severely agitated, or comatose, should be treated with intravenous physostigmine, up to 2 mg, given slowly. Physostigmine is the drug of choice because it is tertiary rather than quaternary ammonium salt, unlike other reversible acetylcholinesterase inhibitors. Therefore, physostigmine is unique in crossing the blood–brain barrier. A second dose of 1–2 mg of physostigmine can be given 15 min later. Vital signs should be monitored carefully, and the patient should be closely monitored for cardiac arrhythmias. A decline in heart rate is good evidence that physostigmine is counteracting the anticholinergic toxicity. Because the action of physostigmine is of short duration compared to that of many anticholinergics, it is sometimes necessary to readminister it in 2 or 3 hours, or even more frequently.

Physostigmine should be given cautiously, however, to avoid cholinergic toxicity. If too much is given, a cholinergic crisis results with bradycardia, increased salivation, diarrhea, and occasionally seizures and respiratory arrest. Cholinergic crisis can be reversed with 0.5–1.0 mg of atropine given intravenously. Medical contraindications to physostigmine include a history of heart disease, asthma, peptic ulcer, diabetes, mechanical obstruction of the bowel or bladder, hyperthyroidism, pregnancy, or a history of a previous allergic reaction to physostigmine. Not every patient with anticholinergic toxicity requires physostigmine. Many patients can be treated with diazepam; and nonpharmacological methods, e.g. supportive reassurance can be used to soothe adverse reactions to hallucinogens (Berger and Tinklenberg, 1979; Granacher et al., 1976).

In addition to physostigmine, the patient with anticholinergic toxicity may need further medical treatment. If the patient is comatose, a urinary catheter should be used to avoid urinary retention, 50 cc of 50% glucose should be administered intravenously in case hypoglycemia has contributed to the coma, and 0.4 mg of naloxone should be given on the possibility that opioids have contributed to the coma. Physostigmine is only useful for the supraventricular tachycardia caused by the anticholinergic syndrome. It is not helpful for the cardiac conduction defects or ventricular tachyarrhythmias. For these cardiac problems, it is often helpful to give intravenous fluids and to alkalinize the blood with sodium bicarbonate or sodium lactate. If the arrhythmias do not respond to alkalinization, lidocaine, phenytoin, and propranolol can be useful, while quinidine or procainamide are contraindicated. Finally, the patient who has attempted suicide with anticholinergic agents or who abuses anticholinergics for their psychoactive effects, should be offered psychiatric evaluation and treatment (Berger and Tinklenberg, 1979; Goldfrank and Meliek, 1979; Granacher et al., 1976).

CLASSICAL HALLUCINOGENS AND CANNABIS

History

Hallucinogens derived from natural substances have been used by numerous cultures for many centuries: The hemp plant, *Cannabis sativa*, in China and Italy; the mushroom, *Amanita muscaria* (fly agaric) in Europe; and the psilicybe mexicana mushroom, peyotl cactus, and *Rivea corymbose* (morning glory) seeds in Pre-Columbian America. The psychological syndromes produced by these substances were essential and central elements in religious ceremonies, healing rituals, and for predicting the future. The substances were probably also used in warfare. The word "assassin" is derived from "Hashshashian," the name of a group that terrorized Persia during the eleventh century. This group is alleged to have committed murder under the influence of hashish, derived from *Cannabis sativa*. The Viking "Beserkers" are said to have prepared for battle by using the mushroom *Amanita muscaria* (Ayd and Blackwell, 1970).

Hallucinogens also have a modern history, beginning with lysergic acid diethylamide-25 (LSD-25). In the 1930's in Basel, Switzerland, Albert Hofmann of Sandoz was working with ergot alkaloids, which were active in smooth muscles and therefore exciting to medicinal chemists. Hofmann was part of the scientific team that obtained the lysergic acid nucleus from ergot alkaloids by alkaline hydrolysis. The group of investigators modified the lysergic acid nucleus in an attempt to obtain more smooth muscle activity. In the process, Hofmann combined lysergic acid with amines in a protein linkage. One of the results, lysergic acid diethylamide-25, was synthesized in 1938 but was put away until April 16, 1943. On this day, Hofmann decided to look at the pharmacological activity of LSD-25, synthesized some more, and accidentally ingested a small amount. Hofmann then described a classical psychedelic experience in his diary. This first description is as graphic as any that followed (Ayd and Blackwell, 1970).

The incredibly low effective doses of LSD (5000 to 10,000 times more active than mescaline) were of great scientific interest to pharmacologists and psychiatrists studying schizophrenia; it now seemed more feasible that undetectable traces of an extremely potent psychoactive substance produced by the body itself could cause schizophrenia. The first synthetic hallucinogen, LSD-25, is unique in potency, but not in its clinical syndrome which is also produced by natural substances (Ayd and Blackwell, 1970).

Since cannabis is the only plant that yields both a psychoactive drug and a useful fiber (hemp), its early history can be traced through references to a plant that yields both. Such references are found in the earliest writings from India, Assyria, and China. The ancient Greeks used alcohol rather than cannabis as an intoxicant, but there are passages in ancient Greek (Herodotus, Dioscorides, and others) and Hebrew writings that describe the cultivation and use of cannabis in surrounding cultures. The references are frequent enough to leave little doubt that throughout Asia and the Near East, cannabis was grown from the earliest known times to the present, both for its fiber and for its psychoactive properties. Cannabis is currently the fourth most popular psychoactive substance worldwide, preceded only by caffeine, nicotine, and alcohol.

The Spanish naturalists, who followed Cortez, wrote of a number of plants that possessed psychoactive characteristics which were known in Mexico but not in Europe. The three main groups were: peyotl cactus (peyote), teonanacatl mushroom, ololiuqui or the seeds of bind weeds, now called morning glory.

Peyote was the first of these substances to be studied. Louis Lewin, a brilliant plant pharmacologist, wrote about peyote in his monograph *Phantastica*, published in 1924. The peyotl cactus was named *Anhalonium lewinii* in honor of Lewin and Heffter's isolation of mescaline in 1896. In 1919, E. Spaeth elucidated the structure of mescaline (trimethoxyphenylethylamine, structurally related to dopamine) and synthesized it. A period of pharmacological research followed, which was summarized in 1920 by K. Beringer and published in 1927 (Ayd and Blackwell, 1970).

In 1936, Richard Schultes, a distinguished botanist from Harvard, learned that the naturalists who followed Cortez had been correct. Mushrooms were still used as hallucinogens in Mexico. In 1955, G. Wasson was probably the first outsider to ingest the "holy" mushrooms and sent some to R. Heim of the National Natural History Museum of Paris. Heim classified the mushrooms and grew some in his laboratory. Wasson also sent them to Albert Hofmann in Basel who, after evaluating them, ate 2.4 g of the *Psilocybe mexicana* and had another remarkable "psychedelic" experience. Soon the active principles psilocybin and psilocin (phosphorylated N,N-dimethyl-4-hydroxytryptamine and N,N-dimethyl-4-hydroxytryptamine, both structurally related to serotonin) were defined, and Hofmann and his group synthesized these substances. In 1963, Hofmann took them to Mexico and gave them in pill form to the Indians from the group who originally had supplied the mushrooms. They were delighted and found no differences between the effects of the mushrooms and the synthetic psilocybin (Ayd and Blackwell, 1970).

Ololiuqui was first described in 1570 by Francisco Hernandez who, in the name of Philip II of Spain, was sent to study the flora and fauna of Mexico. He wrote a scholarly description of the plant and mentioned that its seeds induced "a thousand visions and satanic hallucinations." Shultes reported an unsuccessful attempt to isolate the active principle in 1937, but in 1955, the Canadian psychiatrist, Osmond took 800 *Rivea corymbosa* (morning glory seeds) and had an hallucinatory experience. Wasson sent some seeds to Hofmann and he found a relative of LSD, namely lysergic acid 1-hydroxyethylamide. The syndrome produced by this psychoactive substance is different from LSD-25 and mescaline.

Morning glory seeds are reported to produce tiredness, apathy, a feeling of mental depression, and feelings of unreality and meaninglessness (Ayd and Blackwell, 1970).

The hallucinogen from ancient Europe, *Amanita muscaria*, has proved to be more difficult to characterize pharmacologically. For many years, it was assumed that its active ingredient was the potent and often toxic muscarine, a cholinergic agonist. However, recently, the gamma-aminobutyric acid (GABA) agonist, "muscimol" was also isolated from *Amanita muscaria*, and was shown to be an hallucinogen. Further study will be needed to determine whether muscimol alone is responsible for the use of *Amanita muscaria* as an hallucinogen.

Patterns of Use

Classical hallucinogens such as LSD are most frequently used by middle- and upper-class youth, often college students. A 1972 survey found that somewhat less than 5% of youths over 12 years of age have used hallucinogens. The mid-1960's marked the period of most intense use of the classical hallucinogens. Daily use is uncommon because there is rapid tolerance and because the psychoactive effects are considered to produce a powerful and important experience which consumes both psychological and physical energy. Advocates of hallucinogens claim that these substances produce a very special kind of euphoric experience. Rather than the peaceful withdrawal associated with opiates or the exhilaration produced by amphetamine and cocaine, the classical hallucinogens produce an experience that has been variously described as mystical, religious, or philosophical; they are often thought to provide the user with new insight or greater understanding of himself or some aspect of reality (Berger and Tinklenberg, 1979; Cohen, 1978; Hollister, 1968).

The psychoactive effects of cannabis depend on the concentration of the active pharmacological substances, the tetrahydrocannabinols. Marijuana is a relatively weak preparation, while hashish is stronger. Users describe a biphasic sequence of initial stimulation and euphoria followed by sedation and tranquility. A distortion of time sense, altered thinking patterns, an initial giddiness, increased appetite, heightened sensory awareness, a tendency toward thoughtful reflection, and a comfortable warm feeling are some of the positive aspects of marijuana intoxication described by users. Stronger preparations of cannabis, such as hashish, can produce the mystical, philosophical, and insight euphoria which is similar to the syndrome described by the users of the classical hallucinogens (Harris, 1978; Meyer, 1978).

CLINICAL SYNDROME: CLASSICAL HALLUCINOGENS
HALLUCINOSIS (327.56)
DELUSIONAL DISORDER (327.55)
AFFECTIVE DISORDER (327.57)

The prototype of the clinical syndromes produced by classical hallucinogens, such as lysergic acid diethylamide (LSD) includes perceptual, somatic, and psychological symptoms. Perceptual symptoms can include alterations in colors and shapes, increased auditory acuity, difficulty in focusing on objects and, occasionally, synesthesia, the appearance of sensations in one sensory modality caused by a stimulus in another. For example, the user of LSD may report "seeing" a sound. Somatic symptoms can include drowsiness, dizziness, paresthesias, weakness, tremors, and nausea (Berger and Tinklenberg, 1979; Hollister, 1968).

Personal predisposition seems to render the symptoms of classical hallucinogen ingestion quite variable. Symptoms can include profound but labile alterations in mood, difficulty in expressing thoughts, distorted time sense, dreamlike feelings, and, at times, visual hallucinations. Some individuals report a sense of "universal insight" or feel an emotional connection to all other people or other living things. Advocates of hallucinogens such as LSD see these aspects of the syndrome as positive. The LSD user, however, may also experience unpleasant, frightening images or disturbing, even paranoid, thoughts. Loss of control of coordination and of emotions, or of intellectual function may lead from confusion to anger or panic (Berger and Tinklenberg, 1979; Hollister, 1968).

Transient aberrant behavior caused by hallucinogens can also cause problems. Drug-induced feelings of omnipotence could lead to fatal leaps from high places or to attempts to stop moving cars. Severe panic may also conceivably lead to injury when a user tries to escape terrifying thoughts or sensations. While such events are reported to occur, they are probably not as common as the lay press frequently suggests. Longer reactions with persisting psychosis, prolonged depression, or clouded thinking and judgment with deficient social functioning are also reported. These reactions have not been shown to be a direct pharmacological effect of hallucinogens. In some areas, the mixing of inexpensive psychoactive agents, such as anticholinergic medications, with expensive hallucinogens is a common practice. The so-called "chronic" effects of hallucinogen drug abuse may also be influenced by existing personality problems (Berger and Tinklenberg, 1979).

The clinical symptoms caused by LSD, psilocybin, and mescaline are nearly indistinguishable to users. Dimethyltryptamine (DMT) produces a shorter syndrome with similar symptoms, but visual distortions are more commonly distressing. Several hallucinogens, which are structurally related to amphetamine, and known as "psychotomimetic amphetamines" produce a syndrome which can have characteristics of both the classical hallucinogen syndrome and the syndrome produced by the psychostimulants, amphetamine and cocaine. These methoxylated amphetamines include STP (DOM, 2,5-dimethoxy-4-methylamphetamine), MDA (3,4-methylene-dioxyamphetamine), and 26 other similar compounds (DOM, 1973).

CLINICAL SYNDROME:
CANNABIS INTOXICATION (327.60)
DELUSIONAL DISORDER (327.65)

Cannabis is the general term for psychoactive compounds derived from the hemp plant *Cannabis sativa*. A variety of terms are used for these substances which contain the tetrahydrocannabinols (THC). The concentration of THC, and hence the potency, varies considerably in different preparations of cannabis. *Marijuana* is the term frequently used for relatively weak preparations of cannabis that are smoked or eaten; *hashish* refers to a preparation with a higher concentration of THC (Harris, 1978; Meyer, 1978).

Cannabis, like the classical hallucinogens, can produce panic reactions. Adverse cannabis reactions can occasionally include anxiety, fear, a sense of helplessness, and loss of control. Sometimes delusions, including paranoid thoughts, confusion, depersonalization, temporary amnesia, emotional liability, and hallucinations may also be present, particularly at high levels of intoxication. These more serious adverse psychological reactions are similar to the "bad trips" that are most commonly associated with the use of the classical hallucinogens. However, adverse reactions to cannabis occur less frequently and are often of shorter duration than

those involving such hallucinogens as LSD. Adverse reactions to cannabis are usually associated with high doses or with any dose in an individual who fears adverse reactions or is unprepared for the psychoactive
effects. In individuals with a previous history of a personality or psychiatric disorder, intensification of underlying pathology by cannabis use
has been reported. Disagreement does exist as to whether these reactions
should be attributed to individual premorbid pathology or to a direct
pharmacological effect of cannabis (Berger and Tinklenberg, 1979; Harris, 1978; Meyer, 1978).

Chronic cannabis users are said to develop an "amotivational syndrome" characterized by passivity, decreased motivation, and a preoccupation with taking drugs. The pharmacological role of marijuana in
this syndrome is controversial. Consistent evidence that marijuana in-
duces permanent organic brain changes does not exist. However, preexisting personality traits, social factors, and other drug use, together with
regular cannabis use, could conceivably contribute to some personality
changes, particularly during the formative period of adolescence. Further
study in this area is important as marijuana use becomes more widespread (Harris, 1978; Meyer, 1978).

Management of Adverse Reactions

"Bad trips" is a common name for adverse reactions to hallucinogens.
Lethal overdoses of hallucinogenic drugs used alone are probably rare,
but a fatal outcome can occur when the classical hallucinogen has been
mixed with adulterants, such as sedative-hypnotics or anticholinergics.
The management of the anticholinergic intoxication syndrome is described in an earlier section of this chapter. The general principles for
the treatment of "bad trips" associated with classical hallucinogenic drugs
and cannabis are similar to those for the treatment of adverse reactions
that result from PCP, solvent inhalants, CNS stimulants, and from combinations of these substances. The reader is referred to the section near
the beginning of the chapter on polydrug abuse for the methodology of
managing other adverse drug reactions (Berger and Tinklenberg, 1979;
Greenblatt and Shader, 1975b).

A physical examination can help establish the diagnosis. Because of
the problem of drug contamination, specific physical findings should be
sought. LSD, mescaline, and psilocybin generally produce dilated pupils

and hyperactive reflexes; cannabis does not produce mydriasis, but can cause dilation of conjunctival blood vessels. Signs of other drug effects, such as anticholinergic, sedative-hypnotic, or stimulant toxicity, may also be present because of the tendency of some substance abusers to use multiple drugs. The physician should attempt to reduce the toxic effects of the drug and manage behavioral disturbances as the diagnosis is established. Nonpharmacological interventions are probably best (Berger and Tinklenberg, 1979).

The patient's environment should be arranged to avoid either too little or too much sensory input, since both can cause the hallucinogen user to become more anxious. An uncrowded room with moderate light and sound is recommended. Treating staff should avoid rapid or sudden movements. A treatment method called the "talk down" can be very useful for "bad trips" and cannabis panic reactions. The treating staff or the patient's friends should talk to the patient in a soothing, almost parental manner. The patient is told that he or she is experiencing a reaction that is temporary, and is reassured that disturbing thoughts and feelings will gradually decrease. Some individuals are calmed by being repeatedly oriented to the environment. Others find it helpful to verbalize experiences, since this gives a greater sense of control (Berger and Tinklenberg, 1979; Greenblatt and Shader, 1975b).

In general, the treating staff should be flexible and attempt to find and pursue any topic of conversation that reduces anxiety. As the toxic reaction diminishes, the patient often experiences the ebb and flow of disturbing symptoms. This phenomenon should be anticipated and described by the treating staff, who should be wary of concluding that the adverse reaction has passed, since the patient may be experiencing a transient improvement. Hallucinogens or cannabis-induced adverse reactions usually require only clarifying and supportive treatment. However, in the busy emergency ward, there may be insufficient staff or time for the "talk down" procedure. In these circumstances, medication may be necessary to control anxiety and agitation. Antianxiety drugs such as diazepam (20–30 mg orally if possible since IM absorption can be erratic) or other benzodiazepines, which have a wide margin of safety, are often useful. These medications should be given in the lowest dose sufficient to reduce anxiety and as infrequently as possible (e.g. every 3–6 hours) to reduce agitation to manageable levels without altering and depressing vital signs or causing too much sedation (Berger and Tinklenberg, 1979).

There are several reasons why phenothiazines or other antipsychotic agents should be avoided in the treatment of adverse reactions to hallu-cinogens, cannabis, or multiple drugs. Anticholinergic substances, which may have been taken by the drug user in the form of an adulterant, can interact with phenothiazines to induce anticholinergic toxicity. With many antipsychotics, the margin between effective behavioral sedation and the production of hypotensive reactions is small. The use of such potent drugs for sedation is questionable for any clinical disorder in which the untreated course is usually benign. Antipsychotic agents may also mask a schizophrenic psychosis which could otherwise be detected and treated appropriately. Finally, the immobilizing properties of these drugs and their frequent extrapyramidal reactions are distressing and may increase the patient's feelings of loss of control and helplessness (Berger and Tink-lenberg, 1979).

Uncomplicated adverse reactions to hallucinogens and cannabis rarely require hospitalization. However hospitalization is indicated where im-paired cognitive functions or perceptions last for more than 4 to 6 hours in spite of medication. If there is no need for hospitalization, the patient can be discharged into the care of a responsible person when the patient's cognitive function and vital signs have returned to normal. A patient who lives alone should be helped to find a place with relatives or friends for at least 24 hours. Lethargy, irritability, and depression sometimes characterize recovery from an adverse drug reaction. This alteration in mood should be explained to the patient. A psychiatric evaluation or a drug treatment program should also be offered (Berger and Tinklenberg, 1979).

"Flashbacks" are spontaneous recurrences of thoughts, feelings, and perceptions originally experienced during acute hallucinogen drug intox-ication. The mechanism of these mental events is not clear, but flash-backs are probably psychological in origin. They can occur months after the last drug ingestion when pharmacological actions of the drug would not be expected. Flashbacks are usually triggered by fairly specific psy-chological factors such as certain emotions, thoughts, or environmental events. They are seldom a significant clinical problem. A patient with flashbacks should be advised to refrain from the use of hallucinogens or other psychoactive drugs that may contribute to the difficulty. The fre-quency of flashbacks can be diminished by avoiding precipitants that trigger the phenomenon. Patients can be reassured by the fact that for most people, the flashbacks gradually become less intense, less frequent, and eventually disappear altogether. For some individuals, it may be helpful to use low doses of antianxiety medications (Berger and Tinklenberg, 1979).

TOBACCO

History

Almost 500 years after its controversial introduction to Europe, tobacco remains a topic of considerable debate. The inclusion of tobacco in this chapter is evidence of the recent change in attitude toward its use. Whether tobacco should be classified as a drug of abuse and what criteria are to be used for such a classification are unresolved dilemmas.

Tobacco use is many centuries old and tobacco smoking was traditionally a religious, medicinal, and ceremonial custom of the New World. The earliest evidence of tobacco use is the depiction of a Mayan shaman in the Palenque ruins in Mexico dated from the fifth century (High Times Encyclopedia of Recreational Drugs, 1978). Tobacco played a central role in North American tribal life. Many varieties were available; several were mixed together for flavor, and certain kinds were specific to individual tribes or locations. Tobacco was wrapped in corn husks and smoked by the Tainos of Hispaniola, placed in hollow reeds by the Aztecs, and placed in elbow-shaped pipes by the Plains Tribes in Minnesota. Although most commonly they were smoked, tobacco leaves could be chewed, eaten, drunk as juice as in South America, or snuffed as is still the custom in the Amazon (High Times Encyclopedia of Recreational Drugs, 1978).

Columbus is said to have been responsible for the introduction of tobacco from the Americas to Europe in 1492 (Jarvik and Gritz, 1977). Smoking became popular in Spain, spread rapidly across Europe, and brought in its wake a storm of controversy. The appearance in London of Sir Walter Raleigh's treasures of pipes, tobacco, and leaves from the Americas elicited a vehement condemnation from James I in 1604 (Jarvik and Gritz, 1977). Both rulers and religious leaders were suspicious of the "foreign substance" and denounced the practice of smoking as a source of political unrest, moral decadence, unwarranted pleasures, and a fire hazard. In Turkey and in Germany, public exhibition of smoking was punishable by death, and in Russia, castration was the threatened sentence for smoking (Brecher, 1972; Cohen, 1979b).

The warnings and punishments went mostly unheeded, and in spite of some evidence of medical hazards, efforts to eradicate and expel tobacco from Europe were in vain. Tobacco use spread rapidly through every class and most European cultures where its use was reported to be and is currently experienced as pleasurable, and a fashionable accoutrement to social functions. The popularity of tobacco and its eventual widespread social acceptance stimulated competitive industry, technology, agriculture, and the economy. By the mid-nineteenth century the appearance of the modern slim, mass-produced cigarette combined with more mild vareties of tobacco made smoking easily accessible and available (Cohen, 1979b). At present, the cigarette is one of the most efficient and least expensive device for self-administration of tobacco. Industry, employment, and taxes on the import and export of tobacco have helped to establish tobacco as a source of economic and political power.

PATTERNS OF USE

Smoking is a popular, commonly accepted and widely practiced social act among almost all societies, and by people of all races and social classes. It is a behavior well recognized as a sign of sophistication and a symbol of companionship, acceptance, and attainment of a certain level of maturity. Hence, the image of adulthood, maturity, and freedom currently includes casual, but regular use of tobacco, often combined with alcohol (and sometimes other drugs).

At present, more than 4000 cigarettes are smoked per person each year in the United States (Cohen, 1979b). The principle users up to the present era have been men; advent of the women's liberation movement has changed the female roles and attitudes toward women. The previous stigma of cigarette smoking for women has been lifted, and a rapidly increasing proportion of women smoke as much as men. Smokers constitute 41% of the adult population in the United States, and 25% of adults smoke more than a pack of cigarettes each day (Jaffe and Jarvik, 1978).

Experimentation with smoking usually begins in adolescence, a developmental stage characterized by a vulnerability to image-conforming behaviors. Many teenagers are reported to be steady users of tobacco. They begin in response to the influence and smoking habits of friends, family, significant individuals, and their own changing self-concept, perception of reality, and personality. For example, there is evidence that children of parents who smoke, who are less educated, and who work part-time or not at all are more likely to smoke (Jaffe and Jarvik, 1978). Smokers appear to be more extroverted, impulsive, and antisocial (Jarvik and Gritz, 1977).

Personality traits, the effect of local environmental, peer, and social pressure; heavy advertising; and perhaps innate drug-seeking behavior are all factors that potentially contribute to and influence the extent and frequency of tobacco use. Exactly what proportion or combination of each of these factors determines such behaviors as light, medium, and heavy smoking is at present uncertain.

REASONS FOR SUBSTANCE USE AND ABUSE

Tobacco is a paradoxical substance of abuse, since it seems to act as a panacea for seemingly opposite psychological and physiological states. Smoking provides stimulation for those who are fatigued or bored; it has been subjectively reported and also clinically shown to improve coordination in activities such as routine methodical tasks. Conversely, studies also reveal that smoking acts to "calm the nerves," and acts as a muscle relaxant during periods of stress, allowing individuals under long-term pressure and tension to perform better than average, and even to enhance concentration (Jarvik and Gritz, 1977).

Smoking is also thought to lower anxiety levels, "steady the nerves," and allay anticipated tension in provoking situations such as social functions. The ritual of taking a cigarette, lighting up, and inhaling occupies the hands and is an acceptable introductory behavior. It can also be used as a rebellious gesture, one easily available to teenagers. However, for many, smoking is a pleasurable act in itself. It is an easy habit to acquire, uphold, and maintain, as there is subjective as well as external reinforcement. Unlike other substances of abuse, it is inexpensive, readily available, and an attractive alternative to the other substances in that it does not impair muscle function and coordination. Smoking also has fewer immediate negative medical or psychological consequences or side effects. Physiological effects of smoking, especially initially, include vasoconstriction, increased blood pressure, tremor, tachycardia, nausea, and increased gastrointestinal activity (Jarvik and Gritz, 1977).

The reasons for smoking mentioned above imply some degree of control, flexibility, and choice. However, recent investigations also show evidence that tobacco contains a chemical substance or substances which trigger the desire, need, or craving for regular and continued self-adminstration of that substance. Most studies show nicotine, and to a lesser extent tar, to be the basic pharmacological reinforcers in smoking (Jarvik and Gritz, 1977; Cohen, 1979b; Jaffe and Jarvik, 1978; Jarvik et al., 1977).

Although it remains a controversial topic, nicotine is now widely viewed as an addictive substance. This theory is supported by results from studies in which smokers are given cigarettes with lower tar and nicotine content. These subjects were found to smoke more cigarettes and/or inhale more deeply to maintain a constant level of nicotine in the body as measured in the blood plasma levels. When subjects were given cigarettes high in nicotine content, fewer cigarettes were smoked and the inhalations were not as deep. This suggests that there is an as yet unknown mechanism in the brain which regulates nicotine levels (Jaffe and Jarvik, 1978; Jarvik et al., 1977; Jarvik et al., 1978).

Nicotine has a short half-life in the blood and brain which allows repeated and frequent use without loss of effect. Nicotine from every inhalation reaches the brain from the lung in 7 sec as compared to the 14 sec it takes heroin to flow from arm to brain. Thus heavy smokers maintain their plasma nicotine levels for maximum satisfaction and need by steady daily inhalation of nicotine which floods the brain. The titration hypothesis holds that smokers can control and stabilize their plasma nicotine levels by absorbing nicotine through their choice of cigarette size, quantity, inhalation rate, and depth. The number of high-nicotine level cigarettes smoked decreased among smokers more familiar with medium-nicotine level cigarettes, yet their plasma levels of nicotine were found to be identical with what they had been before. Furthermore, when mecamylamine, a centrally active nicotine antagonist, was administered to subjects, there was a marked increase in the number of cigarettes consumed. The bolus hypothesis states that the brain receives a sharp flooding of a bolus of blood containing high concentrations of nicotine after each inhalation which is quickly absorbed. This immediate absorption enables the smoker to control the plasma nicotine levels, preventing a nicotine withdrawal syndrome (Jarvik and Gritz, 1977; Cohen, 1979b; Jaffe and Jarvik, 1978).

Tobacco: Use or Abuse

The inclusion of tobacco and nicotine under addiction and drug abuse is the subject of much controversy. Dependence (and ultimately addiction) can be viewed as a state where the individual craves a substance, suffers a withdrawal syndrome without it, and cannot stop using it voluntarily. In this light, nicotine can be seen as a substance of abuse. However, as no immediate side effects, intoxication, distress, or behavioral impairments are seen, and tolerance to nicotine is rapid, it is difficult to define criteria for nicotine dependence or nicotine abuse (tobacco dependence or tobacco use disorder) (Jaffe and Jarvik, 1978).

Smokers who are healthy, suffer no impairment, and are at ease with their habit would be difficult to describe and classify as addicted to nicotine. However, smokers who are concerned or distressed about their habitual and compulsive use of tobacco for whatever psychological or physiological reason would qualify for the diagnostic term "tobacco use disorder" (Jaffe and Jarvik, 1978; Jarvik et al., 1977).

Recent research has demonstrated a strong correlation between heavy smoking and major medical disorders such as chronic bronchitis; emphysema; cancer of the lung, larynx, and mouth; and coronary atherosclerosis (Brecher, 1972; Jarvik et al., 1977). Therefore, heavy smokers who are at high risk for developing serious medical disease and/or who are disturbed at their inability to refrain from smoking can be classified as having "tobacco use disorder." Currently, three out of four smokers express their desire to stop smoking. Also to be included in the group qualifying for treatment for tobacco use disorder are those who attempt to stop smoking, but who exhibit severe symptoms of the nicotine withdrawal syndrome (Jaffe and Jarvik, 1978; Jarvik et al., 1977).

The medical consequences of chronic and heavy smoking are confirmed and well-publicized in reports about respiratory types of cancer and other lung and blood vessel diseases (Jarvik et al., 1977). However, to many, these negative consequences are relatively remote, perhaps 30 to 40 years in the future. This is unfortunate considering the immediate positive reinforcement and reward of pleasure that smoking provides.

MEDICAL MANAGEMENT OF BOTH ACUTE AND CHRONIC ADVERSE REACTIONS TO NICOTINE

Several psychological, physiological, and behavioral reactions of varying intensities have been experienced following the cessation of smoking, but these do not appear to comprise a clear-cut recognizable withdrawal syndrome. Symptoms described include mild or severe disturbances in sleep patterns, gastrointestinal distress, changes in heart rate, blood pressure, and pulse, irritability, restlessness, headache, nausea, anxiety, difficulty with concentration and psychomotor coordination, and weight gain. The syndrome is experienced within either hours or days upon cessation and can last up to several months. Toxicity is rarely seen among chronic smokers because of their tolerance to nicotine. Toxicity is usually seen only in nonsmokers who attempt to smoke. Symptoms of toxicity occurring in nonsmokers include diarrhea, vomiting, increased salivation, abdominal cramps, sweating, dizziness, and occasionally faintness and shock; nonsmokers may also demonstrate an allergic reaction (Jarvik and Gritz, 1977).

Some of the "withdrawal" symptoms of tobacco may be physiological responses to the interruption of nicotine consumption, or may represent psychological reactions to the change of many habitual behaviors. But the fact that these symptoms disappear completely and relatively quickly upon resumption of smoking may indicate the existence of a physiological withdrawal syndrome. Severity of withdrawal symptoms correlates with the intensity and frequency of smoking (Jarvik and Gritz, 1977; Jaffe and Jarvik, 1978; Jarvik et al., 1977).

The high relapse rate of smokers is evidence of the extent of the problems involved in the treatment of the tobacco use disorder. It is difficult to select a compatible group of patients for treatment, as each may have differing levels of motivation, different levels of knowledge of the medical consequences, different accompanying medical problems, and disparate degrees of addiction and tolerance to nicotine and tobacco. However, it is not yet clear why such variability exists in individual withdrawal patterns and what roles personality, environmental factors, and stress-response play in the progression of dependence, tolerance, and addiction (Jarvik et al., 1977; Jarvik et al., 1978; Hunt and Bespalec, 1974; Russell, 1977).

Many methods for the prevention of smoking are being used and studied at present: behavioral psychotherapeutic techniques include aversive conditioning, desensitization, and covert desensitization; other psychotherapies include educational therapy, group therapy, supportive therapy, and hypnotherapy (Jaffe and Jarvik, 1978; Jarvik et al., 1977; Hunt and Bespalec, 1974; Russell, 1977). Additional treatments include confrontation, rapid smoking methods, and a combination of one or two of the above with drug therapy. It is interesting to note that the same rate of treatment success is seen with placebos as with drugs. Pharmacological treatment alone is seldom used, but is prescribed to help lessen anxiety, tension, and the craving for nicotine. It is also used to assist variability in mood during the adjustment period of withdrawal, or to act as a replacement for nicotine. Lobeline, a drug which mimics the pharmacological action of nicotine, is prescribed, but has shown only moderate short-term success. Other pharmacological agents have been used, but with little success. These include amphetamine, diazepam, phenobarbital, meprobamate, fenfluramine, and methylphenidate (Jarvik and Gritz, 1977; Jaffe and Jarvik, 1978; Jarvik et al., 1978; Hunt and Bespalec, 1974).

Many of these treatments achieve some measure of success and, interestingly, the success rate in abstinence after cessation of smoking is higher in men than women. The success rate depends on factors such as general motivation, will power, motivation for medical reasons, method of treatment, and compatibility of the subject with the method of treatment. As yet, there is no "cure" for nicotine and tobacco addiction. The most impressive results are seen in educational programs combined with group therapy and support. Although initially successful, there is also very little difference in long-term success rates among methods such as pharmacological treatment, combined medication and psychotherapy, and behavioral therapy. The substitution of nicotine-containing gum and low-nicotine cigarettes, when combined with the above treatments, results in moderate, short-term success (Cohen, 1979a; Jaffe and Jarvik, 1978; Jarvik et al., 1977; Hunt and Bespalec, 1974).

Treatment registers a higher success rate on a short-term basis, with an approximate 70% success rate after the completion of an average six-week course. However, the percentage of nonsmokers declines with time. At the end of a year, 80% of smokers revert to their original habit with respect to quantity and time spent smoking. Roughly 20% of previous smokers remain nonsmokers (Technical Review on Cigarette Smoking as an Addiction, 1979).

Motivation seems to be the biggest factor in determining success and failure rates and more research is needed to determine the most effective method or combination of methods of treatment. The problem with many of the behavioral treatments for the cessation of smoking is that motivation is either too low or is very difficult to sustain since the social aspects of smoking are so comforting. The best method seen so far is abrupt abstinence when motivation is high (Jarvik et al., 1977; Russell, 1977). An additional problem to successful treatment is the attitude of society toward smoking. In contrast to the attitude toward heroin abuse, the common social acceptance of and tolerance in attitude toward smoking and to relapse to smoking make it more difficult for the would-be abstainer.

In this light, there exists an ethical dilemma for the treating physician who smokes. Members of society, including both patient and physician, are aware of the image, social prestige, and the often awesome influence that physicians possess. It would appear crucial for physicians and other educators and influential persons to critically review and evaluate effects their smoking habit and behaviors may have on their patients and to avoid any double standards with regard to the dangers and consequences of cigarette smoking.

CAFFEINE

ESSENTIAL FEATURES

The essential features of *caffeine intoxication* (305.90) are restlessness, nervousness, excitement, insomnia, flushed face, diuresis, and gastrointestinal complaints. Some individuals develop these symptoms with as little as 250 mg of caffeine per day, whereas others require much larger doses. With levels of more than 1 g a day there may be muscle twitchings, periods of inexhaustibility, psychomotor agitation, rambling flow of thought and speech, and cardiac arrhythmia.

HISTORY

Caffeine in the form of coffee, tea, cocoa, and "cola" beverages is currently the most widely used psychoactive substance, followed closely by nicotine and alcohol. Yet, like these substances, the initial reaction to coffee in Europe and the Americas was one of abhorrence and opposition. This was no doubt in response to the alleged "intoxicating" and "hazardous" effects exhibited by consumers of the new beverage.

The explorers of the fifteenth and sixteenth centuries returned from their voyages heavily laden with caffeine. From Arabia and Turkey came the first taste of coffee, originally from Ethiopia and North Africa. Tea was brought from China and, from West Africa came the kola nut which was the source of caffeine later added to the "cola" drinks. The cocoa tree was imported from Mexico and the Central Americas. The ilex plant, the source of the caffeine drink, mate, was brought back from Brazil. In North America, discovery was made of cassine, the tea plant or Christmas berry tree from which Native Americans made a caffeine brew (Brecher, 1972).

The first description of coffee is found among the writings of the Arabian physician, Avicenna, in the tenth century. In the following centuries, coffee with its stimulant properties held the paradoxical position of being revered and ceremoniously used by Moslem Arabs in their religious all-night vigils, and being thoroughly condemned by pious European priests and respectable citizens as "intoxicating" and giving rise to unseemly, overexcited, and blasphemous behavior.

Despite warnings, prohibitions, and punishment, the coffee habit endured and increased. Mankind has long searched for natural stimulants, so coffee became popular, accepted, and valued socially for its ability to stimulate, and for its mellow yet piquant flavor. The introduction of sugar and its combination with coffee may well have sealed the fate of consumers, who responded enthusiastically to the pleasant mixture. This led to strong demands for the import and constant supply of coffee beans. In 1554, the first coffee houses sprang up in Constantinople. Later coffee cults, such as the Bohemians of the 1840's, became popular, their members drinking coffee while discussing political and philosophical issues in stimulating debates (Brecher, 1972).

The ceremonial honor awarded tea and its consumption in China in 350 AD, and much later in England, bears witness to the central role of this beverage in these countries. Documentation of the "aphrodisiac" properties of cocoa and chocolate date from as early as 300 years ago. One famous story describes the consumption of 50 cups of "chocolate" by the Aztec ruler Montezuma in preparation for a lively evening with many of his 700 wives (High Times Encyclopedia of Recreational Drugs, 1978). Of all the caffeine-containing beverages, chocolate caused the greatest suspicion, as it was viewed as an inciter of lustful energy and immoral behavior (Brecher, 1972; High Times Encyclopedia of Recreational Drugs, 1978).

The last major category of caffeine-containing substances includes many over-the-counter medications for headaches and colds, and certain nonprescription stimulants. In addition, a substance derived from the Brazilian herb guarana, which contains caffeine and other possible psychoactive substances, has recently been sold in certain health food stores as a natural stimulant called "Zoom."

The popularity, social acceptance, and extensive use of caffeine-containing beverages may confirm mankind's need for stimulating substances. Coffee is also comparatively inexpensive. Caffeine in coffee, tea, and carbonated cola drinks, has been thoroughly incorporated into the average daily lifestyle. Opinions still differ as to whether caffeine should be categorized as a drug of abuse, despite its obvious pharmacological activity. Many users protest and deny that they are "addicted" to caffeine-containing beverages.

PATTERN OF USE

Coffee, tea, cocoa, cola drinks, and over-the-counter medications with caffeine content are so widely used that a household shelf without one or more of these beverages would be rare indeed. Considering that most caffeine in the United States has to be imported and that coffee constitutes the most common source of caffeine, it is not surprising to discover that in 1972, the United States spent $1.2 billion for 2.8 billion pounds of coffee (Winstead, 1976). Furthermore, in the same year, approximately 34 million pounds of pure caffeine were consumed (Graham, 1978).

Since coffee is the most available source of caffeine, and as the average cup of coffee contains 85 mg of caffeine (range of 50–120 mg, excluding decaffeinated coffee) and the average consumption is 2.25 cups a day, the average daily intake of caffeine is about 190 mg. This, combined with caffeine from other dietary sources and medications, results in an average minimum daily per capita intake of approximately 210 mg of caffeine. This figure can fluctuate between 140 and 800 mg. Naturally, the method of brewing, coffee bean chosen, and number of cups per day varies widely among individuals according to personal habits, mood, activity, and personality characteristics, such as dependency (Graham, 1978).

Caffeine-containing beverages are an essential part of most lifestyles and cultures throughout the world. Along with tobacco, these beverages are a central element of daily meals and ritual intake. Caffeine is used to awaken, to sustain individuals at mid-morning and during the working day, and to give a sophisticated sense of closure after the evening meal.

It takes several years to acquire the taste and habit of coffee or tea drinking, since most children dislike the bitterness of these beverages. Many parents forbid their children's consumption of tea and coffee, yet, inconsistently, they encourage the use of cola drinks. Hot chocolate and cocoa are still recommended and acceptable drinks for children.

The daily intake of caffeine rises with age during childhood and adolescence, with initial intake beginning as young as six to eleven months. Adults over 18 years of age are the heaviest consumers, as are "extroverted" personalities, and those involved in successful, fast-paced professions. Heavy users are oversimplistically characterized as achievers with obsessive compulsive personalities, who are often anxious and/or depressed, and whose active lifestyles require sustained periods of concentration and performance. Heavy caffeine users are frequently users of other substances of abuse, such as alcohol and tobacco. Housewives comprise a large proportion of regular users of caffeine-containing beverages, and students ingest large amounts of coffee as well as over-the-counter caffeine-containing stimulants (Brecher, 1972).

REASONS FOR USE

Caffeine, theophylline, and theobromine are structurally related methylated xanthines, which are available naturally and in synthesized form. As such, they act as CNS and cardiac stimulants, although their intensity and effect on specific organs differ. Pharmacologically, caffeine is preferred as the more potent CNS stimulant, theophylline is used as a coronary artery dilator and diuretic, and theobromine, with the least stimulating activity, is used as a diuretic. Physicians prescribe caffeine for the alleviation of asthma, respiratory problems, headache (including migraine), pain, and fatigue. The usual pharmacological dose of caffeine is about 200 mg (Levenson and Bick, 1977).

Caffeine taken orally is twice as rapidly absorbed as when given intramuscularly, and is evenly distributed throughout the body (including the placenta and fetus) in proportion to tissue water content. In humans, caffeine possesses a half-life of 3 hours and is almost entirely excreted by the kidney, leaving no residue in plasma or day-to-day accumulation (Graham, 1978; Levenson and Bick, 1977). To sustain its pharmacological effects, caffeine must be regularly administered. Chronic long-time use, even of large amounts, seems to be relatively safe and nontoxic, especially when compared to other substances of abuse (Levenson and Bick, 1977). Acute toxicity, however, can occur with hazardous side effects which are discussed below.

The general effects of caffeine are well known from almost universal personal experience. In our performance and success oriented society, the CNS stimulant properties of caffeine are highly valued and appreciated. These include the sensation of increased concentration and energy, enhanced alertness, wakefulness, the alleviation of fatigue and boredom, and of increased work capability. Arousal and alteration of mood seem to occur without changes in the perception of reality (Levenson and Bick, 1977).

Given these relatively mild and pleasant effects, caffeine, most often in the form of coffee, is a welcome habit used to allay dysphoria and low energy levels. Due to its short half-life of three hours, dependency results from the effort to maintain the stimulant effects. Tolerance and psychological dependency do develop over time, to the extent that most people admit their need for the early morning "eye opener," "lift," or "pick-me-up," and the later "keep awake" properties. Thus, caffeine is used widely by long-distance drivers, office workers, students, and others who feel the need for pharmacological stimulation (Brecher, 1972).

In addition, the countless number of over-the-counter stimulant tablets, headache and pain remedies, and allergy relief tablets containing caffeine attest to the popularity of this substance. These nonprescription drugs include Bromoquinine, Sinarest, Dristan, Cope, Excedrin, Anacin, No Doz, Vivarin, and others (see Table 4-2). Caffeine is also found in foods such as coffee-flavored ice-cream, chocolate, and chocolate-flavored foods.

Thus, the craving for caffeine as well as the withdrawal symptoms that can develop at some dosage levels are evidence of the caffeine dependency and are the basis for its inclusion under drugs of abuse. An interesting aspect of caffeine ingestion is the response in nonusers, characterized by nervousness, irritability, sleep disturbance, headache, dysphoria, and anxiety. These side effects are almost identical with those experienced as withdrawal symptoms by regular and/or heavy users. High caffeine intake correlates with high levels of anxiety. It is uncertain whether the high levels of anxiety are the result of caffeine excess or whether anxiety stimulates the need for caffeine and motivates regular coffee ingestion (Brecher, 1972; Graham, 1978; Levenson and Bick, 1977).

It is noteworthy that DSM-III contains no diagnostic criteria for caffeine abuse or dependence.

WITHDRAWAL SYMPTOMS AND TOXICITY

The withdrawal symptoms from caffeine are directly related to dosage, potency, individual sensitivity to caffeine, and the combination of caffeine with other drugs. Withdrawal symptoms are usually relatively mild and include irritability, anxiety, and headache, all of which spontaneously disappear after a few hours (Levenson and Bick, 1977). Caffeine toxicity usually occurs only after extreme and prolonged excessive ingestion of caffeine, requiring a dose of approximately 600–1000 mg (Stillner et al., 1978). The symptoms include headache, disturbances in sleep patterns, gastrointestinal distress, restlessness, irritability, palpitations, arrhythmia, tremor, vertigo, agitation, and anxiety. Extreme cases of acute toxicity can result in convulsions, vomiting, and occasionally hallucinations as in "caffeine-induced delirium" (Levenson and Bick, 1977; Stillner et al., 1978).

Moderate use of caffeine seems safe and even useful for some individuals at times when they wish to stay alert, e.g. while driving. However, a narrow margin exists between comfortable, desirable, and efficient caffeine intake and excess intake or abuse. Caffeine stimulant tablets are so readily available, that many people may be hovering close to the point where hazardous complications may arise, such as while driving. Self-prescription and increased usage of the combination of coffee and caffeine stimulant tablets in times of prolonged stress can be harmful. Caffeine overdose can occasionally produce hypomanic and severely agitated states which can result in brief hospitalizations (Brecher, 1972). In some cases, as few as five 200 mg caffeine tablets have been reported to cause an agitated delirious state (Stillner et al., 1978).

MEDICAL MANAGEMENT

Caffeine toxicity is rarely reported by clinicians or physicians. However, there may be more cases than is first apparent. Caffeine toxicity and chronic heavy caffeine use can be easily misdiagnosed as acute or chronic anxiety, and occasionally can mimic some of the symptoms and signs of diabetic ketoacidosis (Mace, 1978). A careful history can reveal heavy consumption of caffeine and should include reference to additional sources of caffeine, such as over-the-counter medications.

Decreasing the caffeine intake or recommending abstinence will cause the symptoms of toxicity to completely disappear within 48 hours. Mild withdrawal symptoms will spontaneously remit after four to six hours. Pharmacological intervention is rarely necessary, except for the patient with extreme agitation and anxiety in which case diazepam 10 to 30 mg orally can be useful. For the relief of severe withdrawal headaches, when agitation is not a problem, 150 mg of caffeine can be helpful.

The interaction of caffeine and affective disorders is a relatively unresearched area. There are reports that bipolar depressed patients increase their caffeine intake during depressive episodes (Neil et al., 1978). Caffeine, when combined with tricyclic antidepressants and MAO inhibitors can cause increased nervousness, irritability, and anxiety (Neil et al., 1978; Greden et al., 1978). Caffeine, in the form of coffee, seems a natural choice of beverage to alleviate the side effects of increased thirst, dry mouth, and sedation of some tricyclic antidepressants. It can, however, exacerbate mixed depression-anxiety states and increase the likelihood of panic attacks (Winstead, 1976; Greden et al., 1978). The treating physician should be alert to the possibility of an overdose of over-the-counter caffeine stimulants in children. For example, 25 No Doz tablets in a three-year-old can produce emesis, altered states of consciousness, palpitations, photophobia, muscle twitching, miosis, and elevated blood sugar (Mace, 1978). In addition, caffeinism should be considered in the differential diagnosis of anxiety syndromes, particularly among students, intellectuals, entertainers, long distance truck-drivers, waitresses, and night-workers.

It is ironic that the most widely used psychoactive substance has received so little attention from medical researchers. Many psychiatric inpatients consume vast amounts of coffee, as it is one of the few stimulating substances available to them. There is some indication that caffeine may have some, as yet undefined, effects on severe psychiatric disorders, such as schizophrenia (Winstead, 1976; Greden et al., 1978). Research is needed on such effects in addition to the study of drug interactions between caffeine and other medications.

LONG-TERM TREATMENT AND REHABILITATION OF SUBSTANCE ABUSERS

Psychoactive substance abusers do not respond well to long-term treatment and have high relapse rates regardless of the treatment used. However, there are some general guidelines that apply. The physician should always consider the possibility that the patient may be taking the psychoactive substance in an unsupervised attempt to treat a psychiatric disorder. For example, a manic patient may try to reduce hyperactivity with a CNS depressant, while a depressed individual may use psychostimulants in an attempt to relieve dysphoria (Berger and Tinklenberg, 1979). However, most substance abusers do not have psychiatric problems that would respond to specific treatments, but rather show the relatively permanent maladaptive patterns of behavior that are classified as character or personality disorders (see Chapter 16). For some of these patients, hospitalization or at least separation from their drug-taking environment can facilitate treatment (Berger and Tinklenberg, 1979).

It is important that treatment approaches include some focus on the improvement of interpersonal skills, since substance abusers are frequently deficient in social functioning and in their personal relationships. Here a combination of group and individual psychotherapy is sometimes helpful. Programs and workshops which teach the development of vocational skills are often effective, as are treatment modalities that emphasize the development and modeling of coping strategies for future anticipated situations. These can include behavioral modification techniques or traditional insight-oriented therapies. The use of groups that emphasize confrontation or Gestalt sensitivity techniques have yielded mixed results and can be detrimental for some participants. The experiential transfer of useful information from these therapy sessions to actual situations has had little success (Berger and Tinklenberg, 1979).

For reasons that are unclear, the most comprehensive treatment programs for substance abusers are available for opioid abusers, mainly heroin addicts. These programs and their relative success rates may pave the way for the development of programs for abusers of other substances. There are currently five major treatment programs for the opioid abuser. These include methadone maintenance, maintenance with opioid antagonists, therapeutic communities, drug-free programs, and detoxification programs. Of course, most treatment programs combine more than one approach. Other treatment centers offer opioid abusers a choice of more than one treatment technique. No single treatment has proven successful for the majority of opioid abusers who apply for or are recommended for treatment (Berger and Tinklenberg, 1979; Mirin and Meyer, 1978).

Methadone maintenance is the most successful drug treatment for opioid abuse (Mirin and Meyer, 1978; Kissin et al., 1978). Its introduction in the mid-1960's was based on a biochemical hypothesis of relapse to opioid use. This hypothesis states that a return to opioid use was due to a biochemical defect which resulted from chronic opioid use and led to "narcotics hunger." Methadone corrects this hypothesized biochemical defect and thus prevents the "narcotics hunger." The cross-tolerance between methadone and opioids may also explain its success. Methadone in high oral doses has been shown to reduce or even prevent opioid-induced euphoria (Berger and Tinklenberg, 1979; Kissin et al., 1978; Green et al., 1975). Long-term studies of patients on methadone maintenance have not discovered any serious consequences to chronic methadone use (Berger and Tinklenberg, 1979; Kissin et al., 1978; Green et al., 1975). Levo-alpha-acetylmethadol (LAAM) is a long-acting (2–3 days) cogener of methadone which has a pharmacological profile similar to methadone with a longer duration of action, which may make it more practical (Ling and Blaine, 1979).

Critics of methadone maintenance claim it merely substitutes one addiction for another. The illegal administration of intravenous methadone stolen from methadone programs is also a problem. In addition, the investigations that show methadone maintenance to be successful for many opioid abusers have been criticized for using techniques that artificially inflate the success rate (Mirin and Meyer, 1978). However, the user of clinically supervised oral methadone leads a more healthy and safe life than the user of illegal, expensive, and impure heroin (Berger and Tinklenberg, 1979).

Maintenance with opioid antagonists is based on a conditioning theory of opioid dependence and relapse (Wikler, 1965). Former opioid abusers can experience classically conditioned abstinence symptoms, even though they have not recently used opioids, when they return to environments where they have experienced pharmacological withdrawal symptoms in the past. The relief from "conditioned" withdrawal symptoms and the euphoria produced by intravenous opioids would be a powerful reinforcement for relapse to opioid use. Thus, the classically conditioned abstinence syndrome rather than a biochemical defect may be the basis for "narcotics hunger." If opioid use and relapse to opioids use are conditioned behaviors, then these behaviors should be responsive to deconditioning. Thus opioid use should be extinguished or gradually decline if opioid injection no longer relieves the conditioned abstinence symptoms nor produces euphoria (Wikler, 1965). An opioid antagonist taken on a daily basis can prevent both the euphoria and the relief of conditioned abstinence symptoms of the former opioid abuser (Resnick et al., 1979).

Cyclazocine, naloxone, and naltrexone have all been used as opioid antagonists in experimental treatment programs. Cyclazocine has some agonist activity, a slight withdrawal syndrome, and was therefore, less than ideal. Naloxone is a pure antagonist, but unfortunately, when taken orally it is poorly absorbed. Naltrexone is a nearly pure antagonist, is well absorbed when taken orally, and initial clinical trials are promising but still too limited to predict what role naltrexone maintenance will play in the management of opioid addiction (Resnick et al., 1979).

Buprenorphine is a mixed agonist–antagonist, which has been suggested for potential use in treating narcotic addiction. It appears to be acceptable to addicts, is long-acting, produces a low level of physical dependence allowing for easy detoxification, and, most importantly, it blocks the effects of injected narcotics. This potentially useful compound deserves a trial as a maintenance treatment for opioid abusers (Jasinski et al., 1978).

Therapeutic communities are usually full-time residential programs that emphasize group therapies, peer pressure, and patient government. Their goal is to reeducate the former opioid abuser to more adaptive attitudes, and more mature and productive patterns of behavior. Examples of such programs are Odessey House, Daytop, Phoenix House, and other private agencies for the rehabilitation of opioid addicts. The duration of therapeutic community treatment varies from short-term two-month programs to programs that last a year or longer. A continuing problem for therapeutic communities is the large number of opioid abusers who fail to complete the required program (Mirin and Meyer, 1978; Sells, 1979).

Drug-free outpatient treatment programs are frequently offered to opioid and nonopioid substance abusers. These programs vary widely in duration of treatment as well as in program content, processes, and goals.

At one end of the continuum are the relaxed programs that offer informal group discussions, recreational activities, and help with social and vocational problems on request. At the other end are rigorously structured resocialization programs which are comparable to day-time therapeutic communities. Retention of patients in drug-free programs is an even greater problem than in therapeutic communities (Sells, 1979).

Detoxification programs are short-term and their goal is to withdraw the patient from opioids without undue discomfort and, therefore, terminate the opioid abuser's physiological dependence on opioids. The usual program is a 7 to 21-day inpatient detoxification method using oral methadone in gradually decreasing doses. Some do provide a limited amount of counseling, although this is not a primary goal. Outpatient detoxification of opioid abusers using gradually decreasing oral doses of methadone is an experimental treatment that was started in the early 1970's. Outpatient detoxification is less rigorous and longer in duration than inpatient detoxification (Sells, 1979).

To compare the efficacy of these five treatment regimens for opioid abusers is difficult because of methodological issues. Even within each of the five treatment regimens, there is considerable variation in treatment goals, treatment processes, staffing, physical facilities, demands on patient time and effort, duration of treatment, discipline and use of sanctions, degree of individual responsibility required of the patient, and use of patient–peer influence in treatment. Other variations include the use of ancillary rehabilitation services such as vocational training, job placement, family counseling, personal counseling, educational programs, recreational programs, medical services, and individual and group psychotherapy. This makes it extremely difficult to compare the successful rehabilitation rate and method of one program with another. Long-term follow-up is a necessary, but formidable, task to confirm that a former opioid abuser has been successfully treated. Finally, well-designed trials with random assignment are extremely rare in this field (Sells, 1979).

Given these limitations, the outcomes for methadone maintenance and therapeutic communities seem to be most favorable for opioid abusers. Drug-free regimens appear more suited to non opioid substance abusers. Detoxification programs seem to be the least effective. Detoxification is probably best used as an entry procedure for drug-free treatment or as a means of recruitment for other treatment modalities. Thus, there is some evidence that at least two types of treatment have some efficacy in the long-term rehabilitation of opioid abusers. However, even these treatments are effective in less than half of the patients who participate in these programs. The majority of opioid abusers relapse to their former habit either during the treatment program or when the program has been completed. The relapse rate for abusers of other psychoactive substances is even greater (Sells, 1979).

CONCLUSION

Disorders caused by the use of psychoactive substances result in profound problems for society and are a continuing challenge to the medical profession. The careful emergency medical management of patients with substance use disorders often yields dramatic recoveries. Acute organic brain syndromes produced by intoxication by or withdrawal from psychoactive substances usually respond rapidly to treatments based on knowledge of and clinical experience with the pharmacological properties of such substances.

Sadly, long-term treatment and rehabilitation programs for patients with substance use disorders are far less successful than treatments of their acute toxic reactions. Most substance abusers revert rapidly to the dangerous patterns of drug self-administration that initially caused the toxic reactions. The most widespread substance use disorder, tobacco dependence, almost never produces an acute toxic reaction that requires treatment by physicians. Yet, the long-term effects of this disorder, such as increased risk for respiratory system cancer and cardiac disease, make tobacco use disorder one of the most serious threats to the health of society. Thus, there exists an urgent need of medical research to develop new treatment approaches for chronic maladaptive or self-destructive behaviors and lifestyles.

REFERENCES

High Times Encyclopedia of Recreational Drugs. Stonehill Publishing Company, New York. 1978.

Akil H: Opiates: Biological mechanisms. In: Psychopharmacology from Theory to Practice. Barchas, JD, Berger, PA, Ciaranello, RD, and Elliott, GR (eds). Oxford University Press, New York. pp. 293–305, 1977.

Ayd FJ, Blackwell B: Discoveries in Biological Psychiatry. Lippincott, Philadelphia. pp. 218–219, 1970.

Berger PA, Tinklenberg JR: Treatment of abusers of alcohol and other addictive drugs. In: Psychopharmacology from Theory to Practice. Barchas, JD, Berger, PA, Ciaranello, RD, and Elliott, GR (eds). Oxford University Press, New York. pp. 355–385, 1977.

Berger PA, Tinklenberg JR: Medical management of the drug abuser. In: Psychiatry for the Primary Care Physician. Freeman, AM, Sack, RL, and Berger, PA (eds). Williams and Wilkins, Baltimore. pp. 359–380, 1979.

Brecher EM, and the Editors of Consumer Reports. Licit and Illicit Drugs. Little, Brown, Boston, 1972.

Cohen S: Trends in substance abuse. Newsletter, Drug Abuse and Alcoholism, vol VII, #7. 1978.

Cohen S: Inhalants. In: Handbook on Drug Abuse, Dupont, RI, Goldstein, A, and O'Donnell, J (eds). U.S. Government Printing Office, National Institute on Drug Abuse, DHEW. pp. 213–220, 1979a.

Cohen S: On the smoking of cigarettes. Drug abuse and alcoholism newsletter, vol. VIII, No. 5. 1979b.

DOM (STP): Report Series. National Clearing House for Drug Abuse Information, Series 17, No. 1, May 1973.

Ellinwood EH: Amphetamines/anorectics. In: Handbook on Drug Abuse. Dupont, RI, Goldstein, A, and O'Donnell, J (eds). U.S. Government Printing Office, National Institute on Drug Abuse, DHEW. pp. 221–231, 1979.

Goldfrank L, Meliek M: Locoweed and other anticholinergics. Hospital Physician. 8:13–39, 1979.

Graham DM: Caffeine—its identity, dietary sources, intake and biological effects. Nutrition Reviews. 36:97–102, 1978.

Granacher RP, Baldessarini RJ, Messner E: Physostigmine treatment of delirium induced by anticholinergics. Am Fam Physician. 13:999–103, 1976.

Greden JF, Fontaine P. Lubetsky M, Chamberlin J: Anxiety and depression associated with caffeinism among psychiatric inpatients. Am J Psychiat. 135:963–966, 1978.

Green AI, Meyer RE, Shader RI: Heroin and methadone abuse: acute and chronic management. In: Manual of Psychiatric Therapeutics: Practical Psychopharmacology and Psychiatry, Shader, RI (ed.). Little, Brown, Boston. pp. 203–210, 1975.

Greenblatt DJ, Shader RI: Psychotropic Drug Overdosage. In: Manual of Psychiatric Therapeutics: Practical Psychiatry and Psychopharmacology. Shader, RI (ed). Little, Brown, Boston. pp. 237–267, 1975a.

Greenblatt DJ, Shader RI: Bad trips. In: Manual of Psychiatric Therapeutics: Practical Psychopharmacology and Psychiatry. Shader, RI (ed). Little, Brown, Boston. pp. 185–192, 1975b.

Greene MH, Dupont RL: The treatment of acute heroin toxicity. In: A Treatment Manual for Acute Drug Abuse Emergencies. Bourne, PG (ed). U.S. Government Printing Office, DHEW, Washington, D.C. pp. 11–16, 1974.

Harris LS: Cannabis: a review of progress. In: Psychopharmacology: A Generation of Progress. Lipton, MA, DiMascio, A, and Killam, KF (eds). Raven Press, New York. pp. 1565–1574, 1978.

Hollister LE: Chemical Psychoses. C. C. Thomas, Springfield, Ill. 1968.

Hunt WA, Bespalec DA: An evaluation of current methods of modifying smoking behavior. J Clin Psychol. 30:431–438, 1974.

Jaffe JH, Jarvik ME: Tobacco use and tobacco use disorder. In: Psychopharmacology: A Generation of Progress. Lipton, MA, DiMascio, A, and Killam, KF (eds). Raven Press, New York. pp. 1665–1676, 1978.

Jarvik ME, Cullen JW, Gritz ER, Vogt TM, West LJ: Research on smoking behavior. NIDA, Research Monograph Series, #17. DHEW, U.S. Government Printing Office, Washington, D.C., 1977.

Jarvik ME, Gritz ER: Nicotine and tobacco. In: Psychopharmacology in the Practice of Medicine. Jarvik, ME (ed). Appleton-Century-Crofts, New York. pp. 481–495, 1977.

Jarvik ME, Popek P, Schneider NG, Baer-Weiss V, Gritz ER: Can cigarette size and nicotine content influence smoking and puffing rates?. Psychopharmacology. 58:303–306, 1978.

Jasinski DR, Pevnick JS, Griffith JD: Human pharmacology and abuse potential of the analgesic buprenorphine. Arch Gen Psychiat. 35:501–516, 1978.

Kissin B, Lowinson JH, Millman RB: Recent Developments in Chemotherapy of Narcotic Addiction. New York Academy of Sciences. Vol 311, 1978.

Levenson HS, Bick EC: Psychopharmacology of caffeine. In: Psychopharmacology in the Practice of Medicine. Jarvik, ME (ed). Appleton-Century-Crofts, New York. pp. 451–463, 1977.

Ling W, Blaine JD: The use of LAAM in treatment. In: Handbook on Drug Abuse. DuPont, RI, Goldstein A, and O'Donnell J (eds). U.S. Government Printing Office, National Institute on Drug Abuse, DHEW. pp. 87–96, 1979.

Mace J: Toxicity of caffeine. J Pediat. 92:345–346, 1978.

Mahender RA: The management of the narcotic withdrawal syndrome in the neonate. In: A Treatment Manual for Acute Drug Abuse Emergencies. Bourne, PG (ed). U.S. Government Printing Office, DHEW, Washington, D.C. pp. 27–28, 1974.

Martin WR, Haertzen CA, Hewett BB: Psychopathology and pathophysiology of narcotic addicts, alcoholics, and drug abusers. In: Psychopharmacology: A Generation of Progress. Lipton, JA, DiMascio, A, and Killam, KF (eds). Raven Press, New York. pp. 1591–1602, 1978.

Meyer RE: Behavioral pharmacology of marijuana. In: Psychopharmacology: A Generation of Progress. Lipton, MA, DiMascio, A, and Killam, KF (eds). Raven Press, New York. pp. 1639–1652, 1978.

Mirin SM, Meyer RE: Treatment of substance abusers. In: Principles of Psychopharmacology. Clark, WG, and del Guidice, J (eds). Academic Press, New York. pp. 701–720, 1978.

Neil JF, Himmelhoch JM, Mallinger AG, Mallinger J, Hanin I: Caffeinism complicating hypersomnic depressive episodes. Compr Psychiat. 19:377–385, 1978.

Petersen RC, Stillman RC: Cocaine: 1977. NIDA Research Monograph #13. U.S. Government Printing Office, DHEW, Washington, D.C. May 1977.

Petersen RC, Stillman RD: Phencyclidine (PCP) Abuse: An Appraisal. NIDA Research Monograph 21. U.S. Government Printing Office, DHEW, Washington, D.C. August 1978.

Pittel SM, Oppedahl MC: The enigma of PCP. In: Handbook on Drug Abuse. Dupont, RI, Goldstein, A, and O'Donnell, J (eds). U.S. Government Printing Office, National Institute on Drug Abuse, DHEW. pp. 249–254, 1979.

Resnick RB, Schuyton-Resnick ES, Washton AM: Treatment of opioid dependence with narcotic antagonists: a review and commentary. In: Handbook on Drug Abuse. Dupont, RI, Goldstein, A, and O'Donnell, J (eds). U.S. Government Printing Office, National Institute on Drug Abuse, DHEW. pp. 97–104, 1979.

Russell MAH: Smoking problems: an overview. NIDA Research Monograph #17. U.S. Government Printing Office, DHEW, Washington, D.C., December 1977.

Sells SB: Treatment effectiveness. In: Handbook on Drug Abuse. Dupont, RI, Goldstein, A, and O'Donnell, J (eds). U.S. Government Printing Office, National Institute on Drug Abuse, DHEW. pp. 105–118, 1979.

Sharp CW, Brehm ML: Review of Inhalants: Euphoria to Dysfunction. NIDA Research Monograph 15. U.S. Government Printing Office. DHEW, Washington, D.C. October 1977.

Sigell LT, Kapp FT, Fusaro GA, Nelson ED, Pharm D, Falck RS: Popping and snorting volatile nitrites: a current fad for getting high. Am J Psychiat. 135:1216–1218, 1978.

Snyder SH: Catecholamines in the brain as mediators of amphetamine psychosis. Arch Gen Psychiat. 27:169–179, 1972.

Stillner V. Popkin MK, Pierce C: Caffeine-induced delirium during prolonged competitive stress. Am J Psychiat. 135:855–856, 1978.

Technical Review on Cigarette Smoking as an Addiction. Report from the National Institute on Drug Abuse, September, 1979.

Tinklenberg JR, Berger PA: Treatment of abusers of non-addictive drugs. In: Psychopharmacology from Theory to Practice. Barchas, JD, Berger, PA, Ciaranello, RD, and Elliott, GR (eds). Oxford University Press, New York. pp. 387–403, 1977.

Weil A: The Natural Mind. Houghton Mifflin Boston. 1972.

Wikler A: Conditioning factors in opiate addiction and relapse. In: Narcotics, Wilner, DM and Kassebaum, GG (eds). McGraw-Hill, New York. pp. 85–100, 1965.

Winstead DK: Coffee consumption among psychiatric inpatients. Am J Psychiat. 133:1447–1450, 1976.

5 | Schizophrenic Disorders

GEORGE M. SIMPSON and
PHILIP R.A. MAY

The schizophrenic disorders are a heterogeneous group ranging from relatively benign conditions to serious chronic disorders. There is little systematic knowledge about some disorders and a substantial amount regarding others. No single treatment is adequate for any schizophrenic
disorder and therefore an eclectic therapeutic philosophy of treatment
with the emphasis on practical considerations is of prime importance.

We would urge, in general, that no formal treatment be started without a careful and thorough evaluation, i.e. diagnosis in the broad sense
rather than the mere attachment of a DSM-III diagnosis. Deciding on a
course of action usually requires a full and sensitive understanding of the
situation. This is particularly true of psychosocial support and rehabilitation measures, perhaps less true of physical forms of intervention. Even
in the latter case, however, it is wise to remember that the attitudes of
family members as well as the patient may critically influence the outcome of therapy and that these factors should be given thorough consideration *before* starting any therapeutic intervention.

Emergency action may, of course, be necessary in some situations.
And when resources are limited, evaluation and assessment will inevitably be less thorough. This should not become an excuse for ignoring
basic principles; the issue is therapeutic strategy: the proportion of resources that should be devoted to initial and continuing assessment and
evaluation as well as to actual treatment. An impetuous rush to treat
symptoms without a thorough diagnostic evaluation may prevent a firm
diagnosis from being made, and treatment may be unnecessarily prolonged or complicated. *If* possible, a reasonable period of observation
(e.g. a week) should take place before any major treatments are started. It
may be easier to maintain subjects drug-free in an inpatient setting and
indeed we would recommend this during an initial evaluation.

In an outpatient setting the situation is less controllable since close supervision may not be feasible and it may seem difficult to follow these guidelines. Again, absence of hospitalization should not become an excuse for ignoring basic principles. Adequate diagnostic evaluation is a prerequisite for starting any form of "definitive" treatment in an outpatient setting. If the patient's condition is so serious and urgent that therapy cannot await a treatment-free period of outpatient observation, a period of hospitalization may be required to make a diagnosis and to formulate an appropriate treatment plan. We emphasize this point since, for the conditions discussed here, antipsychotics are in most cases the single most potent treatment available. Their efficacy, plus their ease of administration, can easily lead to precipitate and prolonged use, particularly since the difficulty of reducing or withdrawing medication in the community relates to the adequacy of community supports. The point is that if treatment is started badly, without consideration for the complexities involved, it is likely to continue badly.

Patients with any of the psychiatric conditions discussed in this chapter are at high risk of relapse and are affected by potentially positive and/or negative social, family, and environmental interactions. Therefore, even after having performed an initial broad-based diagnostic evaluation, continued observation and evaluation of the patient's condition is essential in order to assess the psychological and social consequences (costs and benefits in the therapeutic as well as the economic sense) of the steps already taken. In addition, careful observation and repeated diagnostic review will be of help in confirming the formal diagnosis. Many times it is not possible to make a valid diagnosis in one interview and occasionally a definitive diagnosis cannot be made even after observation for a week or two. Unfortunately, it is sometimes mandated by law or hospital regulation that a diagnosis must be given within a few days. Clinicians caught in such circumstances must therefore maintain a distinction between *legal* and *clinical* or *therapeutic* diagnostic requirements. In this context, cautious terms such as "diagnostic impression," or "tentative diagnosis" are more consistent with sound clinical practice than premature closure on a final opinion.

The next general point we would like to emphasize is that where there is a range of treatments that are presumed to be reasonably effective, the more benign treatment should, in general, be tried first. This should not, however, be taken as a mandate to start with a "treatment" that is likely to be ineffective just because it seems to be "safe."

The crux of the matter is "therapeutic cost-benefit," weighing the risks and benefits of one treatment against those of all other available treatments and including the risks of nontreatment; of chronicity; of social, occupational, and psychological scarring and desocialization; and of a vicious cycle of effects on the family and other significant persons. In some situations the severity of the disorder will therefore override the lower-order treatments. For example, a placid patient with a brief reactive psychosis (298.80) might be placed in a supportive milieu and given mild sedation; a very excited and assaultive person with a similar diagnosis might, on the other hand, be given an antipsychotic early in treatment.

Optimal treatment should be the aim and optimal is often less than maximal, i.e. the least amount of the treatment should be given that will produce the most benefit, but this principle means we must have definable treatment goals. While the overall goal of treatment is to restore the patient to complete and integrated functioning, this is often impossible. Specific treatment goals of: reducing symptoms and signs of schizophrenia; improving family, social, and sexual relationships; enhancing occupational/educational functioning; fostering appropriate independence; and increased understanding of the illness may be pursued in small combinations and in succession, but seldom simultaneously. It also means that treatments must be carefully described and evaluated.

The indications and efficacy of treatments for schizophrenia remain controversial, particularly for the psychological and social forms of therapy where it is commonly (and erroneously) assumed that more is better and that toxic side effects are nonexistent. An example from pharmacotherapy is simpler to understand. In treating a florid schizophrenic condition, one should use the amount of antipsychotic that is likely to rapidly (e.g. in a two- to four-week period) remove the psychotic symptoms with the least amount of unwanted effects. The optimal dose can best be arrived at by a simple test dose procedure, i.e. giving an appropriate *low* dose of the drug, observing its effects and asking in detail for the patient's subjective response to the drug. From this information the treatment plan can then be modified. In this way we can avoid the oversedating that sometimes results from what appears to be reasonable dosage of an antipsychotic according to cookbook formulas.

Thus, an individualized approach to evaluation and treatment is essential. With this in mind we can discuss the separate diagnostic entities. Before doing so, however, we must point out that there are substantial problems in applying the findings of all previous research to the new DSM-III nomenclature. In theory, changing over to DSM-III invalidates all previous studies that used the old system, since one can no longer be confident that all cases would receive the same diagnosis under the new system. Further, the last two decades have witnessed a decided change in focus in the treatment of chronic schizophrenic conditions. There has been an improvement in the general level of hospital care and changed standards for release into the community; patients are now receiving more attention under better conditions so the previous control group comparisons may no longer be valid. Studies that ignore drug therapy can have little relevance to present-day reality. Moreover, many of the older studies involved chronic institutionalized patients, who, on the one hand, may have been unlikely to improve to any great extent, and on the other hand might have shown some response to nearly any kind of human intervention and nonspecific attention, living as they were in poorly staffed and neglected environments. In a small, well-staffed research ward the placebo response in such subjects is reported to be almost zero (Bishop and Gallant, 1966). Today, when institutions have to a large extent changed for the better and contain a different patient population, the results of many of the early studies may be irrelevant.

For these reasons, unless there are special circumstances, the authors have chosen to base their discussion and conclusions on studies that were completed in the last 20 years and that come within the top two of six categories of the Design-Relevance (D-R) Scale (May and Van Putten, 1974). In such studies the diagnoses would probably be sustained in DSM-III, and the treatment (including drug treatment) would have been reasonably adequately recorded or controlled.

SCHIZOPHRENIC DISORDER (295.)

ESSENTIAL FEATURES

The essential features of *schizophrenia* are the presence of certain psychotic features during the active phase of the illness, characteristic symptoms involving multiple psychological processes, deterioration from a previous level of functioning, onset before the age of 45, and a duration of at least six months.

At some phase of the illness schizophrenia always involves delusions, hallucinations, or certain disturbances in the form of thought. The characteristic symptoms involve disturbance in the content of thought (particularly bizarre delusions), disturbance in the form of thought (for example, loosening of associations, incoherence), altered perception (for example, auditory hallucinations), disturbances in affect (blunting, flattening, or inappropriateness of affect), disturbance in the sense of self (for example, delusions of thought control), disturbance in volition (apathy), disturbance in the relationships to the external world (autism), and disturbance in psychomotor behavior (for example, catatonic symptoms). All these disturbances are seldom present in a single individual.

SCHIZOPHRENIFORM DISORDER (295.40)

ESSENTIAL FEATURES

The essential features of *schizophreniform disorder* are identical with those of *schizophrenia* except that the duration, including prodromal, active, and residual phases, is less than six months but more than two weeks.

Schizophreniform disorder includes all the acute schizophrenic reactions in DSM-II with the exception that *brief reactive psychosis* (298.80) and *atypical psychosis* (298.90) are separated in DSM-III. The acute and florid symptoms, and even clouding of consciousness, that are common in schizophreniform disorder in themselves suggest a good prognosis and of course by definition the disorder lasts no more than six months. However, many patients who initially receive a diagnosis of schizophreniform disorder will later be diagnosed as schizophrenic. In effect, we are unable to separate these two conditions in most of the published literature.

Treatment of these psychotic disorders can be divided arbitrarily into inpatient and outpatient, to emphasize that inpatient treatment presumes the constant availability of skilled care, the patient's removal from the environment in which he became ill, and the possibility for different and more varied treatment modalities. If someone develops a schizophrenic disorder while living at home, one could, with adequate family support, treat the patient at home; formal inpatient milieu therapy is not then an option, but drug therapy becomes almost essential. In an inpatient setting, on the other hand, one can observe closely, confirm the diagnosis, closely monitor the patient's response to milieu and other routine hospital procedures, begin discharge planning and possibly delay drug therapy. Thus, in a broad sense, *milieu therapy* is the first treatment option in an inpatient setting; indeed milieu therapy, or the social interactions of the patient's surroundings, is always provided whether conceptualized as such or not.

MILIEU THERAPY

The concept of a therapeutic milieu can be traced back to the Greco-Roman era, but its modern form owes much to Simmel (1929), Sullivan (1931, 1940), and Main et al. (1946). Their pioneering work and subsequent efforts by, among others, Caudill (1958), Cumming and Cumming (1962), Jones (1953), Stanton and Schwartz (1954), and Wilmer (1958), led to widespread reforms designed to avoid or eliminate the insidious deculturing and deteriorating effects of custodial programs and attitudes (May and Simpson, 1980). Ideally, milieu therapy will "make certain that the patient's every social contact and his every treatment experience are synergistically applied toward realistic, specific treatment goals" (Abrams, 1969). It remains difficult, however, to disentangle the effects of milieu therapy from the effects of removal from a noxious environment plus the passage of time.

In the past, it was often assumed that the good results reported by certain hospitals could be attributed to their better milieu. The good results, however, may be primarily the result of admitting patients with better prognoses (Goldberg et al., 1970).

Recently there has been serious consideration of the possibility that milieu therapy may have toxic, antitherapeutic effects in some cases. Methods appropriate for depressions, neuroses, and character disorders have been indiscriminately applied to schizophrenics, and a number of reports indicate that this may lead to regression or exaggeration of pathological defenses (Spadoni and Smith, 1969; Quitkin and Klein, 1967; Friedman, 1969; Pardes et al., 1972; Goldberg and Rubin, 1964; Van Putten, 1973). Thus, intensely active, highly staffed units may be disruptively intrusive for schizophrenic patients who more often benefit from decreased stimulation and a greater measure of solitude and clear role models.

The introduction of drug therapy also prompts a reappraisal. How much does milieu therapy really add to the treatment of a hospitalized schizophrenic? The evidence is divided as to whether a more intensive level of milieu care improves the results of drug therapy. It is reasonably well established that release rate is increased by milieu therapy and that more patients go to work when they leave the hospital, but that may be a matter of better discharge planning, rather than any difference in patients' post-treatment status. Otherwise, there is little effect of milieu therapy on psychopathology; the results seem to be equally good at all levels of care except under circumstances of virtual neglect or gross deficiency, when a custodial environment is likely to aggravate and even induce withdrawal and social detachment (May and Simpson, 1980). However, it should not be assumed that drugs and psychosocial measures always potentiate each other in all cases (Freedman et al., 1961; Paul et al., 1972; Paul and Lentz, 1977).

Reasonable conclusions from the literature are that (1) drug therapy is, in general, advantageous in any hospital setting; (2) drug therapy is likely to be more effective—at least, in terms of employment and release rate—in a more intensive treatment milieu and less effective when the milieu is grossly deficient; (3) an intensive treatment milieu by itself, without drug therapy, is not generally an adequate substitute for treatment with antipsychotic drugs; (4) nevertheless, in a few cases (usually patients with a schizophreniform disorder characterized by good premorbid adjustment and rapid onset of the first episode of illness), medication may interfere with milieu therapy and other forms of psychosocial treatment (May and Simpson, 1980).

With current psychopharmacologic and psychosocial approaches to therapy, there are still a number of treatment-resistant patients, and long-term hospital milieu care in conjunction with antipsychotics may be the best option. But with the use of modern psychotropic drugs, the hospital can be, for the average schizophrenic patient, essentially a center for relatively brief crisis treatment. Deeper insights or new patterns of social behavior should not be sought before release at the price of the detrimental effects and added cost of prolonged hospitalization, which deprives the patients of the sustaining and satisfying ego-organizing influence of work, family, and friends. The greatest potential for milieu and social therapy may lie on the one hand in specific individual interventions in the hospital to restore the patient's major life role as worker, student, parent, spouse, etc. and, on the other hand, in community-oriented techniques, which include the patient and family in flexible, integrated, and individually prescribed outpatient program. A constricted four-walls approach should be replaced by an expanded concept that considers the patient's milieu after he leaves the hospital.

Current forms of milieu therapy appear to have little specific effect on acute schizophrenic symptoms. Moreover, any nonspecific effects are difficult to separate from the remission of schizophrenic symptoms with the passage of time, improvement being variously reported as ranging from nearly zero up to 30% (Bishop and Gallant, 1966; Clark et al., 1977). A small number of schizophrenic patients remit and most improve after being provided asylum in hospital (Pi et al., unpublished report). Nonetheless, a good milieu may lead to improvement in staff morale, a decrease in the amount of medications used unnecessarily, and reduction in the amount of seclusion and restraint, although this point is not easily proved (Carroll et al., 1980).

To some extent the case for voluntary admission, open doors, democracy, better conditions, and other reforms must rest more on general humanitarian concern and social conscience than on demonstrated therapeutic benefits to the patient (Letermendia et al., 1967). However, what appears to be a generally beneficial reform may be potentially harmful for some patients—witness the current furor over patients "dying with their civil rights on" (Treffert, 1974).

A number of overlapping themes are embodied in current concepts of a therapeutic milieu. Approaches center on the group and focus on social functioning, rather than on psychopathology; they encourage self-reliance and reward the patient for efforts toward social readaptation. The patient is expected to participate in planning his own treatment program, in helping other patients, and in assuming responsibility in ward affairs and the outside world.

Individual milieu approaches focus on transactions between the individual patient and individual staff members. Specific staff attitudes and management tactics toward each patient are prescribed, and the individual patient's daily program is carefully designed to include activities suited to particular goals. In some centers the main goal is to provide the patient with an opportunity to form durable relationships and build in good objects, helping him or her to internalize controls that may eventually lead to autonomous mastery (Freeman et al., 1958).

In examining the literature on milieu therapy, it is important to distinguish among: (1) studies of inpatient hospital treatment; (2) studies of aftercare—that is, treatment for the expatient after he is released from the hospital; and (3) studies of alternative care—that is, outpatient treatment alternatives to inpatient care. It should not be assumed that findings on one of these approaches can be applied to the others.

INPATIENT MILIEU THERAPY

Two first-class studies of inpatient milieu therapy, by Greenblatt et al. (1965) and Hamilton et al. (1963), produced weakly positive results. Two less rigorous studies (Fairweather, 1964; Ludwig et al., 1967) reported positive and negative results respectively. These mixed findings raise considerable doubt as to the effectiveness of in-hospital milieu treatment programs and increased staffing. Those programs that were effective emphasized practical issues of living such as planning for discharge, getting jobs, maintaining an apartment and bank accounts, shopping etc.

BRIEF HOSPITAL CARE

Three excellent studies examined brief hospital care versus regular longer-term hospital care. One (Caffey et al., 1972) indicated that brief hospitalization (21 days) plus aftercare produced as good or better results as a longer stay. After a brief hospital stay, however, patients had more symptoms at the time of discharge than after a longer stay. The second study (Glick et al., 1974; Glick et al., 1975; Glick et al., 1976) indicated that short-term patients functioned better at four weeks than did patients after a longer hospital stay. Little additional advantage in symptom reduction was gained by keeping patients for a longer hospital stay. The long-term group did, however, function significantly better one year after admission, but the differences were only modest and could be attributable to their having received more psychotherapy and more phenothiazines. In the third study; (Herz et al., 1976; Herz et al., 1977; Herz et al., 1979) there were no significant differences in levels of psychopathology at 3 and 12 weeks, but the briefly hospitalized patients were able to resume their vocational roles sooner. There were no significant differences in readmission rates, and short-term patients showed somewhat less psychopathology and impairment in role functioning, e.g. they went back to work sooner and suffered less financial burden.

ALTERNATIVES TO HOSPITAL CARE

This approach includes home care, intensive outpatient care, and day care. Several studies have evaluated these as alternatives to inpatient hospitalization. That this type of approach has not become widespread may attest to conservatism in psychiatry or to the recognition that the enthusiasm generated in special projects of this kind may not carry over into routine practice.

Both Linn et al. (1979) and May and Simpson (1980) reviewed a large number of studies and concurred that the findings of the less rigorous studies are conflicting. The two best studies (Pasamanick et al., 1967; Herz et al., 1971) were both weakly positive—that is, they showed slightly better results from alternative care than from hospital care. Success seemed to depend on active outreach, good extrahospital nursing care, and adequate drug therapy. However, the advantages were rapidly lost when the programs were discontinued.

The work of Stein, Test, and Weisbrod is also relevant (Stein et al., 1979; Test and Stein, 1980; Weisbrod et al., 1980). Virtually without use of the hospital, it was possible to treat, in the community, an unselected group of patients presented for admission. The sustained community living was not gained at the expense of quality of life, level of adjustment, self-esteem, or personal satisfaction with life. Relative to control patients receiving conventional treatment, those in the program showed enhanced functioning in several significant areas, less subjective distress, and greater satisfaction with their lives. However, when intensive treatment ceased, these patients regressed and used the hospital more.

A doctrinaire assumption that short (or no) hospitalization is better for everyone may be counter to individual needs, yet a person should not be admitted to a hospital just because he or she is schizophrenic. Many patients can be successfully treated in other settings. Quite apart from financial savings, the outcome may be better if the secondary gains of patienthood, the losses of status and self esteem, and the social disarticulation that result from hospitalization are avoided.

However, the burdens and hazards involved and the quality of the care and availability of supportive services must be carefully considered. As Wing and Brown (1970) and Grad and Sainsbury (1966, 1968) have pointed out, the burden on relatives and the community imposed by severely impaired patients is rarely negligible. And in this country, there are gross deficiencies in community resources for the treatment, support, and rehabilitation of schizophrenic patients (Hogarty and Goldberg, 1973). Early discharge obviously helps counteract dependence on the institutional way of life. However, the preference for institutional living may have arisen, in part, from an earlier predisposition; some patients will become dependent on any way of life that allows them to be socially inactive, in or out of an institution. Thus, the equivalent of institutionalism outside the hospital can be prevented only by detailed attention to the outside environment.

OUTPATIENT AFTERCARE

The evidence from the literature on outpatient aftercare of schizophrenics is scanty but positive. In, general, the successful programs had focused mainly on problem solving, social adjustment, living arrangements, obtaining employment, and facilitating cooperation with maintenance drug therapy.

Two careful studies (Caffey et al., 1972; Meltzoff and Blumenthal, 1966) had definitely positive results. Another (Linn et al., 1979) examined day program components in more detail, and addressed the question whether a day aftercare program adds to the benefit of antipsychotic drugs alone. Schizophrenic patients referred for day care at the time of discharge from hospital were randomly assigned to several different day care centers to receive day treatment plus drugs or drugs alone. They were tested before assignment and 6, 12, 18, and 24 months later for social functioning, symptoms, and attitudes. Community tenure and costs were also measured. Some centers were found to be effective. All significantly delayed relapse and reduced symptoms. More professional staff hours, group therapy, and a high patient turnover treatment philosophy were associated with poor results. More occupational therapy and a sustained, nonthreatening environment characterized the centers with more successful outcome.

ANTIPSYCHOTIC DRUGS

INTRODUCTION

Perhaps because of the timing of their introduction—when little else had proven effective—perhaps because of their ease and economy of administration, and perhaps because of their extensive research support from government and private industry, antipsychotic (neuroleptic) drugs have received the most systematic and intensive study of all types of treatment used for schizophrenia. Literally hundreds of double-blind placebo controlled studies have been carried out (Davis, 1980). Not only have these shown drugs to be more effective than placebo, but they have also shown a dose–response relationship, such that differences in therapeutic outcome relate to the amount of active drug given (Cole and Davis, 1969). Even if we accept the more optimistic claims of spontaneous remission rates (up to 30%), antipsychotics have doubled that figure, and have reduced the duration of the psychotic episodes even in relatively inactive or unorganized treatment settings.

TREATMENT OF ACUTE EPISODES

As stated earlier, we recommend a drug-free interval (for evaluation purposes) as the first stage of an ideal treatment regimen. We also recognize the impracticability of this approach in some settings, such as outpatient clinics, or inpatient wards with staff shortages, poor morale, or an excess of acutely excited patients. How long should one wait, in the best settings, for a patient to improve before starting pharmacotherapy? In our opinion, schizophrenic patients who show no improvement at the end of one week free of drugs should then receive antipsychotics. While no single modality of treatment has proven universally superior or even adequate for all schizophrenic patients, the most clearly effective, specific, rapid, and economical treatment known at this time comprises the antipsychotic drugs.

There is no consistent evidence demonstrating the superiority of one antipsychotic drug over another. The choice of a specific antipsychotic will depend partly on the psychiatrist's training and experience, partly on the patient's past experience with such drugs (including side effects, therapeutic response, and dosages), and at times on family history of similar illness and drug response. The acceptability of certain side effects for the individual patient often determines the drug choice. Thus, the initial sedation produced by drugs like chlorpromazine and thioridazine may prove advantageous with a young, agitated patient, while the hypotensive or anticholinergic effects of these same medications may prove unacceptable for another patient, elderly and infirm. Table 5-1 lists some common antipsychotic drugs and their usual oral dosages.

Table 5-1.

Common Antipsychotic Drugs and Daily Dosage Range for Adults (MG)

NAME		DOSAGE	
GENERIC	TRADE	ACUTE	MAINTENANCE
Butaperazine	Repoise	15–100	5–50
Chlorpromazine	Thorazine	25–800	40–200
Fluphenazine	Prolixin	5–20	1–5*
	Permitil		
Haloperidol	Haldol	1–100	1–15
Loxapine	Loxitane	20–100	60–100
Molindone	Moban	15–225	15–225
Perphenazine	Lidone	16–64	8–16
Trifluoperazine	Trilafon	10–60	2–20
Thioridazine	Stelazine	300–800	100–300
Thiothixene	Mellaril	6–100	6–50
	Navane		

*Can also be given as decanoate or enanthate injection, 12.5–50 mg weekly to triweekly.

We recommend that, once a specific drug has been selected, a test dose of that drug be administered (1–2 mg/kg of oral chlorpromazine or its equivalent in another antipsychotic drug) and the patient's response be noted over a short period of several hours to a day. This approach gives some idea of the immediate affect of that drug on that patient—for example, marked sedation at low dosage. At the same time, the patient's subjective feelings and early clinical response to the test dose may well predict his later outcome on that drug (May and Tuma, 1976). Of course, this approach may be impractical for an acutely excited patient, who may require immediate use of higher and more frequent doses, or even "rapid tranquilization." This approach refers to the frequent administration of intramuscular antipsychotics over a short period of time to produce a rapid effect on behavior. Donlon et al. (1979) have described a strategy involving injections every 30–60 minutes (Donlon et al., 1979). We prefer the following procedure, which would rarely involve repeating an injection after only 30 minutes.

First, a drug must be selected. It should be kept in mind that chlorpromazine and related phenothiazines produce relatively less extrapyramidal side effects than the more potent drugs, such as haloperidol and thiothixene, but can also produce more hypotension and sedation, though the latter could represent an advantage in an excited or assaultive patient.

Chlorpromazine by injection may be more painful than other drugs. Haloperidol in high doses may produce not only more frequent, immediate dystonias, but also delayed appearance of pseudoparkinsonism or akathisia a few days later.

After a drug is selected for rapid tranquilization, dosage must be decided. In this situation, conversion tables are inadequate guides to "equivalent" doses of antipsychotics, e.g. 100 mg of oral chlorpromazine to about 2 mg of oral haloperidol (Hollister, 1978). In rapid tranquilization, a patient might receive 40–60 mg per day of parenteral haloperidol, whereas one would never give the "equivalent" 2000–3000 mg of chlorpromazine by this route. The lack of feasibility of such high "equivalent" dosages has led many to prefer drugs like haloperidol and thiothixene for rapid tranquilization.

Choosing the initial dose for a given patient will depend on the patient's age, weight, and previous exposure to antipsychotics. Subsequent dosage will depend on clinical observations. Assume, for example, a starting dose of 2½ mg haloperidol or 4 mg thiothixene given intramuscularly. An hour later, direct observation of the patient provides the basis for a decision to repeat the dose, increase it, or postpone a second injection. With little evidence of sedation or other behavioral effects, the dosage might be doubled, followed by reevaluation one hour later, for possible further injections. Obvious drowsiness might delay repeating an injection for an hour or longer. Seldom will the situation require more than three or four injections, totaling more than 20 mg of haloperidol or thiothixene, within the first day. However, much higher doses—for example, 40 mg per day of haloperidol—may be required in occasional difficult cases. Still higher doses—up to 100 mg per day of intramuscular haloperidol—while feasible, may have delayed extrapyramidal side effects that unnecessarily complicate treatment.

The high frequency of dystonic reactions argues against rapid tranquilization as a routine procedure, or as a strategy for patients in whom the gradual use of oral medications may suffice. Despite a lack of evidence that the "prophylactic" use of "antiparkinson" agents prevents extrapyramidal side effects, clinicians who would avoid their use in oral treatment regimens tend to employ such "prophylactic" agents in hopes of preventing the sudden and alarming appearance of these reactions during rapid tranquilization. This, in turn, poses the difficult question of how long to continue the antiparkinson medication. To avoid extrapyramidal withdrawal phenomena, these agents should be tapered off slowly, which generally means that they must be continued for at least three months.

The procedure for rapid tranquilization outlined here relies on individualized dosing, rather than fixed-formula conversions from intramuscular to oral doses. One patient may require only a single injection, while another may need intramuscular medication for days. At the end of the intramuscular injections, one patient, quite sedated, might need daily oral dosage equal to or less than that used parenterally, while another, remaining quite active yet amenable to oral treatment, might receive oral doses two, three, or in rare instances even four times the daily parenteral dose. The procedure recommended here differs from some others in its conservative approach, aiming to limit the amount of antipsychotic administered in order to minimize side effects, while still accomplishing the goal of quieting the aggressive patient.

Maintenance Therapy

There is impressive evidence that continued use of antipsychotics, after remission of the acute phase of the illness, helps prevent relapse. Combining studies to demonstrate the superiority of these drugs over placebo for maintenance of remission results in a kind of statistical overkill; after such an effort, Davis (1980) concluded that the probability that existing findings in favor of antipsychotics are chance events is less than 10^{-100}.

This does not imply that all patients diagnosed as suffering from schizophrenia should remain on drugs indefinitely. Maintenance drug treatment requires a separate decision for each patient, after taking into consideration chronicity of illness, severity of symptoms, and availability of good social support systems. Patients asymptomatic after first episodes of schizophrenia may normally be tapered off drugs within six months. Timing of drug withdrawal may depend on factors such as where the initial treatment took place, e.g. a patient treated for three weeks in the hospital might well continue on similar dosage after discharge, until he has settled into his community, whereupon slow tapering of medication might begin. If symptoms start to reappear, the dosage may be raised again and maintained at a therapeutic level for a longer period of time, e.g. up to one year, before beginning another attempt at medication withdrawal.

The analogy commonly drawn between antipsychotic treatment of schizophrenia and life-long insulin treatment of diabetics is misleading. Some schizophrenics will indeed require continuous maintenance with antipsychotics, but, unlike diabetics, schizophrenics should generally undergo periodic trials of medication withdrawal. This approach not only helps keep antipsychotic dosage at the minimum level necessary to control symptoms, but also recognizes the fact that, as time passes, an increasing number of patients may no longer require drugs.

Relapse following withdrawal of antipsychotics may occasionally occur within a week, but far more commonly occurs after a month or more. Patient and family should be appraised of this, since they can provide an "early warning system" prompting timely intervention in the event of relapse. Well-developed community services able to support and monitor the patient's functioning facilitate effective use of withdrawal trials; lack of such services will promote more rigid regimens. At all times, concern for the possible sequelae of relapse must be weighed against the potential for long-term side effects of antipsychotics, such as tardive dyskinesia.

ANTIPSYCHOTIC DRUG SIDE EFFECTS

Antipsychotic drugs are comparatively safe, having a large therapeutic index (the ratio between therapeutic and toxic dosage). Nevertheless, they produce noticeable side effects in most patients which may be so annoying that patients unilaterally discontinue medication or ask help in reducing their severity. Many common side effects (drowsiness, dizziness as a result of orthostatic hypotension, dry mouth, constipation, and blurred vision) occur in the first few days of treatment and decrease as quickly to tolerable levels. Patients should be assured that they will not suffer distressing levels of side effects indefinitely. Administering all of the day's medication at bedtime times most side effects to occur while the patient will be asleep. If reassurance, single nighttime dosing, and the passage of time do not reduce side effects satisfactorily, decreasing the dose or switching to another antipsychotic may be required. Since almost all patients will experience some annoying side effects with *any* antipsychotic, repeated changes are not recommended.

Some side effects do not respond to the passage of time and other approaches are indicated.

Weight gain can be managed with some increase in caloric expenditure

TABLE 5-2.
COMMON ANTIPARKINSONIAN AGENTS

NAME		ADULT DOSE (mg)	
GENERIC	TRADE	DAILY	SINGLE
Benztropine	Cogentin	0.5–6	1–2*
Biperiden	Akineton	2–6	2*
Diphenhydramine	Benadryl	10–400	10–50*
Procyclidine	Kemadrin	2–20	2–5
Trihexypheridyl	Artane	1–10	1–3

*Parenteral forms available.

through exercise combined with appropriate caloric restriction—with emphasis on avoiding high-calorie beverages used to slake thirst associated with dry mouth.

Extrapyramidal side effects (rigidity, akathisias, dystonias, and parkinsonism) can be alleviated with antiparkinsonian medications (see Table 5-2) given orally for chronic problems or parenterally for acute dystonias. Amantidine is proving to be a useful addition or alternative in situations resistant to the more conventional drugs.

Tardive dyskinesia is best managed by prevention, through minimizing dose and duration of antipsychotic drug treatment. This goal is difficult with patients who become psychotic when medication is stopped. Increasing the antipsychotic sometimes decreases the dyskinetic movements. Such paradoxical improvement in response to an increase in the offending agent provides little reassurance since the dyskinesia is merely further delayed. Research on the problem of tardive dyskinesia is proceeding and some agents (reserpine, choline, deanol, and tetrabenzine among others) have been suggested as possible remedies.

Agranulocytosis and hyperthermia are rare and hepatitis uncommon, but any of these conditions requires immediate cessation of treatment with the antipsychotic involved. If clinical requirements dictate retreatment with an antipsychotic, a different class should be tried.

Seizures are also uncommon. When they occur, control can be maintained with anticonvulsive medications if continued antipsychotic treatment is needed.

Pruritis and photosensitivity are seldom problematic, but can be managed with antihistamines and by protecting skin from sunlight, respectively.

Eye changes are usually benign and reversible (lenticular and corneal pigmentation and epithelial keratopathy), although central chorioretinopathy with daily thioridazine doses greater than 800 mg is well documented. If doses of thioridazine approaching 800 mg per day are required to treat a patient's psychosis, an alternative antipsychotic should be used.

OTHER SOMATIC TREATMENTS

A wide variety of other treatments have been proposed for schizophrenia. Many may be considered peripheral, obsolete, unproven, unprovable, or still experimental. We will discuss only a few of the more well known: electroconvulsive therapy (ECT), beta-blocking drugs, megavitamins, and dialysis. Insulin coma therapy (ICT), mentioned in passing, now belongs to the past. Of all these methods of treatment, ECT probably has the strongest scientific support, and deserves the most detailed consideration.

ELECTROCONVULSIVE THERAPY (ECT)

Despite its early introduction as a treatment for schizophrenia in 1938 (Cerletti and Bini, 1938), ECT still lacks a clear demonstration of efficacy in treating schizophrenia in general and incipient psychosis of undetermined etiology in particular (Klein et al., 1980). Early enthusiasm for ECT in the treatment of schizophrenia (Kalinowski, 1943; Danziger and Kendwall, 1946; Baker et al., 1960)—extending to claims of superiority over antipsychotics (Baker et al., 1958; Baker et al., 1960; Kalinowski, 1975)—has diminished. Among the factors that explain this situation are the cumbersome legal constraints surrounding the use of ECT, the growing popularity of the antipsychotics since their introduction in 1952, and the methodological defects in most clinical studies of ECT (Riddell, 1963; Tourney, 1967).

Methodological problems include reliance on retrospective studies, inadequacy of statistical analyses, failure to specify methods of evaluating treatment outcome, variable diagnostic criteria, uncertain diagnoses, coadministration of drugs with ECT, and inappropriate use of ECT (Abrams, 1975). While recognizing the difficulties of designing and following a "blind" study protocol in administering ECT to schizophrenic patients, recent reviewers have emphasized the need for well-designed, well-controlled research to evaluate whether ECT works as a treatment for schizophrenia or has advantages over other available treatments, at least for a subgroup of schizophrenic patients (Abrams, 1975; Salzman, 1978; 1978; Fink, 1978; Salzman, 1980). However, we will here reconsider some of the available studies, first those with acute, and then those with chronic schizophrenics.

In early, open clinical trials, approximately 75% of acute schizophrenic patients treated with ECT showed improvement, as indicated by discharge from hospital or reduction in schizophrenic symptomatology (Kino and Thorpe, 1946; Kalinowski, 1943; Zeifert, 1941; Baker et al., 1960). Compared with insulin coma therapy (ICT) and psychotherapy, ECT resulted in shorter periods of hospitalization and higher discharge rates (Rachlin et al., 1956). In controlled studies comparing ECT with antipsychotics in acute schizophrenic patients hospitalized for the first time, short-term treatment response proved equivalent (Riddell, 1963; Baker et al., 1960; King, 1980; Childers, 1964; Langsley et al., 1959; May, 1968).

There is little on the effectiveness of combining ECT with antipsychotics. On symptom rating changes, Childers (1964) found significant differences in outcome between ECT alone and ECT plus chlorpromazine, but the ECT-chlorpromazine combination did prove superior to chlorpromazine alone. Smith et al. (1967) found better short-term improvement with ECT plus chlorpromazine than with ECT alone, though there was no difference in long-term outcome. On the other hand, the combination of ECT and antipsychotics may increase the risk of complications or even fatalities (Grinspoon and Greenblatt, 1963; Foster and Gayle, 1955; Bracha and Hes, 1956; Gaitz et al., 1956).

In general, the literature supports the choice of antipsychotics as the initial somatic treatment for acute schizophrenia. However, ECT may have a role with schizophrenic patients who fail to respond to antipsychotics (May, 1968; 1978).

Reports of early, open clinical studies claimed that of patients who do not respond to antipsychotics, 10–20% will respond to ECT (Kalinowski, 1943; Shoor and Adams, 1950). A comparative study of ECT, ICT, and psychotherapy showed no differences in short-term outcome between the treatments (Gottlieb and Huston, 1951). However, few controlled clinical studies of chronic schizophrenics have found ECT to be ineffective, in contrast to results with other modalities in this patient group (Riddell, 1963; Greenblatt et al., 1966; Miller et al., 1953; Brill et al., 1959).

In 1965 May, Tuma, and colleagues published the first of several reports on a study comparing five treatment modalities—individual psychotherapy, antipsychotics alone, antipsychotics plus individual psychotherapy, milieu therapy, and ECT—with a group of "middle prognosis" schizophrenic patients at Camarillo State Hospital. In immediate outcome, antipsychotics with or without psychotherapy proved superior to ECT. On a three-year follow-up (1968), the two drug groups and the ECT group showed no significant differences in time spent hospitalized since original treatment. At five-year follow-up (1976), the ECT-treated group was doing minimally better than the drug-treated groups. At final follow-up (1981), the ECT and drug alone groups tended to have the best outcome and the psychotherapy alone group the worst.

The frequency and number of ECT treatments may relate to the duration of illness in determining outcome for chronic schizophrenic patients; some have claimed that the more chronic the patient, the greater the number of treatments that patient will need to show improvement (Kalinowski, 1943; Baker et al., 1960; Murillo and Exner, 1973). *Regressive ECT*, given at least daily until the patient regresses to a "state of helplessness, apathy, confusion, memory loss, speech alterations and gross disorientation" (Glueck et al., 1957) represented one solution to the question of number of ECT treatments and was recently reexamined. With this treatment, a group of chronic or "process" schizophrenic patients showed a more favorable outcome than a control group which was treated with antipsychotics and psychotherapy (Murillo and Exner, 1973); follow-up after four years (Exner and Murillo, 1977) confirmed these findings.

In conclusion, the limited amount of controlled research available has suggested that, while ECT may produce improvement in some schizophrenic patients, it has shown no clear superiority in efficacy over antipsychotics, which are preferred for other reasons, including the great body of controlled research to support their efficacy. However, as tardive dyskinesia secondary to long-term usage of antipsychotics becomes of increasing concern to psychiatry, ECT—whether routine or regressive—deserves further investigation in some schizophrenics, particularly those who remain psychotic and are refractory to antipsychotic drug treatment.

BETA-BLOCKING DRUGS

The use of such drugs in the treatment of schizophrenia has remained controversial, for more than a decade since propranolol was first claimed beneficial for psychoses, including schizophrenia (Atsmon et al., 1971; Atsmon and Blum, 1978). Further studies, mostly uncontrolled, produced mostly positive results (Cole et al., 1980). Claims of improvement on and relapse off propranolol, reports of improvement in some previously treatment-resistant patients, and positive findings from a double-blind trial (Yorkston et al., 1978), merit attention. However, all of these reports involved patients already on antipsychotics who in addition received high dosages of propranolol—300–3000 mg per day or more—which can produce troublesome side effects (Cole et al., 1980). A more recent double-blind crossover study in chronic schizophrenics maintained on antipsychotics claimed that 50% of such subjects benefited from propranolol (Lindstrom and Person, 1980). It seems reasonable to conclude that this experimental treatment needs further study before it can be recommended for general clinical use.

MEGA-VITAMINS

Enthusiasts continue to recommend and practice this approach, which forms one thread in a lengthy vitamin saga fraught with passionate belief and poverty of proof. Most patients treated with mega-vitamins have actually received antipsychotics combined with a wide variety of vitamins and trace elements in varying amounts. We have seen patients receiving daily doses of over ten substances in addition to their antipsychotics. An appropriately controlled study to assess all these factors exceeds the current bounds of feasibility. The Canadian studies on claims for vitamin therapy of schizophrenia proved unencouraging (Ban and Lehmann, 1975). Moreover, it remains unclear that such treatments are free enough from side effects to support the claim that "at least they are harmless" for clinical use. However, the interest they evoke in some seems likely to last, at least until definitive treatments for schizophrenia emerge.

DIALYSIS

Belief in some endogenous toxin as an etiologic factor in at least some forms of schizophrenia dates back a long time. Transfusion experiments in the treatment of schizophrenia were reported in 1959 (Nicklin et al., 1959); hemodialysis was proposed as a treatment in 1960 (Feer et al., 1960). Technical difficulties and lack of positive clinical reports deterred further interest until the remarkable claims of Wagemaker and Cade (1977) that dialysis had a dramatic therapeutic effect on a few schizophrenic patients. However, later studies have shown less positive results; indeed, Sjostedt et al., as reported by Fogelson et al. (1980), found no effects whatsoever in 13 patients. With the results of controlled studies beginning to appear, enthusiasm for dialysis seems to be waning. Thus, Schulz and colleagues reported on a double-blind evaluation of eight carefully diagnosed schizophrenics. They found no difference between the patients when treated with real and sham dialysis (Schulz, 1981). It seems inappropriate to recommend this treatment for schizophrenia until patient selection criteria are established and until positive results of controlled trials emerge.

PSYCHOTHERAPY

INDIVIDUAL PSYCHOTHERAPY

It is generally held that a relationship can be established with schizophrenic patients in psychotherapy, although it is intensely charged and quite different from that which develops in the treatment of neurosis, in that the schizophrenic often projects his delusional complexes onto the therapist.

A number of widely different psychotherapeutic approaches have been developed and many have assumed that techniques suitable for the treatment of neurotic patients should be applied to psychotics. The confusion between what is good for neurosis and what is appropriate for psychosis has been aggravated by a reluctance to subject hypotheses and techniques to scientific study and controlled comparisons, leading to a widespread overestimation of the indications for and effectiveness of current methods of psychotherapy for schizophrenia.

As Greenblatt observes, everyone believes that human behavior, thinking, and feeling can be profoundly affected by the interaction of one person with another, and much time, effort, and money are expended on individual psychotherapy. Yet it is difficult to obtain convincing proof that individual therapy, as conventionally practiced, is worth the effort. Thoughtful therapists will also wonder whether a few hours of face-to-face verbal interaction each week can really have the impact necessary to affect patients who are deeply embedded in maladaption (Greenblatt, 1972).

We find it helpful to distinguish between formal psychotherapy and psychotherapeutic management. The latter may be defined as the application of psychological understanding to the management and rehabilitation of the individual patient, which often includes establishing a therapeutic relationship, helping the patient to identify and deal with current life problems, and working with his family and significant others. This can lead to a deeper understanding of the individual patient which may in turn guide the therapist in choosing the most effective interventions. As so defined, psychotherapeutic management may occur at any stage of the schizophrenic process.

With schizophrenics, flexibility is essential. The main aim is to convey the idea that the therapist wants to understand the patient and will try to do so and that he has faith in the patient's potential as a human being, no matter how disturbed, hostile, or bizarre he may be at the moment.

Once a relationship has been established, the patient may be willing to let down his "defenses." Some therapists believe that, if the relationship can be sustained, no specialized technical maneuvers are required with schizophrenics, e.g. Bleuler (1950, 1965). Others do more. Some who delve more deeply into the psychosis make intense and persistent attempts to communicate with the patient in primary-process language. Those who see therapy as a learning experience and themselves as ambassadors of reality, make appeals to the intact adult part of the patient's ego to become more realistic.

Some claim, without convincing evidence, that action, posture, and movement interventions that are largely nonverbal may, in some cases, open up another avenue of dialogue, with direct access to material that is relatively inaccessible in the verbal mode (DesLauriers, 1960; Bellak, 1963; May et al., 1963).

The specialized intensive psychotherapies, mostly psychoanalytic in origin, are essentially research techniques that are of great potential value in developing principles for wider application and for the treatment of unusual cases and those patients who fail to respond to other types of intervention. Thus, the individual psychodynamic approach may be of value at present less as a therapeutic technique than as an instrument of investigation (Greenblatt, 1972).

Progress has been made in developing techniques that seem to have been effective in individual cases. There are no well controlled studies supporting the efficacy of these intensive psychotherapeutic approaches and a great expenditure of time and effort is required, making them applicable only to relatively few among the great number of patients for whom help is needed.

We believe that formal psychotherapy, as distinguished from psychotherapeutic management, should be reserved for the outpatient, postpsychotic phase of treatment, when the patient is in better contact with reality and more capable of communicating and understanding. Psychotherapeutic intervention may be most useful in helping the patient deal with real-life problems associated with the illness. Formal individual psychotherapy in the hospital should be considered only if a patient fails to respond to other forms of therapy.

The treatment of schizophrenic patients is always a stressful experience. A perusal of the literature on psychotherapy for schizophrenia gives one some understanding of the massive resistances presented by schizophrenics, of the frustrations and disappointments of working with them, and of the dedication and persistence required (Greenblatt, 1972).

Turning from general clinical impressions to controlled studies, however, the balance of evidence indicates that insight-oriented psychotherapy has limited value for schizophrenic patients who are sick enough to be in a hospital. Moreover, psychotherapy has an adverse effect on some patients, as does drug therapy (Hogarty and Goldberg, 1973; Hogarty et al., 1979).

On the other hand, a series of good studies has shown that *outpatient* individual sociotherapy *plus* drugs is more effective than either treatment alone, though outpatient drug treatment alone is better than outpatient sociotherapy alone. These studies indicate that the effects of drugs and intensive social case work, combined with vocational rehabilitation, are additive. The contribution of drugs to reducing the relapse rate was relatively greater than that of case work; the impact of the counseling became significant only after patients had remained out of the hospital for at least six months (Hogarty et al., 1979).

Thus it is not a matter of *either* drug therapy *or* rehabilitation *or* psychotherapy. All are necessary to achieve optimum results, although the precise plan must vary according to the needs of the individual patient. Therefore, the outpatient treatment plan should usually combine antipsychotic medication with social and occupational rehabilitation and psychotherapy (May and Simpson, 1980).

Hogarty et al. (1979) conclude that the greatest prophylactic effect occurs in the presence of continued medication and supportive therapy. In the absence of medication (i.e. noncompliance), supportive therapy exerts no prophylactic effect. In the absence of supportive therapy, long-acting fluphenazine decanoate alone has only limited success in protecting patients against stimulation from a stressful environment. The most potent predictor of relapse in patients who receive long-acting fluphenazine decanoate is the degree of contention and disagreement in the patient's home at the time of hospital discharge (Hogarty et al., 1979). This finding gains support from the results of British investigators studying the effects of familial expressed emotion (EE) on schizophrenic relapse (Brown et al., 1972; Vaughn and Leff, 1976).

GROUP PSYCHOTHERAPY AND FAMILY THERAPY

Group therapy has an uncertain status in the treatment of schizophrenics. Some patients feel more secure in a group; groups also offer more opportunity for consensual validation, breaking down isolation, and for peer confrontation. "Medication groups" can be helpful, not only in improving cooperation with medication procedures through discussions of side effect and dosage problems, but also in offering an entry into other life problems and family relationships. Informal groups can be supportive and are often less threatening than formal therapy; indeed, patients should be encouraged to form or join informal social and activity groups.

All the experimental studies of inpatient group therapy either took place before 1960 or were confounded by drug treatment. They leave an overall impression that inpatient group therapy aimed at insight and psychological understanding is of little benefit to schizophrenic patients. Group therapy may be more helpful when it focuses on real-life plans, problems, and relationships; on social and work roles and interaction; on cooperation with drug therapy and dealing with its side effects; or on some practical activity related to work or recreation.

The few experimental studies of outpatient group therapy have shown generally positive results, provided that it is combined with drug treatment. Claghorn et al. (1974) compared drug therapy alone with drug therapy plus group therapy. While there was no significant difference in symptomatic improvement, the patients who received group therapy did show more appreciation of their own disability.

O'Brien et al. (1972) compared group therapy with individual therapy in patients who all received concurrent medication. The outcome for group therapy was significantly better, based on both social effectiveness and psychiatric symptom rating scales; rehospitalization rates were not significantly different. The authors speculate that patients receiving group therapy took medication more reliably, since the groups tended to focus on this.

Some therapists deal with schizophrenia as an illness not of the patient alone but of the entire family. In any case, appropriate active involvement with the family and other significant persons is usually essential, both while the patient is in the hospital and after release. The patient may be assisted with the simple problems of everyday life. In addition, there may be deliberate psychotherapeutic work on the conflict-provoking nature of family relationships, and on defective communication, roles, and attitudes.

Goldstein et al. (1978) found that drug treatment (high dose versus low dose) reduced the relapse rate but, more interestingly, that crisis-oriented family therapy further reduced the relapse rate from 10% to 0% in high-dose patients and from 48% to 9% in low-dose patients.

Adequate doses of long-acting fluphenazine and crisis-oriented family therapy had a synergistic effect in reducing relapse during the period of delivery, as well as in preventing relapse over the subsequent five months. Not a single relapse occurred in the group that received both adequate pharmacological and social support. Where both were lacking, the rate of relapse approximated the national average of 45%. Despite these relapse data, however, the analysis of symptom ratings (on the Brief Psychiatric Rating Scale) by Goldstein et al. (1978) failed to disclose a single statistically significant drug effect. Noticeable effects of social therapy on symptoms did emerge independently of drug level during the first six weeks, but were sustained over six months only in the group that received the higher phenothiazine dose. In this sense, the relapse and symptom rating data were in agreement since the best long-term outcome on both measures was found in the high-dose, family-therapy group.

Some excellent research by Brown et al. (1972) and Vaughn and Leff (1967) on outpatient drug therapy and family relationships has focused attention on the need for interventions specifically aimed at certain toxic effects of the family, particularly when the family is hostile, overtly hypercritical, or emotionally overinvolved with the patient. Vaughn and Leff (1976) concluded that the degree of expressed emotion (EE) in the patient's family is a good predictor of posthospital relapse, independent of the patient's previous behavior disturbance and work impairment. They found the best results when drug treatment was given and the family was low in expressed emotion. When expressed emotion was high, drugs to some extent counteracted the toxic effects of the family and lowered the relapse rate. The recurrence rate was highest when expressed emotion was high and drugs were not given.

In schizophrenics with high-EE families, Vaughn and Leff (1976) found a relapse rate of 53% for those on drugs, 92% for those off drugs. When family EE was low, drug treatment made little difference in the relapse rate (15% on drugs, 12% off drugs).

BEHAVIOR THERAPY

A number of studies have used behavioral techniques including immediate positive reinforcements with praise, food, and privileges. These are formalized token economy programs aimed at modifying specific behavior patterns in schizophrenic patients. There is substantial evidence of their effectiveness for this limited purpose. In particular, the two best-designed studies showed positive results with social reinforcement (praise and attention), token reinforcement (tokens), and informational reinforcement (explanations of reasons tokens were given) (Jones, 1978). Token reinforcement of social learning in small groups, and classes (Paul and Lentz, 1977) has proven to be more successful than intensive milieu therapy. Most such studies, however, have been carried out with chronic patients, and the results and techniques may apply only to this group.

Few studies have compared different types of behavioral therapies.

Two studies by Jones (1978) and Cliffe (1974) compared contingent versus noncontingent reinforcement. The results of one study weakly favored contingency and the other strongly favored it, as operant conditioning theory would predict.

Behavior therapy is a relatively new treatment that may well prove worthwhile for certain schizophrenic patients, and may also prove additive in therapeutic effect when combined with more established treatments, but its exact place in the treatment of schizophrenia remains to be determined by more extensive research in a broad range of clinical situations.

SUGGESTED TREATMENT FOR SCHIZOPHRENIA

An outline for an approach to the treatment of schizophrenia is shown in Figure 5-1. We emphasize again the need for careful diagnosis, consideration of the best available setting for treatment, and an attempt whenever possible to observe the hospitalized patient unmedicated for a time. Also whenever possible, a test dose procedure should precede the course of drug therapy, which should in turn employ the smallest dosage sufficient to control symptoms within a reasonable period of time.

Monitoring signs of clinical improvement and side affects will help determine the dosage. The clinician should bear in mind that minimal extrapyramidal side effects (EPS) may be a positive indication of the drug reaching the central nervous system in amounts adequate to affect the basal ganglia and perhaps also those areas of the brain relevant to the symptoms of schizophrenia. Thus, mild deterioration in handwriting has correlated positively with behavioral improvement (Haase, 1959), although marked extrapyramidal effects have shown negative correlations (Simpson et al., 1964). With more agitated patients, requiring more aggressive treatment, gross sedation or EPS may mark the point where no further dosage increase is required.

A trial of a specific antipsychotic should last four to six weeks, given an adequate dosage of the drug, for example up to 1000 mg of chlorpromazine per day or 20–40 mg of haloperidol per day. The length of the trial may vary according to the chronicity of the patient's illness; more chronic patients may show slower and/or less obvious improvement, so that a longer treatment period is needed for clear assessment of drug effects.

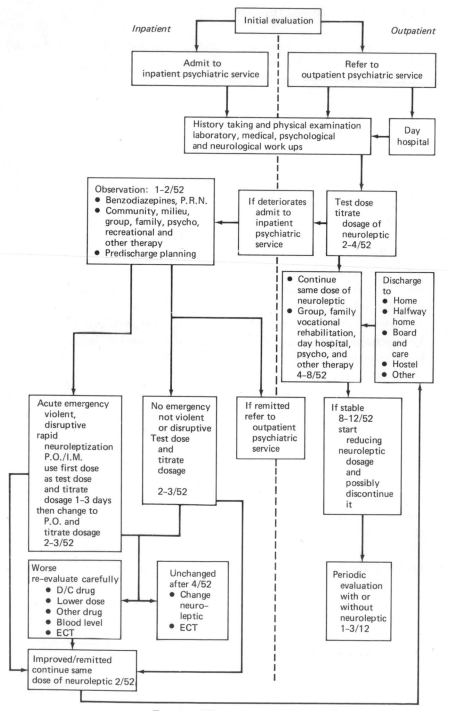

Fig. 5-1. The treatment of a nonaffective psychosis.

In the event of poor response to such a trial, we recommend that the following measures precede a switch to a different antipsychotic: First, check for compliance by pill count and more careful observation of the patient as he actually consumes the medication and immediately thereafter. Second, shift to a liquid vehicle for the medication and monitor for changes in side effects indicative of greater central nervous system effect; this provides a check on both compliance and absorption. Third, give a small, parenteral test dose of the antipsychotic, for example, 50 mg of intramuscular chlorpromazine. Obvious side effects from such an injection suggest noncompliance, poor absorption, and/or rapid metabolism of the drug. In the absence of a compliance problem, where poor absorption or rapid metabolism is suggested, a switch to another antipsychotic is in order. In such cases, keep in mind that the use of long-acting, intramuscular antipsychotics not only avoids problems of compliance, but also eliminates problems of poor absorption and rapid breakdown in the gut or liver.

Questions of compliance and absorption may be answered more quickly by determining the plasma level of the antipsychotic, assayed from a blood specimen drawn about 12 hours after the last dose. The usefulness of plasma-level monitoring of antipsychotics has been questioned in that therapeutic levels have proven difficult to define and none having gained universal acceptance (Cooper, 1978). Nevertheless, the presence of minute amounts of the drug in the blood—for example, less than 10 ng per ml of chlorpromazine—suggests a need for higher dosage or, if the patient already reliably takes a high dosage, for a change to another drug. On the other hand, putatively "toxic" levels, greater than 600 ng per ml, might suggest a trial reduction of dosage before changing drugs, since both clinical and laboratory evidence suggests that too much antipsychotic may worsen psychosis (Simpson et al., 1981). Levels in the "adequate" range of 50–300 ng/ml, without improvement, indicate the need to change drugs. Thus, plasma levels may provide important information in specific situations—where routine and ostensibly adequate treatments fail to produce desired therapeutic effects—though plasma-level monitoring of antipsychotics cannot be recommended as a routine procedure in itself.

A trial of a new antipsychotic after failure with a previous one should closely follow the pattern of the original trial in most respects. As long as positive symptoms of schizophrenia persist, e.g. hallucinations, delusions, or thought disorder, then systematic adjustments of antipsychotic treatment should continue in an effort to control these symptoms. On the other hand, negative symptoms—such as blunted affect, withdrawal, and autism—unless associated with positive symptoms, may show little response even to adequate antipsychotic treatment.

Antipsychotics are best combined with other therapeutic approaches, such as good aftercare, family therapy, day programs, social skills training, adequate living arrangements, and, above all, a flexible treatment regimen. Antipsychotics on their own cannot get a patient a job, a place to live, a way to meet people, or an opportunity to learn new things in a changing world; but they can enable many patients to take advantage of the opportunities that are made available to them. Accomplishing this requires adept use of drugs, with knowledge of and sensitivity to their side effects. It also requires sound knowledge of the natural history of schizophrenia, including alternative courses such as spontaneous remission relapse under stress, or stagnation in chronic defect states, each of which demands a different type of intervention.

PARANOIA (297.10)

Essential Features

The essential feature of *paranoia* is the insidious development of persecutory delusions or delusional jealousy while clear and orderly thinking is preserved. Bizarre delusions, incoherence, or marked loosening of associations (the characteristic symptoms of schizophrenia) are not present. Hallucinations, if present, are not prominent.

Paranoia is an uncommon condition, well recognized in the world literature for its striking content, insidious onset, and often intractable course. Its persistence is, perhaps, related to the onset, i.e. the delusional system usually develops gradually, and while it may influence some aspects of the person's behavior, he or she may continue to function acceptably, or even well in some ways. There is a regrettable paucity of information about paranoia, largely because of the low incidence of this disorder and also because patients with the abovementioned features have usually been included in studies of schizophrenia.

Treatment

In the past, paranoid patients have received various somatic and psychotherapeutic therapies with no great success (Retterstol, 1966). The earlier the disorder is detected and the more apparent precipitants there are, the more likely it is to respond to antipsychotics. For example, an elderly, slightly deaf person who moves to a new neighborhood and is largely on his own may develop ideas of reference, suspicion of neighbors, and ultimately a delusional system which might respond well to antipsychotics and be of short duration (Post, 1973; Raskind et al., 1979). In Europe this would be termed a late paraphrenia (Roth, 1955).

By contrast, rapid improvement is the exception in mid-life paranoid disorders, which tend to be unresponsive to treatment, (Retterstol, 1966). More common would be the development of somewhat haughty attitudes in a relatively efficient person who continues working, although perhaps isolating himself from colleagues at work. Later he would tend to develop a delusional system about his own special powers which are perceived as being reenforced by special messages from important people, with the whole situation going on for years before anyone realizes that something is amiss. We would treat such a condition as if it were schizophrenia.

SHARED PARANOID DISORDER (297.30)

Essential Features

The essential feature of *shared paranoid disorder* is a persecutory delusional system that develops as a result of a close relationship with another person who already has a psychotic (usually paranoid) disorder. The delusions are at least partly shared. In the past this disorder has been termed *folie à deux*. In rare cases more than two persons may be involved (*folie à trois*, etc.).

TREATMENT

The DSM-III definition suggests a benign outcome, at least for the more dependent of the parties involved. This is often correct, i.e. separation by hospitalization and/or treatment of the original delusional subject is often sufficient to set the stage for remission in the other party. It should be stressed, however, that since shared paranoid disorder usually occurs in close relatives, e.g. parent/child or siblings, the potential for the secondary or "infected" person to be vulnerable to the original disorder also exists, whether from heredity or from earlier family influence.

The treatment would therefore be: (a) to separate the two parties; (b) supportive therapy in an appropriate environment, with the results determining whether or not to use (c) drug therapy if frank psychotic symptoms persist in either person.

ACUTE PARANOID DISORDER (298.30)

ESSENTIAL FEATURES

The essential features of *acute paranoid disorder* are persistent persecutory delusions or delusional jealousy of less than six months duration. The onset is usually relatively sudden and the condition rarely becomes chronic. The prototype situation involves culture shock, as in emigration.

TREATMENT

Unfortunately, there are no valid controlled studies of the results of treatment for these conditions. One must rely on clinical intuition and uncontrolled reports (Modlin, 1963; Retterstol, 1970).

A sudden onset often pinpoints the precipitant situation and also the treatment. For example, a husband, guilty after his first extramarital affair, arrives home and notes that the telephone is in an unusual position, and begins developing delusions of jealousy about his wife. If the patient comes to treatment early, psychotherapy with emphasis on a positive, supportive relationship and simple elementary explanation and interpretation may well be sufficient. If psychotherapy does not diminish or relieve the symptoms in a few weeks, antipsychotics are indicated. If there is an associated severe sleep disturbance, the antipsychotic might be given at night in a single dose.

Migrants, and indeed any persons who are uprooted for whatever reason, are particularly prone to acute paranoid disorders. These are perhaps more serious or more difficult to cope with the more the new culture differs from the original one. Nostalgic, dysphoric, hypercritical, sensitive, irritable reactions normally peak around three to six months after the move and usually remit slowly over a period of months, e.g. 6 to 18 months. A sustained paranoid reaction may, however, develop. Early identification of the nature of the problem plus support from people with a similar cultural background who have made a successful adjustment may be helpful (Tyhurst, 1977). If all else fails, returning to the original and more comfortable environment should be seriously considered. Clearly, this is not possible in the case of forced migration, and there are, of course, varying degrees of "force." It has been claimed that forced migration produces a different clinical picture than normal migration (Tyhurst, 1977). Paranoid psychoses in the wake of migration are frequent and Tyhurst suggests combined educational, group, and self-help approaches. However, in persisting paranoid states, these methods may need to be combined with antipsychotics.

References

American Psychiatric Association, Task Force Report 14. Electroconvulsive Therapy, Washington, D.C. 1978.

Abrams GM: Defining milieu therapy. Arch Gen Psychiat. 21:553–560, 1969.

Abrams R: ECT and psychotropic drugs. In: Rational Psychopharmacotherapy and the Right to Treatment. Ayd, FJ Jr. (ed). Ayd Medical Communications, Baltimore. 1975.

Atsmon A, Blum I: The discovery. In: Propranolol and Schizophrenia. Roberts, E and Amacher, P (eds). Liss, New York. pp. 5–38, 1978.

Atsmon A, Blum I, Wijsenbeek H, et al: The short-term effects of adrenergic blocking agents in a small group of psychotic patients. Psychiat Neurol Neurochir. 74:251–258, 1971.

Baker AA, Bird G, Lavin NI: ECT in schizophrenia. J Ment Sci. 106:1506–1511, 1960.

Baker AA, Game JA, Thorpe JG: Physical treatment for schizophrenia. J. Ment Sci. 104:860–864, 1958.

Ban TA, Lehmann HE: Nicotinic acid in the treatment of schizophrenias. Can Psychiat Assoc J. 20:103, 1975.

Bellak L: Methodology and research in the psychotherapy of psychoses. Psychiat Res Rep. 17:162, 1963.

Bishop MP, Gallant DM: Observation of placebo response in chronic schizophrenic patients. Arch Gen Psychiat. 14:479–503, 1966.

Bleuler E: Dementia Praecox or the Group of Schizophrenias. International Universities Press, New York. 1950.

Bleuler M: Conception of schizophrenia within the last fifty years and today. Int J Psychiat. 1:501, 1965.

Bracha S, Hes JP: Death occurring during combined reserpine-electroshock treatment. Am J Psychiat. 113:257, 1956.

Brill NO, Crumpton E, Eiduson S et. al: Relative effectiveness of various components of electroconvulsive therapy. Arch Neurol Psychiat. 81:627–635, 1959.

Brown G, Birley J, Wing J: Influence of family life in the course of schizophrenic disorders. A replication. Brit J Psychiat. 121:241–258, 1972.

Caffey EM, Galbrecht CR, Klett CJ: Brief hospitalization and aftercare in the treatment of schizophrenia. Arch Gen Psychiat. 24:81, 1972.

Carroll RS, Miller A, Ross B, Simpson GM: Research as an impetus to improved treatment. Arch Gen Psychiat. 37:377–380, 1980.

Caudill WA: The Psychiatric Hospital as a Small Society. Harvard University Press, Cambridge, Mass. 1958.

Cerletti U, Bini L: L'Elettroshock. Arch Gen Neurol, Psychiat Psychoanal. 19:266, 1938.

Childers RT: Comparison of four regimens in newly admitted female schizophrenics. Am J Psychiat. 120:1010–1011, 1964.

Claghorn JL, Johnstone EE, Cook TH et al: Group therapy and maintenance treatment of schizophrenics. Arch Gen Psychiat. 31:361–365, 1974.

Clark ML, Costiloe JP, Wood F , Parades A, Fulkerson FG: Butaclamol in newly admitted chronic schizophrenic patients: a modified fixed-dose-range design. Dis Nerv Syst. 38:943–947, 1977.

Cliffe MJ: Reinstatement of speech in mute schizophrenics by operant conditioning. Acta Psychiat Scand Suppl. 50:577, 1974.

Cole JO, Altesman RI, Weingarten CH: Beta-blocking drugs in psychiatry. In: Psychopharmacology Update. Cole, JO (ed). Collamore Press, Lexington, Mass. pp. 43–68, 1980.

Cole JO, Davis JM: Antipsychotic drugs. In: The Schizophrenic Syndrome. Bellak, L and Leb, L (eds). Grune and Stratton, New York, 1969.

Cooper TB: Plasma level monitoring of antipsychotic drugs. Clinical Pharmacokinetics. 3:14–38, 1978.

Cumming J, Cumming E: Ego and Milieu: Theory Practice of Environmental Therapy. Atherton, New York. 1962.

Danziger L, Kendwall JA: Prediction of the immediate outcome of shock therapy in dementia praecox. Dis Nerv Syst. 7:229–303, 1946.

Davis JM: Antipsychotic drugs. In: Comprehensive Textbook of Psychiatry, 3rd ed. Kaplan, HI, Freedman, AM, Sadock, BJ (eds). Williams and Wilkins, Baltimore. 1980.

DesLauriers A: The psychological experience of reality in schizophrenia: Therapeutic implications. In: Chronic Schizophrenia. Appleby, L, Scher, JR, and Cummings, J (eds). Free Press of Glencoe, Ill. pp. 275–302. 1960.

Donlon PT, Hopkin J, Tupin JP: Overview: efficacy and safety of the rapid neuroleptization method with injectable haloperidol. Am J Psychiat. 136:273–278, 1979.

Exner JE, Murillo LG: A long-term follow-up of schizophrenics treated with regressive ECT. Dis Nerv Syst. 38:162–167, 1977.

Fairweather GW (ed): Social Psychology in Treating Mental Illness: An Experimental Approach. Wiley, New York. 1964.

Feer H, Thoelen H, Massine MA et al: Hemodialysis in schizophrenia. Comp Psychiat. 1:338–344, 1960.

Fink M: Efficacy and safety of induced seizures (EST) in man. Comp Psychiat. 19:1–18, 1978.

Fogelson DL, Marder SR, Van Putten T: Dialysis for schizophrenia: review of clinical trials and implications for further research. Am J Psychiat. 137:605–607, 1980.

Foster MW, Gayle RF: Dangers in combining reserpine (Serpasil) with electroconvulsive therapy. JAMA. 159:1520–1522, 1955.

Freedman N, Engelhardt DM, Hankoff LK, Schwartz S, Zobel H: Patterns of verbal group participation in the drug treatment of chronic schizophrenic patients. Int J Group Psychother. 11:60, 1961.

Freeman T, Cameron JL, McGhie A: Chronic Schizophrenia. International Universities Press, New York. 1958.

Friedman MJ: Some problems of inpatient management with borderline patients. Am J Psychiat. 126:299, 1969.

Gaitz CM, Pokorny AD, Mills M: Death following electroconvulsive therapy. Arch Neurol Psychiat. 75:493–499, 1956.

Glick ID, Hargreaves WA, Drues J, Showstack JA: Short or long hospitalization for psychiatric disorders?. Psychopharmacol Bull. 11:35, 1975.

Glick ID, Hargreaves WA, Drues J, Showstack JA: Short versus long hospitalization: A prospective controlled study. III. Inpatient results for non-schizophrenics. Arch Gen Psychiat. 33:78, 1976.

Glick ID, Hargreaves WA, Goldfield MD: Short versus long hospitalization: A prospective controlled study. I. Preliminary results of a one-year follow-up of schizophrenics. Arch Gen Psychiat. 30:363, 1974.

Glueck BC, Reiss H, Bernard LE: Regressive electroshock therapy. Psychiat Q 31:117–136, 1957.

Goldberg A, Rubin B: Recovery of patients during periods of supposed neglect. Brit J Med Psychol. 37:265, 1964.

Goldberg SC, Klerman GL, Cole JO, Davis D, Zeman D: Hospital differences in outcome as a function of patient, ward and hospital characteristics. In: Psychopharmacology and the Individual Patient. Wittenborn, JR, Goldberg, SC and May, PRA (eds). Raven Press, New York. 1970.

Goldstein MJ, Rodnick EH, Evans JR, May PRA, Steinberg MR: Drug and family therapy in the aftercare of acute schizophrenia. Arch Gen Psychiat. 35:1169–1180, 1978.

Gottlieb JS, Huston PE: Treatment of schizophrenia. A comparison of three methods: Brief psychotherapy, insulin coma, and electric shock. J Nerv Ment Dis. 113:237–256, 1951.

Grad J, Sainsbury P: Problems of caring for the mentally ill at home. Proc Roy Soc Med. 59:20, 1966.

Grad J, Sainsbury P: The effects that patients have on their families in a community care and a control psychiatric service. A two-year follow-up. Brit J Psychiat. 114:265, 1968.

Greenblatt M: Introduction. In: Schizophrenia: Pharmacotherapy and Psychotherapy. Grinspoon, L, Ewalt, JR, and Shader, RI (eds). Williams and Wilkins, Baltimore. 1972.

Greenblatt M, Freeman H, Meshorer E, et al: Comparative efficacy of antidepressant drugs and placebo in relation to electric shock treatment. In: Biological Treatment of Mental Illness. Rienkel, M (ed.). L.C. Page & Co., New York. pp. 574–594, 1966.

Greenblatt M, Solomon MH, Evans AS, Brooks GW (eds): Drugs and Social Therapy in Chronic Schizophrenia. C.C. Thomas, Springfield, Ill. 1965.

Grinspoon L, Greenblatt M: Pharmacotherapy combined with other treatment methods. Comp Psychiat. 4:256–262, 1963.

Haase HJ: Correlation between extrapyramidal symptom groups and psychiatric states. In: Psychopharmacology Frontiers, Kline, NS (ed). Little, Brown, Boston. 1959.

Hamilton M, Hordern A, Waldrop FN, Lofft J: A controlled trial on the value of prochlorperazine trifluoperazine and intensive group treatment. Brit J Psychiat. 109:510, 1963.

Herz MI, Endicott J, Gibbon M: Brief hospitalization: 2-year follow-up. Arch Gen Psychiat. 36:701–705, 1979.

Herz MI, Endicott J, Spitzer RL: Brief hospitalization of patients with families. Initial results. Am J Psychiat. In Press, 1982.

Herz MI, Endicott J, Spitzer RL: Brief versus standard hospitalization: The families. Am J Psychiat. 133:795–801, 1976.

Herz MI, Endicott J, Spitzer RL: Brief hospitalization: a two-year follow-up. Am J Psychiat. 134:502–507, 1977.

Herz MI, Endicott J, Spitzer RL, Mesnikoff A: Day versus inpatient hospitalizations: a controlled study. Am J Psychiat. 127:1371–1382, 1971.

Hogarty GE, Goldberg SC: Drugs and sociotherapy in the posthospital maintenance of schizophrenic patients. 1-year relapse rates. Arch Gen Psychiat. 28:54, 1973.

Hogarty GE, Schooler NR, Ulrich R, Mussare F, Ferro P, Herron E: Fluphenazine and social therapy in the aftercare of schizophrenic patients. Relapse analyses of a two-year controlled study of fluphenazine decanoate and fluphenazine hydrochloride. Arch Gen Psychiat. 36:1283–1294, 1979.

Hollister LE: Clinical Pharmacology of Psychotherapeutic Drugs. Churchill Livingstone, New York. p. 159, 1978.

Jones HG: Psychological aspects of treatment of inpatients. In: Schizophrenia: Towards a New Synthesis. Wing, JK (ed). Grune and Stratton, New York. p. 189, 1978.

Jones M: The Therapeutic Community Basic Books, New York. 1953.

Kalinowski LB: Electric convulsive therapy, with emphasis on importance of adequate treatment. Arch Neurol Psychiat. 50:652–660, 1943.

Kalinowski LB: In: Comprehensive Textbook of Psychiatry. Freedman, AM, Kaplan, MI, and Sadock, BU (eds). Williams and Wilkins, Baltimore. 1969, 1975.

King P: Chlorpromazine and electroconvulsive therapy in the treatment of newly hospitalized schizophrenics. J Clin Exp Psychopath. 21:101–105, 1980.

Kino FF, Thorpe FT: Electrical convulsion therapy in 500 selected psychotics. J Ment Sci. 92:138–145, 1946.

Klein DF, Gittleman R, Quitkin F, Rifkin A: Diagnosis and Drug Treatment of Psychiatric Disorders: Adults and Children. 2nd ed. Williams and Wilkins, Baltimore/London. pp. 152–153, 1980.

Langsley DG, Enterline JD, Hickerson GX: A comparison of chlorpromazine and ECT in treatment of acute schizophrenic and maniac reactions. Arch Neurol Psychiat. 81:384–391, 1959.

Letermendia FJJ, Harris AD, Willems JA: Effects on chronic patients of administrative changes. Brit J Psychiat. 113:959, 1967.

Lindstrom HH, Persson E: Propranolol in chronic schizophrenia: a controlled study in neuroleptic-treated patients. Brit J Psychiat. 137:126–130, 1980.

Linn MW, Caffey EM, Klett J, Hogarty GE, Lamb HR: Drug treatment and psychotropic drugs in the aftercare of schizophrenic patients. Arch Gen Psychiat. 36:1055–1066, 1979.

Ludwig AM, Marx AJ, Hill PA, Hermsmeier GI: Forced small group responsibility in the treatment of chronic schizophrenia. Psychiat Q. 41:262, 1967.

Main TF, Bridger H, Bion WR, Dewan MC, Foulkes SH, Davidson S: The hospital as a therapeutic institution. Bull Meninger Clin. 10:66, 1946.

May PR, Tuma AH: Follow-up study of the results of treatment of schizophrenia. In: Evaluation of Psychological Therapies. Spitzer, R and Klein, DF (eds). Johns Hopkins, Baltimore. pp. 256–284, 1976.

May PRA: Treatment of Schizophrenia. Science House, New York. 1968.

May PRA, Simpson GM: Schizophrenia: overview of treatment methods. In: Comprehensive Textbook of Psychiatry/III. Kaplan, HI, Freedman, AM, and Sadock, BJ (eds). Williams and Wilkins, Baltimore. 2:1193–1216, 1980.

May PRA, Tuma AH, Dixon WJ, Yale C, Thiele DA, Kraude WH: Schizophrenia: A follow-up study of the results of five forms of treatment. Arch Gen Psychiat. 38:776–784, 1981.

May PRA, Tuma AH, Kraude W: Community follow-up of treatment of schizophrenia: Issues and problems. Am J Orthopsychiat. 35:754–763, 1965.

May PRA, Van Putten T: Plasma levels of chlorpromazine in schizophrenia. scale of design and outcome for use in literature surveys. Comp Psychiat. 15:267–275, 1974.

May PRA, Van Patten T: Plasma levels of chlorpromazine in schizophrenia. Arch Gen Psychiat. 35:1081–1087, 1978.

May PRA, Wexler M, Salkin J, Schoop T: Nonverbal techniques in the reestablishment of body image and self identity. Psychiat Res Rep. 16:68, 1963.

Meltzoff J, Blumenthal R: The Day Treatment Center. C. C. Thomas, Springfield, Ill. 1966.

Miller DH, Clancy J, Cummings F: A comparison between undirectional current non-convulsive electrical stimulation, alternating current electroshock and Pentothal in chronic schizophrenia. Am J Psychiat. 109:617–620, 1953.

Modlin C: Psychodynamics in management of paranoid states in women. Arch Gen Psychiat. 8:263–268, 1963.

Murillo LG, Exner JE: The effects of regressive ECT with process schizophrenics. Am J Psychiat. 130:269–273, 1973.

Nicklin G, Sacks W, Wehrheim H: Cross transfusion in schizophrenia. Am J Psychiat. 116:334–336, 1959.

O'Brien CP, Hamm KB, Ray BA, Pierce JF, Luborsky L, Mintz J: Group vs individual psychotherapy with schizophrenics: a controlled outcome study. Arch Gen Psychiat. 27:474, 1972.

Pardes H, Van Putten T, Bjork D, Kaufman M: Failures on a therapeutic milieu. Psychiat Q. 46:29, 1972.

Pasamanick B, Scarpitti F, Dinitz S: Schizophrenics in the Community. Appleton-Century Crofts, New York. 1967.

Paul GL, Lentz RJ: Psychosocial Treatment of Chronic Mental Patients. Harvard University Press, Cambridge, Mass. 1977.

Paul GL, Tobias LL, Holly BL: Maintenance psychotropic drugs in the presence of active treatment programs: A "triple blind" withdrawal study with long-term mental patients. Arch Gen Psychiat. 27:106, 1972.

Pi EH, Miller A, Rosenberg MR, Schultz C, Simpson GM: Therapeutic effects of psychiatric hospitalization. Unpublished report. Available from Dr. Simpson, Adult Psychiatric Clinic, Graduate Hall, 1037 Hospital Place, Los Angeles, CA 90033.

Post F: Paranoid disorders in the elderly. Postgrad Med. 53:52, 1973.

Quitkin FM, Klein DF: Follow-up treatment failure. Psychoses and character disorder. Am J Psychiat. 124:499, 1967.

Rachlin HL, Goldman GS, Gurvitz M: Follow-up study of 317 patients discharged from Hillside Hospital in 1950. J Hillside Hosp. 5:17–40, 1956.

Raskind M, Alvarez C, Herlin S: Fluphenazine enanthate in the outpatient treatment of late paraphrenia. J Am Geriatric Soc. 27:459–463, 1979.

Retterstol N: Paranoid and Paranoiac Psychoses. C. C. Thomas, Springfield, Ill. 1966.

Retterstol N: Prognoses in Paranoid Psychoses. C. C. Thomas, Springfield, Ill. 1970.

Riddell SA: The therapeutic efficacy of ECT. Arch Gen Psychiat. 8:546, 1963.

Roth M: The natural history of mental disorder in old age. J Ment Sci. 101:281–301, 1955.

Salzman C: Electroconvulsive therapy. In: Harvard Guide to Modern Psychiatry. Harvard Univ. Press, Cambridge, Mass. 1978.

Salzman C: The use of ECT in the treatment of schizophrenia. Am J Psychiat. 137:1032–1041, 1980.

Schulz SC: Dialysis in schizophrenia: a double-blind evaluation. Science. 211:1066–1068, 1981.

Shoor M, Adams IH: The intensive electroshock therapy of chronic disturbed psychotic patients. Am J Psychiat. 107:279–282, 1950.

Simmel E: Psychoanalytic treatment in a sanitorium. Int J Psychoanal. 10:70, 1929.

Simpson GM, Amuso D, Blair JH, Farkas T: Aspects of phenothiazine-produced extrapyramidal symptoms. Arch Gen Psychiat. 10:199–208, 1964.

Simpson GM, Pi EH, Sramek JJ: Adverse effects of antipsychotic agents. Drugs. 21:138–151, 1981.

Smith K, Surphilis WRP, Gynther MD: ECT-chlorpromazine and chlorpromazine compared in the treatment of schizophrenia. J Nerv Ment Dis. 144:284–290, 1967.

Spadoni AJ, Smith JA: Milieu therapy in schizophrenia. Arch Gen Psychiat. 20:547–547, 1969.

Stanton AH, Schwartz MS: The Mental Hospital. Basic Books, New York. 1954.

Stein LI, Test MA, Knoedler WH: The community treatment of schizophrenia. Unpublished manuscript. Available from L. I. Stein, Dept. of Psychiatry, University of Wisconsin, Center for Health Sciences, 600 Highland Ave., Madison, Wis. 53792.

Sullivan HS: Sociopsychiatric research: its implications for the schizophrenia problem and the mental hygienes. Am J Psychiat. 10:977, 1931.

Sullivan HS: Conceptions of Modern Psychiatry. William Alanson White Foundation, Washington, D.C. 1940.

Test MA, Stein LI: Alternative to mental hospital treatment. III. So. cost. Arch Gen Psychiat. 37:409–412, 1980.

Tourney G: A history of therapeutic fashions in psychiatry. Am J Psychiat. 124:784–796, 1967.

Treffert DA: Dying with their rights on. PRISM. 2:49–52, 1974.

Tyhurst L: Psychosocial first aid for refugees (an essay in social psychiatry). Mental Health Soc. 4:319–343, 1977.

Van Putten T: Milieu therapy: Contraindications?. Arch Gen Psychiat. 29:640, 1973.

Vaughn C, Leff JP: The influences of family and social factors on the course of psychiatric illness. Brit J Psychiat. 129:125, 1976.

Wagemaker H, Cade R: The use of hemodialysis in chronic schizophrenia. Am J Psychiat. 134:684–685, 1977.

Weisbrod BA, Test MA, Stein LI: Alternative to mental hospital treatment. II. Economic benefit-cost analysis. Arch Gen Psychiat. 37:400–405, 1980.

Wilmer HA: Social Psychiatry in Action. C. C. Thomas, Springfield, Ill. 1958.

Wing JK, Brown GW: Institutionalism and Schizophrenia. Cambridge University Press, London. 1970.

Yorkston N, Gruzeline J, Zaki S: Propranolol as an adjunct to the treatment of schizophrenia. In: Roberts, E, Ama cher, P (eds): Propranolol and Schizophrenia. Liss, New York. pp. 69–82, 1978.

Zeifert M: Results obtained from the administration 12,000 doses of Metrazol to mental patients. Psychiat Q. 15:772–778, 1941.

6 | Affective Disorders

ANDREA JACOBSON and
WILLIAM T. McKINNEY

The first part of this chapter is devoted to a discussion of general issues in the treatment of affective disorders. Then each of the DSM-III affective disorders is reviewed separately, with a summary of the essential diagnostic features followed by a review of current clinical practice in the treatment of the disorder. Where treatment has a relevant research base, it is summarized after clinical practice is discussed.

Psychopharmacological methods lend themselves to this approach because of the easy correspondence they often bear to DSM-III categories, e.g. antidepressants to major depression. Psychotherapeutic methods, however, are not usually keyed to specific affective disorders. We have therefore given a general discussion of psychotherapy for depression, presented under the treatment of dysthymic disorder, but certainly relevant to other affective disorders.

First, however, let us consider the more general issues.

THE NECESSITY FOR MORE THAN AN AFFECTIVE DISORDER (AXIS I) DIAGNOSIS IN TREATMENT PLANNING

While this chapter deals with the treatment of disorders, clinicians are concerned with the treatment of patients. The difference between a disorder and a patient is recognized in DSM III's admonition that it is a classification of disorders which individuals have, and not of the individuals themselves. A patient is no more adequately described as "a manic-depressive" than as "the ruptured spleen in the emergency room." Additional information is needed for adequate treatment planning.

Some of this additional information can be found on the other Axes of DSM-III. Axis IV, Severity of Psychosocial Stresses, is particularly relevant. Psychosocial stressors should be described on this Axis in terms of both severity and source, and a list of possible sources of stress is offered. Adequate coding requires a thorough inquiry into the patient's familial, occupational, social, material, and developmental circumstances. Another potent source of stress not specifically mentioned in DSM-III for Axis IV is role conflict. For example, familial and occupational role requirements may be reasonable when considered separately, but incompatible or overwhelming when joined.

Other kinds of information that are important for treatment planning are not included on any of the DSM-III axes. Interpersonal style, for example, is not central to Axis I diagnoses, which are expressed largely in intrapersonal terms. Important characteristics of interpersonal style are not described unless they are so abnormal as to warrant an Axis II character disorder diagnosis. Yet the differences between a dependent, talkative patient and a silent, withdrawing patient can be quite important in treatment planning. Several systems of describing interpersonal behavior exist, among which Benjamin's is notable for its precision, reliability, and face validity (Benjamin, 1979).

In the following discussion of choice of treatment and treatment goals, reference will be made to many kinds of additional information, as explained above.

TREATMENT GOALS

In the central part of this chapter, treatment goals are offered for each disorder. While the goals for treatment of a disorder may validly consist of reducing or eliminating the symptoms of the disorder, immediate symptom removal alone may well not be a sufficient goal for an individual patient. Overt manic symptoms may be adequately relieved by haloperidol and/or lithium, but if this was the fifth manic episode in the life of a patient who recurrently stops taking medications, then just treating the symptoms is clearly inadequate and the cause for discontinuation must be sought and dealt with.

Even long-term symptom removal may not be enough, however. We also need to consider the meaning and function of the symptoms in the patient's life situation. Klein (1976) discusses this issue quite explicitly and gives the following example: "The depression, and later the anger, of the woman trapped in an unsatisfying role . . . may be healthy steps in recognizing and doing something about a dehumanizing situation. In this case a reduction in pain is healthy only when accompanied by a change in role definition freely worked out by the individual woman." To treat just the symptoms of such a depression would be equivalent to turning off a ringing fire alarm and doing nothing about the fire. Teaching a patient whose depression is partially a response to his/her life situation to simply counteract depressive thoughts by self-control methods would deprive the patient of an accurate signal that he/she needs to effect some changes in that life situation. An adequate assessment of psychosocial stressors, as discussed above, should lead naturally to a more complete set of treatment goals that will help avoid a simplistic attack on the disorder or the symptoms alone.

Some clinicians formulate explicit treatment goals; others leave them implicit. In either case one must be sensitive to the patient's aspirations so that the formulation, implicit *or* explicit, is collaborative. In the short run, there may be differences (e.g. physical restraint of a violently manic patient will most likely not be a collaborative goal), but in the long run, if clinician and patient cannot establish common goals, the treatment may flounder.

Both clinician and patient also need to be aware of what have been termed "emergent treatment goals" (Gurman and Klein, 1980). The chief complaint at initial assessment may quickly give way to a more central concern that the patient could not present at first.

In summary, the treatment goals listed for each disorder provide a beginning point in the determination of adequate treatment goals for an individual patient. Psychosocial evaluation and the treatment process itself may determine other important treatment goals.

TREATMENT METHODS

In the discussion of specific affective disorders, treatment methods will be recommended for attaining the treatment goals for that disorder. As we have just noted, however, the goals for a patient may be somewhat different than the goals for the disorder. These different goals may then determine additional or alternative treatment methods. Marital therapy for reduction of marital stress may be added to the lithium maintenance that is intended to reduce the recurrence of affective episodes.

Other factors may modify the treatment of choice. Obviously, the patient's history and preference for mode of treatment may help shape treatment choice. Also, the various treatment modalities are not available everywhere. Cost, unfortunately, will place some treatment methods beyond the reach of some patients.

BIPOLAR DISORDER, MANIC (296.4)

ESSENTIAL FEATURES

The essential feature of *bipolar disorder, manic* is one or more manic episodes. The major finding in a manic episode is a distinct period when the predominant mood is either elevated, expansive, or irritable. In addition, other symptoms are associated with the manic syndrome, such as hyperactivity, pressure of speech, flight of ideas, inflated self-esteem, decreased need for sleep, distractibility, and excessive involvement in activities that have a high potential for painful consequences.

TREATMENT GOALS

For the severely manic patient, the first goal is prevention of harm to the patient, family, or community. Attention can then be turned to more specific goals, the first of which is restoration of normal mood and affect. The acutely manic patient's mood may be markedly elevated, expansive, or irritable (category A of DSM-III diagnostic criteria). Treatment should restore his/her ability to respond with a normal range of affect to the joys and sorrows of daily life. Other goals include the return to normality of whichever criteria from category B were abnormal: increased activity, increased talking, flight of ideas, inflated self-esteem, decreased sleep, distractibility, and reckless judgment.

Since bipolar disorders have a tendency to recur, education and consideration of long-term treatment goals should be introduced into treatment of the acute phase.

Research on mania has, thus far, been unable to evaluate the attainment of all these goals. Some early research focused on how a patient may be brought under control or improved (Entwistle et al., 1962; Rees and Davis, 1965). While this focus on control may at times be the clinician's necessary first concern, it should not be the only concern. As Shopsin (1979) points out:

> merely subduing the manifest belligerence, hostility, anger, irritability, quarrelsomeness, grandiosity, jocularity, unconventional speech and intolerance does not signify sufficient or acceptable control of the manic state; factors such as sleep, a more discreet appreciation of social participation and interaction, general performance . . . are necessary considerations.

Unfortunately, reliable measurement of these less blatant, but still very important, aspects of mania has been difficult. At least two groups have reported difficulty in getting their objective scales to distinguish patients who seem clinically to be quite different—e.g. the patient who is clinically ready for discharge may appear, on objective measures, no different from the one who remains uninhibited, glib, and self-satisfied (Platman, 1970; Shopsin et al., 1975). Thus, in the following discussion, the reader should keep in mind that *treatment* may often mean only treatment of the more florid aspects of mania.

TREATMENTS

Hospitalization

Choice of treatment locale precedes choice of treatment method in severely manic patients. The grandiosity, lack of insight, spending sprees, hypersexuality, irritability, and paranoia that can appear in severe mania threaten the well-being of the patient, his/her family, and the community. These dangers, plus the unreliability of many patients with manic disorder in cooperating with treatment, often make the hospital, with its structure and supervision, the optimal place for treatment. However, grandiosity, lack of insight, and paranoia may lead the patient to refuse hospitalization.

The law of most states now stipulates that patients cannot be committed to hospital care against their will unless their behavior is explicitly dangerous to themselves or others. The symptoms of manic disorder, alone, may or may not provide an adequate legal basis. The first appropriate legal step in some situations is the appointment of a financial guardian if the patient is disposing of funds in what the court finds to be a sufficiently bizarre manner—e.g. passing out hundred dollar bills to strangers in the belief that an infinite supply is available in the patient's bank account. Commitment itself depends on more stringent grounds. Patients may become immediately dangerous to themselves, as in attempting to fly out a third story window under the assumed protection of a divine power. Or patients may be dangerous to others, when irritability and paranoia lead them to physically attack someone "known" to be intent upon their destruction. In clear cases of dangerous behavior, the courts and police will usually intervene.

There are occasions when patients clearly need hospitalization for optimal treatment, but their behavior is not yet dangerous enough for the court to commit the patient for observation or treatment. In such a situation, the clinician can only continue to attempt to encourage adequate outpatient treatment, involving the family or support system so far as possible, and continue to observe the patient for either improvement or worsening to a stage at which commitment is legally possible.

Antipsychotic Drugs

Antipsychotic drugs are prescribed for the acutely manic patient because of their rapid effect in decreasing psychomotor excitement, agitation, aggressiveness, and assaultiveness. They are used to provide immediate control, and they act more rapidly than lithium. Treatment can be initiated with intramuscular haloperidol or chlorpromazine. The intramuscular route assures rapid onset of action and avoids uncertainty about whether the patient actually swallows the pills. For patients who consent to medication but refuse injections, liquid forms of both haloperidol and chlorpromazine are available. As mania decreases, the medication can be given in tablet form.

A major collaborative study supports this use of antipsychotics. (Prien et al., 1972). Four days of chlorpromazine produced a significant reduction in excitement and psychotic disorganization; after a week, grandiosity, hostility, and resistiveness had also decreased. These changes occurred more rapidly than in patients treated with lithium alone. The clinical adequacy, as opposed to statistical significance, of all these changes is not clear from the data, but it does seem clear that a noticeable change occurred. A similarly rapid course of response has been described with the use of haloperidol, in which many behavioral and psychomotor symptoms were controlled in three days (Shopsin, 1979).

Although haloperidol is widely used as the first treatment agent for acute mania, an adequate research literature on its specific therapeutic effects as well as the percentage of patients responding is not available.

Reports on the use of haloperidol have stressed its global efficacy in controlling the unmanageable aspects of severe mania. One study has further specified its effects (Shopsin et al., 1975). Anxiety, tension, mannerisms and posturing, grandiosity, unusual thought content, and excitement all decreased by an amount that seemed both statistically and clinically significant. Other dimensions of mania were also affected, but the clinical significance of these changes is less clear. These less affected aspects included hostility, uncooperativeness, suspiciousness, and conceptual disorganization. The authors themselves noted that even patients who on objective scales were improved sometimes retained inappropriate judgment that did not register on any of their measures, as for example the patient who was discreetly continuing his spending sprees via the ward telephone. They concluded that haloperidol covered over the mania but did not eliminate it. Other authors have disagreed with this evaluation of the limitations of haloperidol.

The percentage of manic patients that improve on antipsychotic drugs is not well documented. Two uncontrolled studies give figures of 83% and 100%, but their response criteria are not clear (Entwistle et al., 1962; Rees and Davis, 1965). In a VA-NIMH collaborative study, 14% of chlorpromazine-treated patients terminated because of poor clinical response, toxicity, or uncooperative behavior (Prien et al., 1972).

In summary, current research demonstrates the value of antipsychotics in rapidly controlling the more florid symptoms of most manic patients. The effects of antipsychotics on subtler aspects of mania are not clear. Their major role is probably to help control flagrant symptoms until lithium can begin to work.

Choice of antipsychotic drug. Haloperidol and chlorpromazine are the most commonly used agents. Thioridazine is usually avoided because of the retinal toxicity which can occur at the high doses sometimes needed for treatment of acute mania. The thioxanthines and other phenothiazines have not been critically evaluated in the treatment of mania. However, clinical experience as well as their pharmacological spectrum suggests that they would be effective.

Haloperidol is frequently preferred to chlorpromazine because of its relative freedom from hypotensive side effects, especially during intensive initial treatment, but this side effect must still be monitored. Chlorpromazine was reported in one study to be less effective than haloperidol on several aspects of mania, but further evidence is needed to establish the superiority of haloperidol.

Lithium. Lithium is clearly valuable and widely used in the treatment of acute mania. It appears to combat the same florid aspects of mania as antipsychotics, but with a slower onset of action. It may also relieve aspects of acute mania untouched by antipsychotics.

Several major reviews have confirmed the efficacy of lithium (Shopsin, 1979; Gerbino et al., 1978; Fieve, In Press). The exact nature of this efficacy is, however, more difficult to determine. Many of the studies reviewed have used either global or vague outcome measures. In the VA-NIMH collaborative study, the most significant changes were in excitement, elevated mood, and grandiosity, the more observable outward signs of mania (Prien et al., 1972). The authors note that their scales were not ideal for detecting changes in underlying mood. Another study demonstrated a similar reduction in grandiosity, hostility, uncooperativeness, unusual thought content, and excitement (Shopsin et al., 1975).

Many studies do not reveal the percentage of patients improving, but only record changes in an entire group's mean score on an outcome measure. However, Johnson and co-workers (1968) have reported a double-blind study in which 76% of patients on lithium responded well. This appears consistent with summaries of many studies, including uncontrolled and single-blind studies, where the composite improvement rate was 60–100% (Shopsin, 1979). We may conclude that while lithium is effective in the majority of patients with acute mania, there is a group of patients who do not respond. Thus, nonresponse to lithium does *not* mean that the patient is not suffering from bipolar disorder as it is currently defined.

It would be most desirable to predict which patients with mania would respond to lithium, and to spare nonresponders the risks and delay of an unsuccessful trial. At present, however, there is no well-established method to predict nonresponders.

Initiation of lithium treatment should be preceded by a careful medical evaluation, including medical history, physical evaluation, and BUN or creatinine and thyroid function, and any other studies as indicated by clinical state (electrolytes, electrocardiogram, etc.) Pregnancy, particularly during the first trimester, is a relative contraindication, and serious renal (Jefferson and Greist, 1979) or cardiac (Jefferson and Greist, 1979a) disease requires close medical supervision and consultation if lithium is to be used. Since lithium has a low therapeutic index, and its toxicity is not reliably predicted from the blood level in a specific patient, users must be carefully monitored clinically for signs of toxicity. Early signs include tremor, nausea, and blurred vision. Later signs include ataxia, slurred speech, nystagmus, hyperreflexivity, vomiting, and changes in consciousness that can progress from confusion and disorientation, lethargy, or excitement, to stupor, coma, and death (Jefferson and Greist, 1978).

Lithium administration is governed by the attempt to produce a therapeutic blood level without incurring toxicity. For acute mania, blood levels of 1.2 mEq and above have been considered appropriate, but there is substantial variability among patients in both therapeutic levels and capacity to tolerate high doses. Lithium is given orally, twice or three times per day. Starting dosages are usually 600–900 mg/day, with increments over several days until a therapeutic level is reached. Blood samples for monitoring blood level should be drawn as near 12 hours after the last evening dose as possible, and *before* the morning dose.

The reader unfamiliar with the details of lithium use is referred to more extensive discussions (Jefferson and Greist, 1977; Baldessarini, 1977; Johnson, 1980).

Electroconvulsive Therapy (ECT)
ECT was formerly used in the treatment of acute mania. With the introduction of successful drug therapy, its use has decreased. There is only a small literature on ECT in bipolar disorder, and there are no well-controlled studies. Open studies and anecdotal reports describe reliable results (Fink, 1979); in the absence of reliable research data, however, ECT is best considered a therapy to be resorted to when antipsychotics and/or lithium are unsuccessful or contraindicated and severe mania requires immediate treatment.

Psychotherapy
Most schools of psychotherapy do not address the treatment of mania. The acutely manic patient, with flight of ideas, pressured speech, and grandiosity, is indeed an unlikely candidate for most psychotherapies. The patient is relatively inaccessible to verbal interaction, and is particularly disruptive in any group psychotherapy. There is a limited psychoanalytic literature concerning these patients (Ginsberg and Marks, 1977). While analysis is clearly no longer a primary treatment method, this literature does contain many insights into therapeutic relationships with these patients which are applicable to nonpsychoanalytic treatment.

BIPOLAR DISORDER, DEPRESSED (296.5)

ESSENTIAL FEATURES

The essential feature of *bipolar disorder, depressed*, is one or more manic episodes and a current main depressive episode. The main finding in a major depressive episode is either depressed mood or loss of interest or pleasure in all or almost all usual activities and pastimes. This disturbance is prominent, relatively persistent, and associated with other symptoms of the depressive syndrome. These symptoms include appetite disturbance, change in weight, sleep disturbance, psychomotor agitation or retardation, decreased energy, feelings of worthlessness or guilt, difficulty concentrating or thinking, and thoughts of death or suicidal attempts.

TREATMENT GOALS

If the patient is severely depressed, the first treatment goal is prevention of suicide. Suicide evaluation is discussed in the section on major depression, p. 201. The other treatment goals are similar to those described for major depression, pp. 201–202. Since bipolar disorder has a known tendency to recur, education and consideration of long-term treatment goals should be part of treatment during the acute phase. After remission of the depressive episode, the clinician must be alert for signs of hypomania.

TREATMENTS

Antidepressants
When a patient who has already been diagnosed as having a bipolar disorder becomes depressed while receiving adequate lithium medication, antidepressants are usually added to the drug regimen. If the patient is not taking lithium when the depression occurs, but appears by history to be suffering from a clear bipolar disorder, many clinicians would start antidepressants and then add lithium.

Research on the efficacy of antidepressants has not, in general, distinguished their action on patients with a bipolar disorder depressed phase, from their action on patients with major depression. There are, to our knowledge, no good studies of the efficacy of tricyclic antidepressants (TCAs) specifically in bipolar, depressed patients. For a discussion of TCAs in major depression, the reader is referred to p. 202. The validity of extrapolating from the studies cited there, many of which included mixed diagnostic groups, to this diagnostic category, is unknown. Monoamine Oxidase Inhibitors (MAOIs) have not been used very much for bipolar, depressed patients. There is a small literature suggesting a combination of lithium and MAOIs for refractory depression (Himmelhoch et al., 1972) but this treatment is not well established. A patient with bipolar disorder who becomes depressed while receiving adequate lithium therapy and does not respond to the addition of tricyclic antidepressants may be a candidate for MAOIs or ECT.

Lithium
Lithium may be effective in the treatment of depressive episodes. A recent, thorough review of the relevant research concluded that "there is suggestive evidence of an antidepressant effect in a certain subgroup of bipolar patients," but also that "more investigation is needed before any serious claims for lithium as an antidepressant can be justified" (Gerbino et al., 1978).

ECT
ECT is reported to have been widely used for this disorder in the past, but there is no well-controlled research on its efficacy. The reader is referred to the discussion of ECT in major depression, pp. 207–208.

Psychotherapies
Most psychotherapeutic discussions of depression do not distinguish bipolar disorder, depressed phase, from other depressions. The psychoanalytic sources mentioned above are an exception to this. The reader is referred to these sources and to the discussion of psychotherapy for major depression below.

Other Treatments
Although some physicians use antianxiety agents to treat the anxiety often present in depression, their use should be conservative and time limited.

While antipsychotic drugs have been advocated for the treatment of depressions accompanied by delusions, there is controversy about whether they should be used alone or in combination with antidepressants.

Summary

The tricyclic antidepressants are generally accepted as the treatment of choice for a depressive episode of bipolar disorder. They may decrease the intensity of the episode and/or shorten the length of the episode. Lithium may also be effective, but in actual practice many of these patients are already being treated with lithium when the depressive episode occurs. The research basis for choosing treatments of the depressive phase of bipolar disorder is weaker than for the treatment of the manic phase, and reliable information is not available on what percentage of patients respond, and in what ways. Empirically, the following steps are appropriate:

1. Be sure lithium levels are in therapeutic range.
2. Reevaluate for situational determinants
3. Add a tricyclic antidepressant
4. Use either MAOI or ECT if not responsive to tricyclics

MAINTENANCE OF REMISSION IN BIPOLAR DISORDER

A patient can be considered to be in good remission under treatment if four to six months have elapsed since the last depressive or manic episode. The clinician and patient must then decide whether to continue treatment, and, if so, how to conduct the treatment. Many patients with bipolar disorder *are* candidates for maintenance treatment, but since a recommendation of long-term medication has important psychiatric, medical, and legal implications, the decisions should be careful and informed on the part of both clinician and patient.

The therapeutic question is, as always, whether the benefits are worth the costs and risks of treatment. In evaluating the benefits of treatment, the clinician must consider the natural history of the disorder, the history of how the disorder has manifested itself in the patient, and the effectiveness of the maintenance treatments available. The natural history of bipolar disorder is discussed in DSM-III. While there is a clear tendency toward frequent recurrence, the period between episodes can vary widely from patient to patient, and in some patients there may be no recurrences. (One manic episode justifies a diagnosis of bipolar disorder, manic episode in DSM-III.) This variability in the natural history of the disorder makes the individual patient's history particularly important. The patient who is experiencing a fifth affective episode in three years is a much stronger candidate for maintenance therapy than the one who is experiencing a second affective episode following an initial episode eight years before. By considering both the natural history of the disorder and the history of the individual patient, the clinician can make an informed estimate of the risk of recurrence in the future. The clinician's estimate of the probability of recurrence must then be weighted by how much the patient (and in some cases the community) wants to avoid such a recurrence. A busy, competitive administrator may care much more about avoiding a moderate depression than would some other people. Hypomania may be so pleasurable to some that the risk of depression seems well worth taking. If the patient does not seriously desire a decrease in affective episodes, the most carefully planned treatment program will probably fail.

When the risk and relative cost of recurrences have been clarified, then the clinician must present the treatment alternatives and describe, insofar as possible, their likelihood of decreasing recurrences and the aspects of recurrences they may decrease. The patient may know what sorts of approaches have worked in the past in his/her own case. Thus, the potential benefit of treatment can be estimated.

Every treatment has its risks, such as adverse drug reactions, and costs. The patient will know how the risks and costs appear in the context of his/her own life. Monthly expenditures for medication may be merely tax deductions, or they may be a heavy strain on a poverty-level budget. Weekly treatment may mean arranging to leave the office for one patient, or for another it may mean finding a babysitter for five young children and taking two crosstown buses in the wintertime. Being a chronic patient may or may not be acceptable. If the costs and risks *as they appear to the patient* are too high, treatment will founder; thus, they need to be realistically assessed and dealt with early in treatment.

In summary, clinician and patient must consider the risks of recurrence if the disorder is untreated, the costs and risks of treatment, and the potential benefits of treatment. The family and/or other relevant persons may need to be included in these considerations.

For the patient with bipolar disorder who has severe recurrences, the decision for lithium maintenance should be straightforward, although often it is not. In other cases, though, collaborative analysis should lead both to better decisions and an increased probability that the patient, having participated in the decision, will participate in the treatment.

The patient's family is often important in planning for treatment during remission. Family members can provide information not otherwise readily available to the clinician, as, for example, in recalling the social and financial costs of a manic episode that the patient no longer clearly remembers. The family's concerns about the disorder, including its possible progression, genetic origins, or even whether they may have caused it, all need to be discussed. Their cooperation with an ongoing treatment program can be important in ensuring compliance with appointments and medication and in recognizing the early symptoms of recurrent manic or depressive episodes.

Treatments

The following discussion of specific treatment methods for bipolar disorder in remission will not be subdivided according to whether the last episode was manic, depressive, or mixed. While these distinctions clearly have implications for the first months after resolution, and perhaps for the longer course as well, clinical research is not yet sufficiently precise to justify making such distinctions here.

Antipsychotics. Antipsychotic drugs are sometimes added to a lithium regimen at the first signs of hypomania in the hope of averting a manic episode. Occasionally, an antipsychotic drug is used with lithium when neither alone suffices. There have been reports of neurological toxicity due to combined lithium and haloperiodol, although these are uncontrolled case reports often involving patients with preexisting neurological disorders.

Antipsychotics are not currently used alone as a routine maintenance medication for bipolar disorder. This is due to the effectiveness of lithium for this purpose (see pp. 198–199), the reluctance of many patients to remain on chronic antipsychotic drugs, and the recognition of tardive dyskinesia as a potential complication of long-term antipsychotic medication.

Antianxiety drugs—not used.

Antidepressants. Antidepressants may be of value in preventing recurrences of depressive episodes in patients with bipolar disorder, particularly if the patient is continuing to have depressive episodes on adequate lithium medication. Many clinicians hesitate to use tricyclic antidepressants alone, when there is a previous history of mania, because a manic episode may be precipitated following resolution of the depression. This risk does not represent an absolute contraindication to their use in combination with lithium, if the patient is monitored carefully for hypomania and adequate lithium levels are maintained.

Research in this area is limited. One phase of the VA-NIMH collaborative study followed 44 bipolar disorder patients for two years after a depressive episode and compared the effects of lithium, imipramine, and placebo (Prien et al., 1973). While the report does not focus on the efficacy of imipramine in decreasing depressive episodes, nevertheless, the frequency of severe depressive recurrences for the three treatment groups was noted: none in the imipramine group, 12% of the lithium group, and 55% of the placebo group had severe depressive episodes. Thus, imipramine clearly decreased the incidence of severe depression, defined in this study as an episode requiring hospitalization or alteration of treatment. The possibility of a residium of less severe depressive episodes even in imipramine-treated patients is suggested by the authors' comment that many patients in the study who did not meet the stringent criteria for recurrence of an affective episode nevertheless "did have periods of mild or moderately severe symptomatology."

The authors also report an increased incidence of mania in patients treated with imipramine alone (67% compared with 33% of placebo-treated patients and 12% of lithium-treated patients).

In summary, tricyclic antidepressants (or MAOIs) are a reasonable choice as additional maintenance medication in a patient who is at substantial risk for severe depressive recurrences even on lithium. The research base for this treatment regimen needs further development. See p. 203 for discussion of clinical use of TCAs, p. 205 for MAOIs.

Lithium. Lithium, as discussed above, is the treatment of choice for acute manic phases of bipolar disorder. Its value in decreasing recurrent manic episodes is also well established, making it the treatment of choice for maintenance. The details of this clinical usage have been well described (Jefferson and Greist, 1977).

Numerous reviews document the efficacy of lithium for this purpose (Davis, 1976; Gerbino et al., 1978; Klerman, 1978). Phase 2 of the VA-NIMH collaborative study (Prien et al., 1973b) followed 205 bipolar disorder patients treated with lithium or placebo for two years after a manic episode. The rate of severe relapse for lithium-treated patients was half the rate for placebo-treated patients. Even with lithium treatment, however, 31% of the patients were hospitalized at least once, and another 12% required a change in medication. Manic or depressive symptoms not severe enough to require a change in medication were not noted. Thus, it is quite clear that lithium is of substantial value in decreasing the number of severe manic episodes, although some patients will continue to have such episodes and many will continue to have less severe manic symptoms.

The value of lithium in decreasing depressive episodes has been increasingly acknowledged by clinicians. However, among reviewers, there is a range of opinion; some believe that lithium has "highly significant prophylactic effects" against depression in bipolar patients (Gerbino et al., 1978) while others believe that the evidence is increasing but not yet conclusive (Klerman, 1978). Review of this literature is complicated by the fact that many studies of lithium prophylaxis did not distinguish between recurrence rates of manic and depressive episodes. Data from remaining studies strongly suggest that lithium decreases depressive recurrences. The VA-NIMH study discussed above, for example, reported a depressive recurrence rate of 12% for patients on lithium, versus 55% for patients on placebo. There were, however, only 17 lithium patients and 9 placebo patients in this phase of the study. More evidence is also needed to establish optimum lithium levels for the prevention of depressive episodes.

In summary, lithium is clearly valuable for the long-term treatment of patients with bipolar disorder in decreasing the frequency and severity of manic episodes and probably also of depressive episodes. Not all well-diagnosed bipolar disorder patients will respond to lithium maintenance therapy, and some may respond only partially. It is currently not possible to predict the responders. The effects of lithium maintenance on hypomanic and milder depressive symptoms is not clear.

Other drug treatments. Carbamazepine (Tegretal), a drug useful in treating temporal lobe epilepsy, has been shown to have antimanic and antidepressant effects in two double-blind controlled studies (Okuma et al., 1979; Ballenger and Post, 1980). Some patients whose mania was not controlled by lithium and neuroleptics improved when carbamazepine was added to their drug regimen. This treatment remains experimental and should not be employed unless other treatments have failed and the physician is experienced in its use.

Psychotherapy. Most schools of psychotherapy do not discuss long-term treatment of patients with bipolar disorder. The psychoanalytic discussion of these patients is mentioned on p. 192. There is an interesting report on group therapy of couples in conjunction with lithium in the treatment of married bipolar patients (Davenport et al., 1977). Comparison of this treatment with lithium alone and referral back to a community clinic suggested benefits in terms of family interaction, monitoring of early affective episodes, and decreased hospitalization. More research is needed to establish the value of this approach.

Summary

The treatment of bipolar disorder in remission begins with a thorough evaluation of the need for maintenance therapy. If it is indicated, lithium is the drug treatment of choice, particularly to decrease manic episodes. Antidepressants may be useful in patients who continue to have depressive episodes while they are on lithium, and antipsychotics may be used to ward off manic episodes that appear to be developing. Psychotherapy may prove useful in maintaining remission, treating the milder aspects of affective episodes during remission of the most disruptive aspects, and supporting the chronically disabled patient. The efficacy of psychotherapy for these purposes has not been demonstrated in controlled research.

MAJOR DEPRESSION, SINGLE EPISODE (296.2X)

ESSENTIAL FEATURES

The essential feature of *major depression, single episode*, is a major depressive episode with no history of a prior major depressive, manic, or hypomanic episode. The major finding in a major depressive episode is either depressed mood or loss of interest or pleasure in all or almost all usual activities and pastimes. This disturbance is prominent, relatively persistent, and associated with other symptoms of the depressive syndrome. These symptoms include appetite disturbance, change in weight, sleep disturbance, psychomotor agitation or retardation, decreased energy, feelings of worthlessness or guilt, difficulty concentrating or thinking, and thoughts of death or suicide attempts.

Treatment Goals

One of the first decisions to be made when a patient has a major depression is whether the patient is suicidal. If so, prevention of suicide becomes the first goal of treatment and takes priority over other goals in determining locale and method of treatment. The determination of suicidal risk is a well-discussed psychiatric topic, and lists of possible risk factors are available (Greist and Greist, 1979).

If a patient is judged to be suicidal, then the locale of treatment must be matched to the degree of suicidality. How closely the patient should be watched must be carefully weighed. If a patient is mildly suicidal, but has a network of supportive friends and family, some hopes for the future, and the capacity to make a firm agreement with the therapist to enter into treatment and contact the therapist or an emergency service if suicidal thoughts increase, then the therapist may reasonably take the risk of treating the person as an outpatient. A more severely suicidal patient, hopeless, eager to die, and one who lacks a social support system should be hospitalized. Once hospitalized, such a patient must still be closely observed. A thorough evaluation of suicide risk, including both current status and past history, will help the clinician take appropriate precautions and decide on a course of treatment.

The issues of suicide evaluation and appropriate treatment become more complicated when the patient is chronically or recurrently suicidal. For these patients, repeated hospitalizations may well be appropriate. With some patients, however, repeated, frequent hospitalizations for suicidal risk may be a sign that the hospitalization provides secondary gain to the patient, family, or others in the patient's social system. When the therapist suspects such a possibility, inclusion of family members or others may clarify the situation and help avoid angry acting-out, by either patient or therapist.

After dealing with the issue of suicide, physician and patient can begin to consider other treatment goals. The dysphoric mood or loss of interest in daily activities that is central to the diagnosis is also central to the treatment. In some depressions, significant family or social stressors are known to contribute to the depression. The effects of these stressors must be alleviated if treatment is to be successful over the long term. Interventions can be made to rearrange the patient's social system and thereby decrease stress, to increase the patient's ability to cope with the stress, or preferably both. A severely depressed woman who has been isolated for several years with three young children and a blind, senile mother-in-law may need antidepressants. But she also needs social and family support to relieve her overburdened situation, as well as help in learning to set limits on the amount of work she can and will do for others.

Tricyclic Antidepressants

TCAs are the drug treatment of choice for most major depressions. Several major reviews have summarized the many double-blind, placebo-controlled studies that support the efficacy of TCAs in depression. Improvement is reported in about 60–70% of patients treated with TCAs compared with 30–40% of those treated with placebos (Klerman and Cole, 1965; Kessler, 1978). However, there are limitations to these studies. Patients with different kinds of depression have sometimes been mixed together. In some cases, depression was not even the primary diagnosis. Among the patients diagnosed as depressed, some were termed psychotic and some neurotic. Diagnostic criteria were often not included in the primary research reports. Thus, it is impossible to sort out from these reviews what percentage of patients with major depression, as defined by the DSM-III category, respond to TCAs. In such a well-defined group it may well be higher than the 60–70% response rate reported for the mixed group. Possible identification of biologic markers of different subtypes of depression which are responsive to different treatments is receiving increasing attention and may yield better outcomes (Carroll et al., 1981).

The specific aspects of depression that improve with tricyclic treatment also need further clarification. Early improvement of sleep patterns, followed by resolution of appetite disturbance and suicidal thoughts, has been reported (Haskell et al., 1975). After these changes, the patient may look more animated to the observer, but continue to feel quite depressed. An effect on mood and activity level may not be seen before two to four weeks of treatment with tricyclics.

Although DSM-III does not provide a separate diagnostic category for severely depressed patients with mood-congruent delusions, clinical experience suggests that these patients may be unusually resistant to treatment with TCAs alone. Reviews of the literature support this impression (Minter and Mandel, 1979; Kantor and Glasman, 1977). Quitkin et al.

(1978) have disagreed, stating that imipramine is effective for delusional patients.

It has been suggested that paranoid delusions imply poorer response to TCAs alone than do somatic or nihilistic delusions (Minter and Mandel, 1979; Minter and Mandel, 1979a). This remains to be confirmed, as does the proposed separation of delusional major depression into a depressive component responsive to antidepressant therapy and a delusional component responsive to antipsychotic therapy (Nelson and Bowers, 1978).

Pending further research, a reasonable treatment of choice for delusional major depression is either ECT or a combination of antidepressant and antipsychotic medication.

Clinical Use of TCAs

Choice of drug. Although numerous TCAs are on the market, there is no clear evidence for the superiority of any one. As in other areas of clinical psychopharmacology, the clinician may have to choose among the TCAs largely on the basis of side effects. The choice is also determined by past response or lack of response to a particular TCA, especially in patients but also in family members.

Imipramine is the TCA in longest use. Amitriptyline and imipramine are the most well-researched. Since amitriptyline has the greatest sedative and anticholinergic side effects, some clinicians have proposed its preferential use in agitated depression, but this has not been conclusively established by research. Desipramine, nortriptyline, and protriptyline have less sedative and anticholinergic side effects. Doxepin may have somewhat less cardiotoxicity, but this is not well established (Jefferson and Greist, 1979a).

Some current research is aimed at predicting which TCA a patient is most likely to respond to. TCAs affect at least two neurotransmitters; serotonin and norepinephrine. There is a hypothesis that serotonergic TCAs (e.g. amitriptyline) work best in patients with low pretreatment levels of the serotonin metabolites (5-HIAA), and that noradrenergic TCAs (e.g. desipramine) are best for patients with low pretreatment levels of the norepinephrine metabolites, (MHPG). While some studies support this hypothesis (Goodwin et al., 1978), others do not (Coppen et al., 1979). The clinical value of the hypothesis remains to be determined.

Monitoring plasma levels. It is well established that after the same dose of a TCA, different patients may show a ten- to twenty-fold variation in

Table 6-1.
Representative Tricyclic Antidepressants

Generic Name	Trade Name	Usual Starting Dose (mg/day)	Maximum Daily Dose (mg)
Tertiary amines			
Amitriptyline	Elavil, Endep Etrafon	25 to 75	300
Imipramine	Tofranil	25 to 75	300
Doxepin	Adapin, Sinequan	25 to 75	300
Trimipramine	Surmantil	25 to 75	300
Secondary amines			
Desipramine	Norpramin, Pertofrane	25 to 75	300
Nortriptyline	Aventyl, Pamelor	20 to 40	200
Other tricyclics			
Protriptyline	Vivactil	10 to 20	60
Amoxapine	Asendin	50 to 100	600

plasma levels, with some of the variation possibly related to genetic factors or to the use of other CNS-active drugs (Kessler, 1978). Many patients on standard doses do not have adequate blood levels.

The interpretation of plasma levels is not, however, entirely straightforward. Nortriptyline, for example, may show a "therapeutic window" phenomenon, in which levels both above and below this range are associated with a poor clinical response (Asberg, 1974). Imipramine, on the other hand, has not been shown to have such a therapeutic window.

The main clinical indication for checking plasma levels has in the past been nonresponse to an apparently adequate TCA trial in order to ascertain that the lack of response is not due to poor absorption or rapid metabolism of the drug. Plasma-level determination is not well enough established to "fine tune" doses, but it may be helpful in checking compliance, providing a rough idea of magnitude of overdose, managing pharmacological and psychological side effects, and, for drugs with a therapeutic window, being certain that the dose is neither too high or too low.

Dose and dosage schedule. Tricyclic antidepressants are given in low initial dose followed by regular increases (see Table 6-1). In determining

TABLE 6-2.
SIDE-EFFECTS OF TRICYCLIC ANTIDEPRESSANTS

	FREQUENT	INFREQUENT
Sympathomimetic	Tachycardia	Agitation
	Tremor	Insomnia
	Sweating	Aggravation of psychosis
Anticholinergic	Blurred vision	Aggravation of glaucoma
	Constipation	
	Urinary hesitancy	Paralytic ileus
	Fuzzy thinking	Urinary retention
		Delirium
Cardiovascular	Orthostatic hypotension	Delayed cardiac conduction
	Electrocardiogram abnormalities	Arrhythmias
		Cardiomyopathy
		Sudden death
Neurological	Paresthesias	Seizures
	Electroencephalogram alterations	
Allergic/toxic		Cholestatic jaundice
		Agranulocytosis
Metabolic/endocrine	Weight gain	Gynecomastia
	Sexual disturbances	Amenorrhea

the rate of dosage increase, the therapeutic benefit of quickly reaching an effective level must be balanced against side effects. In older patients with decreased metabolism, lower initial doses are appropriate, as is a slower increase in dosage. The final upper limit will be determined by either the appearance of intolerable side effects, the appearance of a therapeutic response, or the upper limit of safety for the particular TCA.

The reader is referred to detailed discussions (Greist and Greist, 1979; Hollister, 1978) of possible contraindications (e.g. arrhythmias, seizures, glaucoma, and others) and of the various side effects, including sedative and anticholinergic ones (see Table 6-2). A single evening dose may reduce the prominence of the side effects and, in a patient with insomnia, make good use of the sedative effects.

Monoamine Oxidase Inhibitors (MAOIs)
The MAOIs are sometimes used in the treatment of major depression when a trial of one or perhaps two different categories of TCAs has

TABLE 6-3.

TREATMENT: MONOAMINE OXIDASE INHIBITORS

GENERIC NAME	TRADE NAME	USUAL STARTING DOSE	USUAL THERAPEUTIC DAILY DOSE
Phenelzine	Nardil	15 mg t.i.d.	60–90 mg
Isocarboxazid	Marplan	10 mg b.i.d.	30 mg
Tranylcypromine	Parnate	10 mg b.i.d.	30 mg

proven ineffective. The most widely used MAOI is phenelzine. Although it is often given in a dosage of 30–45 mg/day, this may be only marginally effective for most adult patients (Robinson et al., 1978). Many adult patients may require 60–90 mg/day for good effect (see Table 6–3 for MAOI dosage suggestion). Dietary restrictions are necessary, especially for foods containing large amounts of tyramine (Robinson et al., 1963). Drug effect is often detectable by 14 days, sometimes as early as seven days, and substantial improvement is usually noted by four weeks, although positive response may occur even later.

Research on the MAOIs has been more limited than on the tricyclic antidepressants and has tended to include mainly outpatients. Klein suggested that MAOIs are especially useful for "atypical depression." This phrase refers not to an unusual type of depression, but rather to a depression with symptoms different from those that have been termed vegetative signs of endogenous depression: weight loss, sleep loss, crying spells, psychomotor retardation. Patients with atypical depression are said to show more anxiety, a variety of somatic complaints, and "neurotic signs" such as phobias, hysterical personality, and self-pity (Robinson et al., 1978). It is possible, but not yet firmly demonstrated, that these are the patients who respond best to MAOIs.

The response of such patients to MAOIs was characterized in one study as improvement in either physiological symptoms (anxiety, somatic complaints) or observable psychomotor symptoms (retardation, agitation, irritability) (Robinson et al., 1973). Subjective and ideational symptoms (depressed mood, guilt, suicidal ideation, nihilistic ideation, psychic anxiety, phobic anxiety) tended not to improve.

In summary, it is fairly well documented that MAOIs are more effective than placebo in some depressed patients. There is some suggestion that patients with predominantly somatic, motor symptoms are helped more than other depressed patients. While these patients are sometime said to be suffering from "atypical depression," it must be noted that the DSM-III category *atypical depression* (296.82) refers to a residual group of depressions of several different sorts, and *not* specifically to these patients.

Antipsychotics

In the 1960s antipsychotics were suggested as the treatment of choice for anxious or agitated depressions. Subsequent research has not supported this proposal. Antipsychotics are now recommended for major depression only as a temporary supplement to control psychosis or marked agitation until other treatments take effect, or as an alternative treatment for agitated depression unresponsive to antidepressants (Greist and Greist, 1979).

Stimulants

There is no evidence from controlled studies for long-term benefits of treatment with stimulants, and numerous bad side effects can occur (Greist and Greist, 1979).

Lithium

Lithium is not a widely accepted pharmacological treatment for major depression. While it is probably effective in some cases, it is not as often effective as with bipolar disorder, depressed phase and even that use is not firmly established (Jefferson and Greist, 1977). There are some preliminary suggestions that lithium levels must be kept high to be effective in the treatment of major depression, (above 1.0 mEq/l) (Jefferson and Greist, 1977). The patient must be monitored closely for toxicity at these levels. At present, lithium should be considered for use in the treatment of major depression only when more established methods have failed.

Electroconvulsive Therapy (ECT)

Following the introduction of ECT in the late 1930's by Cerletti and Bini, it soon became a standard somatic therapy for a variety of psychiatric illnesses. It has tended to be underutilized or overutilized, depending on the orientation of the clinician.

At the time ECT was introduced, modern-day methods of conducting clinical trials were not prominent; therefore, ECT has not been subjected to as many rigorously controlled studies as have antidepressant drugs. There are obvious problems with doing such studies, yet there have been several interesting approaches. The following summary statements can be made regarding the role of ECT in the treatment of major depressions.

1. A number of well-done studies as well as clinical experience strongly suggest the efficacy of ECT in severe depression. It is at least as effective as tricyclic antidepressants and in some cases it is more effective.

2. It is not clear yet whether there are subgroups of depressives that respond only to ECT and not to antidepressant drugs. There have been controversial findings about the possible ECT specificity in delusional depressives.

3. If, for reasons of convenience, patient acceptability, or other factors, drugs are tried first, it should be kept in mind that some patients with major depressions who do not respond to drugs may respond to ECT.

4. No "dose–response curve" has been determined for ECT. There is no evidence that extending the course of therapy beyond the recommended number of treatments will yield better clinical results and prevent relapse. Most patients require six to nine treatments.

5. Virtually all studies point to the equal therapeutic efficacy of unilateral ECT (nondominant hemisphere) in comparison with bilateral ECT. Also, it has been shown to produce less memory disturbance as a side effect.

6. The mortality rate with modern techniques is minimal (.008% to .05%) (Turek and Hanlon, 1977; Fink, 1979). However, ECT is a specialized treatment technique and should be used only by psychiatrists with demonstrated skills who use it regularly.

Such brief summary statements can scarcely do justice to this complicated topic. The reader is referred to a recent task force report of the American Psychiatric Association for further information on electroconvulsive therapy (American Psychiatric Association) (1978) and to Fink (1979). Squire (1977) has reviewed the ECT and memory loss issue.

Psychotherapy
Psychotherapy of depression is discussed primarily under dysthymic disorder (pp. 214–225). In a relatively homogeneous group of patients diag-

nosed as having a primary major depression by RDC criteria (which are quite similar to DSM-III criteria), a comparison of interpersonal psychotherapy (see p. 218) with TCA treatment suggested equal overall effectiveness (DiMascio et al., 1979). The TCA dosage used, however, may not have been sufficient for optimal results in all patients. Significant effects on overall depression appeared by the fourth week of psychotherapy, with apathy and anxiety/depression sometimes improved in the first week. While the authors do not discuss the clinical significance of the changes, the quantitative difference after psychotherapy seems large enough to be clinically noticeable.

Combination of Somatic and Psychotherapeutic Treatment
A combination of antidepressants and some form of psychotherapy is common in the current treatment of patients with major depression. The type and frequency of psychotherapy vary. Many clinicians believe that patients do better with both psychotherapy and antidepressant drugs than with either alone. There is research support for this belief. DiMascio et al. (1979) found greater overall improvement when acute major depression was treated with both amitriptyline and interpersonal psychotherapy. Not only was the difference between combined and single treatment substantial, but also the percentage of patients completing the 16-week treatment was noticeably higher with the combined treatment (67% of patients receiving both treatments vs. 48% for psychotherapy alone, 33% for drug therapy alone, and 30% in a nonscheduled treatment-on-demand group).

Most clinicians do not combine ECT and psychotherapy, believing that the transient organicity often produced by ECT interferes with psychotherapy.

MAJOR DEPRESSION, SINGLE EPISODE: RECOVERY PHASE

The issue here is the proper treatment of patients in whom the signs of major depression are remitting. The course of recovery from depression is known to be uneven, with brief returns of dysphoria, suicidal ideation, marital stress, etc. What kind of treatment should such a patient receive, and for how long?

It is important to distinguish the patient who experiences a relapse during the recovery phase from the patient with true recurrent depression. This distinction is reflected in the choice between the DSM-III categories major depression, single episode, and major depression, recurrent. While DSM-III itself does not suggest how to distinguish relapses from recurrences, one criterion that has been offered elsewhere is that a true recurrence must be preceded by a symptom-free interval of 6 to 12 months (Klerman, 1978). Relapses then, would refer to the return of symptoms during the 6- to 12-month recovery phase following the initial episode.

Treatment Goals

The goals of treatment in the recovery period include both the original and emergent goals, and the prevention of relapse. Klerman (1978), summarizing 11 studies, concluded that 65% of depressed patients experience some degree of relapse within the first year if they are untreated or receiving only placebo during that period. It is not possible to predict which patients will relapse, nor how severe the relapse would be.

Antidepressant drugs. Current clinical practice is to continue TCAs at a maintenance dose level for 6 to 12 months after an adequate response has occurred and then slowly taper off the dose.

Recent reviews support the value of this continuation therapy (Quitkin et al., 1976; Klerman, 1978). Various studies report that the relapse rate, usually defined as readmission or need to alter treatment, can be reduced 20 to 50% by continuation therapy. In a typical study, for example, the relapse rate was reduced from 50% to 22% (Mindham et al., 1973).

It would be ideal to be able to predict which patients need this continuation therapy, and thus avoid the unnecessary treatment (drug and psychotherapy) of many patients. One study suggested that patients who, despite a good response to antidepressants, still felt they had some remaining symptoms were the ones who most benefited from the continuation therapy (Mindham et al., 1973). Another study comparing amitryptyline and placebo has supported an eight-month period of continuation treatment (Coppen et al., 1978). The individual patient's history of recovery from any previous depression, as well as the risks of recurrence inherent in his/her psychosocial situation, may help determine whether continuation therapy is indicated.

Since most of the relevant literature deals with relapse as the outcome measure, it is not known whether continuation therapy is of benefit to patients in eliminating less extreme recurring manifestations of depression during the recovery phase.

In summary, tricyclics have been shown to help prevent a major relapse in some patients recovering from a major depressive episode, and they may benefit other patients in subtler ways. In view of the low risk of this limited period of extended usage, continuation therapy is recommended after a simple episode of major depression.

Lithium. Since lithium is not a common treatment for the acute phase of major depression, its use in the recovery phase has not been defined.

ECT. Some clinicians give ECT-treated patients a few more ECT treatments immediately after remission of the major depression, in hope of stabilizing the remission. The value of this practice is not established.

Psychotherapy. Generalizations cannot be readily made about psychotherapy during the recovery phase. Both type and duration of therapy depend on the specific issues involved with a given patient, and the diagnosis itself does not dictate one or another form of therapy. Research in this area is very limited.

MAJOR DEPRESSION, RECURRENT (296.3x)

ESSENTIAL FEATURES

The essential feature of *major depression, recurrent* is a major depressive episode in an individual who has had a previous major depressive episode but has never had a manic or hypomanic episode. Since these patients may be vulnerable to future episodes of major depressions, one of the goals of therapy must be the ultimate decrease in such episodes.

ANTIDEPRESSANTS

There is no well-defined clinical practice regarding the use of TCAs in recurrent depression. An increasing number of clinicians simply maintain patients on chronic medication. Others try, after each episode, to discontinue the drug after an adequate continuation phase (see above) and watch closely for recurrence.

Research in this area provides limited evaluation of either the benefits of long-term use of TCAs or the medical/psychological risks. A major collaborative study (Prien et al., 1973) suggested that rehospitalization decreased when imipramine was taken for up to two years after an acute depression by patients with a history of previous major depression, but the study was not double-blind. Experience and research with MAOIs have been much more limited, but there does seem to be a poorly defined subgroup of patients with recurrent depression for whom MAOIs are the treatment of choice (see pp. 205–207).

LITHIUM

The use of long-term lithium maintenance in the treatment of unipolar depression is a topic of current dispute. Research is active, but the results thus far have been controversial. A major review concluded that lithium is effective in unipolar patients (Davis, 1976), and a collaborative study indicated that it is as effective as imipramine over a two-year period in preventing rehospitalization (Prien et al., 1973). There is, however, a shortage of prospective, placebo-controlled studies with random patient assignment. Many of the studies that have been conducted may be dealing with patients who have unusually severe recurrent depression (Davis, 1976), and data on male patients with recurrent depression are inadequate (Quitkin et al., 1976). Thus, while there is evidence that lithium maintenance is of some benefit to patients with recurrent depression, both the APA Task Force and other reviewers (Klerman, 1978; Quitkin et al., 1976) have concluded that a definitive statement on its value cannot yet be made.

CYCLOTHYMIC DISORDER (301.13)

ESSENTIAL FEATURES

The essential feature of *cyclothymic disorder* is a chronic mood disturbance of at least two years' duration, involving numerous periods of depression and hypomania, but not of sufficient severity and duration to meet the criteria for a major depressive or manic episode (the full affective syndrome). The depressive and hypomanic periods may be separated by periods of normal mood lasting as long as several months at a time. Or they may be intermixed or alternating.

TREATMENT

The treatment of cyclothymia is not well-defined by clinical experience, and research until quite recently had been almost nonexistent. Attempts have been made to specify the relation of cyclothymic to bipolar disorder (Akiskal et al., 1977); and the occurrence of cyclothymic disorder in adolescence (Gallemore and Wilson, 1972) and in association with drug and alcohol abuse (Flemenbaum, 1974) has been discussed. However, it has not been a well-defined disorder. Its frequency may have been underestimated in the past, and it may have been confused with personality or thought disorders, rather than being recognized as an affective disorder.

The notion that cyclothymia exists on a continuum with bipolar disorder suggests the possibility that lithium may help in some patients. The data in this regard are not firm but suggest a beneficial effect in some patients. The criteria for this disorder rule out symptoms that would suggest the use of antipsychotic drugs, and the value of antidepressants is unclear.

The role of the various psychotherapies has not been studied, but Akiskal's report of "life events of a tempestuous nature in well over 75% of these patients" (Akiskal et al., 1977) would suggest the need to evaluate the patient's work and family situations, and consider psychotherapeutic intervention.

DYSTHYMIC DISORDER (or DEPRESSIVE NEUROSIS) (300.40)

ESSENTIAL FEATURES

The essential feature of *dysthymic disorder* is a chronic disturbance of mood involving either depressed mood or loss of interest or pleasure in all or almost all usual activities and pastimes, but not of sufficient severity to meet the criteria for a major depressive episode (full affective syndrome). For the diagnosis in adults, two years' duration is required; for children and adolescents, one year is sufficient. Normal periods may last a few days to a few weeks. The depressive periods involve some of the milder features of a major depressive episode. Frequently, there is a superimposed major depressive episode that may be the occasion for the patient to seek treatment.

Dysthymic disorder, as defined in DSM-III, may overlap several previous DSM-II categories. Similarly, a disorder classified in DSM-II as a depressive neurosis might meet DSM-III criteria for a dysthymic disorder, a major depression, or an atypical depression depending on its particular clinical presentation. Thus, conclusions from previous research and clinical experience organized around the DSM-II system can only be tentatively extrapolated to dysthymic disorder.

TREATMENT

Antidepressants. It is conceivable that a patient classified under dysthymic disorder would have superimposed symptoms of sleep disturbance, crying, and feeling slowed down and would be appropriate for an antidepressant trial. An adequate literature specific to dysthymic disorder does not yet exist.

Lithium. Not usually used. No relevant research.

ECT. Not indicated.

PSYCHOTHERAPY

The following discussion of psychotherapy of depression is being presented under treatment of dysthymic disorder in the belief that this is the closest equivalent to what the various schools of psychotherapy have had in mind when they refer to "depression." It is possible, however, that some authors have been referring to disorders that would be classified in DSM-III as atypical depressions, adjustment reactions, or even major depressions. Thus, the following section on psychotherapy should be read for its relevance not only to dysthymic disorder, but also to other forms of depression.

Before proceeding to a review of some of the major schools of psychotherapy, we will first discuss a few general issues regarding psychotherapy and depression.

Countertransference

Countertransference is a continuing issue in the treatment of depressed patients, particularly severely depressed patients. Depressed patients bring their hopelessness and despair into therapy, and the therapist may be affected. If the depression improves slowly, or not at all, the therapist may feel guilty, angry, and/or helpless. After seeing several severely depressed patients in a day, the therapist may feel quite drained and eventually may become unwilling to work in the future with similar patients. Suicidal patients can evoke particularly difficult countertransferences (Maltsberger and Buie, 1974).

One safeguard against such difficulties is the therapist's continuing awareness of these feelings and their relation to his or her own psychodynamics. A suffering patient may mobilize the therapist's fantasy of being able to heal and earn gratitude, deftly and single-handedly; or may stir up the therapist's anger at the existence of suffering. An abiding awareness of these reactions will help the therapist maintain the patience and satisfaction with small gains that are necessary for conducting psychotherapy with severely depressed patients. At the same time, the therapist must avoid overstepping his/her role and trying to do all the work for an apparently weak patient. The interested reader may enjoy Menninger's long list of subtle signs of harmful countertransference (Menninger and Holzman, 1973). Consultation with a colleague may also be helpful in this work.

Women and Treatment of Affective Disorders

Because the incidence of depression is approximately twice as high in women as in men, special consideration of their assessment and treatment is necessary. Many issues can interfere with a woman's receiving appropriate and beneficial psychiatric treatment. These issues have been discussed at length elsewhere (Weissman and Paykel, 1974; Scarf, 1980); here we will mention only a few.

Getting a good history of sources of stress has been discussed above as a necessary component of treatment planning. This task is often made more difficult in the case of women with affective disorders by what might be termed "cross-cultural ignorance," in which the therapist is unaware of the daily life conditions and social forces affecting the patient.

Failure to correctly identify sources of stress can lead to treatment that is ineffective or even damaging to the patient. Women have traditionally been responsible for the happiness of the home and when the family is unhappy, the women, believing themselves responsible, may seek psychiatric help for themselves (Klein, 1976). If the problems are primarily marital/family issues, treatment should be directed at the entire marital/family system. Treating the woman alone may reinforce her inappropriate guilt and related depression. Individual treatment may also be deleterious to marital/family relationships (Gurman and Klein, 1980). In general, it is best for the size of the unit in treatment (individual, couple, or family) to correspond to the sources of stress (and of strength). When the couple or family is needed but not available for treatment, the therapist treating the patient individually should help the patient recognize the external stressors she is experiencing, as distinguished from her intrapsychic struggles. This approach is also necessary when societal forces are the external stressors, e.g. sexism, racism.

These cases in which a woman's depression is secondary to marital/family disturbances must, of course, be carefully distinguished from cases in which the depression is primary and the disturbances in the family system are secondary to it.

In summary, one must try to gain a realistic understanding of the life situations and social roles of women patients, and also to determine the appropriate unit of treatment: individual, marital, or family. The same considerations hold for men, but the authors feel that the common male therapist–female patient dyad requires special awareness of womens' roles.

Attention must be paid, therefore, to sex-specific obstacles that might block appropriate and effective psychotherapy for women. The role of women in the mental health system has been discussed at length, e.g. Chesler (1976) and has been treated in a novel (Piercy, 1976). Here we will mention only a few issues.

A therapist's model of psychological well-being is very important to the patient, even when the model is not explicitly presented to the patient. Unfortunately, models of psychological health may carry sexist biases. Developmental models may focus on male development, with addenda for female development, so that female experience is seen as a variant of and departure from the more standard, male development.

Therapists have been reported to use quite similar words to describe healthy *men* and healthy *people*, but a rather different set of words to describe healthy *women* (Broverman et al., 1970). Some of the attributes ascribed specifically to healthy women include passivity, easily hurt feelings, dependency, submissiveness, and being easily influenced. While a therapist who encourages these attributes in a depressed woman may merely be echoing the values of the larger culture, nevertheless passivity and dependency are hardly qualities whose development is likely to help a depressed woman. Similarly, the discouragement of what the therapists in this study reported to be particularly masculine attributes (e.g. assertiveness, decisiveness) could work directly against the interests of a depressed woman. Thus, a traditional model of psychological health can lead to psychotherapeutic interventions that can be harmful to depressed women in psychotherapy. Even one of the more positive of traditional female virtues, compassion for others, may not be appropriate for development in therapy. As Klein (1976) has pointed out, many women have entirely too much self-denying "compassion" and rather need to be encouraged to make their self-concern explicit.

One frequently mentioned goal of therapy with depressed patients is an increase in self-esteem. Some psychotherapists have approached this goal by trying to improve the patient's view of how well he/she is performing. Patients will be taught to notice and praise themselves for accomplishments, and not condemn themselves for failures.

Some feminist therapists note that for many women the problem is not unrealistic, lowered evaluation of what they are actually doing, but an unrealistically elevated idea of what it is possible to do. This principle of unrealistically high ideals is familiar in general psychiatry in the treatment of obsessive-compulsive neurosis. But many apparently nonobsessive women carry unattainable ideals, and the role of cultural influences must be considered. Therapy with some women will include making a realistic evaluation of their total role requirements and lowering the ideals they hold for themselves. Measured against these realistically lowered ideals, their current performance may be sufficient to generate self-esteem.

Another issue to be considered with regard to self-esteem is the source. If a woman is so other-directed as to base her self-esteem entirely on the opinion of others, this self-esteem may appear intact at a given time in psychotherapy, but actually be fragile and quite vulnerable to criticism from others.

Psychoanalysis

While formal psychoanalysis is now a less prominent treatment method for seriously depressed patients, many of its theoretical constructs and techniques have been incorporated into current long and short-term psychotherapy. A clear and thorough discussion of these techniques is available (Menninger and Holzman, 1973). Short-term psychotherapy may sometimes be the major treatment method for dysthymic disorder. Enelow (1977) has discussed the development out of psychoanalysis of insight-oriented and process-oriented psychotherapies. There is, to our knowledge, no methodologically sound research on the use of these therapies in depression.

Interpersonal Psychotherapy

Interpersonal psychotherapy contains elements of both supportive and psychodynamic therapy. This school of thought assumes that the development of depression occurs in a social and interpersonal context and focuses on improving the patient's social and interpersonal functioning. Symptom resolution and social adjustment are the main concerns in interpersonal therapy; no claims are made for enduring personality change (Weissman et al., 1974). A manual for this therapy has been written, discussing selection and treatment of specific problem areas (grief, role transitions, interpersonal deficits, or interpersonal disputes).

Two controlled studies of interpersonal therapy with depressed patients have been published (DiMascio et al., 1979; Weissman et al., 1974). The latter involved 150 recovering depressed women who had already responded to amitriptyline therapy. They were treated during recovery with TCA, placebo, or no pill and interpersonal psychotherapy or no psychotherapy, in a 2×3 factorial design. It is not clear whether these women would best be described as suffering from major depression or dysthymic disorder. After eight months of treatment, women receiving interpersonal psychotherapy showed improved social adjustment *if* they had remained in the study and had not relapsed. Interpersonal psychotherapy did not decrease relapse rate though it did improve social functioning.

Short-term Psychotherapy

By "short-term psychotherapy," we refer here only to those brief therapies that developed within the psychodynamic tradition. Malan (1979) and Sifneos (1972) are among the proponents of such therapies.

Malan and Sifneos agree that short-term psychotherapy should be offered only to those patients who have a definable focus for treatment. Sifneos requires that the patient "be able to voice a specific chief complaint" while Malan requires that "the patient's *life problem* can be clearly identified, and this offers a clear-cut theme or *focus* for therapy." This kind of requirement speaks against the use of these psychotherapies with very chronically depressed patients who have no such focus.

Patients must also be psychologically minded enough to respond to interpretations, and this must be evaluated at the initial interview. And they must be motivated to work on their difficulties from a psychological perspective. These requirements would eliminate very apathetic patients, both those with major depression and accompanying retardation and those who appear to have extremely passive personalities.

Sifneos makes his requirements more stringent by adding the stipulations that the patient must be of above-average intelligence, "have had at least one meaningful relationship with another person during his lifetime," and fulfill detailed criteria of motivation. This stringency is consistent with the explicitly anxiety-provoking nature of the psychotherapy proposed by Sifneos.

Once patients are accepted into treatment, it proceeds in accordance with psychodynamic principles. Malan (1979) discusses the treatment of depression at great length. He proposes that one of the central issues in depression is the need to express instinctive impulses at the apparent expense of someone deeply needed or loved. So far as we know, there has been no well-controlled research on short-term therapy of depression.

Behavioral Therapy

There are many different behavioral therapies for depression, and several recent reviews can be consulted for a comprehensive discussion of these therapies (Hollon, 1980; Rehm and Kornblith, 1979). Here we will mention only two behavioral therapy approaches: social skills training and self-control techniques.

Social skills training. Lewinsohn (1975) proposes that a low rate of positive reinforcement causes depression. The guiding principle for the treatment of depression then becomes "to restore an adequate schedule of positive reinforcement for the individual through altering the level, the quality, and the range of the patient's activities and interactions." Intermediate goals include increasing the patient's activity level, reducing ruminations, self-condemnatory statements, and complaints, inducing affect that is incompatible with depressed affect, and enhancing the patient's ability to act in the interpersonal world in such a way as to receive positive reinforcement. Once the level of positive reinforcement is increased, it is hypothesized that the depression will lift. This causal connection remains hypothetical, as Lewinsohn clearly acknowledges.

Self-control techniques. In this approach the role of reinforcement in depression is viewed somewhat differently. It is proposed that while normal people are able to maintain responses even when not receiving immediate reinforcement, depressed persons lack the necessary "self-control" to do this. Three processes are central to this concept of self-control:

Self-monitoring is the ability to observe accurately the relations between situations, behaviors, and consequences, rather than attend selectively only to either negative events or immediate consequences rather than delayed consequences.

Self-evaluation consists of setting reasonable goals and monitoring one's progress toward them, rather than setting impossible goals and berating oneself for inevitable failure.

Self-reinforcement consists of appropriate praise and criticism given oneself, rather than the excessive self-punishment hypothesized in depression. Therapy for depression, then, consists of explaining the role of these components of self-control and giving behavioral assignments to increase normal, rather than depressed, self-monitoring, self-evaluation, and self-reinforcement (Fuchs and Rehm, 1977).

Fuchs and Rehm (1977) have reported that depressed women treated with self-control training improved both in specific self-monitoring skills and in general measures of depression. Two of their measures of depression, however, were self-reports, which are questionable for patients who have probably been taught specifically not to regard themselves as depressed. It has also been suggested that self-monitoring alone is more effective than the entire treatment package (Hollon, 1980). Self-control behavior therapy, then, is clearly defined theoretically and research has begun to substantiate or refute its hypotheses.

Cognitive Therapy
In recent years there has been increasing interest in more cognitively oriented approaches to the treatment of several kinds of depressions. This therapy is directed at the depressed person's negative self-perceptions and lowered self-esteem. It challenges negative self-images verbally and also engages the patient in a series of graded tasks at which the patient can succeed and thereby observe his/her own achievement (Beck, 1976).

The details of this approach are beyond the scope of this chapter.

Systematic comparisons of the cognitive approach with other therapies are underway, though some studies have already been done (Rush et al., 1978; Rush et al., 1977). Some of the principles of cognitive therapy have begun to find their way into clinical work with depressed patients. The approach appears to be particularly useful in depressed persons whose negative self-images are especially strong.

Supportive Therapy

As its name indicates, supportive therapy aims to *support* patients, strengthen their defenses, and prevent them from getting worse during the healing process.

Some aspects of supportive therapy for depression have been succinctly summarized by Schuyler (1974):

1. an explanation relating the patient's physical symptoms to depression
2. assurance that the patient's illness is self-limiting and that he or she will get well
3. explanation of the patient's illness to the family and enlistment of their aid in managing the patient
4. acceptance of the patient despite his or her rejection of the therapist
5. encouragement of direct methods of self-expression of the patient's feelings
6. emphasizing to the patient that he or she should not embark on any major psychologic or social changes during the course of the illness
7. fostering in the patient of understanding, hope, and appropriate planning for the near future
8. protection of the patient by anticipation of the risk of suicide
9. providing the patient with a well-structured daily program, if necessary.

The words used here—explanation, assurance, encouragement, acceptance, fostering, protection, providing—are all consistent with the basic nurturant and educational stance of supportive therapies. The supportive therapist teaches patients about their situation, but avoids increasing anxiety through confrontation.

Supportive therapy as described by Schuyler is no simple matter. Enlisting the aid of a depressed person's family is no small task. From the viewpoint of a family therapist, it may be a central issue. Encouraging depressed patients to express their feelings is a major therapeutic task. And fostering an understanding of the near future, with its necessary precondition of understanding the present, would be an acceptable goal for most long-term therapies, not to mention major religions. Indeed, for many of the severely or chronically disturbed patients for whom supportive therapy is often recommended, even to establish a relationship represents a substantial achievement. So the challenge of supportive therapy is not to be underestimated.

Group Psychotherapy

Group therapies are as varied as individual psychotherapies, ranging from psychoanalytic to behavioral to Gestalt. Yet it is possible to define common elements of many group psychotherapies (Yalom, 1975; Levine, 1979). Group therapy is particularly useful in providing patients with the opportunity for a corrective recapitulation of the primary family group, the development of socialization techniques, interpersonal learning, and an experience of group cohesiveness (Yalom, 1975).

Criteria for group referral, Yalom notes, have tended to be exclusive (e.g. no patients with sociopathic disorder) rather than inclusive. The factors that have been suggested as predictors of good response to group therapy are similar to presumed predictive factors for other forms of psychotherapy: motivation for change, realization of deficiences in self-understanding and sensitivity to others, and belief in the treatment method. Many patients with depressive disorders are considered appropriate for group referral if their depression is not so deep as to produce retardation and immobility. The patient's interpersonal history must also be considered. While many patients will express some anxiety about group referral, the patient who is acutely anxious and has a history of painful or paralyzing group experiences is not a good candidate for group therapy. The individual must also be matched to the particular group that has openings, and should be able to identify in important ways with at least one other member (Levine, 1979).

There is little research or even published discussion on the treatment of depression by group psychotherapy. Stein (1975) has proposed that some types of depression, particularly chronic depression associated with strong masochistic tendencies, are particularly well suited to group psychotherapy.

Covi et al. (1974) compared group psychotherapy with biweekly brief supportive therapy in patients receiving imipramine, diazepam, or placebo. Weekly group therapy showed no advantage over supportive therapy, though there may have been problems with the choice of outcome measures.

Family Therapy

Family therapy aims at changing the family, and so its concerns can at times be oblique to the concerns of individual diagnosis and treatment, as exemplified in DSM-III and in this book. As Beels and Ferber (1973) have said:

> This goal of changing the family system of interaction is family therapy's most distinctive feature, its greatest advantage, and, especially to those who come to it from other disciplines, its greatest stumbling block.

Family therapists rarely discuss treatment of depressed individuals. They do, however, frequently treat families which contain one or more depressed individuals.

Several theories have been offered about families in which serious depression occurs (Slipp, 1976; Hogan and Hogan, 1975). Here we will discuss primarily the assessment of families containing a depressed member. The clinician's goal in this context is to gain an understanding of the relationship between the individual's depression and the family dynamics by interview of all family members.

Family problems separate from the depression of the identified patient need to be recognized by the therapist, even when the family cannot directly acknowledge them. A knowledge of principles of the family life cycle and the stresses normally encountered in each stage will help the therapist recognize a family stuck in its own development. The clinician who knows the normal family developmental tasks of early marriage may more easily recognize that the couple whose presenting complaint is the wife's recurrent depressions (which have incidentally caused them to postpone having a child) may actually be experiencing extreme ambivalence about parenthood and also may not have resolved issues of individuation and intimacy in early marriage. Work on these underlying issues may alleviate the depression.

The emotional dynamics of the family may need to be explored. The clinician needs to know if affection and anger are clearly expressed and resolved between all members of the family. The appropriate autonomy and intimacy needs of each member may or may not be met in the family system. Depression in one member can be the final common pathway for many repetitive and futile family emotional dynamics. The family that cannot tolerate anger and individuation may develop a depressed teenager who occasionally acts out his/her anger at not being permitted to proceed in developing autonomy, but then returns to passive, hopeless depression. Treatment aimed at enlarging the family's capacity for tolerating anger and autonomy may be the most efficient way of helping the teenager.

Thus, family therapy requires an assessment of many factors that are not included in DSM-III diagnostic criteria. At the same time, individual diagnosis must not be neglected. The therapist must recognize that a primary affective disorder in one family member can easily disturb family dynamics.

We will not attempt to summarize here all the approaches to family therapy. Although this is a young therapy, it has already differentiated into many forms, just as individual psychotherapy did. A discussion of psychoanalytic and objective relations, intergenerational experiential approaches, systems, and behavioral approaches is available (Gurman and Kniskern, 1978). As treatment proceeds, the therapist must, while maintaining a family perspective, also remain aware of the severity of depression manifesting in any one member, and the consequent suicidal risk. Skill and experience are required to know when to treat a suicidal gesture as a family event and when, while maintaining this perspective, to hospitalize the person who made the gesture. The therapist must also remain aware of the possibility that as one member recovers from an affective disorder, family homeostatic forces in some instances may push another member toward the recently vacated position of patient.

Regardless of whether the therapist chooses to treat primarily the identified patient or the entire family, several principles regarding the family remain important in the treatment of affective disorders:

1. Family assessment should be part of the evaluation.
2. A family may need considerable support when one of its members has a major affective disorder.
3. Family members need to be absolved of "blame" for "causing" the depression.
4. Family forces need to be aligned so as to increase treatment compliance.

Couples Therapy

Couples therapies also vary widely, and recent reviews of psychoanalytic, behavioral, and systems theory perspectives are available (Paolino and McCrady, 1978). When a depressed patient is married or living with another person, couples therapy may be recommended for a variety of reasons. Marital discord is a frequently cited stressor among depressed patients, although one must be careful to distinguish whether the depression caused the marital discord or vice versa. Inclusion of the marital partner permits the therapist to observe the patient "in action."

Couples therapy requires assessment of factors not included in DSM-III. Much of the discussion of family therapy applies to couples therapy.

Little research is available on the effect of couples therapy on an individual patient's depression.

SUMMARY

Psychotherapy and antidepressant drugs must both be considered for dysthymic disorder. Antidepressants alone are indicated for a minority of patients, probably those with disturbances in vegetative functions and good premorbid functioning. The psychotherapies appear to benefit social and family functioning, and, in some approaches, specific depressive symptoms as well. But much more research is needed to clarify the benefits of psychotherapy and to specify who needs what type of psychotherapy and at what stage of the illness. For many patients, a combination of antidepressant medication and psychotherapy may provide the best treatment.

Although a duration of two years is required to make the diagnosis of dysthymic disorder, there are some patients whose depression is more longstanding. In one study, forty women were followed for four years after a depressive episode (Bothwell and Weissman, 1977). At the end of this time, 26% were as depressed as they had been originally. When a patient has been depressed this long, his or her social and work worlds are usually quite intertwined with the depression. Psychotherapeutic attention to these areas, both as causes and effects of the depression, is necessary. The relation between chronic depressions, "characterological depressions," and dysthymic disorder is not clear. Dysthymic disorder may prove to include a wide variety of disorders (see Yerevanian and Akiskal, 1979, for a detailed discussion).

ATYPICAL BIPOLAR DISORDER (296.70)

This is a residual category for affective disorders that have some manic features (e.g. hypomania) but do not fulfill the criteria for bipolar disorder or cyclothymic disorder. Major depressive episodes may have occurred in the past, but no full manic episodes. Some clinicians will know this group as "bipolar II."

General statements about treatment of such patients are made with difficulty and cannot currently be based on any research. Depending on the degree of hypomania, one might wish to use maintenance lithium. This would be particularly true if the patient has had recurrent depressive episodes. On the other hand, the hypomania may be relatively mild and of short duration and there may not be a history of recurrent depressions. In this situation the approach might be to follow patients closely in supportive psychotherapy and help them set limits on their hypomanic behavior. Short-term use of neuroleptics might also be considered.

In both of the above instances it is important to maintain close contact with significant others in the patient's life so that hypomanic behavior does not escalate unbeknown to the therapist.

ATYPICAL DEPRESSION (296.82)

Since this is a residual and varied category, no comprehensive summary of treatments can be offered. In general, the reader is advised to consult the discussions of whatever specific affective disorder(s) the atypical depression most closely resembles.

There has been discussion in the literature of a subgroup of depressed patients who may respond preferentially to MAOIs. The term "atypical depression" (not synonymous with the DSM-III meaning of this term) has been used to refer to conditions with neurotic and phobic components that lack some of the traditional depressive signs. One study of outpatients with "persistent and significantly disabling depressive symptomatology" and a history of nonresponse to TCAs or benzodiazepines, noted that phenelzine was particularly helpful in decreasing irritability, hypochondriasis, agitation, and psychomotor agitation (Robinson et al., 1978). These authors discuss the possibility of identifying a MAOI responsive group, but note that it still remains to be seen whether, even for such a subgroup, MAOIs are superior to TCAs.

Another proposed subgroup consists of patients who respond to rejection with abrupt onset of intense dysphoria, hostility, lethargy, and sense of futility (Gallant and Simpson, 1975). Liebowitz and Klein (1979) offer diagnostic criteria for this "hysteroid dysphoria." Chronic MAOI maintenance therapy may decrease the abruptness and frequency of the dysphoria.

SCHIZOAFFECTIVE DISORDER (295.70)

DSM-III describes *schizoaffective disorder* as an illness in which the clinician is unable to make a differential diagnosis with any degree of certainty between *affective disorder* and either *schizophreniform disorder* or *schizophrenia*. Two examples of cases (given in DSM-III) that may be appropriately diagnosed as schizoaffective disorder are:

> (1) an episode of affective illness in which preoccupation with a mood-incongruent delusional dominates the clinical picture when affective symptoms are no longer present.
> (2) an episode of illness in which there is currently a full affective syndrome with prominent mood-incongruent psychotic features, but inadequate information about the presence of previous nonaffective psychotic features makes it difficult to differentiate between schizophrenia or schizophreniform disorder (with a superimposed atypical affective disorder) and affective disorder.

This disorder is so poorly defined that providing specific treatment recommendations would be premature. The category has no diagnostic criteria and is currently a residual category for psychotic disorders with an affective component that do not meet the criteria for affective disorder, schizophreniform disorder, or schizophrenia. Dunner and Rosenthal

(1979) discuss some of the conceptual difficulties in this area and note the importance of not under-using lithium because of reclassification of patients from bipolar disorder to schizoaffective disorder.

Potentially useful pharmacological agents include antipsychotics, antidepressants, and lithium, with the most prominent symptoms usually determining the agent which is tried first. More than one agent may be necessary, sequentially or concurrently, before a good effect is seen. Minimal controlled research has been done on schizoaffective disorder but a thorough review of the controversy is available (Procci, 1976).

REFERENCES

American Psychiatric Association, Task Force Report 14. Electroconvulsive Therapy, Washington, D.C. 1978.

Akiskal HS, Djenderedjian AH, Rosenthal RH, Khani MK: Cyclothymic disorder: validating Criteria for inclusion in the bipolar affective group. Am J Psychiat. 134:1227–1233, 1977.

Asberg M: Plasma nortriptyline levels—relationships to clinical effects. Clin Pharmacol Therapeutics. 16:215–229, 1974.

Baldessarini RJ: Chemotherapy in Psychiatry. Harvard U Press, Cambridge, Mass. 1977.

Ballenger JC, Post RM: Carbamazepine in manic-depressive illness: a new treatment. Am J Psychiat. 137:782–790, 1980.

Beck AT: Cognitive therapy and the emotional disorders. International Universities Press, New York. 1976.

Beels C, Ferber A: What family therapists do. In: The Book of Family Therapy, Ferber, A, Mendelsohn, M and Napier, A (eds). Houghton Mifflin, Boston. 1973.

Benjamin LB: Structural analysis of differentiation failure. Psychiatry. 42:1–23, 1979.

Bothwell S, Weissman MM: Social impairments four years after an acute depressive episode. Am J Orthopsychiat. 47:231–237, 1977.

Broverman IK, Broverman DM, Clarkson FE, Rosenkrantz P, Vogel SR: Sex-role stereotypes and clinical judgments of mental health. Cons. a Clin Psychol. 34:1–7, 1970.

Carroll BJ, Feinberg M, Greden JF, Tarika J, Albala AA, Haskett RF: A specific laboratory test for the diagnosis of melancholia. Arch Gen Psychiat. 38:15–22, 1981.

Chesler P: Women and madness. Doubleday, New York. 1976.

Coppen A, Ghose K, Montgomery S, Rama Rao VA, Bailey J, Jorgensen A: Continuation therapy with amitriptyline in depression. Brit J Psychiat. 133:28–33, 1978.

Coppen A, Rao VAR, Ruthven CRJ, Goodwin BL, Sandler M: Urinary 4-hydrozy-3-methoxyphenylglycol is not a predictor for clinical response to amitriptyline in depressive illness. Psychopharmacology. 64:95–97, 1979.

Covi L, Lipman RS, Derogatis LR, Smith JE, Pattison JH: Drugs and group psychotherapy in neurotic depression. Am J Psychiat. 131:191–198, 1974.

Davenport Y, Ebert MH, Adland MC, Goodwin FK: Couples group therapy as an adjunct to lithium maintenance of the manic patient. Am J Orthopsychiat. 47:495–502, 1977.

Davis J: Overview: Maintenance therapy in psychiatry. II. Affective disorders. A J Psychiat. 133:1–13, 1976.

DiMascio A, Weissman MM, Pousoff BA, Nen C, Zwilling M, Klesman G: Differential symptom reduction by drugs and psychotherapy in acute depression. Arch Gen Psychiat. 36:1450–1456, 1979.

Dunner DL, Rosenthal NF: Schizoaffective states. Psychiatric Clinics of North America. 2:441–448, 1979.

Enelow AJ: Elements of psychotherapy. Oxford University Press, New York. 1977.

Entwistle C, Taylor R, MacDonald I: The treatment of mania with haloperidol ('Serenace'). J Ment Sci. 198:373–375, 1962.

Fieve R: Chapter—overview of therapeutic and prophylactic trials with lithium in psychiatric patients. In press.

Fink M: Convulsive Therapy: Theory and Practice. Raven Press, New York. pp. 39, 218. 1979.

Flemenbaum A: Affective disorders and "chemical dependence": lithium for alcohol and drug addiction?. Dis Nerv Syst. 35:281–285, 1974.

Fuchs CZ, Rehm CP: A self-control behavior therapy program for depression. J Cons. Clin. Psychol. 45:206–215, 1977.

Gallant DM, Simpson GA (eds.): Depression—behavioral, biochemical, diagnostic, and treatment concepts. Spectrum, New York. 1975.

Gallemore JL, Wilson WP: Adolescent maladjustment or affective disorder?. Am J Psychiat. 129:120–125, 1972.

Gerbino L, Oleshansky M, Gerson S: In: Psychopharmacology: A Generation of Progress, Lipton, MA, DiMascio, A and Killam, KF (eds). Raven Press, New York. 1978.

Ginsberg G, Marks IM: Cost-benefit analysis of treatment of neurosis by nurse-therapists. Psychol Med. 1977.

Goodwin FK, Cowdry RW, Webster MH: Predictors of drug response in the affective disorders; toward an integrated approach. In: Psychopharmacology: A generation of Progress, Lipton, MA, Dimascio, A and Killam, KF (eds). Raven Press, New York. 1978.

Greist JH, Greist TH: Antidepressant Treatment: The Essentials. Williams and Wilkins, Baltimore. 1979.

Gurman AS, Klein MH: The treatment of women in marital and family conflict: recommendations for outcome evaluation. In: An Assessment of Research on Women and Psychotherapy, Brodsky, AM and Hare-Mustin, RT (eds). Guilford Press, New York. 1980.

Gurman AS, Kniskern DP: Research in marital and family therapy: progress, perspective, and prospect. In: Handbook of Psychotherapy and Behavior Change (revised edition), Garfield, SL and Bergin, DE (eds). Wiley, New York. 1978.

Haskell DS, DiMascio A, Prusoff B: Rapidity of symptom reduction in depression treated with amitriptyline. J Nerv Ment Dis. 160:24–33, 1975.

Himmelhoch JM, Detre T, Kupfer PJ, Swartzburg M, Byck R: Treatment of previously untreatable depressions with tranylcypromine and lithium. J Nerv Ment Dis. 155:216–220, 1972.

Hogan P, Hogan BK: The family treatment of depression. In: The Nature and Treatment of Depression, Flach, FF and Draghi, SC (eds). Wiley, New York. 1975.

Hollister LE: Treatment of depression with drugs. Ann Int Med. 89:78–84, 1978.

Hollon SD: Status and efficacy of behavior therapies for depression: comparisons and combinations with alternative approaches. In: Behavior Therapy for Depression, Rehm LR (ed). Academic Press, New York. 1980.

Jefferson JW, Greist JH: Primer of Lithium Therapy. Williams and Wilkins, Baltimore. 1977.

Jefferson JW, Greist JH: Lithium intoxication. Psychiatric Ann. 8:458–468, 1978.

Jefferson JW, Greist JH: Lithium and the kidney. In: Psychopharmacology Update: New and Neglected Areas, Davis, JH, Greenblatt, D (eds). Grune and Stratton, New York. 1979.

Jefferson JW, Greist JH: The cardiovascular effects and toxicity of lithium. In: Psychopharmacology Update: New and Neglected Areas, Davis, JM and Greenblatt, D (eds). Grune and Stratton, New York. 1979a.

Johnson G, Gershon S, Hekinian LJ: Controlled evaluation of lithium and chlorpromazine in the treatment of manic states. An interim report. Comp Psychiat. 9:563–575, 1968.

Johnson FN: In: Handbook of Lithium Therapy, Johnson, FN (ed). University Park Press, Baltimore. 1980.

Kantor SJ, Glasman DH: Delusional depressions: natural history and response to treatment. Brit J Psychiat. 131:351–360, 1977.

Kessler K: In: Tricyclic antidepressants: mode of actions and clinical use in psychopharmacology: a generation of progress, Lipton, MA, DiMascio, A and Killam, KF (eds). Raven Press, New York. 1978.

Klein MH: Feminist concepts of therapy outcome. Psychother Theory Res Pract. 13:89–95, 1976.

Klerman G: Long-term treatment of affective disorder. In: Psychopharmacology: A Generation of Progress, Lipton, MA, DiMascio, A and Killam, KF (eds). Raven Press, New York. 1978.

Klerman GL, Cole JO: Clinical pharmacology of imipramine and related antidepressant compounds. Pharmacol Rev. 17:100–141, 1965.

Levine B: Group Psychotherapy: Practice and Development. Prentice-Hall, Englewood Cliffs, N.J. 1979.

Lewinsohn PM: Behavioral study and treatment of depression. In: Progress in Behavior Modification, Hersen, M, Ersler, RM and Miller, PM (Eds). 1:19–65, 1975.

Liebowitz MR, Klein DF: Hysteroid Dysphoria. Psychiatric Clinics of North America. 2:555–576, 1979.

Malan DH: The Frontier of Brief Psychotherapy: An Example of the Convergence of Research and Clinical Practice. Plenum, New York. 1971.

Malan, DH: Individual Psychotherapy and the Science of Psychodynamics. Butterworth, Boston. 1979.

Maltsberger AT, Buie DH: Countertransference hate in the treatment of suicidal patients. Arch Gen Psychiat. 30:625–633, 1974.

McLean PO, Ogston K, Grauer L: A behavioral approach to the treatment of depression. J Behav Therapy Exp Psychiat. 4:323–330, 1973.

Menninger KA, Holzman PS: Theory of Psychoanalytic Technique. Basic Books, New York. 1973.

Mindham RS, Howland C, Shepherd M: An evaluation of continuation therapy with TCA in depressive illness. Psychol Med. 3:5–17, 1973.

Minter RE, Mandel MR: A prospective study of the treatment of psychotic depression. Am J Psychiat. 136:1470–1472, 1979.

Minter RE, Mandel MR: The treatment of psychotic major depressive disorder with drugs and electroconvulsive therapy. J Nerv Ment Dis. 167:726–733, 1979a.

Nelson C, Bowers MB: Delusional unipolar depression. Arch Gen Psychiat. 35:1321–1328, 1978.

Okuma T, Inanaga K, Otsuki S: Comparison of the antimanic efficacy of carbamazepine and chlorpromazine: a double-blind controlled study. psychopharmacology. 66:211–217, 1979.

Paolino TJ, McCrady BS: Marriage and Marital Therapy. Brunner/Mazel, New York. 1978.

Piercy M: Woman on the edge of time, Fawcett, Greenwich, Conn. 1976.

Platman S: A comparison of lithium carbonate and chlorpromazine in mania. Am J Psychiat. 127:351–353, 1970.

Prien R, Caffey E, Klett C: Comparison of lithium carbonate and chlorpromazine in the treatment of mania: report of the VA/NIMH collaborative study group. Arch Gen Psychiat. 26:146–153, 1972.

Prien R, Klett CJ, Caffey E: Lithium carbonate and imipramine in prevention of affective episodes: a comparison in recurrent affective illness. Arch Gen Psychiat. 29:420–425, 1973.

Procci WR: Schizoaffective psychosis: fact or fiction? Arch Gen Psychiat. 33:1167–1178, 1976.

Quitkin F, Rifcin A, Klein DF: Prophylaxis of affective disorders. Arch Gen Psychiat. 33:337–341, 1976.

Quitkin F, Rifkin A, Klein DF: Imipramine response in deluded depressive patients. Am J Psychiat. 135:806–811, 1978.

Rees L, Davis B: A study of the value of haloperidol in the management and treatment of schizophrenic and manic patients. Int J Neuropsychiat. 1:263–266, 1965.

Rehm LP, Kornblith SJ: Behavior therapy for depression: a review of recent developments. In: Progress in Behavior Modification, Hersen, RM, Eisler, RM, Miller, PM (eds). 7:277–321, 1979.

Robinson DS, Nies A, Ravaris CL, Ives JO, Bartlett D: Clinical psychopharmacology of phenelzine: MAO activity and clinical response. In: Psychopharmacology: A Generation of Progress, Lipton, MA, DiMascio, A and Killam, KF (eds). Raven Press, New York. 1978.

Robinson DS, Nies A, Ravaris CL, Lambourn KR: The monoamine oxidase inhibitor phenelzine in the treatment of depressive-anxiety states. Arch Gen Psychiat. 29:407–413, 1973.

Rush AJ, Beck AT, Kovacs M, Hollon S: Comparative efficacy of cognitive therapy and pharmacotherapy in the depressed outpatient. Cog Therapy Res. 1:17–39, 1977.

Rush AJ, Hollon SD, Beck AT, Kovacs M: Depression: must pharmacotherapy fail for cognitive therapy to succeed. Cog Therapy Res 2:199–207, 1978.

Scarf M: Unfinished Business: Pressing Points in the Lives of Women. Doubleday, Garden City, New York. 1980.

Schuyler D: The depressive spectrum. Jason Aronson, New York. 1974.

Shopsin B: Manic Illness. Raven Press, New York. 1979.

Shopsin B, Gerson G, Thompson H, Collins P: Psychoactive drugs in mania: a controlled comparison of lithium carbonate, chlorpromazine, and haloperidol. Arch Gen Psychiat. 32:34–42, 1975.

Sifneos P: Short-term therapy and emotional crisis. Harvard U Press, Cambridge, Mass. 1972.

Slipp S: An intrapsychic-interpersonal theory of depression. J Am Acad Psychoanalysis. 4:389–409, 1976.

Squire LR: ECT and memory loss. Am J Psychiat. 134:997–1000, 1977.

Stein A: Group psychotherapy in the treatment of depression. In: The Nature and Treatment of Depression, Flach, FF and Daghi, SC (eds). Wiley, New York. 1975.

Turek I, Hanlon T: The effectiveness and safety of electroconvulsive therapy (ECT). J Nerv Ment Dis. 164:419–431, 1977.

Weissman MM, Klerman GL, Paykel ES, Prusoff B, Hanson B: Treatment effects on the social adjustment of depressed patients. Arch Gen Psychiat. 30:771–777, 1974.

Weissman MM, Paykel ES: The Depressed Woman. University of Chicago Press, Chicago. 1974.

Yalom I: Theory and Practice of Group Psychotherapy. Basic Books, New York. 1975.

Yerevanian BI, Akiskal HS: "Neurotic", Characterological, and Dysthymic Depressions. Psychiatric Clinics of North America. 2:595–618, 1979.

7 | Anxiety Disorders

ISAAC MARKS

In the management of phobic and obsessive-compulsive disorders, behavioral psychotherapy is probably the treatment of choice in most cases, whereas other approaches are currently indicated for the treatment of general anxiety states, post-traumatic stress disorder, and atypical anxiety disorder. Phobic and obsessive-compulsive disorders will be discussed first. Then the management of anxiety disorders will be considered in two sections according to those where behavioral management is the main treatment approach and those where it is not.

PHOBIC AND OBSESSIVE-COMPULSIVE DISORDERS

Essential Features

The essential feature of a *phobic disorder* is persistent and irrational fear of a specific object, activity, or situation that results in a compelling desire to avoid the dreaded object, activity, or situation (the phobic stimulus). The fear is recognized by the individual as excessive or unreasonable in proportion to the actual dangerousness of the object, activity, or situation.

The essential feature of *agoraphobia* (300.22 and 300.21) is a marked fear of being alone, or being in public places from which escape might be difficult or help not available in case of sudden incapacitation. Normal activities are increasingly constricted as the fears or avoidance behavior come to dominate the individual's life. In the most common form of agoraphobia there is a history of panic attacks.

The essential feature of *social phobia* (300.23) is a persistent, irrational fear of, and compelling desire to avoid, situations in which the individual

234

may be exposed to scrutiny by others. There is also the fear that the individual may behave in a manner that will be humiliating or embarrassing.

The essential features of *obsessive-compulsive disorder* (300.30) are obsessions or compulsions. Obsessions are recurrent, persistent ideas, thoughts, images, or impulses that are ego-dystonic, that is, they are not usually experienced as voluntarily produced, but rather as thoughts that invade consciousness and are experienced as senseless or repugnant. Compulsions are repetitive and seemingly purposeful behaviors that are performed according to certain rules or in a stereotyped fashion. The behavior is not an end in itself, but is designed to produce or to prevent some future event or situation. The act is performed with a sense of subjective compulsion, coupled with a desire to resist the compulsion (at least initially). The individual generally recognizes the senselessness of the behavior, although this may not be true for young children.

TREATMENT GOALS

The major goals are to reduce phobic and obsessive-compulsive behavior to the extent that it no longer interferes with the patient's everyday functioning and to help the patient improve social adjustment that has been impaired by these problems. The aim is not to abolish all anxiety or rituals in the presence of their evoking stimuli, but to reduce them to a level at which the patient can tolerate them and to develop coping skills that will enable the patient to nip in the bud any future tendencies to recurrence.

Personality change is not an aim of treatment, although relief from formerly crippling phobic or compulsive problems often produces ripples of improvement in social adjustment which help the development of new interpersonal skills and make wider gains in personality functioning possible.

TREATMENTS

Although a generation ago phobic and obsessive-compulsive disorders were generally considered resistant to therapy, they can now be predictably and effectively treated by a form of behavioral psychotherapy called "exposure." In this form of treatment the patient is repeatedly brought into prolonged contact with those situations which usually evoke distress until discomfort in their presence subsides. Cooperative patients can be treated successfully in from 1 to 30 sessions of about 90 minutes each, the mean in one series being eight sessions for phobics and eleven for compulsive ritualizers (Marks et al., 1977). Recently, the trend has been to allow patients to increasingly take over their own management as "self-exposure homework" with the help of relatives as cotherapists, and in one series of agoraphobics substantial gains were made with a mean therapist time per patient of only 3.5 hours (Jannoun et al., 1980). With exposure treatment, the patient need not consume much of the psychotherapist's time, as the methods can be used just as effectively by suitably trained nurses (Marks, 1977).

The subtypes of phobic disorders listed in DSM-III do not affect the kind of behavioral treatment given: the presence of panic attacks does not alter the management. In general, the simpler, more focal phobias can be treated more rapidly than more diffuse problems like widespread agoraphobia. Long duration of the disorder, however, does not necessarily make exposure treatment more difficult. Patients with phobias or rituals of many years standing can often be treated as rapidly as those in whom the problem has only been present for a short time.

Interestingly, Freud himself can be listed among the pioneers of exposure therapy. In 1919 he stated in *Lines of Advance in Psychoanalytic Therapy* (Jones, 1955):

> One can hardly ever master a phobia if one waits till the patient lets the analysis influence him to give it up . . . one succeeds only when one can induce them through the influence of the analysis to . . . go about alone and struggle with the anxiety while they make the attempt.

This observation was neglected when modern psychoanalytic thinking came to focus instead on the idea that phobias and obsessions result from intrapsychic or interpersonal conflicts that must be resolved before treatment can be effective. The thesis of the behavioral psychotherapist, on the other hand, is that it is not necessary to use analysis to induce patients to struggle with the anxiety—it is only necessary that they face the anxiety and do so repeatedly until it becomes manageable. If the patient is motivated and cooperative, as most are, exposure therapy generally succeeds in its goal, provided the patient has been appropriately selected and treated. Without exposure, however, these patients are not likely to improve.

Selection of patients is described on pp. 253–255. It will suffice at this point to emphasize that the clinician should be satisfied before embarking on treatment that the patient is willing and motivated to go through with it and to experience discomfort when necessary. Not only is it unethical to use exposure therapy against the patient's will, but one runs the risk that the patient may become worse rather than better if he or she leaves therapy before it is completed; and an unwilling patient is far less likely to complete treatment than one who is cooperative.

For reasons that are not yet clear—with repeated exposure to the stimuli which evoke anxiety and/or panic—the patient gradually comes to tolerate them, and the phobic and obsessive-compulsive responses fade away. Contrary to what might be expected, only rarely do patients become more sensitized to a situation through clinical exposure. Such sensitization occurs in perhaps 3% of all patients, again for unknown reasons. The question of why exposure to certain stimuli sometimes produces phobias and at other times cures them is a prime theoretical issue which is not yet resolved.

Exposure treatment can take many forms. For purposes of illustration, imagine a man who has a height phobia. He is quivering with fear at the bottom of a 20-foot ladder, placed upright against a stack of books in a library. At the top of the stack is a book entitled, *How to Overcome Your Fear of Heights*. Our goal is to help the man climb the ladder to obtain the book. One approach is to ask the man to close his eyes, relax, and imagine himself putting his foot on the first rung of the ladder, then to take his foot down and relax again. We can repeat this sequence several times until the image inspires no anxiety, after which the man can be asked to imagine himself standing on the first rung, and putting his foot on the second rung, and so on. This process is termed *desensitization in fantasy* or *systematic desensitization*. If we ask the man to perform the same maneuvers in real life instead of in fantasy, the terms used are *desensitization in vivo* or *contact desensitization*.

An alternative strategy would be to ask the man to close his eyes and imagine himself standing at the top of the ladder—looking down, swaying in fear, feeling dizzy and terrified—and to continue imagining this until he feels better. This approach is *implosion*, or *flooding in fantasy*. There is also the approach of *flooding in vivo*. In our hypothetical situation this would mean grabbing the patient by the scruff of the neck and thrusting him to the top of the ladder—with his permission, of course—where he would sweat out his fear until it went away.

The term *desensitization* indicates a relatively slow exposure and *flooding* a very rapid exposure to the evoking stimulus (ES). When the speed of approach to stimulus is less headlong, but still rapid, we speak of *rapid exposure*. If desensitization is like wading into a swimming pool slowly from the shallow end, then flooding is like jumping into the deep end.

In any of these approaches one can first demonstrate to the patient what it is he has to do, and this too has several variations. Preceding our height-phobic patient up the ladder would be termed *modeling*. *Operant conditions* or *shaping* means praising the patient at each step he takes up the ladder. If we ask our patient to close his eyes and imagine himself persuading another person with a height phobia that it is good for him to go up the ladder, this would be a form of *cognitive rehearsal*. If the patient is asked to say to himself, "This isn't so bad; I can really tolerate this fear," the term used is *self-regulation*.

The therapeutic strategy required for each patient has to be worked out on an individual basis. The task of the therapist is to search for those situations that evoke phobias or rituals and then to persuade the patient to remain in contact with them until he gets used to them. The search for evoking stimuli (ES) is conduced by asking the patient relevant questions and can be aided by using simple questionnaires, such as those in the book, *Living with Fear* (Marks, 1978a). The management principles and assessment forms to be used by the patient are also in that book. There is no need for elaborate tests in the search for the ES; the patient's thoughts are relevant only to the extent that they indicate which cues might be critical for the therapist to incorporate into the exposure program. The patient's physical state may contribute to a decision about which approach to behavioral psychotherapy should be taken. When high anxiety is medically undesirable, as in patients with serious heart disease, severe asthma, or ulcerative colitis, one of the slower forms of exposure treatment should be used. When patients are physically fit, severe anxiety is neither physically nor mentally dangerous, and no restrictions need be placed on the type of behavioral treatment employed (see pp. 255–256).

The prospective patient should, in advance, agree to carry out homework assignments that will bring him into contact with discomforting stimuli. He should understand and agree that, under certain circumstances, relatives may need to be involved as co-therapists. For example, when the evoking stimuli are present mainly in the patient's home, as is common in obsessive compulsive states, the treatment may require several sessions at home in order to ensure that improvement is transferred from the clinic setting to the real life situations where the problem is most bothersome.

The following is a typical explanation given to a patient before treatment begins. In this case it is directed to an agoraphobic:

> We find from past experience that a good way of getting over your fear is to allow yourself to confront the very situations you have tended to avoid, but the confrontation should be for quite long periods of time—several hours is better than a few minutes. We will help you go into these situations in the beginning and then gradually fade ourselves out of the treatment sessions. Eventually, we will expect you to do it by yourself. For example, you had somebody escort you here because you couldn't make the trip alone. We will ask you within two or three sessions to come to the clinic alone.
>
> Of course, you will experience quite a bit of anxiety, especially in the beginning. You may even panic and feel that you must rush out of the situation; but the one thing you mustn't do is rush out, because that will only make your phobia worse. You will learn that if you just stay there, in that frightening situation, the panic will go away—usually in less than 20 minutes, sometimes a little longer. But if you can persuade yourself to stay in the situation, and the great majority of patients like you can, the next time you try, it will be much easier.
>
> In between sessions with us, we will ask you to engage in what we call homework tasks. We will ask you to lay out a series of goals that you know you have to achieve in order to overcome your phobia. You might choose to go into a crowded part of town every day and stay there in the crowds for at least an hour. At the same time you can go into the supermarket and perhaps for a walk in the park. We will ask you to record your goals and achievements in a diary and record what your anxiety rating was, so we both can see it go down from a maximum of 8 to maybe 6 or 5 in the course of a couple of tries. You will bring your diary to each session, and we will use it to help plan the next phase of therapy. Members of your family can help you with your homework, if you wish. They can act as your co-therapists.
>
> We won't cure you absolutely. There will be a tendency for some recurrence of the fear from time to time, but we will teach you the coping strategies that will enable you to stop avoiding fearsome situations.

After all this has been discussed and the patient has agreed to participate in the program, understanding the commitment it requires, the first step is to work with him or her to establish concrete goals and to rank them in order of importance. The definition of goals must be as specific as possible. For example, "I want to spend two hours a week shopping alone at the nearest mall" is a well-defined goal for an agoraphobic; "I want to be able to get out and go about by myself" is less well-defined and thus has less likelihood of successful achievement. Similarly, "I want to get rid of my hang-up about dirt" is a generalized statement that a compulsive might make, but "I want to be able to touch the garbage can every day without washing my hands afterwards" is a tangible goal for which success or failure can be quantified. It is usually most effective to start with the most severe problem since those at the bottom of the hierarchy often disappear by the time the more important goals are reached.

Therapy is then divided into two parts: therapist-assisted exposure sessions, such as those already discussed, and homework. The latter maintains exposure and generalizes improvement in the natural environment.

When possible, as it usually is in the families of cooperative patients, a family member is recruited as cotherapist. The husband or wife, for example, is asked to initial each day's diary entries, witnessing that the tasks were completed.

An essential part of the homework is that the family *not* reward phobic or ritualistic behavior. It is counterproductive to reassure those who ritualistically ask for reassurance. The illness phobic who constantly asks for reassurance, hoping to be told he is not sick, does have his anxiety reduced by such reassurance, but only briefly—the anxiety flares up again a short time later. What he must do is learn to tolerate the idea of illness just as most other people do. Withholding the reassurance deprives him of his fix, so to speak. Addiction to reassurance can be broken only by withdrawal.

Learning not to reply to requests for reassurance can be surprisingly difficult for family members. Relatives may have had years of training to answer, "Yes, you're all right, you're doing fine." Repeated rehearsal in the presence of the therapist and patient can help them to unlearn the response—and help the patient learn that the denial of reassurance is part of the treatment.

For illness phobics the primary care physician must be brought into the picture. He needs to learn to withhold examinations and tests unless they are necessary for genuine medical reasons. Like family members, the physician should withhold reassurance until the patient is able to tolerate the discomfort of not being certain whether he is ill.

Compulsive hoarding can be treated by encouraging patients to get over their fear of throwing things away lest vital information be missed. A therapist may accompany the patient to his home and together they will slowly throw away ten-year-old newspapers to let the person get used to the idea that even if information has been lost it does not matter. It is amazing how reluctant a hoarder can be to throw away decomposing scraps of food or a broken chair which has no hope of being repaired. With gentle encouragement, however, a hoarder might be taught to part with many objects and to clear the living space at home so that visitors can be entertained once more.

Compulsive slowness presents special problems. The lives of such patients and their families can be crippled because the patients may take several hours to get dressed or undressed, have a bath, or cross the road. The problem can at times be helped by "time and motion" treatment. This involves prompting and pacing the patient in progressively more rapid sequences of behavior, with modeling of these when necessary until eventually he is able to complete his actions in normal times. As an illustration, a man who takes three hours to get up and ready for breakfast would be given a stopwatch and asked first to complete these tasks within 2¾ hours while being advised which actions to cut out so that he can speed up. Then he will be encouraged to complete his actions in 2½ hours, 2¼ hours, and so on until he eventually takes no longer than the average person, say half an hour. The patient can take home a tape recording of the therapist's instructions to play at the appropriate times as a reminder. Results with this approach can be encouraging in some patients are utterly bored by the thoughts and cease to be troubled by tical.

Obsessive thoughts without rituals (obsessive ruminations) respond much less predictably to behavioral methods than do rituals. Two procedures that have been used are thought stopping and prolonged exposure. Both have had limited success, but at the moment there is no clear guide to effective treatments of obsessive ruminations. It could be argued that thought stopping is a form of exposure to obsessive thoughts in repeated brief sequences or that it can be construed as an exercise in self-regulatory coping whereby the patient learns to control his or her own thoughts. In this procedure the patient is asked to induce a rumination which is then interrupted by a loud noise such as the patient and therapist shouting *stop*. This is done repeatedly while the shout is gradually faded to a whisper and then to a subvocalization, until finally the patient can achieve control merely by thinking *stop*. Another way of *interrupting* the thought is by snapping an elastic band on the wrist. Prolonged exposure, or satiation, is accomplished by setting aside specific periods of time for deliberate ruminations up to several hours a day until the patients are utterly bored by the thoughts and cease to be troubled by them. Over time, the duration is steadily shortened until the ruminations no longer interfere with other functioning. Patients for whom this approach is successful often find it difficult to ruminate for the prescribed treatment period and are relieved when the rumination sessions are shortened.

Most patients can be treated on an outpatient basis. In the author's unit, only about 10% require inpatient treatment—those who need to be gotten off excessive alcohol or drugs, or who live too far away to come regularly during the early stages of treatment. Others may have relatives who need to be admitted with them to facilitate cotherapy after discharge.

Occasionally, dramatic cures are effected in one or two sessions; explaining the principle of exposure treatment sometimes leads the patient to apply treatment to himself without further help from the therapist. These cures, however, are the exception. In addition to conducting exposure sessions at the clinic, the therapist should be prepared to see the patient frequently, reviewing the homework tasks and making suggestions as to the next phase. He should have time to escort the patient into the evoking situation at each session, staying with him for the first few exposures, then gradually fading into the sidelines and acting simply as monitor.

In the behavioral treatment of phobias and obsessions, the therapist does not spend much time talking with the patient about conflicts "underlying" the problem. Many therapists who have a psychoanalytic background are afraid that treating patients in this way will lead to symptom substitution or worsening of interpersonal relationships. In fact, the evidence runs quite the other way. Patients who improve in phobic or obsessive-compulsive behavior as a result of exposure therapy tend also to improve in other aspects of social adjustment.

Experimental evidence has shown that continuous exposure for two hours leads to better results than does exposure for four nonsequential half-hours (Stern and Marks, 1973). For this reason, patients treated at the Bethlam-Maudsley Hospital tend to have treatment sessions lasting an hour and a half or more, and it is not uncommon for sessions to last three or four hours, especially if they take place in the patient's home. Occasionally, the therapist has even stayed with the patient and his family over a weekend. This willingness to restructure work habits and to be flexible about the place of treatment is a departure for most health care professionals, but can lead to considerable savings in the total treatment time.

Treatment Controversies

Desensitization exposure in fantasy was the commonest behavioral treatment for phobias 15 years ago. It was shown to produce significant improvement in phobic patients in at least 10 controlled studies (reviewed by Marks, 1971). In four studies improvement after exposure in fantasy or in vivo was found to be maintained for 4–9 years after treatment (Marks, 1971; Emmelkamp and Kuipers, 1979; Munby and Johnston, 1980; McPherson and Brougham, 1980), although 15% of patients who were followed up required further treatment for depressive episodes during which phobias were temporarily aggravated. Desensitization in fantasy produces equally good outcome with and without muscular relaxation and taped desensitization has had results comparable to treatment given by live therapists.

Ten years ago much interest centered on the relative merits of desensitization versus flooding in fantasy. The apparent superiority of flooding over desensitization turned out to be attributable less to the fantasy components of treatment than to the fact that exposure in vivo which followed both the desensitization and the flooding in fantasy was probably more vigorous after the latter.

The value of prolonged live exposure was suggested by uncontrolled studies (Watson et al., 1971; Watson et al., 1972) of ten specific phobic patients who improved after treatment for an average of six hours each, spread over two to three afternoons. A subsequent controlled study (Stern and Marks, 1973) found that in vivo exposure was better than fantasy exposure and that two continuous hours of in vivo exposure of agoraphobics yielded significantly greater reduction of phobias than did four half-hour sessions separated by 30-minute rest periods. This finding was replicated in compulsive ritualizers by Rabavilas et al. (1976).

A logical therapeutic development was to use prolonged exposure in groups to save time and possibly enhance potency through social cohesion and observational learning. Group treatment in which exposure is carried out by several patients accompanied by a single therapist has proved to be useful for agoraphobics and social phobics (reviewed by Marks, 1979). Saving of therapist's time gives a clear advantage to group over individual exposure in vivo when this is practical, though there is little evidence that group treatment is more effective.

Even more savings in therapist's time might accrue from use of home-based self-help methods of treatment. It has become increasingly apparent that much behavioral treatment consists of teaching patients what to do between treatment sessions, as in structuring their exposure homework exercises. The value of this approach has been verified experimentally (Jannoun et al., 1980). Until recently, most behavioral treatments employed a therapist to assist the patient in confronting the evoking stimulus until habituation occurred. Theoretically, there is no reason why the patient should not do this without the therapist. In one study that explored this thesis, agoraphobics were seen by therapists three times during six weeks, each time for only 15 minutes. During these sessions, "treated" patients were asked to expose themselves to phobic situations as much as possible and to record their reactions in a diary; control patients were asked only to keep a diary of important emotional events, and exposure was not mentioned. Patients given exposure instructions improved significantly more than the controls (McDonald et al., 1978).

A second study employed a random assignment crossover approach (Greist et al., 1980). Phobic and obsessive compulsive patients were instructed in advance that they would receive a week each of two contrasting approaches to see which would be better for them. In one treatment condition patients were to confront the phobic situations for as long as possible, until anxiety died down, and to record these confrontations in a diary. In the other treatment condition they were to avoid all discomforting stimuli so that they could have a complete rest from tension. At the end of the two contrasting therapy weeks, they would receive whichever treatment had proved to be the more effective. The results were unequivocal. Despite similar expectations about each approach before treatment, phobics and ritualizers improved significantly during their week of exposure and worsened slightly during their week of avoidance. When, after the experiment, patients again received exposure treatment, improvement resumed. This was evidence that commonly given instructions to avoid phobia-inducing or ritual-inducing situations may be antitherapeutic.

Self-exposure treatment, either alone or with the help of family members, can be useful when monitored by mail (Mathews et al., 1980).

In another study (Jannoun et al., 1980), self-exposure treatment proved to be more successful than nonexposure treatment. Agoraphobic patients were assigned at random either to home-based exposure homework or to home-based nonexposure homework devoted to the solving of stressful problems in general. The patient and cotherapist friend or family member were seen five times over four weeks and were given relevant self-help instruction manuals and daily diaries to fill in. In the exposure group the manuals concerned programmed practice of exposure in vivo. In the nonexposure group the manual concerned general problem-solving methods and the patient and cotherapist were asked to discuss sources of stress and to try out solutions to decrease anxiety, but there was no need to go out unless they were willing to do so.

Impressive results were obtained for an expenditure of only 3½ hours of therapist's time per patient. Two therapists using exposure in vivo, obtained substantial improvement in phobias and in general anxiety and this gain was maintained at a six-month follow-up. In contrast, with nonexposure problem-solving, one therapist got no improvement at all while the other therapist obtained as much reduction in phobias and in anxiety as was obtained from exposure. Exposure was a more reliable approach independent of therapist differences, although it is of considerable interest that some therapists can reduce phobias using the nonexposure approach, which raises the issue of when exposure can be regarded as a way of teaching wider coping skills. Another nonexposure approach, the use of antidepressants, can also sometimes decrease phobias and rituals (see below).

Mathews et al. (1980) have suggested that whether the patient decides to approach or to avoid the discomforting situation depends on a balance between incentives (e.g. the need to buy something, to meet friends) and anticipated cost (e.g. fear of panic, embarrassment). One can therefore decrease avoidance either by increasing incentives (e.g. to please the therapist) or by decreasing cost (e.g. decreasing expectation of panic). One might shift the balance by exposure or perhaps in some patients by decreasing levels of general anxiety.

Currently, enthusiasm for "cognitive" behavioral methods outstrips demonstration of their value in clinical populations. Cognitive therapists identify patients' thoughts which might be increasing their anxiety and teach patients to change these thoughts by modifying their attitudes and rehearsing positive self-instruction. So far, cognitive therapy of clinical phobias has been examined in three controlled studies (Emmelkamp, 1979; Williams and Rappaport, 1980). In none of these studies did self-instructional methods enhance the effectiveness of exposure in vivo.

Another approach, which is now beginning to fade, is the use of biofeedback. Two controlled studies in patients with simple phobias demonstrated that although patients can learn to decrease their tachycardia significantly by means of biofeedback during exposure in vivo, this maneuver has little practical benefit because other physiological responses and subjective anxiety do not subside more rapidly as a result of controlling the heart rate (Nunes and Marks, 1975; Nunes and Marks, 1976).

Interpersonal difficulties complicating phobias or rituals do not contraindicate exposure treatment (see Marks, 1979 for review). Similar degrees or improvement have been obtained in low-assertive versus high-assertive agoraphobics, and the amount of marital satisfaction before treatment did not affect outcome (Emmelkamp, 1979). Like Jannoun et al. (1980), Emmelkamp found that exposure treatment was more reliably effective than a generalized approach such as training in assertiveness. In the only controlled study of the issue to date, it was found that when marital discord coexisted with phobic-obsessive problems, contract marital therapy did not significantly help phobic-obsessive problems but did improve the marital interaction, whereas exposure ameliorated both the phobic-obsessive difficulties and the marital discord (Cobb et al., 1980). The authors concluded that exposure treatment is still the preferred approach even when marital discord complicates rituals or phobias.

The role of response prevention in the treatment of ritualizers is still problematic. During exposure treatment, instructions are usually given to patients to refrain from engaging in rituals between treatment sessions (i.e. "do not wash until mealtime even though you feel contaminated"). To some extent response prevention can be regarded as a means of prolonging exposure and it is not yet clear whether response prevention is of itself therapeutic. In a controlled investigation of this issue, Robertson (1979) found that one-hour daily supervision of response prevention was as good as response prevention round the clock and that the one-hour group was actually slightly better at 2–4 years follow-up. Whether response prevention itself contributes beyond its automatic effect of prolonging exposure remains to be seen.

There is now a large literature attesting to the lasting efficacy of exposure treatment. In brief, phobics have been found to maintain improvement as long as four to nine years after desensitization in fantasy. Many studies of exposure in vivo have demonstrated improvement lasting at least six to twelve months. Four studies of obsessive-compulsive ritualizers, with one- to three-year follow-up, all showed durable improvement after exposure in vivo (Figs. 7–1 and 7–2) (Marks, 1981).

Should anxiety be kept low during exposure treatment? Several years ago it was thought that relaxation procedures were necessary to inhibit anxiety while the patient was in contact with the phobic stimulus. It has since been found that relaxation training is a redundant element in the therapeutic package. A controlled clinical study of this point was carried out by Benjamin et al. (1972) with chronic phobic patients who were asked to imagine phobic images while in either a relaxed or a neutral affective state. During two consecutive sessions, relaxed patients indeed had significantly less skin conductance activity between phobic images than did patients who had not been relaxed and were more aroused. However, contrary to expectation, arousal between images did not correlate with increased anxiety either during or after treatment. Nor did relaxation increase the speed with which patients lost their fear during sessions or the extent of improvement at the end of treatment.

In subsequent studies it was found that relaxation without exposure is not helpful for rituals (Marks et al., 1975; Marks et al., 1980). Compulsive rituals did not improve after 15 sessions of muscle relaxation, but were reduced significantly after 15 sessions of exposure in vivo. Indeed, relaxation has come to be considered so inert a factor in the treatment of phobias and compulsions that it is now reliably used as a psychological placebo control for other treatments under investigation.

Studies have also been carried out to test the validity of implosion, which is based on the opposite concept that for improvement to occur, anxiety must be maximally aroused during exposure until the patient is so exhausted that he cannot experience any more emotion. This viewpoint was once paraphrased by Stampfl (1967) as follows: "He who has lived in a cesspool for a few days in his mind will not worry later about a bit of dirt on his hands." But controlled clinical studies to support the approach were lacking and subsequent work has shown that the deliberate evocation of anxiety does not add to the therapeutic effect of exposure.

In a study of phobics during fantasy exposure, Mathews et al. (1974) found that high anxiety yielded no better results than low anxiety. As for in vivo exposure, Hafner and Marks (1976) studied chronic agorapho-

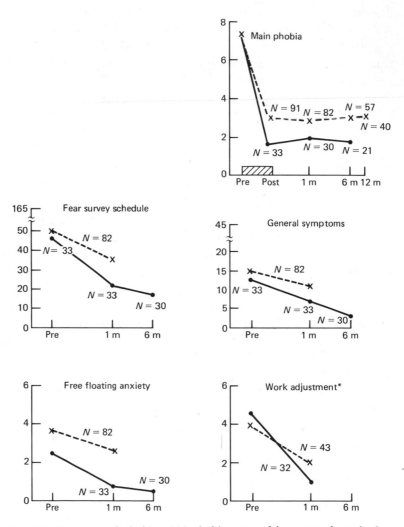

Fig. 7-1. Outcome of phobics: 124 phobics treated by nurse-therapist improve up to one year after exposure *in vivo*. Gains occur not only in main phobia and other fears (FSS), but also in general neurotic symptoms and in work adjustment. Highest scores = maximum pathology. ×---×, first training program for nurse-therapists; ●—●, second training program for nurse-therapists; * therapist rating: patients with initial scores 0–1 omitted. (Redrawn from I.M. Marks, Cure and care of neuroses, *Psychological Medicine*, p. 632, 1979)

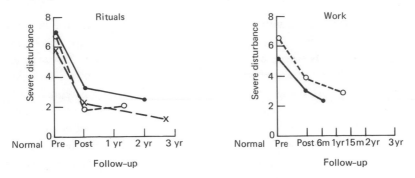

Fig. 7-2. In three different countries 57 compulsive ritualizers show comparable improvement up to three years after exposure *in vivo*. Gains generalize to work adjustment. Lower score = improvement. ●—●, study in London by Marks *et al.* (1975) (*N* = 20); ○---○, in Philadelphia by Foa and Goldstein (1979) (*N* = 21); ×---×, in Athens, by Boulougouris (1977) (*N* = 16). All three studies used measures of Marks *et al.* (1975). (Redrawn from I.M. Marks, Cure and care of neuroses, *Psychological Medicine*, p. 633, 1979)

bic patients exposed continuously to their real phobic situations under high- or low-anxiety conditions for three hours a day over four days. For example, patients were asked to shop in crowded supermarkets or ride in crowded trains until they felt better about being in these situations. To produce a high anxiety state, the therapist kept mentioning how bad the patients looked and enumerated all the catastrophes that might befall them. In the low-anxiety condition, the therapist kept offering reassurance, although of course all anxiety could not be eliminated. The high-anxiety patients did indeed experience significantly more discomfort than the low-anxiety group, but this did not affect treatment outcome on any measure.

At least four other well-controlled experiments have subsequently confirmed that the level of anxiety during exposure does not predict outcome in phobic patients (Marks, 1977). Although heightened anxiety is a common but not universal concomitant of rapid exposure treatment, it may not be an active ingredient of change, but rather an unfortunate by-product of the treatment itself.

Thus, the evidence on arousal level suggests that phobias and obsessions improve with exposure whether the patients are relaxed, neutral, or anxious during treatment.

Unlike arousal level, duration of exposure is an important variable. As noted earlier, the general rule is that longer is better (the experiments on duration were done with chronic patients; the optimum time of exposure might well be less for those whose phobias are of more recent onset). Presumably this is true because longer exposure gives whatever processes are at work more time to take effect. One may hypothesize, for example, that patients are being given enough time to develop self-regulatory strategies to control their emotions or to reach critical levels of habituation.

Other studies suggest that phobias and rituals are reduced more efficiently by in vivo than by fantasy exposure. The optimum strategy is probably to rely primarily on in vivo exposure, resorting to fantasy exposure only for very special situations—such as unobtainable phobic stimuli like thunderstorms—or when the patient's physical condition contraindicates the risks of marked anxiety.

Except for antidepressants, the utility of drugs combined with behavioral treatments for phobic-obsessive disorders has been overstated (Marks, 1980). Cumbersome procedures like the inhalation of carbon dioxide or intravenous injection of sedatives have little to commend them. Oral drugs are preferable for ease and economy of administration as well as greater safety. Several trials of beta-blockers have found that while these reduce heart rate during exposure treatments, at follow-up there is either no significant enhancement of the effect of exposure or a tendency for patients on beta-blockers to do slightly worse (Marks, 1981). The use of small doses of benzodiazepines like diazepam neither helps nor hinders exposure treatment; large doses appear to be counterproductive, perhaps representing a chemical avoidance of exposure. Patients should receive no more than 7.5 mg of diazepam or an equivalent dose of other benzodiazepine, and preferably less, during exposure treatment.

Antidepressants seem worthwhile for some patients with phobic-obsessive problems, although there is no clear-cut evidence yet that such drugs potentiate behavioral treatments, or that they directly reduce phobias and obsessions rather than act indirectly by improving mood. Several controlled studies have shown that the tricyclic, imipramine, and the monoamine oxidase inhibitors, phenelzine and isocarboxazid, are significantly better than placebo in agoraphobics, social phobics, and school phobics, as long as the drug continues to be taken. The same applies to clomipramine for compulsive ritualizers. There is general agreement that these antidepressants take from 5 to 10 weeks to exert their maximum effect and that there is a strong tendency to relapse when patients stop taking the drugs, even after they have been given in adequate dosage for 8–12 months continuously.

Most of the relevant studies have not sufficiently examined the relationship of depressed mood to the utility of antidepressants in phobic-obsessive disorders. It may be that phobic and obsessive inpatients have more depression than untreated phobics and obsessives in the community, that this depression is partly an independent problem, and that antidepressants are only indicated for the depressed mood. When this issue was addressed in two independent studies of compulsive ritualizers (Thoren et al., 1980; Marks et al., 1980; see also Figs. 6.1 and 6.5 of Marks, 1981) clomipramine proved effective only when depressed mood had been present at the start; the drugs had little effect in the absence of such depressive mood. This point immediately became obvious when patients in the highest quartiles of scores on depressed mood at the start of treatment were contrasted with those in the lowest quartiles (the middle 50% were omitted from the analysis by Marks et al. (1980). For ritualizers without depression, exposure in vivo remains the treatment of choice.

Analyses of this kind are not yet available for phobics, not even from the latest two double-blind controlled drug trials in agoraphobics (Sheehan et al., 1980; Zitrin et al., 1980).

For example, the sample of Sheehan et al. (1980) was divided into two groups according to initial scores on five vegetative signs of depression (decrease libido, anorexia, insomnia, constipation, early morning awakening), which means that mid-range patients were included in the analysis; this could have obscured the antidepressant effect noted by Marks et al. and Thoren et al. (1980). Moreover, as vegetative signs of depression were uncommon in the sample of Sheehan et al., 1980 a stronger analysis would have tested for the effect of depressed *mood* of a nonvegetative kind. Even without inclusion of nonvegetative depressed mood, there was a clear antidepressant effect of imipramine and phenelzine in the patients of Sheehan et al., 1980, as a highly significant improvement from drugs versus placebo was noted on their two measures of depression (Zung Depression Scale and SCL-90 Depression Subscale, their Tables 3 and 4). It is interesting that 98% of their patients reported feeling "blue" before treatment began (their Table 2).

The drug effect found by Sheehan et al. (1980) was not only antidepressant and antiphobic, but also generally "patholytic," as their patients improved on every measure, including SCL subscales of psychoticism, hostility, and interpersonal sensitivity, as well as work and social adjustment. This global improvement was also found with clomipramine, which improved depression, rituals, and social adjustment, in contrast to exposure in vivo, which improved rituals, but not mood (Marks et al., 1980). The drug effect took 10–14 weeks to reach maximum in the three studies concerned (that of Thoren et al., 1980 terminated at five weeks). It could be regarded as delayed "anxiolysis" as much as delayed "antidepressant" effect, and no one has yet studied the long-term symptom profile of action of benzodiazepines in such patients. It is still unknown how much benzodiazepines and antidepressants overlap in their actions in phobic-obsessive and anxiety disorders when given over long periods of time.

Zitrin et al. (1980) correlated initial depression ratings (Brief Psychiatric Rating Scale) with outcome of measures other than depression, and did not report the outcome of depression in the manner described by Sheehan et al. (1980) for agoraphobics and by Marks (1975), and Thoren et al. (1980) for ritualizers. It is possible that depressed mood might well have improved in the patients of Zitrin et al. (1980) quite as much as did their panics and phobias. Although Zitrin et al. (1980) found weak relationships between initial depression and worse phobic outcome, the opposite was noted for "spontaneous panic," though this was not significant (their Table 8). No comparison was made between patients who had been in the highest and the lowest quartiles of scores for depressed mood before treatment (omitting 11 patients in the middle range of "slight" initial depression, see Zitrin, 1980, p. 68).

Notwithstanding the apparently generalized effects of antidepressants, the analysis of Marks et al. (1980) suggests that pretreatment level of "depressed mood" and of free floating anxiety (Mawson et al., 1981) is a better predictor of drug effect than the pretreatment level of rituals, and the same may yet be found to hold true for phobias. In the latest study of outpatient agoraphobics by Marks (In Press), imipramine was no better than placebo up to 28 weeks follow-up despite adequate plasma levels. Patients in both groups had self-exposure homework and improved substantially and similarly in rituals, mood (including spontaneous panics), and social adjustment. Pretreatment mood was only marginally depressed in these patients, substantially less than in the inpatient ritualizers of Marks et al. (1980).

"Depressed mood" might itself turn out to be too broad a category of analysis. Detailed item analyses of the "depression" questionnaires used in these studies might permit a more fine-grained identification of which focal problems, if any, are relieved by antidepressants. The time is ripe to study the detailed *symptom* (as opposed to syndrome) profiles of the actions of anxiolytic and antidepressant drugs, among others, in generalized anxiety disorders, neurotic depression, and phobic obsessive-compulsive disorders over several years, including at least a year after drug withdrawal, to allow a better pharmacological dissection than traditional nosology has hitherto permitted. Such research might force us to reexamine the traditional distinctions made between anxiety, panic, and depression and perhaps develop a more meaningful classification of symptoms.

The claim has been made that imipramine is specifically indicated for reducing the panic attacks that afflict some agoraphobics (Klein, 1964; Zitrin et al., 1978). This proposal should be tested by careful measures of the drug's effect on panic attacks independent of its effect on depression. Klein and Zitrin et al. (1980) report neither mean values for depression nor the relationship between absolute measures of panic and depression before and after treatment. These authors clearly recognize the importance of exposure for overcoming avoidance and anticipatory anxiety, since the benefits they attribute to antidepressants in such situations are restricted to amelioration of panic attacks alone (Zitrin et al., 1980). However, the latest study by Marks employing the Klein-Zitrin measure of spontaneous panic in agoraphobics, found that it improved significantly and equally with imipramine and with placebo during treatment by exposure homework.

PRECONDITIONS FOR TREATMENT

The standard treatment for phobic-obsessive disorders is prolonged exposure in vivo to those situations which evoke the phobias or rituals until discomfort subsides. It is critical to select patients carefully, otherwise this approach is of little use. There are ten selection criteria (Marks, 1978a):

1. The patient should not have serious depression; if it is present, antidepressant treatment should be given first.
2. If the patient is drinking alcohol to the point of being drunk frequently or is taking high doses of sedative drugs (e.g. 40 mg or more of diazepam daily), these have to be reduced to acceptable levels (1½ oz. pure alcohol or 7.5 mg diazepam or the equivalent

daily) or preferably discontinued altogether before exposure treatment can begin. The patient can be hospitalized if necessary for drying out. Alcohol dependence is not uncommon among phobic-obsessives (Mullaney and Trippett, 1979), but in my experience such patients can often be successfully weaned from alcohol and treated by exposure.

3. Physical disorders such as cardiovascular disease, asthma, peptic ulcer, or ulcerative colitis might be aggravated by high anxiety and may require that exposure treatment be carried out gradually.

4. Patients' fears or rituals must be triggered by specific situations, people, or objects to be suitable for exposure treatment, otherwise they should be treated as for generalized anxiety states (300.01, 300.02), see p. 259.

5. It must be possible to define the patient's problems precisely through observations, otherwise behavioral treatment is not feasible. Examples of general statements that *do not* lend themselves to a behavioral approach are "I want to be cured, to get better," and "I am a bundle of nerves." Precisely defined problems that can be treated behaviorally would be, for example, "I panic whenever I go out of doors alone, and so I stay indoors unless I have an escort," or "I worry about dirt and germs so that I wash my hands all day and cannot work."

6. Not only should the patient's problems be precisely definable, they should generate specific goals which the patient wishes to achieve in treatment. An example of a less preferable goal would be "I want to become more sociable," whereas a well-defined and more attainable goal would be "At least once a week I want to visit friends or go to a party or reception and stay to the end." Similarly, "I want to lose my fear of air travel," is far less preferable than, "I want to fly from New York to Los Angeles and back."

7. Patients are less likely to cooperate in a potentially difficult treatment program unless overcoming their problems will make a tangible difference in their lives. A patient should be able to list the gains that would result from successful treatment. For an agoraphobic, these might be: "We will be able to go on vacation together for the first time in five years," "I will be able to take a job again," or for a compulsive ritualizer: "I will be able to hug my children again without worrying that I am infecting them with germs," "I will be able to do the cooking, clothes washing, and vacuuming again."

8. As most of the treatment consists of self-exposure exercises, patients must be willing to invest the time and effort necessary to overcome their worries. Even if their timetable is already overcrowded, they must agree to daily practice and if necessary give up some other activity in order to concentrate on dealing with the problem.

9. For some patients the self-management program will also need to recruit relatives or friends as cotherapists to help map out the program, sign the homework diaries, praise the patient for progress he or she has made, and help plan the next steps. If relatives continually participate in the patient's rituals and reassure him, they need to be brought into treatment to learn to stop contributing to such maintenance of the pathology.

10. Occasionally a cotherapist would be useful, but is absent. This might make treatment more difficult but not necessarily impossible.

STRATEGY FOR TREATMENT

This can be divided into five steps (Marks, 1978b):

1. The patient needs to be committed to working hard with the therapist, and if there is doubt about this, a written commitment (contract) to do so is sometimes helpful.

2. The patient should write down the specific problems and goals to be tackled in treatment, revising them as might be necessary.

3. The patient tries to identify the sensations he or she has when frightened, e.g. "I want to scream or run away," "I freeze in my tracks," "I tremble and shake."

4. The patient can be offered a list of tactics for coping with anxiety and discomfort to choose from during the exposure tasks. The patient should bring these coping tactics into play as soon as fear is sensed, and should choose whatever tactics he or she personally finds helpful. Among these tactics are slow, steady, deep breathing in and out; alternate tensing and relaxing of muscles; and, paradoxically, imagining the worst possible thing that could happen to oneself.

5. A timetable can be prepared for exposure of the patient to stimuli that evoke phobias or rituals, with recording immediately thereafter of what happened and revision of plans each week in the light

of progress achieved. The diary in Table 7-1 is an example of the kind of record that is needed. It pays special attention to the duration of exposure sessions, details of the tasks performed during the sessions, anxiety self-ratings during these tasks, and coping tactics used to deal with this anxiety. The patient also includes plans for future sessions in the diary and the cotherapist monitors progress.

General rules for exposure therapy are that goals should be made explicit before each session, enough time (up to several hours if need be) should be allowed to achieve these goals by the end of the session, and details of what transpired during the session should be recorded. Longer sessions are preferable to shorter sessions. Setbacks should be expected and the patient should be prepared to deal with them. The advent of fear should be a "bellringer" for bringing coping tactics into use.

Modifiers of standard course of treatment. If real situations are not readily available for exposure in vivo (e.g. for thunderstorm or flying phobics), the patient can instead be asked to imagine frightening scenes and these could be stimulated by the use of slides, films, books, or simulators such as flight simulations for flying phobics.

In the presence of severe depression, exposure should be stopped and antidepressant drugs like tricyclics or MAOIs given until the patient's mood has improved, after which exposure treatment can begin again. Mild depression is not a contraindication to continuing exposure.

If the patient is not compliant and avoids the cues that evoke phobias or rituals, then a treatment contract can be tried whereby the patient signs a written agreement to each step in treatment. If the patient remains persistently noncompliant after understanding what is required, then behavioral treatment should be discontinued.

A small number of patients do not habituate at all despite continuing exposure to appropriate cues, absence of covert or overt avoidance, absence of depression, and full compliance. Such total nonhabituation is apparent within the first two weeks of exposure treatment and would suggest that exposure should be discontinued. Usually patients who are going to improve show good signs of progress within the first few days. For nondepressed patients who are not compliant with or don't habituate to exposure, there is little to offer at the present time.

Side effects requiring treatment. Anxiety during exposure is common and does not require special measures. Nightmares and mild depression on nights following exposure sessions sometimes occur and usually clear up

TABLE 7–1

DIARY RECORD OF EXPOSURE TASKS

Day	Date	Session Began	Session Ended	The exposure task I performed was:	(0 = complete calm, 100 = absolute panic) My anxiety during the task was:	Comments, including coping tactics I used:	Name of co-therapist if any: *J. Smith* (Co-therapist's signature that task was completed)
				Example from an agoraphobic			
Sunday							
Monday							
Tuesday							
Wednesday		2:30 p.m.	4:30 p.m.	Walked to local supermarket and surrounding shops, bought food and presents for family, had coffee at drug-store	75	Felt worse when shops were crowded, practiced deep-breathing exercises	J. Smith (husband)
Thursday		10 a.m.	11:30 a.m.	Walked to local park, sat there for 1/2 hour till I felt better, then caught a bus downtown and back home	70	Felt giddy and faint, practiced imagining myself dropping dead	J. Smith
Friday		2 p.m.	4 p.m.	Rode a bus downtown and back 3 times till I felt better about it	60	Worst when bus was crowded— did deep-breathing exercises	J. Smith

Plan for next week: Repeat exposure exercises in bus, park and shops every day until my anxiety is no higher than 30. Thereafter start visits to my hairdresser, and short surface train journeys.

Saturday							
Sunday							
Monday							
Tuesday							
Wednesday							

Source: I.M. Marks, *Living with Fear*, McGraw-Hill, New York, 1978, pp. 258–259.

with continuing treatment. If they become more troublesome, then exposure could concentrate on less stressful cues until the patient is used to them, after which more difficult items can be confronted.

The criterion for adequate response is sufficient reduction of discomfort or rituals in the presence of the evoking stimuli. Reduction of anxiety from the start to the end of each session is usually a good indicator of progress. A decrement rather than a disappearance of anxiety is the goal; few patients lose *all* traces of anxiety, even after considerable gains.

If relapse occurs, its potential cause needs to be determined. This could be an intercurrent depressive episode which may require antidepressant drug treatment, or noncompliance, reasons for which would need to be reviewed and dealt with, or new life stress which has to be managed. Brief booster treatments of exposure may be needed on occasion. Generally, however, improvement in patients has been maintained in the two to four years of follow-up after exposure which has been recorded now with hundreds of patients.

ANXIETY STATES

ESSENTIAL FEATURES

The essential features of *panic disorder* (300.01) are recurrent panic attacks that occur at times unpredictably, though certain situations may become associated with a panic attack (e.g. being in situations from which a graceful and speedy exit is not feasible). Panic attacks are manifested by the sudden onset of intense apprehension, fear, or terror, often associated with feelings of impending doom. The most common symptoms experienced during an attack are dyspnea, palpitations, chest pain or discomfort, choking or smothering sensations, dizziness, vertigo, feelings of unreality, paresthesias, hot and cold flashes, sweating, faintness, trembling and fear of dying, going crazy or doing something uncontrolled during the attack.

The essential feature of *generalized anxiety disorder* (300.02) is generalized, persistent anxiety of at least one month's duration, without the specific symptoms that characterize *phobic disorder* (phobias), *panic disorder* (panic attacks), or *obsessive compulsive disorder* (obsessions or compulsions).

The essential feature of *post-traumatic stress disorder* (acute 308.30, chronic 309.81) is the development of a set of characteristic symptoms following a psychologically traumatic event that is generally outside the range of usual human experience. The characteristic symptoms involve reexperiencing the traumatic event; numbing of responsiveness to, or reduced involvement with, the external world; and a variety of autonomic, dysphoric, or cognitive symptoms. The traumatic event can be reexperienced in a variety of ways, such as painful, intrusive recollections of the event, or recurrent dreams or nightmares. In rare instances there are dissociativelike states. Diminished responsiveness to the external world usually begins soon after the traumatic event. The symptoms of excessive autonomic arousal may include hyperalertness, exaggerated startle response, and difficulty falling asleep.

TREATMENT GOALS

Unlike phobic and obsessive-compulsive disorders, anxiety in these conditions is mainly nonsituational, free floating, and not triggered by any particular stimuli. As yet there is no good evidence that for treatment it is necessary to distinguish between anxiety states, panic disorder, generalized anxiety disorder, and atypical anxiety disorder. Until such evidence is available, panic attacks are best regarded as clonic events likely to occur in the setting of chronically high anxiety such as that continuously found in agoraphobia and anxiety states and often also in atypical anxiety disorder. Treatment goals are to reduce the target anxiety, discomfort, or other complaints which patients wish to have treated. Vulnerable features in the personality theoretically indicate the need to improve problem-solving skills, but this is not often possible.

TREATMENTS

Anxiety management training (also known as stress immunization, stress inoculation, and other terms from cognitive behavior therapy) is currently fashionable for these conditions and follows similar lines to those described above under coping tactics during exposure for phobic-obsessive problems. So far, these methods have not been tested adequately in controlled studies of clinical populations. Just as there is a lack of evidence for the value of behavioral psychotherapy for such conditions, so it is with other psychotherapies, including dynamic modalities. Controlled studies of students indicated that systematic dynamic psychotherapy by experienced psychotherapists was no better for anxiety-depression than was counseling given by untrained workers (Strupp and Hadley, 1979). Both types of workers achieved only slightly more than *a waitlist control condition* in helping patients cope with crises. Counseling probably has more of a role to play than intensive psychotherapy, because of its lower cost.

For these disorders the use of antianxiety agents such as benzodiazepines is ubiquitous, and there is widespread evidence of their palliative value (Lader, 1980). However, the effect of these drugs tends to wear off a few hours after their use is discontinued, and addiction is not uncommon with prolonged use. Because it can be difficult to differentiate between anxiety states and other affective disorders (DSM-III categories 300.40 and 296.82, for example) antidepressant drugs are worth considering in patients who have depressed mood. Whether antidepressants have any advantage over exposure for panic disorder remains to be tested. There is little evidence that ECT is of any value for these conditions. There is some support for very limited use of psychosurgery in highly selected patients with chronic anxiety states in whom all other treatments have failed. Two retrospective controlled studies found that modified leucotomy was associated with significantly more anxiety reduction than were other treatments in a matched control group, both in agoraphobics and in obsessive-compulsive ritualizers (Marks et al., 1968; Tan et al., 1971).

There is a large literature on post-traumatic stress disorders describing the role of abreacting traumatic events, and abreaction has been induced by a variety of drugs given by inhalation, injection, or orally; by hypnosis; and by more straightforward suggestion. It is sometimes said that for the results of abreaction to be worthwhile the abreacted material should be integrated into the patient's awareness and linked with other material he has discussed. It is clear that abreaction is often followed by relief of distress, but that in many cases the problem remains unaltered, and a few patients seem to be sensitized by abreaction (Bond, 1952). Controlled studies to sort out these issues remain to be done.

TREATMENT CONTROVERSIES

There is little systematic work to guide the clinician in managing this group of anxiety disorders, and sparse evidence that any method has more than a short-term effect in clinical populations. Antianxiety drugs are largely palliative but in some cases may be the best we can offer. As noted on pp. 252–253, the evidence remains to be collected over several years to see if the symptom relief effects of anxiolytics and antidepressants in phobic-obsessive patients indeed warrant the traditional labels for such drugs or if our concepts need to be revised.

Some controlled work indicates that morbid grief, which might be regarded as one form of post-traumatic stress disorder, can be mitigated by preventive bereavement counseling in high-risk widows (Raphael, 1977). This approach contains an element of guided mourning, which a controlled investigation has found to have a small though significant beneficial effect compared to supportive counseling (Mawson et al., 1981). Other studies suggest that preparatory counseling and stress immunization procedures reduce postoperative stress in children and adults, but work of this kind is at too early a stage to make general recommendations.

SUMMARY OF TREATMENTS FOR ANXIETY STATES AND FOR POST-TRAUMATIC AND ATYPICAL ANXIETY DISORDERS

The standard course of treatment would be to elicit precipitants where present, to deal with these where possible, and to give brief counseling and palliate with antianxiety drugs, unless the anxiety is thought to reflect depressive mood, in which case antidepressant drugs can be considered. Behavioral methods enjoy no clear advantage. Some regard abreactive methods as useful for post-traumatic stress disorders. Crisis coping and counseling are useful when appropriate. For morbid grief, bereavement counseling which contains an element of guided mourning might be indicated. Criteria for adequate response are remission of the anxiety signs and symptoms, particularly when off medication. Addiction syndromes may develop, especially with benzodiazepines, in which case controlled withdrawal from medication is necessary. When antidepressant drugs seem beneficial the tendency is to regard the problem as depressive, and the drugs may need to be continued for years.

OVERALL SUMMARY

Phobic and obsessive-compulsive disorders are treatable by behavioral psychotherapy with exposure to the stimuli which evoke phobias and rituals until the distress subsides. Of the many forms of exposure which are possible, prolonged exposure in vivo seems the most effective, and good outcome has been reported in many studies up to several years follow-up. Improvement tends to generalize to aspects of social adjustment formerly handicapped by the disorder. Recent trends have been to place increasing responsibility for treatment on the patient by having him carry out self-exposure homework with the help of relatives as cotherapists when necessary. Clear delineation of treatment goals and monitoring of progress toward them is an integral part of therapy, which can only be carried out in patients who wish to have treatment and are cooperative. Large amounts of alcohol or antianxiety drugs are counterproductive in such patients. Antidepressants are indicated where there is depressive mood, but avoidance usually requires management by exposure. Antidepressants are ineffective in overcoming anticipatory anxiety and avoidance, which must be managed by exposure.

In anxiety states and post-traumatic stress disorder, behavioral methods enjoy no clear advantage. Management is by a judicious mixture of crisis coping, brief counseling, palliative anxiolytics, and antidepressants. The status of abreactive methods for post-traumatic stress disorders is untested. For morbid grief, bereavement counseling with guided mourning can be useful.

REFERENCES

Benjamin S, Marks I, Huson J: Active muscular relaxation in desensitization of phobic patients. Psychol Med. 2:381, 1972.

Bond DD: The Love and Fear of Flying. International Universities Press, New York. 1952.

Cobb J, McDonald R, Marks IM, Stern R: Marital versus exposure therapy: psychological treatments of co-existing marital and phobic-obsessive problems. Behavior Analysis and Modification. 4:3–6, 1980.

Emmelkamp P&G: Paper to European Association Behavior Therapy. Paris. September 1979.

Emmelkamp PMG, Kuipers ACM: Agoraphobia: a follow-up study 4 years after treatment. Brit J Psychiat. 134:352–355, 1979.

Greist JH, Marks IM, Berlin F, Gourney KA, Nashirvani H: Avoidance versus confrontation of fear: a test of the exposure hypothesis of fear reduction. Behav Ther. 11:1–14, 1980.

Hafner J, Marks IM: Exposure in vivo of agoraphobics: the contributions of diazepam, group exposure and anxiety evocation. Psychol Med. 6:71–88, 1976.

Jannoun L, Munby M, Catalan J, Gelder M: A homebased treatment programme for agoraphobia: replication and controlled evaluation. Brit J Psychiatry. 33:101–105, 1980.

Jones E: The Standard Edition of the Complete Psychological Works of Sigmund Freud. Hogarth Press, London. 17:159–168, 1955.

Klein DF: Delineation of two drug-responsive anxiety syndromes. Psychopharmacologia. 5:397, 1964.

Lader M: Depressions: a fresh approach to assessment defines treatment. Modern Medicine. 25:63–64, 1980.

Marks IM: Behavioral psychotherapy. Review I: obsessive-compulsive disorders. Review II: sexual disorders. Am J Psychiat. 138:584–592, 1981 and 138:750–756, 1981.

Marks IM: Phobic disorders 4 years after treatment. Brit J Psychiat. 118:683–688, 1971.

Marks IM: Behavioral treatments of phobic and obsessive-compulsive disorders: a critical appraisal. Chapter in: Progress in Behavior Modification. Hersen, M, Eisler, RM, Miller, PW (eds), Academic Press, New York. 1975.

Marks IM: Phobias and obsessions. Chapter in: Experimental Psychopathology. Maser, J and Seligman, M (eds.), Wiley, New York. 1977.

Marks IM: Living with Fear. McGraw-Hill, New York. 1978a.

Marks IM: Behavioral psychotherapy of adult neurosis. In Handbook of Psychotherapy and Behavior Modification, 2nd ed. Garfield, S and Bergin, AE (eds.). Wiley, New York. 1978b.

Marks IM: Cure and Care of Neurosis. Psychol Med. 9:629–660, 1979.

Marks IM: Drugs combined with behavioral psychotherapy. Chapter in: International Handbook of Behavior Modification and Behavior Therapy, Bellack, AS, Hersen, M, and Kazdin, AE (eds.), Plenum Press, New York. 1980.

Marks IM: Cure and Care of Neurosis. Wiley, New York. 1981.

Marks IM, Gelder MG, Edward JG: A controlled trial of hypnosis and desensitization for phobias. Brit J Psychiat. 114:1263, 1968.

Marks IM, Hallam RS, Connolly J, Philpott R: Nursing in Behavioral Psychotherapy. Royal College of Nursing Research Series. Henrietta Place, London W1. 1977.

Marks IM, Rachman S, Hodgson R: Treatment of chronic obsessive-compulsive neurosis by in vivo exposure. Brit J Psychiat. 113:271, 1975.

Marks IM, Stern RS, Mawson D, Cobb J, McDonald R: Clomipramine and exposure for obsessive-compulsive rituals. Brit J Psychiat. 136:1–25, 1980.

Mathews AM, Jannoun L, Gelder M: Self-help methods in agoraphobia. Paper to European Association Behavior Therapy, Paris. Behavior Therapy. 1980.

Mathews AM, Johnston DW, Shaw PM, Gelder MG: Process variables and the prediction of outcome in behavior therapy. Brit J Psychiat. 125:256–264, 1974.

Mawson D, Marks IM, Ramm E, Stern RS: Guided mourning for morbid grief: a controlled study. Brit J Psychiat:138, 1981.

McDonald R, Sartory G, Grey SJ, Cobb J, Stern R, Marks IM: The effects of self-exposure instructions on agoraphobic outpatients. Behav Res Ther. 17:83–85, 1978.

McPherson FM, Brougham L: Maintenance of improvement in agoraphobic patients treated by behavioural methods. 4-Year follow-up. Behaviour Research and Therapy. 18:150–152, 1980.

Mullaney JA, Trippett CJ: Alcohol dependence and phobias: clinical description and relevance. Brit J Psychiat. 135:565–573, 1979.

Munby M, Johnston DW: Agoraphobia: long-term followup of behavioral treatment. Brit J Psychiat. 137:418–427, 1980.

Nunes J, Marks IM: Feedback of true heart rate during exposure in vivo. Arch Gen Psychiat. 32:933, 1975.

Nunes J, Marks IM: Feedback of true heart rate during exposure in vivo: partial replication with methodological improvement. Arch Gen Psychiat. 33:1346–1350, 1976.

Rabavilas AD, Boulougouris JC, Stefanis D: Duration of flooding session in the treatment of obsessive-compulsive patients. Behav Res Ther. 14:349–355, 1976.

Raphael B: Prevention intervention with the recently bereaved. Arch Gen Psychiat. 34:1450–1454, 1977.

Robertson JR: 24 hour versus 1 hour daily response prevention for rituals. Unpublished manuscript. 1979.

Sheehan DV, Ballenger J, Jacobsen G: Treatment of endogenous anxiety with phobic, hysterical, and hypochondriacal symptoms. Arch Gen Psychiat. 37:51–59, 1980.

Stampfl TC: Implosive therapy: the theory, the subhuman analogue, the strategy and the technique. 1. The Theory. In: Armitage, SG (ed). Behavior Modifications Techniques in the Treatment of Emotional Disorders, Battle Creek, Michigan. V.A. Publication. pp. 22–37, 1967.

Stern RS, Marks IM: A comparison of brief and prolonged flooding in agoraphobics. Arch Gen Psychiat. 28:210, 1973.

Strupp HH, Hadley SW: Specific versus non-specific factors in psychotherapy. Arch Gen Psychiat. 36:1125–1136, 1979.

Tan E, Marks IM, Marset P: Bimedial leucotomy in obsessive-compulsive neurosis: a controlled serial inquiry. Brit J Psychiat. 118:155–164, 1971.

Thoren P, Asberg M, Cronholm B, Jornestedt L, Traskman L: Clomipramine treatment of obsessive-compulsive disorder: I. A controlled clinical trial. Arch Gen Psychiat. 37:1281–1285, 1980.

Watson JP, Gaind R, Marks IM: Prolonged exposure: a rapid treatment for phobias. Brit Med J. 1:13, 1971.

Watson JP, Gaind R, Marks IM: Physiological habituation to continuous phobic stimulation. Behav Res Ther. 10:269, 1972.

Williams LW, Rappaport JA: Exposure with and without cognitive therapy in agoraphobics. Paper to American Psychological Association, Montreal. September 1–5, 1980.

Zitrin CM, Klein DF, Woerner MG: Behavior therapy, supportive psychotherapy, imipramine and phobias. Arch Gen Psychiat. 35:307–316, 1978.

Zitrin CM, Klein DF, Woerner MG: Treatment of agoraphobia with group exposure in vivo and imipramine. Arch Gen Psychiatry. 37:63–72, 1980.

8 | Somatoform Disorders

SOMATIZATION DISORDER (300.81)
Herbert Ochitill

ESSENTIAL FEATURES

The essential features of *somatization disorder* are recurrent and multiple somatic complaints of several years' duration for which medical attention has been sought but which are apparently not due to any physical disorder.

TREATMENT GOALS

There are several interrelated objectives in the treatment of somatization disorder (also known as Briquet's syndrome). The clinician attempts to reduce the frequency, intensity, and persistence of the diverse symptomatology of these patients. Thereby, the patient's use of the health care system and risk of superfluous diagnostic and therapeutic activity are reduced. Treatment is directed at minimizing the disturbance of family life, social relations, and vocational ability created by the disorder. The psychiatrist hopes to increase the patient's appreciation of relations among his somatic complaints, life setting, and psychological response. The patient is assisted in developing alternative coping strategies in the face of life changes.

Treatment

A review of the treatment approaches to somatization disorder requires strict inspection of each description of the involved patient population, because all such populations do not clearly demonstrate the diagnostic criteria given in DSM-III for those with somatization disorder. There have been several difficulties in making a judgment regarding the characteristics of the patient group: nosologic terms have had diverse and changing meanings; many studies describe patients in terms of categorical levels only; information about longitudinal course is minimal or nonexistent. Rather than reviewing treatment approach and outcome of dissimilar patient groups considered under the rubric "hysteria," I have selected studies in which it was likely that the patient group reflected the criteria defining somatization disorder in DSM-III.

Various opinions exist as to who ought to manage the patient with chronic somatization. There is sentiment in some quarters that the nonpsychiatric physician is well-placed to provide sufficient management of such cases, i.e. those elements necessary to improve the patient's condition can be supplied by the physician. Goodwin (1969) noted that the physician ". . . by reassurance, direct advice and permitting the patient to talk freely, may help produce behavioral change that will improve the patient's social adjustment, if not diminish the flow of medical complaints." Indeed, the fact that the patient asks for medical treatment of a somatic complaint implies a key treatment role for the nonpsychiatric clinician. This issue has been raised regarding all of the somatoform disorders.

Individual Psychotherapy
Investigation of individual psychotherapy has uncovered major difficulties. Guze and Perley (1963) followed patients with Briquet's syndrome over a six- to eight-year period. While all were offered individual psychotherapy, only a small minority began and most asserted that therapy was irrelevant or ineffective. Only four patients engaged in psychotherapy for a period of months—and only one lasted a full year. The authors suggested that psychotherapy had no short- or long-term influence and they concluded that "refusal to accept a psychiatric approach appears to be a characteristic of this disorder." This finding is consistent with the observation that patients who define their illness in "bodily terms" tend to do poorly in psychotherapy (Stone et al., 1961).

Behavioral Therapy

Kass et al. (1972) studied a behavioral therapy approach in five hospitalized single women (ages 17–25) with hysterical (histrionic) personality disorder. While their histories did not clearly describe somatization disorder, they acknowledged psychological distress and disturbed interpersonal relations. Only one of the five had chronic physical complaints which she voiced when discouraged or frustrated. None had a history of excessive visits with physicians or unusual amounts of medication, surgery, or hospitalization. Therapy combined elements of a behavioral and a group approach. The patients lived together in the ward, were expected to define the maladaptive behaviors of each other, and played an active part in the selective reward and punishment of behavior. Behavioral techniques included operant conditioning, desensitization, assertiveness training, role-playing, and psychodrama. The patient with somatic complaints remained in the hospital 28 days. She continued in a periodic group experience for six months following discharge. On discharge and at 18-month follow-up, the patient demonstrated marked reduction in somatic complaints and other behaviors and had made striking gains at work and in her social relations.

The study of Kass et al. (1972) is too limited in scope to draw conclusions. No study of behavioral treatment in patients with well-defined somatization disorder has been done, so that the area is open to further investigation.

Group Therapy

Slavson (1955) contended that patients who have a "compulsive and continual" need to speak of physical complaints impede the progress of a therapeutic group. Yalom (1970) suggested that group therapy drop-outs demonstrate greater evidence of "somatization of conflicts" with persistent somatic complaints and an inclination to ascribe dysphoria to physical factors.

Despite such concern, several decades ago Brody (1959) treated three middle-aged women with psychoanalytically oriented group therapy, after they had been referred, somewhat unwillingly, from nonpsychiatric physicians. The three had undergone a total of 18 major and minor surgical operations and their physicians believed they had received "unnecessary operations." The group met for 90 minutes each week over a period of three years with one patient a less than constant participant. There is no mention of concurrent treatments, although one patient used sedatives and tranquilizers. The author reported that when the sessions stopped temporarily one summer, the patients' visits to the medical clinic increased. Brody described decreasing depressive and somatic symptoms during the course of the therapy. Although two further operations occurred during the period of group meetings, the therapist observed resistance to surgical "opportunities" among the patients. This uncontrolled study involved patients with documented medical disturbance and, in two cases, the suggestion of other mental disorders. Four other patients entered and quit the group. Study design also compromised the value of the investigation.

More recently, Valko (1976) described a group of psychiatric outpatients who had experienced years of intermittent, disturbing physical symptoms which prompted frequent visits to physicians and the use of several medications. Some patients had not responded to individual therapy. The group met weekly for 90 minutes with the simple intent of getting the patients to talk to each other. Although individual appointments were discouraged, brief discussions with one or two patients often took place following group meetings. During an average stay of five months in the group, six middle-aged female patients experienced improved family relations, fewer physical complaints at home, reduced medication use, less frequent emergency medical visits, and fewer visits to the psychiatric clinic. Two of the six could not sustain these gains and required continued group sessions. The four patients available for follow-up one to two years after the group had begun were able to maintain a reduction of medication, improved mood, and increased self-confidence.

Though deficient in design, these studies of group therapy suggest a positive effect of treatment. These findings deserve substantiation from soundly designed future investigations. Although specific indications for group treatment have not been established, it may be tried as the initial approach, or it may find use with patients when other therapies prove ineffective.

Family Therapy
There has been no formal exploration of family therapy with this disorder. In recent years, the family approach has been effectively employed in the management of a variety of organic conditions such as bronchial asthma and diabetes (Minuchin et al., 1975). It is conceivable, though

untested, that family therapy will prove useful in treating somatization disorder.

Somatic Therapy

Little sound evidence exists as to the efficiency of somatic treatments. There has been brief comment on the use of electroconvulsive treatment. Guze and Perley (1963) noted that two patients with somatization disorder received electroconvulsive therapy during psychiatric hospitalization. While treatment reduced crying spells and depressive feelings, somatic complaints and other behavior did not improve. In a chart review comparing psychiatric inpatients with and without somatization disorder, Bibb and Guze (1972) noted that depression was the most frequent reason for psychiatric admissions of both groups of patients. Electroconvulsive therapy did not reduce the frequency and intensity of chronic somatic complaints.

Peters (1974) described an open, uncontrolled study of 20 patients with head or back pain of unknown etiology seen in an outpatient neurology clinic who demonstrated Feighner's criteria for "probable" hysteria. Both the neurological and general physical examinations were normal. Patients had not found relief from "traditional" or "standard" (undescribed) treatment. All were given six months of chlordiazepoxide followed by six months of chlorpromazine with route and dosage undescribed. Five patients reported considerable symptomatic improvement with chlordiazepoxide while sixteen patients reported considerable improvement with chlorpromazine. The study is seriously limited by inadequate description of the patients, their illness history, past and current treatment, and the lack of rigorous design.

Scallet et al. (1976) reported on a controlled prospective study of electrosleep with twenty psychiatric outpatients with somatization disorder in which electrosleep had no lasting benefit.

Treatment Controversies

Debate continues over the treatment roles of the psychiatric and nonpsychiatric clinician. By necessity, the nonpsychiatric practitioner will see a substantial number of these patients. A sensitive and concerned clinician may reduce the morbidity of this chronic, polysymptomatic disorder. Whether the psychiatrist's particular skills and experience offer significant added benefit remains moot. In fact, many of these patients will not accept psychiatric referral. Much of the work cited above involved patients who may not have had somatization disorder as defined in DSM-III. In addition, those patients who accepted psychiatric treatment may represent a select subgroup which is not representative of the disorder as a whole.

It has been proposed that the clinician who provides advice, reassurance, and opportunity for expression can promote substantial change in the patient with somatization disorder. While clinical experience suggests that such interaction may be effective in some cases, there is little, if any, well conceived investigative work to support these assertions. Some clinicians continue to explore the uses of group therapy in treating this disorder.

SUMMARY

Currently, there are no well designed studies of the treatment of somatization disorder. Clinical experience suggests that a small minority of patients with somatization disorder accept psychiatric treatment. Thus, the nonpsychiatric care provider is often the most likely and accepted therapeutic agent.

There is evidence to suggest that individual psychotherapy is ineffective among those willing to engage in treatment. Behavioral and family treatment remain untested. Study of group therapy indicates preliminary evidence of positive outcome with patients seen in a psychiatric treatment setting.

There has been no convincing evidence that somatic treatment is efficacious. Electroconvulsive treatment has reduced concurrent affective symptoms without amelioration of chronic somatic complaints.

CONVERSION DISORDER (300.11)
(HYSTERICAL NEUROSIS, CONVERSION TYPE)
Herbert Ochitill

ESSENTIAL FEATURES

The essential feature of *conversion disorder* is a clinical picture in which the predominant disturbance is a loss of or alteration in physical functioning that suggests physical disorder but which instead is apparently an expression of a psychological conflict or need.

TREATMENT GOALS

In treating conversion disorder, the clinician attempts to reduce symptoms, alter psychological elements responsible for symptom formation, facilitate greater independence of the patient from the health care system, lessen social and vocational disability, and encourage changes in the patient's environment. Objectives are influenced by the therapist's theoretical orientation, the therapeutic modality, the clinical setting, the interests and abilities of the clinician, and the qualities and self-defined difficulties of the patient.

TREATMENT

Before the treatment of conversion disorder is discussed specifically, findings from a few of the most extensive studies of the course of conversion symptoms will be reviewed.

Age at onset of symptoms has been associated with prognosis (Ljunberg, 1957; Slater and Glithero, 1965); there is a tendency for earlier age at onset to be associated with a better prognosis. Acute onset is also a favorable prognosticator. There has been some evidence that specific symptoms among conversion disorders have a distinctive pattern of relapse and remission (Carter, 1949). Aside from the symptom pattern, Ljunberg's investigation noted an association between abnormal or "deviating" personality as judged by the author's interview and poor prognosis. On seven- to eleven-year follow-up of patients with "hysteria," Slater and Glithero (1965) noted that a majority experienced a course reflective of a basic organic process.

Individual Psychotherapy

Among the psychotherapies which have been employed to treat conversion disorders, psychoanalysis has played a role of considerable importance.

Fenichel (1945) noted fifty years after the publication of *Studies in Hysteria* that "conversion hysteria is the classical subject matter of psychoanalysis . . . the psychoanalytic method was discovered, tested and perfected through the study of hysterical patients . . . it is the psychoanalytic therapy of hysteria that continues to yield the best therapeutic results." More recently, clinicians (Marmor, 1953; Zetzel, 1968) have reviewed the assumptions about personality structure, sources of pathogenesis, and therapeutic outcome. The combination of overt conversion symptomatology and a serious character disorder has come to be understood as an exceedingly difficult therapeutic challenge.

Beyond the collective claims of clinical case descriptions, more extensive investigation of the patient, therapist, and process variables which determine the therapeutic outcome would be of considerable value. Several of the psychoanalytic institutes and clinics have reported reviews of clinical activity. Drawing meaningful conclusions from such reports is hampered by the following: lack of standardized, multidimensional patient descriptions and outcome criteria; lack of controls or comparative groups; little or no description of principles of patient assignment when there are differences in the treatment offered; and rare follow-up information.

Fenichel (1930) reported ten years' experience from the Berlin Psychoanalytic Institute involving 105 cases of conversion hysteria. Seventy-four patients continued in therapy for at least six months. Of the 74, 46 were "cured" or "much improved" while 28 were "improved" or without change. Weber et al. (1967) reported on approximately 1000 patients treated at Columbia Psychoanalytic Clinic, more than half of whom were treated with psychoanalysis while the remainder received psychoanalytically oriented psychotherapy. The entire group began therapy with 11% of the patients demonstrating conversion symptoms; 7% of patients experienced such symptoms at the termination of therapy. Despite this less than dramatic reduction of symptoms, patients experienced a shift in the "primary problem area" during the course of treatment from symptoms to personal relations.

Clinicians have practiced supportive psychotherapy for cases in which there was brief symptom duration without a previous history of conversion, evidence of prominent environmental precipitants, presence of a severe personality disorder, or in work with symptomatic children and adolescents. Excluding those with a severe personality disorder, case reports suggest a relatively rapid, symptomatic improvement for patients in these categories.

Family Therapy

There is no systematic documented work using a primary family system approach to the treatment of conversion disorders; such treatment would consider a conversion symptom in an individual family member to be a marker of a dysfunctional family system and treatment would be directed at changes in the function of the entire system. Previously, the clinician approached the family as a source of information, helped the family to understand that the patient has an emotional disorder, received the family's support for the treatment plan, and tried to reduce the "secondary gain" of the symptom.

Behavior Therapy

Behavior therapists have continued to expand their contribution to the treatment of conversion disorders. Case reports have included outpatient and inpatient treatment utilizing instruction and systematic contingent reward, punishment, or inattention. Enduring success has been reported with patients who were disabled for years despite other therapeutic approaches (Munford et al., 1976; Liebson, 1969).

There is a continued need for controlled, prospective studies. The reviews of clinical practice which follow are limited by meager patient description, lack of controls, unclear rationale for allocation of treatment, use of a mix of treatment methods, lack of independent assessment of patients and, in some of the work, the report of immediate outcome only.

Carter (1949) reviewed the treatment outcome and long-term course of 100 patients with a diagnosis of acute "hysteria." Treatment, including behavioral elements, yielded mixed immediate and long-term results for several types of conversion disorders.

Lazarus (1963) studied treatment outcome for a cohort which included 27 patients with conversion or dissociative symptoms. Behavioral treatments which, at times, involved ancillary use of hypnosis, medication, or multiple therapists resulted in marked improvement or recovery of 19 (71%) patients following the average of 14 treatment sessions.

Dickes (1974) reported on the comparative efficacy of a behaviorally oriented "special regimen" for the inpatient treatment of 16 patients. All received milieu and group therapy. The author noted that the "special regimen" resulted in greater immediate symptomatic improvement.

Hypnosis

Hypnosis has played a modest ancillary role in treatment. Hypnosis offers the opportunity for greater understanding of the patient, emotive abreaction, dramatic (often transient) symptom relief, and powerful expectation of therapeutic change in some patients. Frankel (1978) noted that hypnotizability does not ensure significant, lasting therapeutic benefits and asserted that 20–30% of individuals are "minimally responsive" to hypnotic induction. Clinically, hypnosis has been most often applied when immediate symptom relief is sought. It is also employed as a psychotherapeutic adjunct.

There is no explicit systematic work on combinations of psychotherapy. Without clear specifications for use of various combinations, application has been determined by the judgment of the clinician. Combinations that do appear in case reports include: supportive psychotherapy, family counseling and behavior therapy; and individual, group, and behavior therapy.

Somatic Therapy

Pharmacotherapy has been reported in single cases in which the effective use of antipsychotic medication and, in one instance, lithium have been noted. The latter case (Van Putten and Alban, 1977) is intriguing since the patient had a very long history of conversion symptoms which had not responded to various treatments and in which response to lithium could be contrasted with lack of placebo response.

There have been two reviews of the use of electroconvulsive treatment (ECT). These reports of clinical activity lack controls and adequate description of the patients or the indications for treatment. Milligan (1946) studied treatment outcome for 41 inpatients who generally had long-standing symptoms. Up to four convulsions daily resulted in marked symptomatic improvement in all but one patient during an eight-month follow-up period. Sands (1946) found only temporary symptomatic improvement, at best, among 30 patients with conversion and dissociative symptoms who received ECT.

Walter et al. (1972) studied the use of a combination of somatic treatments; the authors used a tranquilizer or sedative, such as methaqualone, nitrazepam, or chlorpromazine in combination with ECT and antidepressant medication. Patients were admitted with severe, long-standing symptoms usually unresponsive to ECT or antidepressants. Patients were chosen on the basis of prior treatment failure or the need for immediate symptom relief. Thirty-nine percent of patients showed symptomatic recovery or marked improvement.

Various combinations of somatic and psychotherapy have been used. Clinicians have employed minor tranquilizers or sedatives to enhance the suggestive elements of psychotherapy. Commonly, barbiturates have been used to assist recall of traumatic events and associated feelings, and to facilitate symptom improvement. Bratfos et al. (1967) reported a controlled study of supportive psychotherapy and a minor tranquilizer. Thirty-seven psychiatric inpatients with a collection of anxiety, conversion, and depressive symptoms said to be severe and long-standing were treated in a double-blind study of tybamate. Patients were given a week of tybamate and a week of placebo. Tybamate showed no significant advantage over placebo for the reduction of conversion symptoms.

TREATMENT CONTROVERSIES

Controversy continues over the choice of appropriate treatment objectives for each patient. Some clinicians argue that nothing short of personality reorganization is adequate; others assert that efforts beyond symptom elimination are superfluous. Although the assertion of symptom substitution has never been systematically documented, some clinicians continue to believe that symptomatic treatment only encourages the appearance of new forms of psychopathology. The lack of inclusive, long-term outcome data hinders clarification of the controversy.

Review of the use of ECT has yielded conflicting results. Differences in technique and outcome measures may partially account for differences in efficacy.

SUMMARY

Studies suggest that age at onset, acuteness of onset, personality, and existent organic processes influence the course of conversion disorders. The work on prognosis emphasizes the potential for misapplication of psychiatric treatment where organic disturbance predominates.

Regrettably, psychiatric treatment of conversion disorders is without the benefit of adequate empirical substantiation. Few well-designed studies are available to assist the clinician in making a treatment decision.

The particular utility of psychoanalysis and psychoanalytically oriented psychotherapy has not been well established. The claim that these approaches discourage symptom recurrence by treating the sources of symptom formation remains debatable. A survey of clinical activity suggests that these treatments may reduce the patient's relative concern regarding the symptoms although it is unclear whether this change alters the patient's disability level.

Supportive psychotherapy is likely to be used with patients felt to have an especially good or poor prognosis. Therapy research has not described the selective advantage of supportive psychotherapy over no or minimal contact.

Large-scale reports of behavior therapy mix behavioral methods with other treatments, making assessment of behavior therapy difficult. Case reports, although sometimes impressive in the treatment of chronic disturbance, provide no specific indications for behavior therapy. By definition, the patient with an exclusive interest in symptom reduction may be especially receptive to behavior therapy.

Reports of the efficacy of somatic treatment have not been encouraging. The very few studies on pharmacotherapy offer little promise. Studies of electroconvulsive treatment have yielded variable results.

PSYCHOGENIC PAIN DISORDER (307.80)

Carl J. Getto and Herbert Ochitill

Essential Features

The essential feature of *psychogenic pain disorder* is a clinical picture in which the predominant feature is the complaint of pain, in the absence of adequate physical findings and in association with evidence of the etiological role of psychological factors.

It should be noted, however, that this definition actually encompasses two distinct clinical interpretations. On the one hand, it defines a group of patients who persistently complain of pain in the absence of *any* physical findings, and for whom psychosocial factors are felt to be wholly etiologic. These patients are viewed as not having "real" organic (pathophysiologic) pain, but rather, the pain is an expression of an underlying psychological or social problem.

An alternative interpretation of the psychogenic pain disorder views all chronic pain in a multidimensional way. That is, chronic pain actually has several components—organic, psychological, and social.

Pinsky's (1978) description of the chronic intractable benign pain syndrome defines the characteristics of these patients:

1. They have ongoing pain, not due to neoplastic disease and have no significant ongoing pathophysiological mechanisms that would explain their ongoing pain.
2. They have had most, if not all, standard medical/surgical treatment without lasting success.
3. They have a relatively fixed mechanical-organic belief structure with regard to bodily functions.
4. Their chronic pain has become the central focus to their thoughts, behavior, and social relationships.
5. They may have ancillary problems involving opioid or hypnotic drug dependency.
6. These patients have a life history of inability to form any psychological view of life problems.
7. As a group these patients tend to exhibit symptoms consistent with "alexithymia," that is, they have constricted emotional functioning, impoverished family life and difficulty verbalizing their emotions.
8. In general they are fearful and distrustful of psychiatry and psychotherapy.

This multifactorial conceptualization of chronic pain patients represents a recent development in the treatment of chronic pain. The following discussion will be based on this interpretation of chronic pain since it encompasses and enlarges upon the more narrow definition offered in DSM-III.

On one level, treatment of psychogenic pain disorder aims at ameliorating the patient's pain, i.e. the patient's reported distress becomes a treatment target. On another level, however, the clinician intervenes to reduce the consequent disability of pain. The disability is manifested by medication dependence, frequent health clinic visits, unnecessary diagnostic evaluation and treatment, and impaired social and vocational activity. Increased understanding of these patients and recent therapeutic developments have promoted a shift away from treatment of the pain per se. When the pain is associated with another psychiatric disorder, treatment addresses the associated disturbance.

TREATMENTS

Several authors, including Engel (1959) and Blumer (1975) have commented on the hesitation of psychogenic pain patients to accept treatment in a psychiatric setting. Therefore, treatments which are solely psychiatric in nature (i.e. individual psychotherapy) and are given outside of a multidisciplinary program tend to be applicable to a minority of pain patients, and then seem to have only limited effectiveness.

The recognition that chronic pain is really a biopsychosocial illness has prompted the institution of a *multidisciplinary approach* to the evaluation and treatment of chronic pain disorders. Multidisciplinary pain clinics combine the expertise of anesthesiology, neurology, internal medicine, psychiatry and psychology, physiatry, and sociology among other specialties. The advantages of such a multidisciplinary approach for psychiatrists include:

1. "Legitimizing" the role of the psychiatrist and allowing the patient to view psychologic aspects of chronic pain within the context of medical illness.
2. Providing the psychiatrist with thorough knowledge of the patient's physical condition.
3. Allowing integrated treatment planning, which alleviates the feeling on the part of the patient that psychiatric treatment is an "afterthought."
4. Allowing integrated multidisciplinary treatment.
5. Effective treatment. Psychological intervention within a multidisciplinary framework seems to be much more effective than if given outside such an integrated program. The outcome statistics of multidisciplinary inpatient programs, which incorporate a variety of psychological interventions, support this.

Individual Psychotherapy
There has been little systematic study of the efficacy of individual psychotherapy. The available information is derived from retrospective sur-

veys of clinical activity without the advantage of prospective, controlled studies. Reports often include patients with other mental disorders and, typically, treatment is inadequately described.

Ziegler et al. (1960) identified 75 psychogenic pain patients seen via referral to a psychiatric consultation service. The authors cited case material which depicts the tendency for pain to coexist with "some evidence of depression." When the pain is clinically predominant, it is especially difficult to decide if an affective disorder causes the pain. The authors reported little impressive therapeutic outcome with these patients. Patients persistently regarded their difficulties as exclusively physical and "most refused psychotherapy on a tentative trial basis." That minority accepting psychiatric treatment, particularly as inpatients, "did relatively well."

Tinling and Klein (1966) described 14 patients referred from a medical service with intractable pain, no substantiation of organic dysfunction, and evidence of psychogenic elements. Psychiatric treatment was advised particularly if the patients associated pain with difficulties in living. These patients expressed depressive affect and demonstrated difficulty with aggressive feelings. The authors echoed prior concern about the difficulties of treatment; many of the patients regarded psychiatric referral as rejection and were not motivated to seek psychiatric help.

Blumer (1975) reviewed his experience with 27 patients, most of whom had made extraordinary efforts to receive neurosurgical relief for acute exacerbations of severe, long-standing psychogenic pain. Again, patients often resented entry of the psychiatrist, which usually occurred after all somatic studies were complete or were not expected to yield substantial results. The author acknowledged that these patients "are usually not good candidates for psychotherapy." Supportive psychotherapy was helpful for some, especially when a person important to the patient endorsed the effort to identify difficult life changes, express feelings, and minimize discussion of pain.

Walters (1961) reported his experience with 430 of his private patients referred after multiple diagnostic evaluations and therapeutic trials. Over one-quarter of these patients had intractable pain, while two-thirds were referred from medical specialists or general practitioners and had "intercurrent and incidental" pain. A majority of patients had other psychiatric disorders. Although Walters noted that three-quarters of these patients showed considerable symptomatic improvement, the report did not distinguish treatment outcome for patients with psychogenic pain disorder. Treatment was not adequately described and included various treatment combinations.

Group Therapy

Group therapy has become the primary psychotherapeutic approach in many multidisciplinary treatment programs. Pinsky and Malyou (1979) used group therapy extensively within the context of an inpatient multidisciplinary treatment program. Their psychotherapeutic approach combines elements of transactional analysis, psychodrama, psychodynamics, and cognitive therapy. Treatment goals include: (1) changing the experience of pain; (2) eliminating or reducing the dysphoria of chronic pain; (3) modifying dysfunctional pain behaviors (e.g. seeking surgery, continuing the sick role in patient's family); (4) helping the patients assume responsibility for pain reduction; (5) enhancing the patient's ability to enjoy life. This type of therapy has been instrumental in the success of this and other multidisciplinary treatment programs (Hendler, 1981).

Herman and Baptiste (1981) reported on 75 patients treated with outpatient group therapy. Therapy included education, group discussion, and relaxation. Patients were taught to distinguish between neutral and painful sensations, and to substitute relaxation for pain behavior. The consequences of pain behavior were analyzed and alternative coping strategies were examined. Group discussion allowed for ventilation of feelings, mutual support, and learning adaptive alternatives to pain behavior. The patients also received much positive reinforcement from the other group members. Results included reduction in depression, pain perception, and analgesic intake. Furthermore, the numbers who found employment increased significantly.

Behavior Therapy

Inpatient, multidisciplinary pain treatment units have become a standard approach to the treatment of chronic pain. These units are based on a behavioral treatment approach described by Fordyce (1973). Fordyce conceptualized chronic pain as a set of pathologic behaviors which are exacerbated and maintained by environmental influences. The pain behavior of the chronic pain patient is reinforced by rest (inactivity), money (compensation and disability), medications, and the attention of the patient's family and the medical system. In order to treat such behavior (i.e. pain), contingencies can be managed such that the patient is reinforced for healthy behavior rather than for pain behavior.

Fordyce et al. (1973) described the treatment of 36 patients who had

had pain an average of seven years and had failed to respond to usual medical treatment. Treatment took place in an inpatient unit of a medical rehabilitation center. Patients were hospitalized for four to twelve weeks and then continued treatment as outpatients for an average of three weeks.

The treatment goals and interventions can be summarized as follows:

GOAL	INTERVENTION
1. Decrease medication usage	a. Medications given on a time-contingent basis rather than a demand basis.
	b. Medications were gradually decreased over the course of treatment.
2. Increase physical activity	a. Patients were given individualized physical therapy programs.
	b. Activity in physical therapy was increased in gradual stages.
	c. Rest was contingent on activity performed, not on pain behavior.
	d. Patients were reinforced (by attention) for activity performed, not for pain behavior.
3. Decrease pain behavior	a. Patients received a neutral response from staff for pain behavior.
	b. Nonpain behavior ("healthy behavior") was positively reinforced with staff attention, praise, etc.
4. Generalize the gains made to the patients' home environment	a. Patients' families participated in treatment program, and were taught to reinforce nonpain behaviors rather than pain behavior.

Results at time of discharge indicated that the group experienced a 50% increase in "uptime"—time spent sitting, standing, and walking. Exercise tolerance also increased significantly. The patient group experienced a dramatic, significant decrease in the medications that were taken; most patients were taking little or no medication at the time of discharge. After 22 months of follow-up, the patients had maintained their gains.

Since Fordyce's initial description of the pain management unit, this treatment approach has been refined by many other clinicians. The following is a summary of the elements that are common to pain treatment units:

1. Evaluation and treatment are multidisciplinary.
2. The programs are predominantly inpatient programs lasting 4–12 weeks.
3. Goals of treatment include: increasing activity, decreasing medication, decreasing pain behavior, decreasing dysfunction in the patient's life, increasing cognitive mastery over pain, decreasing utilization of the medical system, decreasing the subjective experience of pain.
4. Treatment approaches include a combination of: physical therapy, occupational therapy, recreational therapy, group psychotherapy, individual psychotherapy, family therapy, vocational counseling, medical detoxification, relaxation therapy, biofeedback, hypnosis, and antidepressant medication.
5. Treatment utilizes the principles of learning theory and cognitive ego psychology.

Treatment outcomes differ among the various programs. However, in reviewing studies involving several hundred patients, it is clear that statistically, 60–80% of the patients who enter these programs will experience significant improvement (increased activity, decreased medication use, decreased pain behavior, return to work, decreased use of medical facilities), and this improvement will be maintained by the majority over a three to five-year follow-up. Furthermore, these gains will be maintained even if the subjective experience of pain (subjective report of pain) does not change!

It would appear that the multidisciplinary inpatient approach (combining both somatic therapy and psychotherapy) is the treatment of choice for chronic pain patients. Outpatient programs are being developed in order to provide a similar therapeutic effect without the expense of hospitalization.

Somatic Treatment

Clinical observation and psychological testing have consistently found that patients with chronic pain are depressed. Since it is usually difficult, if not impossible, to determine whether the depression is the result or the etiology of the chronic pain, antidepressants have been used to treat the pain.

Okasha (1973) studied the effect of tricyclics in patients with "psychogenic headache." Using a double-blind design, he administered doxepin 75 mg/day, amtriptyline 75 mg/day, diazepam, 6 mg/day, or placebo to 80 patients. He found that pain, depression, and anxiety decreased significantly in those patients treated with doxepin or amitriptyline, but not with diazepam or placebo.

Turkington (1980) studied 59 patients with pain secondary to diabetic neuropathy. All of these patients were significantly depressed prior to treatment. When treated with imipramine or amitriptyline in doses of 100 mg per day, all of the patients experienced complete relief of depression and pain within 12 weeks. While it may be difficult to achieve 100% effectiveness in clinical practice, this study is well designed and points to the usefulness of tricyclic antidepressants in the treatment of certain specific chronic pain syndromes.

Lindsay and Wyckoff (1981) reported on the use of tricyclic antidepressants in patients with chronic pain complaints and depression. Eighty-three percent of the 116 patients studied obtained significant relief of depression and pain after treatment with usual antidepressant doses of tricyclic antidepressants.

Other authors have reported equally successful results combining tricyclic antidepressants with neuroleptics; Taub and Collins (1974), Duthie (1977), Sherwin (1979) have treated a variety of chronic pain syndromes using amitriptyline 75 mg/day plus either fluphenazine (3–4 mg/day), or perphenazine (2–8 mg/day) or trifluoperazine (2–4 mg/day). However, it would appear from comparison of the studies that the treatments are essentially equal in effectiveness and the combination offers no advantage over the tricyclic alone.

Mixed results have been reported in the treatment of psychogenic pain with electroconvulsive therapy (Sands, 1946; Milligan, 1946; Boyd, 1956). Workers have reported that long-standing severe cases of pain without clinical evidence of depression have shown complete, rapid symptom relief. Often, it is unclear what, if any, prior psychiatric treatment has been received by the patient and follow-up is brief or not described.

Bradley (1963) described 16 patients with symptoms of depression and a primary complaint of severe, localized pain which generally preceded the onset of depression by two to five years. With treatment by ECT alone or in combination "with antidepressant drugs and phenothiazine tranquilizers," these patients "experienced relief" from depression. Partial pain relief occurred only in cases where the depression had exacerbated prior pain. The study suffered from the lack of blind, unbiased outcome assessment. There was no specification of the drugs, dosage, duration of treatment, and proportion of patients who received ECT alone. Follow-up data were incomplete. It appears that ECT may be indicated for those patients who are severely incapacitated by the combination of chronic pain and depression, and who have failed to respond to reasonable trials of antidepressants. More current studies, however, would be useful to further document the effectiveness of this treatment approach.

TREATMENT CONTROVERSIES

The relationship between depression and chronic pain has prompted a great deal of interest. As noted above, depression is a common finding in chronic pain patients. Conversely, pain complaints are common symptoms in depressed patients. Tricyclic antidepressants are effective in the treatment of both. Can one conclude that the two syndromes are linked in some basic, possibly biochemical way? While some clinicians view chronic pain as a "depressive spectrum disease," other researchers would interpret neurochemical (endorphin) data as indicating that the syndromes of depression and chronic pain are expressions of an underlying neurochemical defect. The data currently available suggest that any patient with chronic pain should receive a trial of antidepressants, even if the patient does not appear to be seriously depressed. The tricyclic antidepressants would be the drugs of first choice because of their relative safety and efficacy as illustrated in the previously cited studies.

Inpatient pain units appear to be the most effective treatment for chronic pain syndromes. However, these programs are amalgams of a variety of treatments. It is not clear which of the treatments are most effective, or whether any subgroup of patients would respond equally well to the treatment given outside of an inpatient treatment program. Specificity between a specific treatment approach and a specific patient population has not been demonstrated.

At the present time, the treatment of choice for chronic pain syndromes involves the use of tricyclic antidepressants and comprehensive, multifaceted inpatient treatment programs. It is not at all clear what is "curative" about either of these approaches, and further research is clearly indicated. Furthermore, it is not clear whether chronic pain is best treated by the primary care physician, the specialist (psychiatrist, anesthesiologist, neurologist, surgeon, etc.), or by a new subspecialist—the "algologist," who is thoroughly trained to treat all of the facets of chronic pain. The fact that such a subspecialty is endorsed by many clinicians now active in the field indicates the future significance of this area.

HYPOCHONDRIASIS AND ATYPICAL SOMATOFORM DISORDER (300.70)
Robert Kellner

ESSENTIAL FEATURES

The essential feature of *hypochondriasis* is a clinical picture in which the predominant disturbance is an unrealistic interpretation of physical signs or sensations as abnormal, leading to preoccupation with the fear or belief of having a serious disease.

According to DSM-III, *atypical somatoform disorder* is a residual category to be used when the predominant disturbance is the presentation of physical symptoms or complaints not explainable on the basis of demonstrable organic findings or a known pathophysiologic mechanism and apparently linked to psychological factors.

In planning rational treatment of hypochondriasis, it seems important to explore the patient's psychopathology and to base treatment strategies on the findings, since important differences exist between the beliefs and attitudes of different hypochondriacal patients.

Various theories have been offered to explain the phenomena of somatization and hypochondriasis. Distinctions between functional somatic symptoms, conversion phenomena, and hypochondriacal preoccupations have not always been clearly made; one reason appears to be that functional somatic symptoms and hypochondriacal preoccupation often co-exist. Kenyon (1965) surveyed the theories on the psychopathology of hypochondriasis; most of these assume a repressed complex and view the symptoms as a defense or manifestation of a subconscious conflict. At present, there is little evidence to suggest that psychotherapy based on these theories is more effective than the apparently less time-consuming direct treatment of the more manifest features, such as the fear of illness or the belief of being ill.

In this section, hypochondriasis and atypical somatoform disorders are discussed together because many patients with somatic symptoms which can be classified as atypical somatoform disorders also have hypochondriacal tendencies; further, hypochondriasis appearing alone and not as part of another syndrome seems a rare and extreme form of a common disorder (Kenyon, 1964; Ladee, 1966). This section consists of two parts: a survey of the common psychopathologies found in patients with hypochondriacal features; and suggestions for treatment.

COMMON PSYCHOPATHOLOGY OF HYPOCHONDRIASIS

Somatic symptoms. Somatic symptoms are extremely common (Kellner, 1965; Mayou, 1976); approximately 60% of a normal population experiences at least one somatic symptom in any one week (Kellner and Sheffield, 1973). Several mechanisms have been described by which somatic symptoms can be produced in the absence of physical disease or persistent structural damage to tissues. For example, overactivity of the autonomic nervous system can affect most parts of the body, causing symptoms such as the irritable bowel syndrome (Chaudhary and Truelove, 1961); increased tension in voluntary muscle can cause tension headaches or neck pain (Sainsbury and Gibson, 1954). Excessive psychoendocrine activity, such as increased secretion of epinephrine, leads to characteristic symptoms; minor physical disorders such as soft tissue injuries or subclinical infections can produce transient symptoms which often remain undiagnosed unless special methods of investigations are used.

Somatic symptoms can apparently become a focus for hypochondriacal preoccupations. Psychiatric patients with somatic symptoms, for example depressed patients, tend to have more hypochondriacal preoccupations than psychiatric patients without somatic symptoms (Burns and

Nichols, 1972). Similarly, psychiatric patients with hypochondriacal features have more somatic symptoms than other psychiatric patients (Pilowsky, 1967).

Anxiety and depression. There is a complex relationship between anxiety, depression, somatic symptoms, and hypochondriasis. The order of importance and the interplay of these several features varies with each individual.

There is an association of anxiety, depression, and somatic symptoms on the one hand (Kellner et al., 1972) and anxiety, depression, and hypochondriasis on the other (Spear, 1966). An elevated score on the hypochondria scale of the MMPI (a scale which consists largely of somatic symptoms) is one part of the "neurotic triad" (elevated scores of the hypochondria hysteria and depression scales) (Gough, 1946). In a factor analysis of depressed hypochondriacal patients, Bianchi found one of the factors to be "anxiety" (Bianchi, 1973). Similarly, neurotic patients have a high incidence of anxiety, depressive, and somatic symptoms and a greater proportion of these patients believe that they suffer from a physical illness than do normals (Kellner and Sheffield, 1973). Several studies show that patients with somatic complaints for which no organic cause could be found scored higher on anxiety and depression than normal subjects without such complaints. In controlled drug trials, antianxiety and antidepressant drugs tend to reduce the severity and incidence of somatic symptoms more than placebo. Anxiety tends to lower pain threshold in pain experiments (Merskey and Evans, 1975; Bronzo and Powers, 1967; Shiomi, 1977).

Misunderstanding of the nature of the symptoms, conviction of disease, and failure to benefit from reassurance. These are cardinal features of hypochondriasis and the main criteria for labeling a patient as hypochondriacal. They can exist in varying degrees. The average person may be concerned about a persistent pain, but he is usually reassured by the physician's explaining that he is physically healthy. A more anxious individual who is overly concerned about his health may need repeated reassurances, and even then may not be convinced until the pain or discomfort has subsided. A hypochondriacal patient's anxiety is either not assuaged by reassurance or the effects of reassurance are short lived.

Fear of illness. Worry over illness is common. About 10% of normal people and over 40% of neurotic patients replied in a questionnaire that they were worried that they may have a serious illness (Kellner and Sheffield, 1973).

Fear of illness as the manifestation of a phobia (Ryle, 1948) appears to be qualitatively different from worry about illness or the belief of suffering from an illness. Unlike phobias of external origin such as agoraphobia which produces fear only in certain situations, the fear of illness is a phobia of internal origin (Marks, 1969) from which the patient cannot escape. Illness phobias were found in a factor analysis of hypochondriasis in depressed patients (Bianchi, 1973).

Fear of death may exacerbate or cause hypochondriacal fears; the fear may be of the process of dying or of the idea of emptiness or nothingness after death. At other times a patient's belief that he is ill coincides with the fear of dying. Burns and Nichols (1972) found that 90% of patients suffering localized chest pain without discoverable organic cause believed they were in imminent danger of death.

Predisposing and precipitating factors in functional somatic symptoms. Several predisposing and precipitating factors have been described in functional somatic symptoms; some of these are associated with hypochondriasis and suggest how previous experiences can influence a patient's focus of attention. For example, Appley and Hale (1973) found that children's functional symptoms tend to mimic those of another family member. Kellner (1963, 1966) found that symptoms of distress, including somatic functional symptoms, were reported more often after physical illness of the patient or of the patient's family. Kreitman et al. (1965) found that the somatic symptoms of depressed adult patients tended to resemble the symptoms of their mothers. Bianchi (1973) found a family illness factor in a factor analysis of hypochondriacal depressives. Parkes (1972) found that functional somatic symptoms of bereaved adults resembled the symptoms of the terminal illness of a relative. In depressed patients with functional chest symptoms, Burns and Nichols (1972) found a high incidence of a history of respiratory tract disease in both the patient and his family, as well as a history of recent bereavement, with the patient having witnessed the death with a great emotional impact.

Iatrogenic factors. Some hypochondriacal patients were told by their physician that they suffered from a physical illness and were treated for a physical illness for several years. Subsequent examinations revealed that the patients' abnormalities were innocuous. Apparently functional symptoms and minor laboratory abnormalities led the physician to the wrong conclusion that the patient had a physical illness and the patient accepted the physician's judgment. In a study of adults with functional chest symptoms, Cope (1969) concluded that in one-third of the patients there was an "iatrogenic influence." Likewise, Ruesch (1951) stated that of adult patients with somatic functional symptoms 13% were "definitely iatrogenic."

Selective perception. Hypochondriacal students were found to be more sensitive to the two-flash fusion task than other students, which suggests that hypochondriacs may also be more sensitive in perceiving sensation originating in their bodies (Hanback and Revelle, 1978). Among the many factors which influence perception are the intensity of the stimulus and the motive. Anxiety is apparently an important motive which makes an individual attend to a certain part of his body and perceive sensations which previously were below the level of consciousness. For example, in a study by Wheeler et al. (1958) patients were told after a small chest film that they had to return for a large film because something might be wrong with their hearts; heart symptoms were induced or aggravated in 8% of the patients studied. A history of having had a physical illness or of witnessing a physical illness in others apparently contributes to the awareness of physical disease and increases one's attention and selective perception of sensations from an organ or a part of the body.

Learning. The habitual perception of somatic symptoms apparently improves with learning. Adam (1967) found that experimental subjects could be taught to perceive changes in the movement of the stomach which they were unaware of previously. Autonomic activity can be conditioned to signals which can occur below the level of awareness; Lacey et al. (1955) demonstrated this by conditioning heart rate to cues subjects were not aware of. It seems likely that when subjects repeatedly practice selective attention and selective perception, motivated by the fear of having an illness, they improve their skill in detecting sensations which previously would have remained below the level of awareness.

PSYCHOTHERAPEUTIC TREATMENT STRATEGIES

There are no adequate controlled studies on the psychotherapy of hypochondriasis. The recommendations presented here are tentative; they are based on uncontrolled studies and on studies of psychotherapeutic techniques which appeared to be effective under similar conditions, for example, psychophysiological disorders with or without hypochondriacal preoccupations. The recommendations are based, in part, on published research and, in part, on work which awaits publication, including a long-term uncontrolled study of individual psychotherapy with hypo-chondriacal patients.

The aims of psychotherapy can be summarized as follows: to persuade that the conviction of disease is false and to allay the fear of illness and death; to improve the understanding of the nature of the symptoms and to achieve relief from somatic distress, as well as from anxiety and depression.

Persuasion. Devising methods which convince the patient that his symptoms are innocuous seems crucial to progress. Many patients believe that they suffer from a progressive or dangerous illness which is being neglected because it has not been diagnosed and treated. Unless this conviction changes, it will reinforce a part of the psychopathology which is responsible for his somatic symptoms and other phenomena.

Explanatory therapy. Most patients do not understand the relationship between emotions and somatic symptoms. There have been no controlled studies of hypochondriasis which compared the effects of traditional insight therapy with those of explanatory therapy. Patients with somatic preoccupations tend not to respond well to traditional insight psychotherapy (Rosenberg, 1954; Stone et al., 1961). Several studies suggest that explanatory therapy aids recovery. In an uncontrolled study of patients with lower backache without organic cause, Sarno (1977) found that a large proportion of subjects recovered after an explanation of their condition. Draspa (1959) treated adults with muscular pain (for which no organic cause could be found) with a combination of psychotherapeutic techniques. The treatment was focused on the somatic symptom and included explanation; treated patients had significantly better outcome than patients in the control group. In a study by Appley and Hale (1973) children with abdominal pain were treated with simple psychotherapy and explanation by their pediatrician. When they reached adult life these children were reported to have improved more than a comparable group of children who were not treated with supportive psychotherapy and explanation.

While it is likely that different strategies are appropriate in patients with psychosomatic diseases (Kellner, 1975), it appears that explanatory therapy can help some patients with psychosomatic diseases who also have hypochondriacal fears. Chappell and Stevenson, in their controlled study of psychotherapy of chronic peptic ulcer patients (many of whom were hypochondriacal), found a combination of explanatory therapy and cognitive exercises remarkably effective (Chappell and Stevenson, 1936).

The findings also suggest that cognitive exercises with instructions to deliberately change overlearned habits of thinking (what has since been called the "internal dialogue" or "automatic thinking") may be also helpful in hypochondriacal patients (Beck, 1976; Meichenbaum, 1977).

Accurate information. Explanation of the nature of the symptoms should be as accurate as possible. There is evidence from research in psychophysiology that accurate information about the relationship of a threatening stimulus and its somatic consequences can influence several phenomena including the severity of autonomic responses and the degree of subjective distress and behavior. Schachter and Singer (1962) found that experimental subjects who were accurately informed about the nature of an injection (epinephrine) showed fewer changes in behavior than uninformed or misinformed subjects. Accurate information also apparently can affect the conditioning of the autonomic nervous system. Lacey and his colleagues found that subjects who were informed about a stimulus to be followed by electric shock had a gradual decrease in heart rate, whereas subjects who were uninformed developed a classical conditioning curve with an increase in heart rate (Lacey et al., 1955).

Among the information which can be given to hypochondriacal patients are the findings that somatic symptoms are exceedingly common, that only a very small proportion of somatic symptoms are caused by serious organic disease, and that most of these symptoms have an excellent prognosis. Sequences reported by the patient, such as somatic discomfort and worry about illness which may, in turn, exacerbate somatic symptoms, may be emphasized by the therapist since understanding this cycle may be helpful to the patient.

Repeated explanation. There is research evidence that patients frequently either forget information or remember it inaccurately (Ley and Spellman, 1967). Because psychophysiological relationships may be difficult for the patient to grasp or to remember, it appears more effective to give a small amount of information at any one time and to repeat it. The fact that he may be frightened and in pain may preclude even a knowledgable patient from understanding the physician's explanation.

Relatively innocuous terms used by a previous physician can be misunderstood. A patient, having been told by his physician that he suffers from sinusitis, catarrh, or chondritis, may believe that this condition is responsible for his symptoms. Yet, the patient's current symptoms are either obviously unrelated to his physical abnormality or the abnormality is trivial and couldn't be responsible for his distress.

If the patient had been given an incorrect physical diagnosis by a previous physician, repeated explanations of the true nature of the symptoms are necessary as a form of counterpropaganda since the patient must be persuaded that the previous diagnosis was in error.

Selective perception. The principles of selective perception probably need to be discussed with the patient. Initially nonmedical examples appear to be helpful because it may be easier for the patient to be objective about these. For example, the therapist might explain that the continuous noise of a fan is less likely to be heard than the noise of one which starts and stops; if one is anxious about a visitor's arrival, he is likely to hear footsteps in the hall when ordinarily he would not be aware of them. Repeated medical examples can be given: selective perception can be demonstrated by instructing the patient to attend to sensations from one part of his body, such as the pressure on his buttocks while sitting, the sensation from his tongue resting on the floor of his mouth or the pressure of his belt or collar. It can be explained that concern about one part of the body can make this part the focus of attention leading to new perceptions. An anecdotal example might describe another patient who is distressed over a vague ache around his heart, while ignoring a swollen, badly sprained ankle because he is not concerned about the injury assuming it will heal.

Learning. A constant awareness of sensation in one part of the body can be explained to the patient as being a result of learning and can be likened to the piano tuner who learns to recognize pitch with great accuracy or the painter who learns to discriminate between subtle hues of color in a way impossible for a layman. It is important for the patient to understand that, just as learning to perceive these symptoms took a long time, so will unlearning this habit; that initially, unlearning will frequently be unsuccessful and that his symptoms will recur for some time with almost their original intensity.

Acceptance and empathy. Research evidence indicates that acceptance and empathy by the therapist are important variables in successful client-centered psychotherapy (Truax and Carkuff, 1964; Truax et al., 1965; Truax and Wargo, 1966). There is no evidence available that these attributes are equally effective in the management of hypochondriacal patients. However, several patients who recovered after psychotherapy reported that they believed that their previous physician had misunderstood them, that he did not take their conditions seriously, and that he showed his impatience and apparently either suspected or actually told them that they were faking. Other patients reported that the psychotherapist's understanding of their predicament contributed greatly to relief of their anxiety and their trust in him.

Treatment of anxiety. Anxiety appears to be an integral part in the vicious cycle of somatic symptoms which lead to hypochondriacal concern which in turn increases anxiety and its concomitant autonomic and voluntary nervous system activity resulting in more somatic symptoms, and so on. Several of the psychotherapeutic strategies described here are aimed at removing a link in this chain by reducing anxiety. There is evidence from controlled studies that antianxiety drugs reduce somatic symptoms (Uhlenhuth et al., 1980), but there are no controlled studies with hypochondriacal patients. Clinical experience shows that hypochondriacal patients have taken antianxiety drugs for years with apparently little or no effect on the hypochondriasis.

Antianxiety drugs should be prescribed if there is distressing generalized anxiety. When there is no coexisting general anxiety state, an antianxiety drug may be prescribed (preferably a benzodiazepine) in the largest dose which the patient can tolerate without substantial side effects, and which he should take only at the times he feels distressed. The patient should be told that while this medication is *not* going to relieve his physical discomfort, it may help him to relax. Once he is relaxed, it should be easier not to pay attention to his physical discomfort and, as a result, he may succeed in focusing on other matters.

There is a tendency for physical symptoms and hypochondriacal preoccupations to lessen, even without psychotherapy, when a patient attends a clinic (Kellner and Sheffield, 1971); this may be the consequence of a gradual decrease in anxiety. However, in patients who have had pain or somatic discomfort with hypochondriacal fears or panic attacks for an extended period, it seems to take a long time for the association of somatic symptoms and the thought of illness and attacks of anxiety to weaken. Apparently only with time does the fear associated with somatic symptoms gradually becomes extinguished. The therapist's patience is tested on many occasions when the patient acts as though he has had no psychotherapy, becomes extremely anxious, and reverts to his irrational beliefs when his somatic symptoms recur. Repeated unqualified assurances that the symptoms are benign seems to reduce anxiety at least briefly and may aid in recovery.

Suggestion. The extent to which suggestion is effective in the treatment of somatic functional complaints is not clear. In experimentally induced pain, waking suggestion is effective (Barber and Hahn, 1962; Hilgard et al., 1974). There is also evidence that various therapeutic interventions can have placebo effects (Shapiro, 1971). Preferably suggestion should be coupled with accurate information about the patient's condition as in the following example: "If you manage to remain relaxed and manage to think of something else, the discomfort will be less noticeable than if you panic and start worrying." Similar sequences of events which the patient had previously described can be repeated as a suggestion. If the patient is indeed physically healthy, the excellent outlook for his future should be repeatedly emphasized. Aside from imparting accurate and crucially important knowledge, this information will likely have a suggestive effect.

Physical examinations. A large proportion of patients who have pain for which no organic cause is found believe that they have a physical illness which their physician has failed to discover (Mayou, 1976; Burns and Nichols, 1972; Pilowsky, 1967; Spear, 1966). At present, the role of repeated physical examinations remains unknown. The fact that most hypochondriacal patients have had many physical examinations and laboratory investigations, apparently without beneficial effect in relieving their symptoms, suggests that in many patients examination is not therapeutic. One such study of *chronic* hypochondriacal patients found that *one* physical examination with appropriate laboratory investigations and one session of explanatory therapy did not relieve symptoms significantly (Kellner and Sheffield, 1971). However, other studies suggest that even one physical examination will relieve symptoms, concern, and preoccupation with illness in many patients who have somatic symptoms of recent onset (Cope, 1969; Sarno, 1977; Thomas, 1978). Isolated reports cite dramatic improvements after one physical examination with explanation, albeit at times without follow-up. Ryle (1948) described a patient with various symptoms whom he suspected was suffering from fear of cancer. He told her, "I am glad to tell you that there are no signs of cancer or any serious disease." "Thank you," came the prompt reply, "That is all I wanted to know." Another patient who had lumbosacral pain after a blow to his back believed that he had cancer; he slept badly, lost 14 pounds and had seen several physicians whose reassurance was ineffective. One examination, a simple explanation and reassurance apparently cured him. Cope (1969) reports on patients who, upon coming to the physician's office were placed in a wheelchair by a cautious nurse. After one examination and a reassuring explanation, these patients left the office smiling and confident, saying, "That's all I wanted to know" or "I am glad it wasn't my heart."

The hypochondriacal patient believes that either the previous examinations were inadequate or that in the meantime he acquired a new illness. A case can be made that repeated physical examinations combined with unqualified assurance and a simple explanation will reduce anxiety each time and thus promote recovery. A physical examination and a simple explanation such as, "it is a cramp, these can last for a long time and can be very unpleasant, but they tend to get better" can save a great deal of time and formal psychotherapy.

The findings of an uncontrolled study of hypochondriacal patients who had been treated with the methods described here, including repeated physical examinations, suggest that with each examination came some temporary relief. Later these patients reported that at times they did not panic when they experienced pain and found it easier to be comforted by the examination and reassurance which was initially effective for only a very short while (study awaiting publication). Several of these patients eventually made a complete recovery. There appears to be no danger that the patient will develop new fears because of repeated examinations, nor will he suspect that the physician is not sure himself because he needs to examine the patient again. Since most patients are already very concerned about their physical health, it is unlikely that the idea of physical disease can be implanted into their minds merely by examination. On the contrary, many patients resent that their complaints have been dismissed by previous physicians who apparently believed that the symptoms did not merit another examination, while the patient believed that his serious disease was being neglected once more. Patients usually see physical examinations and laboratory investigations as evidence of thoroughness and care. Several of these patients said that they felt less helpless because they knew that their new physician (the psychiatrist) took their complaints seriously, that he made certain that no illness had developed since the last examination and that he was always readily available.

Sometimes patients telephone in a state of panic, convinced that they are dying or their symptoms are unbearable. In this situation we found an emergency appointment with a physical examination and the kind of assurance and explanation described above to relieve symptoms rapidly. Often reassurance by telephone is adequate. If the therapist is not available, a colleague who knows the patient's history and agrees with the therapist's strategy can respond to telephone calls. This availability does not appear to create undue dependence on the physician or psychiatrist because, with time, the patient calls less frequently and with successful therapy he reaches the stage when he regards many somatic symptoms as trivial and of no concern.

If a psychiatrist is not confident about his skills as a physical diagnostician or if the therapist is not a physician, he should work in close cooperation with a physician who supports this approach and has the temperament to tolerate the patient's unreasonable fears. If the therapist is a psychiatrist, he should probably carry out the physical examination whenever possible, establish himself as the patient's physician, and use other specialists only for consultations. Evidence from a controlled study of group psychotherapy of patients with bronchial asthma shows that it may be preferable to have only one therapist. When an internist treated the patient's asthma and conducted group psychotherapy under the supervision of a psychiatrist, he achieved results superior to those of the supervising psychiatrist who conducted therapy with another group but did not examine the patients nor prescribe drugs for asthma (Groen and Pelser, 1960). Although this phenomenon has been demonstrated in only one study of patients with psychosomatic disease, it is conceivable that a similar phenomenon occurs with hypochondriacal patients who have psychophysiological symptoms. It seems that the rapport established between the patient and the physician who treats him for his physical complaints adds to the physician's psychotherapeutic effectiveness.

Disease phobias. Hypochondriasis and disease phobia often coexist to varying degrees. In DSM-III both are classified under hypochondriasis. The main difference appears to be that the patient with hypochondriasis is convinced that he suffers from a physical disease, whereas the patient with disease phobia dreads disease, seeks reassurance, and often realizes that his fears are irrational. In hypochondriasis, once the patient is convinced that he does not suffer from a physical illness and has an understanding of the nature of the condition, the intensity and frequency of his attacks of panic and somatic symptoms tend to wane and the period of freedom from symptoms gradually lengthens, although frightening recurrences with severe symptoms are the rule rather than the exception. In the phobic patient, reassurance usually offers only temporary relief; there is a tendency to recovery when the phobia coexists with an affective or an anxiety disorder; then the phobia may wane as these disorders improve (Schapira et al., 1970). Although disease phobia should be distinguished from the idea of contamination, which may be a symptom of obsessive-compulsive disorder, perhaps the two conditions should be treated in a similar way (see Chapter 7).

Kumar and Wilkinson (1971) treated four cases of phobias of internal stimuli, including illness phobias, by thought stopping. The patient was interrupted by the therapist with a shout, *Stop*, when the undesirable thought occurred; later the patient was instructed to rehearse silently the order *Stop* to himself, and to substitute a desirable thought each time the undesirable thought occurred. O'Donnell (1978) treated a patient with cancer phobia with implosion and hypnosis. Marks recommends flooding or satiation in imagery or exposure to photographs of pathological specimen in cases of disease phobia (Marks, 1978). The present author successfully treated several patients who had disease phobia with strategies similar to those described above. There is, at present, inadequate evidence to determine the most effective treatment of disease phobia, or to predict which of the opposite approaches of examination with explanatory therapy, thought stopping or flooding is likely to help a given patient. Consequently, one should try one treatment and, if it proves ineffective after an adequate trial, switch to the other treatment.

Fear of death. If hypochondriacal preoccupations are caused by fear of dying, psychotherapy which aims at the hypochondriacal preoccupation is less likely to be successful. There are no controlled studies of the treatment of this condition, only isolated case histories. It appears to be important to establish the source and nature of the patient's fears, whether they are specific, i.e. the fear of funerals, the fear of the process of dying, or the vague fear of not being. For specific phobias, techniques of exposure to fantasied scenes or actual items feared are described in the section on the treatment of phobias (see Chapter 7).

If the fears are vague and concern topics such as emptiness or nonexistence after death, psychotherapy should probably be aimed at these ideas. An attempt should be made to bring about a realization that one of the preconditions of contentment is a more robust and stoic attitude to the inevitable fate of man. Frequent discussions of the topic may have an effect similar to exposure. Perhaps coaching to bring about deliberate changes in thinking by using cognitive methods might be effective (Beck, 1976; Meichenbaum, 1977). If the patient is religious, the aid of a minister of his church who is interested in counseling should be sought; his views on religious and philosophical issues may be more convincing to the patient than those of a physician.

Insight. It is not known whether or not insight into the role of the predisposing and precipitating factors of hypochondriasis is essential for recovery. If having had an illness or having witnessed a dramatic illness or death of a friend or relative has precipitated the hypochondriasis, the patient might profit from an explanation that preoccupation with the possibility of acquiring the same disease can lead to anxiety and the heightened awareness of bodily sensation. If witnessing the death of another person was a particularly traumatic experience, repeated discussion of the event (a form of exposure) and working through with catharsis is probably helpful. If the frightening affect remains associated with the image of death, reexposure to the traumatic image or event may be an effective treatment. If the hypochondriasis is part of an atypical grief reaction, psychotherapy dealing with the grief should be the first therapeutic strategy (Raphael, 1975).

Traditional insight psychotherapy. Many patients with hypochondriacal preoccupation or functional somatic symptoms recover from this syndrome only to reveal other psychopathology. This does not appear to be a symptom substitution; rather, it seems that the conflicts which were relatively unimportant while the patient was preoccupied with his hypochondriacal fears and somatic symptoms have now acquired a greater importance in his life. These patients will need additional psychotherapy for their disorder. In other patients who appear to be initially hypochondriacal and present with somatic complaints, it soon becomes apparent that neurotic conflicts or environmental stress are largely responsible for their distress and for some reason the somatic symptoms were presented to the physician first. These patients may benefit from psychotherapy; often the somatic symptoms appear to be of relatively little concern to the patient and remit as psychotherapy progresses.

Residual somatic symptoms. Sometimes after psychotherapy, the patient has abandoned his conviction of disease or his fear of illness, yet, distressing residual somatic symptoms linger, usually in the form of pain. These symptoms should be treated by direct methods such as biofeedback for tension headaches (Budzynski et al., 1973) or by psychotherapeutic strategies which are appropriate for physical pain or psychalgia.

Chronic invalidism. Some patients in whom hypochondriasis has been present for a long time appear to have adapted to the life of an invalid. The methods described here may be inadequate to deal with the habit of being ill or, perhaps, with the advantages of being an invalid; additional treatment approaches will have to be adopted which alter the patient's habits, attitudes, motives, and goals (Wooley et al., 1978).

Dysmorphophobia. The belief of being deformed, is seen more often in the offices of plastic surgeons than psychiatrists. Many of these patients are found on follow-up to have either schizophrenia or severe nonpsychotic disorders (Hay, 1970; Connolly and Gipson, 1978). At present, there are no adequate studies to evaluate whether one kind of psychotherapy is more effective than another in the treatment of this disorder.

Drug Treament

Antianxiety drugs. Benzodiazepines tend to decrease somatic symptoms in anxious patients and therefore may be useful in some patients with atypical somatoform disorders. There are no controlled studies of their effect in the treatment of hypochondriacal patients. Clinical experience suggests that, by themselves, these drugs are ineffective in hypochondriasis unless other disorders coexist. Their use in conjunction with psychotherapy has been described above.

Propranolol has been found to decrease somatic symptoms in anxious patients and also has some antianxiety effects (Cole et al., 1979). It is not known whether the effects on somatic symptoms are substantially different from those of benzodiazepines if the doses of the drugs are individually adjusted. Propranolol can be tried when the effects of benzodiazepines have been inadequate or when the somatic symptoms appear to be caused by stimulation of the beta-adrenergic receptors, as in tachycardia. One controlled study found tybamate to be more effective in reducing somatic symptoms than emotional symptoms in anxious neurotic patients (Rickels et al., 1968). Tybamate may be tried as an alternative if the somatic symptoms are troublesome, and the patient is in need of medication and has not responded to other antianxiety drugs.

Antidepressants. There is no evidence that antidepressants are effective in hypochondriasis or atypical somatoform disorders unless the patient is also depressed. Some patients with severe, usually conspicuous depressions with endogenous features have hypochondriacal delusions. These patients apparently do not respond to psychotherapy and the hypochondriacal delusions remit when the patient recovers from the depression.

Antipsychotics (neuroleptics). There is no evidence that antipsychotics have a place in the treatment of hypochondriasis or atypical somatoform disorders. Pimozide has been used in a small, uncontrolled study of dysmorphophobia; however, the patients who improved appeared to have been schizophrenic (Riding and Munro, 1975).

Prognosis

Hypochondriacal patients are generally believed to have a poor prognosis (Ladee, 1966). An uncontrolled study of individual psychotherapy, in which the treatment strategies outlined here were used, included 36 patients whose hypochondriasis had lasted for six months or longer. Of eleven patients who had had symptoms for over three years, four were symptom free or improved at the end of treatment; of 25 patients with symptoms for more than six months but less than three years, 19 (76%) were free from symptoms or improved (study awaiting publication). Similar figures were reported by Brown (1936) and less favorable outcomes by Kenyon (1964) and Ladee (1966). It is difficult to evaluate the effectiveness of a treatment method from uncontrolled studies because of the various biases which intrude. However, in contrast with the generally pessimistic outlook for this disorder, the findings suggest that the prognosis is good in a substantial number of patients and the outcome of treatment can be gratifying.

Conclusions and Recommendations

At present, there are no controlled studies of the treatment of hypochondriasis and atypical somatoform disorders and too few uncontrolled studies available to decide which is the most effective psychotherapeutic strategy for the majority of patients. There is evidence to suggest that patients with functional somatic symptoms do not respond as well to traditional insight psychotherapy than do patients with predominantly affective symptoms. There is evidence to suggest that in patients with functional somatic symptoms, direct psychotherapy, including explanation and reassurance, is effective in treating the somatic symptoms, fears, and beliefs. One controlled study showed patients with severe, chronic peptic ulcer, many of whom were also hypochondriacal, to be helped by directive psychotherapy which consisted largely of explanation and cognitive exercises. It is likely that these techniques are also helpful in hypochondriasis. The results of uncontrolled studies with hypochondriacal patients suggest that multifocal psychotherapy consisting largely of physical examination, explanation, reassurance, and education achieves a good outcome in a large proportion of patients.

Drug treatment alone appears to be ineffective in the treatment of hypochondriasis unless the syndrome is part of another disorder. Antianxiety drugs tend to reduce somatic symptoms in anxious patients and are probably helpful in hypochondriasis and in atypical somatoform disorders when combined with psychotherapy.

SUMMARY

The treatment of hypochondriasis and atypical somatoform disorders are discussed together because hypochondriasis appears to be the extreme manifestation of a common condition which is a syndrome of functional somatic symptoms with concern about illness or with hypochondriacal beliefs. There have been no well controlled studies of psychotherapy of hypochondriasis. There are several uncontrolled studies and one controlled study of psychotherapy of patients with somatic functional symptoms which included patients who would probably be classified as having atypical somatoform disorders.

A part of the research on the psychopathology of hypochondriasis and functional somatic symptoms has been reviewed. Treatment strategies are suggested which are based in part on studies of psychotherapy of patients with functional somatic symptoms or psychosomatic disease and in part on the research findings on the psychopathology of hypochondriasis. The suggested treatment strategies include: explanatory therapy, persuasion of the patient as to the innocuousness of his condition, accurate information about emotional stimulus and somatic response, unlearning of selective perception, cognitive exercises, treatment of anxiety, repeated physical examinations in patients with recurrent fears that they have developed a new disease or that their physical disease has been overlooked. Illness phobias, which may coexist with hypochondriacal beliefs, may perhaps be successfully treated with exposure or thought stopping. Traditional psychotherapy may be tried for psychopathology revealed after remission of hypochondriacal fears and beliefs.

There are no controlled drug studies of hypochondriasis. Clinical impressions suggest that drug treatment alone is ineffective unless hypochondriasis is part of another syndrome. Antianxiety drugs have been found to reduce somatic symptoms in anxious neurotics and are likely to be helpful in patients with atypical somatoform disorders who are anxious, as well as in anxious hypochondriacal patients if used in conjunction with psychotherapy. Propranolol reduces the severity of somatic functional symptoms; there is no conclusive evidence at present to show that its effects are preferable to those of benzodiazepines. One controlled study with anxious neurotics found tybamate more effective in reducing somatic symptoms than emotional symptoms.

REFERENCES

Adam G: Interception and Behaviour. Akademiai Kiado, Budapest. 1967.

Appley J, Hale B: Children with recurrent abdominal pain: how do they grow up. Brit Med J. 3:7–9, 1973.

Barber TX, Hahn KW: Physiological and subjective responses to pain-producing stimulation under hypnotically suggested and waking-imaged "analgesia". J Abnorm Soc Psychol. 65:411–415, 1962.

Beck AT: Cognitive Therapy and the Emotional Disorders. International Universities Press, New York. 1976.

Bianchi GN: Patterns of hypochondriasis: a principal components analysis. Brit J Psychiat. 122:541–548, 1973.

Bibb RC, Guze SB: Hysteria (Briquet's syndrome) in a psychiatric hospital: the significance of secondary depression. Am J Psychiat. 129:224–228, 1972.

Blumer D: Psychiatric considerations in pain. In: The Spine. Rothman RH and Simeone FA (eds). Saunders, New York. 1975.

Boyd DA: Electroshock therapy in atypical pain syndromes. Lancet. 76:22–25, 1956.

Bradley JJ: Severe localized pain associated with the depressive syndrome. Brit J Psychiat. 109:741–745, 1963.

Bratfos O, Linjaerde O, Salvesen C: Symptomatic relief of neurotic symptoms with tybamate: a double-blind, placebo-controlled study. Acta Psych Scand. 43:282–285, 1967.

Brody S: Value of group psychotherapy in patients with polysurgery addiction. Psych Quart. 33:260–283, 1959.

Bronzo A, Powers G: Relationship of anxiety with pain threshold. J Psychol. 66:181–183, 1967.

Brown F: The bodily complaint: a study of hypochondriasis. J Ment Sci. 82:295–358, 1936.

Budzynski TH, Stoyva JM, Adler CS, Mullaney DJ: EMG biofeedback and tension headache: a controlled outcome study. Psychosom Med. 35:484–496, 1973.

Burns BH, Nichols MA: Factors related to the localization of symptoms to the chest in depression. Brit J Psychiat. 121:405–409, 1972.

Carter AB: The prognosis of certain hysterical symptoms. Brit Med J. 1:1076–1079, 1949.

Chappell MN, Stevenson TI: Group psychological training in some organic conditions. Ment Hyg. 20:588–597, 1936.

Chaudhary NA, Truelove SC: Human colonic motility: a comparative study of normal subjects, patients with ulcerative colitis, and patients with the irritable colon syndrome. Gastroenterology. 40:1–36, 1961.

Cole JO, Altesman R, Weingarten C: Beta-blocking drugs in psychiatry. McLean Hosp. 4:40–68, 1979.

Connolly FH, Gipson M: Dysmorphophobia—A long-term study. Brit J Psychiat. 132:568–570, 1978.

Cope RL: The psychogenic factor in chest pain. Texas Med. 65:78–81, 1969.

Dickes RA: Brief therapy of conversion reactions: an in-hospital technique. Am J Psychiat. 131:584–586, 1974.

Draspa LJ: Psychological factors in muscular pain. Brit J Med Psychol. 32:106–116, 1959.

Duthie AM: Use of phenothiazines and tricyclics in the treatment of intractable pain. South African Med J. 51:246–247, 1977.

Engel GL: Psychogenic pain and the pain-prone patient. Am J Med. 26:899, 1959.

Fenichel O: Berlin Psychoanalytic Institute Report 1929–30. 1930.

Fenichel O: The Psychoanalytic Theory of Neurosis. Norton, New York. 1945.

Fordyce WE, Fowler RS, Lehmann JF, DeLateur BJ, Sand PL, Trieschmann RB: Operant conditioning in the treatment of chronic pain. Arch Phys Med Rehab. 54:399–408, 1973.

Frankel FH: Hypnosis and related clinical behavior. Am J Psychiat. 135:664–668, 1978.

Goodwin DW: Psychiatry and the mysterious medical complaint. JAMA. 209:1184–1888, 1969.

Gough HG: Diagnostic patterns on the Minnesota Multiphasic Personality Inventory. J Clin Psychol. 2:23–37, 1946.

Groen JJ, Pelser HE: Experiences with, and results of, group psychotherapy in patients with bronchial asthma. J Psychosom Res. 4:191–205, 1960.

Guze SB, Perley MJ: Observations on the natural history of hysteria. Am J Psychiat. 119:960–965, 1963.

Hanback JW, Revelle W: Arousal and perceptual sensitivity in hypochondriacs. J Abnorm Psychol. 87:523–530, 1978.

Hay GG: Dysmorphophobia. Brit J Psychiat. 116:399–406, 1970.

Hendler N: Group therapy with chronic pain patients. Psychosomatics. 22:333–340, 1981.

Herman E, Baptiste S: Pain control: mastery through group experience. Pain. 10:79–86, 1981.

Hilgard ER, Ruch JC, Lange AF, Lenox JR, Morgan AH, Sach LB: The psychophysics of cold pressor pain and its modification through hypnotic suggestion. Am J Psychol. 87:17–31, 1974.

Kass DJ, Silvers FM, Abroms GM: Behavioral group treatment of hysteria. Arch Gen Psychiat. 26:42–50, 1972.

Kellner R: Family Ill Health, An Investigation in General Practice. Travistock Publications and C C Thomas, London and Springfield. 1963.

Kellner R: Neurosis in general practice. Brit J Clin Pract. 19:681–682, 1965.

Kellner R: Psychiatric ill health following physical illness. Brit J Psychiat. 112:71–73, 1966.

Kellner R: Psychotherapy in psychosomatic disorders. A survey of controlled studies. Arch Gen Psychiat. 32:1021–1030, 1975.

Kellner R, Sheffield BF: The relief of distress following attendance at a clinic. Brit J Psychiat. 118:193–195, 1971.

Kellner R, Sheffield BF: The one week prevalence of symptoms in neurotic patients and normals. Am J Psychiat. 130:102–105, 1973.

Kellner R, Simpson GM, Winslow WW: The relationship of depressive neurosis to anxiety and somatic symptoms. Psychosomatics. 13:358–362, 1972.

Kenyon FE: Hypochondriasis: a clinical study. Br J Psychiat. 110:478–488, 1964.

Kenyon FE: Hypochondriasis: a survey of some historical, clinical and social aspects. Br J Med Psychol. 38:117–133, 1965.

Kreitman N, Sainsbury PK, Costain WR: Hypochondriasis and depression in outpatients at a general hospital. Brit J Psychiat. 111:607–615, 1965.

Kumar K, Wilkinson JCM: Thought stopping: a useful treatment in phobias of internal stimuli. Brit J Psychiat. 119:305–307, 1971.

Lacey JI, Smith RL, Green A: Use of conditioned autonomic responses in study of anxiety. Psychosom Med. 17:208–217, 1955.

Ladee GA: Hypochondriacal Syndromes. Elsevier, Amsterdam, London, and New York. 1966.

Lazarus AA: The results of behavior therapy in 126 cases of severe neurosis. Behav Res Ther. 1:69–79, 1963.

Ley P, Spellman MS: Communicating with the Patient. Staples Press, Worcester and London. 1967.

Liebson I: Conversion reaction: a learning theory approach. Behav Res Ther. 7:217–218, 1969.

Lindsay PG, Wyckoff M: The depression pain syndrome and its response to antidepressants. Psychosomatics. 22:571–577, 1981.

Ljunberg L: Hysteria: a clinical, prognostic and genetic study. Acta Psych Neurol Scand. 112:1–162, 1957.

Marks IM: Fears and Phobias. Academic Press, New York, 1969.

Marks IM: Living with Fear. McGraw-Hill, New York, London. p. 113, 1978.

Marmor J: Quality in the hysterical personality. J Am Psychoanal Assoc. 1:656–675, 1953.

Mayou R: The nature of bodily symptoms. Brit J Psychiat. 129:55–60, 1976.

Meichenbaum D: Cognitive-Behavior Modification. An Integrative Approach. Plenum Press, New York and London. 1977.

Merskey HA, Evans PR: Variations in pain complaint threshold in psychiatric and neurological patients with pain. Pain. 1:59–72, 1975.

Milligan WL: Psychoneuroses treated with electrical convulsions. Lancet. 2:516–520, 1946.

Minuchin S, Baker L, Rosman BL, Liebman R, Milman L, Todd TC: A conceptual model of psychosomatic illness in children. Arch Gen Psychiat. 32:1031–1038, 1975.

Munford PR, Reardon D, Liberman RP, Allen L: Behavioral treatment of hysterical coughing and mutism: a case study. J Cons Clin Psychol. 44:1008–1014, 1976.

O'Donnell JM: Implosive therapy with hypnosis on the treatment of cancer phobia: a case report. Psychotherapy, Theory, Research and Practice. 15:8–12, 1978.

Okasha H: A double-blind trial for the clinical management of psychogenic headache. Brit J Psychiat. 113:181–183, 1973.

Parkes CM: Bereavement. Studies of Grief in Adult Life. International Universities Press, New York. p. 114, 1972.

Peters J: The neurologist's use of rating scales, EEG and tranquilizers in dealing with hysterical symptoms. Behav Neuropsych. 6:1–12, 85–6, 1974.

Pilowsky I: Dimensions of hypochondriasis. Brit J Psychiat. 113:89–93, 1967.

Pinsky JJ: Chronic intractable benign pain: a syndrome and its treatment with intensive short-term group psychotherapy. J Human Stress. pp. 17–21, 1978.

Pinsky JJ, Malyou AK: The eclectic nature of psychotherapy in the treatment of chronic pain syndromes. In: Chronic Pain: Further Observations from the City of Hope. Crue, BL (ed). SP Medical Publications, New York. pp. 321–327, 1979.

Raphael B: The management of pathological grief. Aust. N.Z. J Psychiat. 9:173–180, 1975.

Rickels K, Hesbacher P, Vandervort W: Tybamate—a perplexing drug. Am J Psychiat. 125:320–326, 1968.

Riding J, Munro A: Pimozide in the treatment of monosymptomatic hypochondriacal psychosis. Acta Psychiat Scand. 52:23–30, 1975.

Rosenberg S: The relationship of certain personality factors to prognosis in psychotherapy. J Clin Psychol. 10:341–345, 1954.

Ruesch J: Chronic Disease and Psychological Invalidism. A Psychosomatic Study. University of California Press, Berkeley and Los Angeles. 1951.

Ryle JA: The twenty-first Maudsley lecture: nosophobia. J Ment Sci. 94:1–17, 1948.

Sainsbury P, Gibson JG: Symptoms of anxiety and tension and the accompanying physiological changes in the muscular system. J Neurol Neurosurg Psychiat. 17:216–224, 1954.

Sands DE: Electro-convulsion therapy in 301 patients in a general hospital. Brit Med J. 2:289–293, 1946.

Sarno JE: Psychosomatic backache. J Fam Pract. 5:353–357, 1977.

Scallet A, Cloninger CR, Otimer E: The management of chronic hysteria: a review and double-blind trial of electrosleep and other relaxation methods. Dis Nerv Syst. 37:347–353, 1976.

Schachter S, Singer JC: Cognitive, social and physiological determinants of emotional state. Psychol Rev. 69:379–399, 1962.

Schapira K, Kerr TA, Roth M: Phobias and affective illness. Brit J Psychiat. 117:25–32, 1970.

Shapiro AK: Placebo effects in medicine, psychotherapy, and psychoanalysis. In: Handbook of Psychotherapy and Behavior Change: An Empirical Analysis. Bergin, AE and Garfield, SL (eds). Wiley, New York. pp. 439–473, 1971.

Sherwin D: A new method for treating headaches. Am J Psychiat. 136:1181–1183, 1979.

Shiomi K: Threshold and reaction time to noxious stimulation, their relations with scores on Manifest Anxiety Scale and Maudsley Personality Inventory. Percept Mot Skills. 44:429–430, 1977.

Slater ET, Glithero E: A follow-up of patients diagnosed as suffering from "hysteria". J Psychosom Res. 9:9–13, 1965.

Slavson SR: Criteria for selection and rejection of patients for various types of groups psychotherapy. Int J Group Psychother. 5:3–30, 1955.

Spear FG: An examination of some psychological theories of pain. Brit J Med Psychol. 39:349–351, 1966.

Stone AR, Frank JD, Nash EH, Imber SD: An intensive five-year follow-up study of treated psychiatric outpatients. J Nerv Ment Dis. 133:410–422, 1961.

Taub A, Collins WF: Observations on the treatment of denervation dysesthesia with psychotropic drugs. In: Advances in Neurology, Bonica, J (ed). Raven Press: New York. pp. 309–315, 1974.

Thomas KB: The consultation and the therapeutic illusion. Brit Med J. 1:1327–1328, 1978.

Tinling DC, Klein RF: Psychogenic pain and aggression: the syndrome of the solitary hunter. Psychosom Med. 28:738–748, 1966.

Truax CB, Carkuff RR: The old and the new: theory and research in counseling and psychotherapy. Personnel and Guidance J. 42:860–866, 1964.

Truax CB, Carkuff RR, Kodman F: Relationship between therapist offered conditions and patient change in group psychotherapy. J Clin Psychol. 21:327–329, 1965.

Truax CB, Wargo DG: Psychotherapeutic encounters that change behavior: for better or for worse. Am J Psychother. 20:499–520, 1966.

Turkington RW: Depression masquerading as diabetic neuropathy. JAMA. 243:1147–1150, 1980.

Uhlenhuth EH, Glass RM, Kellner R, Habberman SJ: Relative sensitivity of clinical measures in trials of antianxiety agents. In: Quantitative Techniques for the Evaluation of the Behavior of Psychiatric Patients. Burdock, EJ and Gershon, S (eds). Marcel Dekker, New York. 1980.

Valko RJ: Group therapy for patients with hysteria (Briquet's disorder). Dis New Syst. 37:484–487, 1976.

Van Putten T, Alban J: Lithium carbonate in personality disorders: a case of hysteria. J Nerv Ment Dis. 164:218–222, 1977.

Walter CJ, Mitchell-Heggs N, Sargant W: Modified narcosis, ECT and antidepressant drugs: a review of techniques and immediate outcome. Brit J Psychiat. 120:651–662, 1972.

Walters A: Psychogenic regional pain alias hysterical pain. Brain. 84:1–18, 1961.

Weber JJ, Elinson J, Moss LM: Psychoanalysis and change. Arch Gen Psychiat. 17:687–709, 1967.

Wheeler EO, Williamson CR, Cohen ME: Heart scare, heart surveys, and iatrogenic heart disease. JAMA. 167:1096–1102, 1958.

Wooley SC, Blackwell B, Winget C: A learning theory model of chronic illness behavior: theory, treatment and research. Psychosom Med. 40:379–401, 1978.

Yalom ID: The Theory and Practice of Group Psychotherapy. Basic Books, 1970.

Zetzel ER: The so called "good" hysteric. Int J Psychoanal. 49:256–260, 1968.

Ziegler FJ, Imboden JB, Meyer E: Contemporary conversion reactions: a clinical study. Am J Psychiat. 6:901–909, 1960.

9 | Dissociative Disorders

GENE COMBS, JR. and
ARNOLD M. LUDWIG

This chapter includes the following DSM-III dissociative disorders: psychogenic amnesia, psychogenic fugue, multiple personality, depersonalization disorder, and atypical dissociative disorder. Although they are classified as separate disorders in DSM-III, their treatment is best considered from a common perspective, and therefore they will be considered together here.

ESSENTIAL FEATURES

The essential feature of a *dissociative disorder* is a sudden, temporary alteration in the normally integrative functions of consciousness, identity, or motor behavior. In *psychogenic amnesia* (300.12) there is a sudden inability to recall important personal information. In *psychogenic fugue* (300.13) there is sudden, unexpected travel away from home or customary work locale with assumption of a new identity and an inability to recall one's previous identity. In *multiple personality* (300.14) there exist within the individual two or more distinct personalities, each of which is dominant at a particular time. In *depersonalization disorder* (300.60) there are one or more episodes of depersonalization that cause social or occupational impairment. Depersonalization disorder is not diagnosed if the symptom of depersonalization is secondary to any other disorder or if it is not associated with social or occupational impairment. *Atypical dissociative disorder* (300.15) is a residual category for individuals with apparent dissociative disorder who cannot be diagnosed as having one of the specific dissociative disorders.

Treatment Goals

Dissociation is not necessarily bad. It is to some degree a feature of everyday life. We all forget things. It is, in fact, necessary to stay unconscious of most things most of the time so that we can attend to the few activities that demand or attract our conscious attention. Every time we switch from one state of consciousness to another, from waking to sleeping, from day-dreaming to attention, from meditating to working a crossword puzzle, we leave behind one set of memories and attitudes and pick up another. Dissociation is a concomitant of any change in state of consciousness, and the ability to experience altered states of consciousness has been of value to mankind in healing, in gaining new knowledge, and in various social functions (Ludwig, 1966).

In some conditions dissociation becomes a problem. To function fully, people need to be able to shift fluidly from one state of consciousness to another. Rigidly walling off some memories and emotions, sealing them away from the scanning gaze of attention, may cause problems in day-to-day living. This inordinate and inflexible dissociation is what we are called on to treat. We must remember in treating these conditions that they represent an extreme of a normal spectrum of behavior, and that some ability to dissociate is necessary in normal people.

This chapter deals only with the treatment of dissociation per se. It is imperative to remember that dissociation rarely exists as a person's sole problem. Most often it is only the visible tip of a much larger and more complex iceberg of difficulties. This is especially true with multiple personalities and prolonged fugue states. We urge a very careful review of what is left once the dissociative disorder has been dealt with. The person will often have a severe personality disorder, a crippling neurosis, an organic brain syndrome, or some other trouble that will need longer and more definitive treatment.

The literature on treatment of dissociative disorders is scant. There are no controlled studies, and few that look at long-term outcome in any systematic way. Several authors have followed sizeable groups of people with amnesia and have reported their experiences and the impressions they formed in working with those people (Kennedy and Neville, 1957; Sargant and Slater, 1941; Abeles and Schilder, 1935; Kiersch, 1962). The literature on treatment of multiple personality is almost entirely composed of single case studies. The suggestions in this chapter, drawn from our own clinical experience and from the published experience of other clinicians, do not rest on uncontestable scientific fact. What we offer is an attempt at a synthesis of the opinions of competent clinicians who have worked long hours with these patients in trying to evolve useful treatment strategies.

The goal in treating dissociation is to render it more flexible and less absolute, bringing the pathologically separated awarenesses of the patient into closer accord. With acute, stress-related amnesia this often is accomplished over the course of an hour or two. In chronic dissociative disorders like multiple personality, which have been manifested daily for years, rapid success cannot be expected. In such cases, the interim goal of helping the patient live a more satisfactory life becomes important. As daily existence becomes more fulfilling, the need to dissociate should diminish.

TREATMENT APPROACHES

Drug Therapy

Sedative-hypnotic drugs. Intermediate and short-acting barbiturates, usually given intravenously, have been extensively used in the treatment of dissociative amnesia. Sargant and Slater (1941) strongly advocated their use. Barbiturate-assisted interviews seem most helpful in acute stress-related amnesia, and most authors agree that they work best soon after a dissociative episode. Their effectiveness diminishes as the time between the episode and the interview increases. It seems possible that dissociative states are maintained by specific cortical inhibitory pathways and that sedative-hypnotic drugs specifically oppose the action of the inhibitory neurons in those pathways (Ludwig, 1972).

Stimulant Drugs. Kennedy and Neville (1957) found that the addition of intravenous methamphetamine stimulated the affect and loquacity of patients undergoing barbiturate-assisted anamnesis. This procedure has received a certain amount of clinical acceptance, but is by no means as widely used as barbiturate interviews.

Psychotherapy

Psychodynamic Therapy. Most work published on the psychotherapy of dissociative states has been psychodynamic. The following techniques have been identified as useful in symptom removal.

1. *Tincture of time.* Many dissociative states resolve spontaneously once the person has been removed from the stressful situation that brought on the dissociation. It is probably worthwhile to give any person suffering from an acute dissociative disorder some time in a quiet, benign, and supportive environment. This may alleviate the need for any further treatment.

2. *Discussion, support, and persuasion.* In many cases it seems that simply taking a thorough history is all the help a patient needs in regaining lost memories. All too often busy therapists, especially in crisis intervention situations, forget how healing it can be for people to tell their own story as completely as they can to a patient and understanding listener. The listener can help by asking the right leading questions and by persuading the speaker to keep trying when the going is rough.

3. *Associative anamnesis.* When support and persuasion alone are not sufficient, some clinicians (Kennedy and Neville, 1957; Parfitt and Gall, 1944) try to help the patient remember through an associative technique, usually focusing on the remembered events surrounding the amnesia and having the patient freely associate to those events. Parfitt and Gall (1944) claim excellent results with the following method:

> During the first interview the amnesia is played down by concentrating on the general life-story, and reassurance is given . . . that recall will be obtained at the next session. At this session one starts with the last thing remembered and confidently persuades the patient to tell what happened in absolute chronological order. His attention is repeatedly forced back if he attempts to jump events or evade the issue with (vague statements). . . . Usually the recall is rapid, the majority in less than half an hour, but the physician must be prepared for a much longer interview.

The patient's feelings must be borne in mind with this and all the other suggested techniques. Good rapport must be maintained. If the patient feels unduly coerced or demeaned, especially early on, all attempts at therapy will fail. Angrily insinuating that patients are not trying hard enough or that they are lying will only force them to defend their dissociations more rigidly. Any other response would publicly damage their already shaky self-esteem.

4. *Suggestion.* Most authors agree that suggestion is a powerful tool in dealing with dissociative states. As with any powerful tool, it has

as much potential for harm as for good, so that we need to be careful *what* we suggest to people who dissociate easily. It seems that the more easily people dissociate, the more impressed they are by suggestion. Any "bad" behavior unwittingly suggested by the therapist is just as likely to be adopted as is any consciously suggested "good" behavior. This makes it mandatory that we be as aware as possible of our feelings and aims with these patients.

Some therapists have evolved elaborate rituals of suggestion to help in the recovery of dissociated material. Grunewald (1971), for instance, uses the following technique in suggesting that two dissociated subpersonalities (A and B) begin to merge with one another in a patient's dreams:

> At night when A is asleep her guard against you (B) will be lowered and you will be able to speak to her. Tell A everything we have discussed, especially how desirable it is that you become one person. Upon awakening A will know that she has dreamt. She will have a vivid memory of the dream and a strong wish to report its contents to me the next time we meet.

5. *Hypnosis.* Hypnosis has been an important and effective tool in working with dissociative disorders. Kennedy and Neville (1957) give a concise description of its most basic use in these disorders:

> Amnesic patients are easy to hypnotize . . . Under hypnosis the patient is made to relive known incidents in his past and to produce a sort of running commentary. During this there is usually considerable emotional abreaction. . . . When the emotion has subsided the patient is kept talking and told to wake up, when he discovers that he is recounting past events and that his amnesia is at an end.

Various kinds of long-term therapy have been advised for chronic dissociative disorders. Group therapy (Bowers, 1971) and extended family therapy (Beal, 1972) have been recommended as especially useful adjuncts to individual therapy in difficult cases of chronic dissociation.

Behavior Therapy

It would not be difficult to recast most of the techniques listed under *psychodynamic therapy* in behaviorist language. However, we rarely find ourselves thinking in terms of conditioning and reinforcement with simple cases of amnesia. When the symptom proves difficult to remove with support, suggestion, hypnosis, or drugs, we do find it useful to step back and look at the larger pattern within which the symptom exists, searching especially for the environmental reinforcers of the symptom. If and when clear-cut rewards for the symptom (such as money, attention, and relief from unwanted responsibilities) can be identified, we can begin to map out strategies that will provide reinforcement in a healthier direction.

TREATMENT CONTROVERSIES

The most heated controversy in the treatment of dissociative disorders concerns the high suggestibility of patients who dissociate and how physicians ought to behave in the face of that suggestibility. Thus, while several authors (Kennedy and Neville, 1957; Abeles and Schilder, 1935; Kiersch, 1962; Ludwig, 1972a; Brandsma and Ludwig, 1974; Allison, 1974) use hypnosis quite freely in their therapy, others (Parfitt and Gall, 1944; Grunewald, 1971; Bowers, 1971) warn that it may positively reinforce the symptom by giving it too much credence.

This debate is especially intense over which aspects of multiple personality deserve attention. Many people believe that some cases of multiple personality have been unnecessarily created in suggestible patients by overly enthusiastic and undertrained therapists. Even more clinicians believe that lengthy, hypnotically assisted searches for more and more personality fragments tend to encourage further fragmentation, prolonging the task of therapy. On the other hand, it cannot be denied that hypnosis is a rapid and powerful way to establish contact with the dissociated parts of a given personality, making it possible to begin the work toward integration. Grunewald (1971) presents a balanced approach to the problem:

> Hypnosis, while commonly used in such cases for contact with the dissociated personality, is thought to be contraindicated . . . because it may be interpreted by the patients as a sanction of the dissociative process. The result tends to be a further splitting off of personality fragments. However, a working knowledge of the dynamics of hypnosis and of hypnotherapeutic techniques can make a unique contribution to the therapy of dual or multiple personalities.

The "unique contribution" that Dr. Grunewald refers to is the experienced and skillful use of suggestion and charisma in the treatment process.

There is some controversy over the efficacy of barbiturate-assisted interviews. In a recent experiment Dysken (1979) found that both amobarbital and normal saline, when administered intravenously, were moderately useful in obtaining new information from patients. However, they found no significant difference in the clinical usefulness of amobarbital over normal saline. This tends to support other authors (Parfitt and Gall, 1944) who have felt that the only advantage of barbiturate-assisted interviews is symbolic and ritualistic.

There has been some controversy over whether persons should be held legally responsible for what they do in a dissociated state. Although this does not directly relate to therapy, therapists are often called on to give testimony. Kiersch (1962) reviewed 32 cases of alleged amnesia where legal charges were pending. He found that the patients were lying about their memory lapses in 21 of these 32 cases. That is, at a later date they said, without coercion, that they had been greatly exaggerating their difficulties with memory. A large element of exaggeration was thought to exist in nine of the remaining cases. Basing their statement on similar findings, Parfitt and Gall (1944) assert that psychogenic amnesia should never be a defense for any crime whatsoever.

TREATMENT SPECIFICS

When faced with a dissociative disorder, the first task is to ascertain whether it is acute or chronic. Brief spells of amnesia and short fugue states are much more easily treated than are cases where dissociation has become the standard weapon in a person's armamentarium of coping devices.

Before beginning psychological treatment of any amnesia, we must be sure that the mechanisms maintaining that amnesia are largely psychological. A careful history, physical examination, and appropriate laboratory studies must be done to rule out physical causes of amnesia. Once causes such as concussion, transient global amnesia, and toxic/metabolic organic brain syndromes have been ruled out, we can begin psychological treatment.

The first medicine for treating an *acute* dissociative state is *tincture of time*. The patient should be given some time to "pull himself together" in a structured, supportive environment such as the hospital or, in some instances, the family home. Many cases of amnesia remit spontaneously under such conditions.

If the dissociative episode persists, our next remedies are *discussion,* *support,* and *persuasion.* A detailed history should be taken, using a style that capitalizes on the interviewer's powers of *suggestion,* always bearing the patient's self-esteem in mind. An *associative anamnesis,* patiently and repetitively focusing the patient's attention back to the first and last remembered events around the period of dissociation,· is useful in this sort of interview. Such an approach is most likely to be successful if it is not time-limited and if the patient understands that it will last "for as long as it takes."

If the dissociation persists after one's best try at this type of interview, an interview under hypnosis should be attempted. If the clinician is not comfortable with hypnosis, if the patient proves to be a poor subject, or if the hypnosis does not succeed in recovering the lost memories, a *barbiturate-assisted interview* should be done.

By this point most cases of acute dissociative amnesia will have been resolved. If the missing memories still have not been recovered, a careful reassessment of the patient's physical, especially neurological, condition should be undertaken. Has a chronic subdural hematoma been missed? Has the patients suffered a hippocampal infarct? Has the patient been poisoned in some way? Careful re-thinking of these kinds of possibilities should be undertaken before going further with psychological treatment.

If the amnesia persists and is thought to be psychologically maintained, it will be necessary to take a larger view of the situation in which it exists, looking for present and past environmental reinforcers of the dissociation. Does the patient receive some sort of financial gain in maintaining the amnesia? Has someone in the patient's circle of family or friends ever suffered from amnesia? Is the patient's family more attentive and affectionate since the amnesia appeared than they were before? To the extent that such environmental reinforcers can be identified, the clinician will be able to map out a treatment strategy that circumvents or counterbalances them.

It will occasionally happen that no clear reinforcers can be identified or that although they can be identified, nothing can be done to weaken their effect. In such cases we should assume a supportive role, helping the patient to live more creatively even though the tendency to dissociate persists. As the sufferer is helped toward a happier and more fulfilling life, the need for reliance on such a primitive defense as dissociative amnesia should diminish.

The basic approach to the treatment of chronic dissociative disorders, most of which present as multiple personality, is the same as for acute disorders, but the time frame is quite different and the sequence of steps is not so orderly. It is unrealistic to assume that a person with a well-established pattern of dissociating under stress will adopt a totally new pattern over the course of two or three interviews. The fundamental goal remains reintegration of the dissociated parts, but it takes great patience and considerable skill to accomplish the task. People who adopt chronic, intermittent dissociation as a lifestyle are psychological toddlers. They are highly suggestible and willing to comply (over the short run) with almost any strongly suggested behavior in order to win attention or affection. This means that we must be cautious about what verbal and nonverbal suggestions we give to the patient. An inordinate interest in the patient's various dissociated personalities can carry the message, "You are more interesting to me as a multiple personality than you are as a normal person." This encourages the patient to develop even more exotic symptoms in the pursuit of even more attention from the therapist. On the other hand, a flat refusal to accept the various dissociated parts of the person as valid can destroy the therapeutic alliance. We find the following suggestions, adapted from Bowers (1971), to be helpful in keeping one's balance amidst the many upheavals that can mark the course of treating a multiple personality:

1. Help each subpersonality to understand that he/she is missing something as a dissociated side of the total person.
2. If it feels necessary to call each subpersonality by a specific name, make it clear that you do so only for the purpose of having a convenient label. Make it clear that you do not accept each "self" as having any rights to individual and irresponsible autonomy.
3. Listen to each subpersonality with equal empathy and concern.
4. Encourage each subpersonality to accept and understand each other subpersonality, to realize that each is incomplete as long as it stays separate from the others.
5. Use hypnosis only if you are experienced and well-trained, both as a hypnotist and therapist. It is probable that undisciplined hypnotic intervention can further separate the subpersonalities, increase fugue states, and evoke new subpersonalities, thus prolonging the therapeutic task. When expertly and judiciously used, however, hypnosis can serve as a powerful constructive tool.

We must remember that dissociation does not occur in a vacuum. Any work done toward reintegration of a dissociated person must proceed hand-in-hand with supportive therapy, couple and/or family therapy, environmental manipulation, and other interventions aimed at decreasing the daily stress in the patient's life and helping him or her to deal with the remaining turmoil more resiliently.

SUMMARY

The dissociative tendency may serve either adaptive or maladaptive functions for the individual. When clinically maladaptive, treatment intervention becomes necessary.

The absence of controlled treatment and long-term follow-up studies precludes definitive statements about specific treatment interventions. Recommended treatment approaches derive mostly from clinical experience. For most acute dissociative reactions, three categories of treatment—psychotherapy, behavior therapy, and drug therapy—are available. Most reactions will resolve in response to the systematic, step-wise therapy described above. Chronic dissociative states require a much more complicated and intensive treatment approach.

In all dissociative states, resolution of the immediate problem may not be necessary to address those psychological, familial, and environmental factors that reinforce the maladaptive use of dissociative episodes for coping with conflict and stress.

REFERENCES

Ables M, Schilder P: Psychogenic loss of personal identity. Arch Neur Psychiat. 34:587–604, 1935.

Allison B: A new treatment approach for multiple personalities. Am J Clin Hypn. 17:15–32, 1974.

Beal EW: Use of the extended family in the treatment of multiple personality. Arch Gen Psychiat. 26:298–310, 1972.

Bowers MK: Therapy of multiple personality. Int J Clin Exp Hypn. 19:57–65, 1971.

Brandsma JM, Ludwig AM: A case of multiple personality: diagnosis and therapy. Int J Clin Exp Hypn. 22:216–233, 1974.

Dysken MW: Clinical usefulness of sodium amobarbital interviewing. Arch Gen Psychiat. 36:789–794, 1979.

Grunewald D: Hypnotic techniques without hypnosis in the treatment of dual personality. J Nerv Ment Dis. 153:41–46, 1971.

Kennedy A, Neville J: Sudden loss of memory. Brit Med J. 2:428–433, 1957.

Kiersch TA: Amnesia: A clinical study of ninety-eight cases. Am J Psychiat. 119:57–60, 1962.

Ludwig AM: Altered states of consciousness. Arch Gen Psychiat. 15:225–234, 1966.

Ludwig AM: Hysteria: A neurobiological theory. Arch Gen Psychiat. 27:771–777, 1972.

Ludwig AM: The objective study of a multiple personality. Arch Gen Psychiat. 26:298–310, 1972a.

Parfitt DN, Gall C: Psychogenic amnesia: The refusal to remember. J Ment Sci. 90:511–531, 1944.

Sargant W, Slater E: Amnesic syndromes in war. Pro Roy Soc Med. 34:757–764, 1941.

10 | Gender Identity Disorders and Transvestism

RICHARD GREEN

TRANSSEXUALISM (302.5X)

ESSENTIAL FEATURES

According to DSM-III, the essential features of *transsexualism* are a persistent sense of discomfort and inappropriateness about one's anatomic sex and a persistent wish to be rid of one's genitals and to live as a member of the other sex.

TREATMENT GOALS

Transsexualism is a unique phenomenon for the clinician in that the patient makes the diagnosis and outlines the desired course of therapy. The treatment request may include an urgent demand for contrasex hormones and surgical sex reassignment. The clinician's overriding strategy is to do the reversible before the irreversible. Requests for treatment involve, utlimately, *irreversible* procedures. Caution is demanded at every juncture.

An important consideration is to verify the "diagnosis." Throughout the course of treatment, at least before any surgical intervention, alternative diagnoses must be considered. These should be explored so that both patient and therapist become convinced of the appropriate diagnosis. In this way persons who more properly fit the syndromes of transvestism or ego-dystonic homosexuality can be separated from transsexuals.

The patient should experience, as genuinely as possible, life in the

320

opposite sex role and pass socially in that role. This trial-by-living process has been called the "real life test" (Money, 1978). Persons may have unrealistic expectations of what cross-sex living will bring to them. They may be mistakenly ascribing gender role conflicts to more general life conflicts.

Fantasies of flight into an idealized new existence must be tempered before an irreversible intervention is carried out. This is easier said than done. In some job settings, it may not be possible for the transsexual to switch gender role and maintain the same occupational standard. This may result in economic hardship. In some locales, cross-dressing, particularly for anatomic males, is illegal and can result in harassment. Sometimes a letter from the treating physician carried by the individual can be of help; in other circumstances it might be advisable for the individual to live in a jurisdiction in which cross-dressing does not disturb the public peace or the private morals of legislators and police officers.

Another treatment goal during this phase is to temper exaggerated sex-typed mannerisms and other behavioral characteristics that render the individual a caricature of the desired sex role. Appropriate social skills training may be required. It is imperative that the patient first learn to "pass" inconspicuously in his or her new role.

The decision for or against surgery is not the end of treatment planning. Those for whom surgery appears indicated may require considerable additional counseling for adjustment to their new role after surgery. This will include continuing follow-up for surgical complications as well as support for new sexual and social behaviors. Here, too, unrealistic fantasies must be dealt with.

For those denied surgery it is important to dissuade "surgeon shopping." If it is the consensual feeling among the clinicians responsible for the patient's welfare that surgery is not in his or her best interest, considerable effort should be expended to help the patient understand the reasons for this decision. The person should be diverted from seeking another surgical center with looser criteria.

TREATMENT

It is becoming increasingly clear that, for a period of at least one and preferably two years before deciding on surgical sex reassignment, and while experiencing the "real life test," patients presenting as transsexuals should be engaged in psychotherapy. The treatment is not designed to change the patient's mind, or to "cure" the transsexual disorder. Rather, it is intended to promote realistic insight into the rationale for seeking sex reassignment and as clear-sighted a realization as possible of the potential life course following reassignment. Either individual or group therapy is useful, groups being comprised of other "transsexuals" in a comparable life situation. To insure candor during the course of these psychotherapy sessions, it is best that the clinician conducting the therapy not have primary responsibility for the ultimate decision regarding sex reassignment. Other clinicians should enter into that final decision.

It is during this period of psychotherapy that patients who more properly fit the diagnosis of transvestism or ego-dystonic homosexuality can be separated out. Some individuals may find that their transvestic behavior is no longer gratifying and may wish for more complete feminization. Whether this would indeed promote better life fulfillment will need to be explored. In addition, some very feminine male homosexuals and very masculine female homosexuals who have considerable conflict, perhaps of a religious derivation, over their homosexual orientation may seek the transsexual "solution," that is, labeling the orientation heterosexual (Hellman et al., 1981).

Hormonal administration should be under the supervision of an endocrinologist. The decision for referral to an endocrinologist, however, should come from the behavioral clinician. Before hormone therapy begins, a thorough evaluation should have established a presumptive diagnosis of transsexualism to the clinician's satisfaction. While hormone treatment has generally been considered fully reversible, this is an oversimplification, particularly for the female-to-male transsexual. Some of the effects of androgen, such as a deepening voice and hirsutism, are not reversible. However, cessation of menses is reversible and clitoral hypertrophy, although not reversible, may not present any problem. For the male given estrogens there may be sufficient breast development to require reduction mammaplasty, should he decide to reverse course. Testicular atrophy and loss of potency should be restorable. There is no voice change and little change in body hair. There is, however some current concern that estrogen may accelerate atherosclerosis, particularly in the coronary arteries.

The frequently exaggerated mannerisms, demeanor, and dress of persons in the initial phases of preparing for sex reassignment present a different type of problem. Female-to-male transsexuals may adopt an exaggerated swagger and hypermasculine behavior. More commonly, in male-to-female transsexuals there is exaggerated "femininity," with excessive use of cosmetics, jewelry, and perfume, plus overdressing. The novice transsexual may appear in midafternoon dressed for opening night at the opera.

Clinicians should offer grooming advice to help patients blend in with persons of the desired sex role rather than stand out, perhaps grotesquely. Some treatment centers (e.g. Stanford University) developed grooming units that provided guidance in gestures, manners of sitting and walking, and the use of cosmetics.

In the event that after the "real life test" of one to two years, there is a consensus between the behavioral clinicians and the patient that surgical sex reassignment is in the patient's best interest, then a variety of surgical interventions can be considered. These are beyond the scope of this chapter, but the interested reader is referred to the proceedings of a symposium on transsexualism (Laub and Green, 1978).

TREATMENT CONTROVERSIES

The treatment of transsexualism remains one of the most controversial areas of psychiatry. For decades surgery was not available in the United States, and American transsexuals went to North Africa, Europe, or Mexico for sex reassignment. Two medical centers in California treated a small series of patients in the 1950's and early 1960's but it was not until the mid-1960's that large-scale university programs were instituted. In 1966 both The Johns Hopkins Hospital and the University of Minnesota Hospitals launched their widely publicized programs and shortly thereafter many other university and private medical centers followed. By the early 1970's the question of *whether* sex reassignment surgery should be performed had been largely replaced by the question *on whom* should it be performed?

It became increasingly apparent that the syndrome of "true transsexualism," as described by Benjamin (1966) and reported in the popular autobiographies of postoperative persons such as Christine Jorgensen, was not universally found among applicants for sex reassignment, after careful exploration. In fact, when centers stopped basing decisions for sex reassignment on whether the patient fit the classic transsexual picture, what emerged were more candid and varied clinical pictures which included elements of transvestism and ego-dystonic homosexuality. Thus, three subgroups of patients emerged who were able to pass the "real life test" before surgery.

Since surgical intervention has a rather short history in controlled research settings in the United States, follow-up on the hundreds of patients who have undergone sex reassignment is limited. Before discussing these limited data, however, it is worth noting Pauly's earlier review of the world literature (Pauly, 1974). In some 200 operations on male-to-female and female-to-male transsexuals, good outcomes outnumbered the bad by approximately 9 to 1. However, it is difficult to evaluate these findings because of the unstandardized criteria for outcome, the possibility of overlap of subjects in more than one publication, and the fact that at a time when such surgery was not professionally accepted it would have taken a heroic psychiatrist or surgeon to publish poor results.

Preliminary follow-up results from several U.S. medical centers with sex-reassignment programs are now finding their way into scholarly publications (e.g. Laub and Green, 1978). Interpretations of these data are not entirely consistent (see below) but the consensus is that, in carefully selected patients, sex-reassignment surgery has improved the quality of life of the transsexual and rarely results in disappointment for having undergone this dramatic intervention.

The most extensively followed and described series of patients comes from Stanford University. That program reported on more than 80 of 100 patients operated on during recent years. The great majority have done well and only a few have regretted the surgery. Most have reported better social adjustment and psychological well being. So far, there does not appear to be any great difference in outcome between those previously anatomic males who fit the classic transsexual history and those who had elements of transvestism or ego-dystonic homosexuality. However, long-term results may provide some distinctions. Results from the University of Minnesota program also point to generally favorable outcome, although some patients did not respond well to surgical intervention (Satterfield, 1981). Results from Europe are also generally positive. Walinder (1967) reported that the general level of life adjustment in 13 patients was substantially improved after surgery.

One recent widely publicized report from Johns Hopkins raises a discordant interpretation (Meyer and Reter, 1979). However, this report has been attacked for methodologic reasons which in the view of many researchers invalidate the authors' conclusion that surgery is no better than psychotherapy or letting the patient evolve without surgery or psychotherapy. The main criticisms have been that: (1) half the sample of surgical patients was lost to follow-up and clinical experience indicates that patients with better results disappear into the general community, and (2) the study was not an experiment. There was no random assignment of patients to the surgical or nonsurgical group but rather those patients who met the criteria for surgery were granted surgery and those who did not meet the criteria were denied surgery. Thus, the lack of significant difference between the two groups at follow-up may reflect the clinical skills of the Hopkins group in selecting the proper patients for surgery. It has also been pointed out (Walker, 1979, personal communication) that for the surgical group the baseline for making comparisons between the pre- and postoperative state was just before surgery rather than at the time that cross-gender living and hormonal administration began. Most beneficial changes occur at the beginning of cross-gender living. Thus, by not including those behavior changes a bias is introduced against finding a significant positive change. Further, Fleming et al. (1980) have noted that "the most serious failing of the study" has to do with outcome variables. These are considered to be "arbitrary" and "cryptic."

An alternative type of treatment, described by Barlow et al. (1979), consists of behavior therapy aimed at reversing the atypical sexual identity. In this approach, aversion conditioning to achieve a same-sex sexual orientation, training in sex-appropriate motor skills and general demeanor, plus social skills training of a heterosexual nature have changed the transsexual picture in a few patients. It is the exceptional transsexual, however, who is willing to undergo these complex behavioral interventions. Most clinicians have found that those who present with the transsexual picture are highly motivated for hormone therapy, cross-gender living, and sex-reassignment surgery, and will not accept a program designed to change their mind about sex change. This does not negate the findings of Barlow et al. but suggests that behavior therapy may be applicable only to a small number of individuals with the diagnosis of transsexualism.

Older objections to sex-change surgery originated primarily from psychoanalysts. They emphasized that the complex psychodynamics of transsexualism cannot be treated by purely symptomatic therapy, and that hormones and surgical amputation of the phallus are not responsible treatments for unresolved oedipal conflicts and castration anxiety (but represent "collusion with delusion"). Such arguments have not prevailed. On the one hand, there do not appear to have been any reversals of transsexualism by psychoanalytic therapy, and, on the other, the concerns over the dire anticipated effects of a "symptomatic" approach to "psychotic" behavior, have generally not been realized.

Remaining needs in evaluating the outcome of treatment for transsexualism are: (1) consensus among all treatment centers, here and abroad, on the valid indicators for surgery in the anatomic male and female; (2) a standardized means of evaluating and treating the preoperative transsexual; (3) standardized instruments for evaluating postoperative adjustment; (4) a means of evaluating those individuals for whom surgery has been denied and of continuing to provide them with required support; and (5) an international registry of transsexuals, so that full populations can be studied, rather than biased samples. Naturally, every caution must be maintained in any such registry to protect the patients' privacy and the confidentiality of the physician–patient relationship (Green, 1977).

SUMMARY

Transsexualism is a unique disorder in that the patient makes the diagnosis and has already decided on a treatment course. Major responsibilities of the clinician include imparting realistic expectations of what "sex-change" will bring and dissuading persons for whom surgery would appear to be unwise. The overriding treatment strategy is to make reversible interventions before anything irreversible is done. The person requesting sex-reassignment surgery should be required to live as fully as possible in the desired gender role, for at least a year and preferably two, before surgery. Follow-up reports of postoperative patients so far generally indicate improved psychosocial adjustment in carefully selected patients.

GENDER IDENTITY DISORDER OF CHILDHOOD
(302.60)

ESSENTIAL FEATURES

The essential features of *gender identity disorder of childhood* are a persistent feeling of discomfort and inappropriateness in a child about his or her anatomic sex and the desire to be, or insistence that he or she is, of the other sex. In addition, there is a persistent repudiation of the individual's own anatomic attributes.

TREATMENT GOALS

The treatment goals for gender identity disorders of childhood are controversial. They engage issues of sex role stereotyping, the contemporary move away from such stereotyping toward more androgynous child-raising patterns, and the relationship between childhood sex-typed non-genital behaviors and later sexuality including homosexuality.

Male and female children must be considered separately because the implications of the atypical sex-typed behaviors may differ, as well as the degree of social conflict during childhood. The extent of intrapsychic conflict may be more comparable.

First, let us consider males. There are several target behaviors and symptoms for which treatment may be given. The primary one is the strong wish by the boy to be a girl. Not only does this result in intra-psychic conflict, but it spills over into overt behaviors that cause the child social distress. Indeed, should this wish to be of the other sex endure, its ultimate outcome may be transsexualism, with the extraordinary degree of intrapsychic and social conflict that endures, at least to the time of surgical sex reassignment during adulthood. Other target behaviors include "feminine" gestures and mannerisms that are spotted by the peer group and result in teasing and ostracism. These boys walk, gesture, run, and throw a ball differently than their male age-mates.

Another source of conflict for these boys is peer group composition, which is almost exclusively female. This, too, results in considerable teasing and retards the development of a balance of social skills. Thus, another goal of treatment is to encourage more balance between the sexes in the peer group. An aversion to rough-and-tumble play and sports may also result in social rejection. The therapist's strategy regarding the latter is more complex as there may be innate differences in the ability of these boys to perform such behavior, and zealous attempts to push them into these activities may subject them to considerable stress. Rather, the treatment goal should be to find a level of participation in male-type activities that is comfortable for the boy and helps reduce social conflict.

For girls, the primary concern is to uncover the motivations for the strong desire to be male. If this can be understood and the girl can come to accept being female, then little attention, if any, need be paid to the boyish aspects of behavior since they do not result in stigmatization. If the intrapsychic conflict of wanting to be male is resolved, the behavior may change. If the wish to be of the other sex persists into adolescence, the issue of female-to-male transsexualism arises.

Some clinicians have stated that a treatment goal is prophylaxis against later homosexuality (Rekers and Lovaas, 1974). The merits of this position will be discussed below.

TREATMENTS

A variety of treatment approaches have been utilized, primarily with boys. They have included psychoanalytic therapy, token economy behavior modification approaches, group therapy of children, concurrent therapy of children and parents (be it behavior modification, group, or psychoanalytic treatment), and individual role modeling therapy that is not insight-oriented.

The analytic therapies (Sperling, 1964; Greenson, 1966) have looked toward traditional psychodynamic mechanisms such as unresolved oedipal conflicts, fear of castration, and the lack of adequate separation and individuation of the male child from his female parent. The behaviorist approach (Rekers and Lovaas, 1974; Rekers, 1975) has been a detailed attack on individual cross-sex-typed behaviors, be they toy preferences, lack of aggressivity, or "feminine" mannerisms. These have been highly structured, selective reinforcement programs, sometimes extending into the home and school with the assistance of parents and teachers as surrogate therapists.

In group therapy several boys with the same behavioral picture meet with a male therapist in an attempt to increase social skills while interacting with other boys, and to promote identification with the male therapist. Concurrently, both mothers and fathers meet in groups with a male–female cotherapy team so that the parents can share common concerns about their sons' behavior and experiences in attempting to help them (Green and Fuller, 1973).

In the one-to-one supportive and role modeling approach (Green et al., 1972), a male therapist and the young boy meet and try to understand the reasons why the boy wants to be a girl. The therapist explains the irreversibility of anatomic sex, highlighting the positive aspects of being anatomically male. He tries to find activities that will interest the boy and will not set him apart from male age-mates. He hopes to see some emerging degree of identification with himself. In addition, the therapist works with the parents, attempting to understand subtle ways in which they may be reinforcing "feminine" behavior. A considerable effort is made to enhance the quality of the father–son relationship when, as is often the case, the two are alienated. The therapist stresses to the father the unique nature of his son's interests, particularly if the father has been trying to make "a man" of his boy, pushing him toward rough-house play and sports. The goal is to find activities that can be mutually enjoyable for father and son. One such activity that has met with success is the YMCA's Indian Guides Program, a group father-son program that deemphasizes sports and rough-and-tumble play.

For the female child with a gender identity problem, treatment methods have not been described in detail. This is partly because very few such female children are seen by clinicians since girls labeled as "tomboys" do not experience the social conflict of boys who are regarded as "sissies" (Green et al. 1980). One treatment strategy (Green, 1974, unpublished data) has been to utilize a female therapist who is herself a professional, highly competent woman. This therapist, a student in a combined M.D./Ph.D. program, was especially gifted in athletics and quite content with being female. The aim, again, was to understand the source of the conflict over being female and to provide a role model engaged in activities the girls initially thought were the sole province of males. In a later effort with a small number of similar girls (Green and Williams, unpublished), the focus has been understanding the child's goals and pointing out, through example, that such goals are possible for females as well as males. In addition, the parents are strongly encouraged to continue this approach outside the treatment sessions and to help make the distinction between the wish to be of the other sex and the wish to participate in activities commonly associated with the other sex. Thus, the "tomboy" who is perfectly content with her anatomic sex, but prefers many of the activities conventionally considered "masculine," should not experience either intrapsychic or social conflict.

TREATMENT CONTROVERSIES

Those wedded to the conviction that all children should be raised strictly without sex-role typing are critical of treatment interventions with these children. They assert that therapists are reinforcing societal sexism and not allowing the child maximal growth. In response to this criticism, therapists have stressed that these children are not androgynous, but rather are stereotypically cross-sexed in their behavior. They point out, for example, that the boys' behavior, if it were manifested by girls, would be distressing to those who idealize androgyny because it is stereotypically feminine. Therapists also point out that a child's desire to be of the other sex is a source of intrapsychic conflict which, if enduring, can result in decades of anguish culminating in sex-reassignment surgery. Thus, potential future conflict must be considered.

Irrespective of how one sees the future development of these children, the argument can be made for intervention since the children who are referred to psychotherapists are experiencing considerable distress. The boys are loners, teased and ostracized; the girls are also unhappy. Those who advocate treatment argue that it would be irresponsible to turn away the children and their distressed parents out of allegiance to the higher ideal of a society without sex-role stereotypes. The treatment goal is not to convert the boy into an "all-American male," but rather to impart more balance in psychosexual development where previously skewed development has produced conflict.

The diagnostic criteria for this disorder make it clear that these are exceptional children. The boys are not those who occasionally experiment with what society considers to be "feminine" behaviors. The girls are not conventional "tomboys," but rather female children who are desperately unhappy being female.

The behaviorist approach mentioned above (Rekers, 1975) has been criticized as being designed for strict positive reinforcement of stereotypically masculine behaviors including overt aggressivity.

Modifications in the various treatment approaches can be made according to the age of the child. The older child usually has a broader understanding of the social matrix in which he or she lives and of what adolescence will bring. He or she may elect not to modify certain behaviors. The child may be content with his or her anatomic sex and may understand the social consequences for the atypical behaviors. This should be fully explored and support can be given for living in a role that may be socially deviant.

The possibility of a homosexual outcome brings up the question raised earlier as to whether a treatment goal during childhood should be prophylaxis against later homosexuality. Most therapists would answer no. It need not be stressed to anyone familiar with the criteria for diagnosis of ego-dystonic homosexuality in DSM-III that homosexuality *per se* is no longer considered to be a mental disorder. It should also be clear to anyone familiar with the literature on the psychosocial adjustment of matched groups of heterosexual and homosexual men and women that there are no significant differences with respect to life adjustment, other than the sex of partner preference (Saghir and Robins, 1973). Furthermore, there is at present no evidence that treatment intervention in children with gender identity disorders has an effect on later sexual orientation. No large-scale studies have been published comparing treated and untreated children with respect to later sexual orientation or life adjustment.

SUMMARY

A gender identity disorder of childhood is most clearly diagnosed when the child is profoundly unhappy over being of the sex to which he or she was born. This intrapsychic conflict is accompanied in the male by social conflict arising out of sex-atypical behavior, including preferential cross-dressing, a female peer group, preferential role playing as a girl, and "feminine" mannerisms. The goals of treatment are to help the child accept and be content with the sex to which he or she was born, and to reduce social conflict, notably for the boy. This may be accomplished by correcting false childhood beliefs about the rigidity of sex roles and by working with the child and parents to reduce behaviors that result in stigmatization, as well as by promoting interests in new activities.

Treatment must also engage the parents who may, in overt or covert ways, be encouraging conflict-inducing behaviors. Also, parents of an older child or young adolescent who remains different from most same-sex peers need support in understanding their atypical child. What is most needed by the child is a continuing bond with the parents. Fathers, especially, may require considerable assistance, particularly those with boys whose behaviors did not fulfill expectations of how a son was going to be. They should not feel that they have failed in their role as father nor feel guilty for having not provided "enough" contact for the growing boy. Rather they should find ways of engaging in mutually enjoyable activities with their sons so that a positive relationship exists into adolescence, and beyond. Mothers and fathers, both, should they become concerned about existing homosexual behaviors, can be helped to reconcile this so that alienation does not ensue. Alienation leaves the child with a burden and loneliness and rejection that can result in truancy and runaway behavior.

TRANSVESTISM (302.30)

ESSENTIAL FEATURES

The essential feature of *transvestism* is recurrent and persistent cross-dressing by a heterosexual male that during at least the initial phase of the illness is for the purpose of sexual excitement.

TREATMENT GOALS

Treatment goals are somewhat difficult to articulate since the vast majority of transvestites never seek psychiatric help (Prince and Bentler, 1972). Those who do usually do so because of conflict with their spouse over cross-dressing, concern over its effects on young children, particularly boys, or perhaps the inability to attain penile erection without cross-dressing. Some transvestites, however, consult therapists because of strong feelings of guilt over their behavior which they consider to be sick, sinful, or both.

Working through feelings of guilt, shame, or sinfulness about a behavior over which the man may have little control can be important, as can enhancing sexual potency without the use of a fetish. It is helpful to meet with the transvestite's spouse, discuss the meaning of the behavior, provide support, and promote a compromise so that the needs of both marital partners are met without a specific attempt to eliminate the transvestic behavior. Isolating young children from the cross-dressing, until at least school age where some understanding of the behavior may be verbalized, may allay parental concerns about the potential for influencing early psychosexual development. An effort can be made to eliminate cross-dressing when it is clear from a thorough evaluation that the quality of life would be significantly improved and that the individual is motivated to end the behavior. It is when the individual's quality of life would be significantly enhanced and his life goals more readily met that intervention aimed at eliminating cross-dressing is warranted. This is the case when the cross-dressing is compulsive and limits the individual emotionally, socially, vocationally, and sexually.

TREATMENT

Psychoanalytic and insight-oriented therapies have not proven successful in eliminating transvestic behavior. This conclusion is acknowledged by Stoller (1976), himself a psychoanalyst. Indeed, the only reports of successful elimination of cross-dressing behavior with reasonable follow-up have come from behavior therapists. The usual behavioral method is the aversive pairing of electrical shocks to the wrist with the fantasy or act of cross-dressing (Marks and Gelder, 1969). (See Chap. 7 for a discussion of aversion therapy.)

An entirely different approach is to support the transvestic behavior, if it is acceptable to the transvestite and his wife, through enrollment in a transvestite social organization. Here transvestic men dressed in women's clothes meet with their partners in a socially supportive setting, beyond the awareness of their young children if they have any.

In helping a wife understand the nature of her husband's behavior, it may be necessary to distinguish transvestism from homosexuality, relieving the wife of any anxiety she may have about the latter. Reassurance, based on what little data exist, that the husband's behavior does not appear to have any significant influence on a child's psychosexual development, can also be helpful.

An important aspect of treatment for transvestites of any age is to help them avoid self-destructive behavior. This is particularly true for adolescents who may be painfully maintaining their cross-dressing secret. Sometimes, in a "cry for help," they will shoplift women's attire. Or men, struggling with the impulse to reveal themselves publicly, may emerge on their neighborhood streets conspicuously cross-dressed, resulting in embarrassment or ridicule. More modulated ways of self-expression should be encouraged. The young adolescent may need considerable psychological support. If worried about homosexuality, he should be informed that transvestites are typically heterosexual. He should also know that while most adult transvestites recall the onset of their cross-dressing during early adolescence or before, this does not mean that all young adolescents who cross-dress become adult transvestites. The fact is, that we do not know the natural course of fetishistic cross-dressing in the young adolescent, and this can be reassuring to the patient. There is a good possibility that the behavior will disappear as female sexual partners become available if it was serving as a surrogate in the absence of such partners.

TREATMENT CONTROVERSIES

There are ethical objections to aversive therapy for any kind of sexual behavior, including transvestism. But the important point here would seem to be the motivation to stop cross-dressing. If it is strong and well-informed, then the nature of the therapy should be fully explained before the patient makes the final decision to proceed. On the other hand, there are those who object to supportive therapy, such as encouraging enrollment in social groups of other transvestites, for patients who are not motivated to stop the behavior. They would rather see the cross-dressing eliminated since it is a "perversion."

Should children at any age see their father cross-dressed? Pertinent data are not available; however, those transvestites who have been studied do not report learning their transvestism from their fathers. Furthermore, some older children have witnessed the metamorphosis of their transsexual parent from one sex role to the other, including cross-dressing, without any apparent gross effect on their psychosexual development (Green, 1978).

As for the transvestite who is impotent if he does not cross-dress, it may be possible through orgasmic reconditioning to enhance potency (Marquis, 1970). This technique usually involves initially fantasizing cross-dressing while masturbating and then switching to a conventional heterosexual fantasy just before orgasm. Gradually, heterosexual fantasy is introduced earlier in the masturbatory sequence.

The behaviorists who view the early temporal association between sexual arousal and some aspect of women's attire also have a plausible explanation. They are on slightly better theoretical grounds in that it appears possible to "decondition" the fetishistic association. However, because it is possible to "decondition" the behavior does not mean that the behavior was originally "conditioned." Treatment outcome does not explain etiology.

It is curious that fetishistic cross-dressing seems to be an almost exclusively male phenomenon. In the world literature only three female cases are reported, one in a book by Stekel published in the 1930's, and three recently by Stoller (in press).

Since there is much greater latitude for cross-dressing by women than men, it has been suggested that the forbiddenness of this behavior for men is what makes it special. Yet this does not explain why *this* forbidden behavior should become sexually arousing. Possibly greater sensory and visible feedback of sexual arousal from the erect male genital sets the base for conditioning associations to a variety of inanimate objects.

Finally, some transvestites may request "female" hormones. The individual's motivation to take hormones should be thoroughly explored and the possibility of an emerging diagnosis of transsexualism should be considered. It may be possible to have an endocrinologist prescribe dosages that will give the male some additional feeling of being a woman, perhaps providing a degree of gynecomastia and at the same time not resulting in loss of potency. It should be kept in mind, however, that there is growing evidence of accelerated coronary arteriosclerosis in persons receiving estrogens. The decision for hormone therapy in the married transvestite should be made jointly by the patient, physician, and sexual partner.

SUMMARY

The minority of transvestites who consult psychiatrists do so for a wide variety of reasons. These include feelings of guilt over cross-dressing, diminished potency in the absence of cross-dressing, marital conflicts over cross-dressing, the desire for "female" hormones to become more "feminine," and the wish to either eliminate the cross-dressing or more comfortably integrate it into their lives. Thus, treatment strategies are varied. Among the methods used are aversion therapy to "decondition" the cross-dressing, psychotherapy to deal with feelings of guilt, marital counseling, exploration of transsexual ideation, and promotion of social support systems including enrollment in transvestite organizations. Only thorough exploration of the patient's motivations can guide the therapist in choosing the most helpful intervention.

REFERENCES

Barlow D, Abel G, Blanchard E: Gender identity change in transsexuals. Arch Gen Psychiat. 36:1001–1007, 1979.

Benjamin H: The Transsexual Phenomenon. Julian Press, New York. 1966.

Fleming M, Steinman C, Bockneck G: Methodological problems in assessing sex-reassignment surgery: a reply to Meyer and Reter. Arch Sex Behav. 9:451–456, 1980.

Green R: Ethical issues and requirements for sex research with humans: confidentiality. Designated Discussion In: Ethical Issues in Sex Therapy and Research. Little, Brown, Boston. 1977.

Green R: Sexual identity of 37 children raised by homosexual or transsexual parents. Am J Psychiat 135:692–697, 1978.

Green R, Fuller M: Group therapy with feminine boys and their parents. Int J Group Psychother. 23:54–68, 1973.

Green R, Neuberg D, Finch S: Sex-typed motor behaviors of "feminine" boys, conventionally masculine boys, and conventional girls. Sex roles. Accepted for publication, Plenum, 1980.

Green R, Newman L, Stoller R: Treatment of boyhood transsexualism. Am J. Psychiat. 26:213–217, 1972.

Greenson R: A transvestite boy and a hypothesis. Int J Psychol. 47:396–463, 1966.

Hellman R, Green R, Gray J, Williams K: Childhood sexual identity, childhood religiosity, and homophobia as influences in development of transsexualism, homosexuality and heterosexuality. Arch Gen Psychiat. 38:910–915, 1981.

Laub D, Green R: The fourth international conference on gender identity. Dedicated to Harry Benjamin. Arch Sex Behav. 7:243–415, 1978.

Marks I, Gelder M: Aversion treatment in transvestism and transsexualism. In: Transsexualism and Sex Reassignment, Green, R and Money, J (eds). Johns Hopkins Press, Baltimore. 1969.

Marquis JN: Orgasmic reconditioning: changing sexual object choice through controlling masturbatory fantasies. J Behav Exp. 36:1010–1015, 1970.

Meyer JK, Reter DJ: Sex reassignment: follow-up. Arch Gen Psychiat. 36:1010–1015, 1979.

Money J: In: Fourth international conference on gender identity. Dedicated to Harry Benjamin. Laub, D and Green, R (eds). Arch Sex Behav. 7:243–415, 1978.

Pauly I: Female transsexualism. Arch Sex Behav. 3:487–526, 1974.

Prince V, Bentler P: Survey of 504 cases of transvestism. Psychol Rep. 31:903–917, 1972.

Rekers G: Stimulus control over sex-typed play in cross-gender identified boys. J. Exp Clin Psychol. 20:136–148, 1975.

Rekers G, Lovaas O: Behavioral treatment of deviant sex-role behaviors in a male child. J Appl Behav Anal. 7:173–190, 1974.

Saghir M, Robins E: Male and female homosexuality. Williams and Wilkins, Baltimore. 1973.

Satterfield S: Data presented at 7th International Gender Dysphoria Symposium. Lake Tahoe, Nevada. 1981.

Sperling M: The analysis of a boy with transvestite tendencies. Psychoanal Study of the Child. 19:470–493, 1964.

Stoller R: Transsexualism in women. Arch Sex Behav. In Press.

Stoller R: Gender identity. In: The Sexual Experience, Sadock, B, Kaplan, H and Freedman, A (eds). Williams and Wilkins, Baltimore. 1976.

Walinder J: Transsexualism. Academiforlaget, Goteborg. 1967.

11 | Paraphilias and Ego-dystonic Homosexuality

ISAAC MARKS

ESSENTIAL FEATURES

The essential feature of the Paraphilias is that unusual or bizarre imagery or acts are necessary for sexual excitement. Such imagery or acts tend to be insistently and involuntarily repetitive and generally involve either: (1) preference for use of a nonhuman object for sexual arousal, (2) repetitive sexual activity with humans involving real or simulated suffering or humiliation, or (3) repetitive sexual activity with nonconsenting partners.

The Paraphilias included here are, by and large, conditions that traditionally have been specifically identified by previous classifications. Some of them are extremely rare; others are relatively common. Because some of these disorders are associated with nonconsenting partners, they are of legal and social significance. Individuals with these disorders tend not to regard themselves as ill, and usually come to the attention of mental health professionals only when their behavior has brought them into conflict with society.

The specific Paraphilias described here are: (1) *fetishism* (302.81), (2) *transvestism* (302.30), (3) *zoophilia* (302.10), (4) *pedophilia* (302.20), (5) *exhibitionism* (302.40), (6) *voyeurism* (302.82), (7) *sexual masochism* (302.83), and (8) *sexual sadism* (302.84). Finally, there is a residual category, *atypical paraphilia* (302.90), for noting the many other Paraphilias that exist but that have not been sufficiently described to date to warrant inclusion as specific categories.

The essential features of *ego-dystonic homosexuality* (302.00) are a desire to acquire or increase heterosexual arousal, so that heterosexual relationships can be initiated or maintained, and a sustained pattern of overt homosexual arousal that the individual explicitly states has been unwanted and a persistent source of distress.

338

This category is reserved for those homosexuals for whom changing sexual orientations is a persistent concern, and should be avoided in cases where the desire to change sexual orientations may be a brief, temporary manifestation of an individual's difficulty in adjusting to a new awareness of his or her homosexual impulses.

Generally individuals with this disorder have had homosexual relationships, but often the physical satisfaction is accompanied by emotional upset because of strong negative feelings regarding homosexuality. In some cases the negative feelings are so strong that the homosexual arousal has been confined to fantasy.

TREATMENT GOALS

Paraphilias and ego-dystonic homosexuality are unconventional sexual behaviors which henceforth will be referred to, for the sake of brevity, as "deviant" behavior. The term is not intended pejoratively, only to denote that statistically the behavior in question is uncommon.

Patients usually come for treatment of unconventional sexual behavior because of the adverse social consequences which these occasion, e.g. conflict with the law or the spouse. While in theory one could try modifying the attitude of the law or the spouse, this would be generally either impractical or would take so long that it would be inhumane to withhold help from the deviant patient who is suffering meanwhile. Accordingly, a reduction of the unconventional sexual urges becomes a primary treatment goal. In many of these patients conventional sexual behavior is perfectly adequate and in them treatment can be aimed primarily at reduction in unconventional desires, wherever possible with the assistance of the regular sexual partner as a cotherapist.

In those patients where unconventional sexuality is accompanied by sexual dysfunction (e.g. premature or failure of ejaculation, failure of erection, vaginismus, or anorgasmia), then this dysfunction too becomes a target of treatment. Sometimes reduction of sexual dysfunction alone leads to a decrease in unconventional sexual desires. At other times the reverse occurs. Research so far gives no guide as to the optimum strategy in patients who have both sexual dysfunction and unconventional sexual desires, i.e. whether outcome is better if one first treats one or the other or both simultaneously.

It is not usually possible to abolish *all* deviant desires, only to significantly reduce their strength and the frequency of acting on them, which in itself is often sufficient to ameliorate the adverse social consequences which brought the patient to treatment in the first place. Some patients will have interpersonal skill deficits which will require treatment in their own right by social skills training or other appropriate methods. Generally one cannot effect far-reaching personality change, but worthwhile improvement in personality assets can often be produced.

TREATMENT

Before embarking on a program to manage paraphilia or ego-dystonic homosexuality as the main problem, it is necessary to check that the deviant behavior in question is not simply a manifestation of another disorder such as schizophrenia, depression, mania, or interpersonal difficulties. Exhibitionists often expose when depressed or tense after an argument with a wife, a boss, or some other interpersonal frustration and the deviant behavior can be used to reduce tension as well as serve a sexual function. Other deviants may experience their urges especially when depressed or anxious. In such patients reducing the depression, anxiety, or interpersonal tension can by itself diminish the deviant impulse, without attention to heterosexuality or the deviance. A case in point of the author's is a sadistic patient who lost his deviance after aversion treatment. He had a history of depression in earlier years and in the two years after aversion therapy developed further transient depressive episodes. During these episodes the sadistic fantasies would return, only to disappear again after the depression remitted with tricyclic antidepressant drugs. Similarly, a manic-depressive transvestite stopped cross-dressing when his mood swings were controlled with lithium (Ward, 1975). On the same theme, a patient referred to the author for exhibitionism turned out to have severe post-traumatic brain damage with dysarthria and memory loss.

Where it is clear that treatment of the deviance in its own right is worthwhile in order to help the patient lead a fuller life, then experimentally validated approaches to management are indicated. So far, these are mainly behavioral. While there are numerous case reports describing the treatment of deviance by psychoanalytic and other psychodynamic methods, their lack of support by controlled studies makes them difficult to evaluate (Rosen, 1979), whereas several behavioral approaches have been tested and found to be useful, although many questions remain to be answered.

The behavioral management of deviance follows similar principles, whatever the type of deviance, with one exception to be dealt with later. It makes little difference whether the behavior to be changed is fetishism, transvestism, zoophilia, pedophilia, exhibitionism, voyeurism, masochism, sadism, or homosexuality. The general principles are to reduce the deviance, increase heterosexuality (or adult homosexuality where the goal in a pedophiliac might be to increase the patient's liking for an older same-sex partner), and to reduce precipitating factors such as boredom or interpersonal friction with partners by appropriate social training. The only type of deviance which leads to a different management decision is transsexualism, which is not readily responsive to behavioral or any other psychotherapeutic management (Marks et al., 1970). The only well-documented improvement of transsexualism with follow-up is a startling cure by exorcism reported by Barlow et al., 1977; this technique is not recommended as a routine—it has also had its failures (Ross and Stalstrom, 1979).

When heterosexual anxiety is present (heterophobia) then reduction of this in a sexual skills training program is indicated (see Chapter 12). When heterosexual anxiety is so great that the patient cannot even go out with the opposite sex, then social skills training (Stravynski and Shahar, 1980) might be desirable first, focusing on establishing relationships with the opposite sex.

Decreasing deviant behavior usually involves some kind of aversion plus self-regulatory methods, and the trend in recent years has been to arrange treatment so that the bulk of it is carried out by the patient learning self-management approaches, with the therapist acting as guide and monitor.

Aversive methods can take many forms. The aversive stimulus can be paired with any type of deviant cue, including fantasies, photographs, slides, narratives, or real-life situations. The timing of the aversive stimulus can vary from the moment of contact with the deviant cue (either immediate or delayed) to only after erections or other signs of arousal appear to the deviant cues. The aversive stimulus can be given once or many times, and regardless of whether the patient's behavior or erection ceases. Aversion can be paired with relief stimuli (usually heterosexual) at the moment the aversive stimulus ceases. Reinforcement can be partial or complete.

Many aversive stimuli have been used. Chemical aversion was widely used until a few years ago but has fallen into disfavor because, compared with electric aversion, it is more cumbersome, less precise, and potentially dangerous. In addition, fewer trials are possible, it cannot be self-administered, and it must be given in a medical setting. *Electric aversion* has been studied more than any other form. It has been given by classical conditioning, avoidance conditioning, backward conditioning, and aversion relief. Recently, electric aversion has been increasingly self-administered as part of a self-regulatory approach.

Covert sensitization is often used. This form of aversion utilizes the patient's fantasies as noxious stimuli instead of an external agent such as injection or shock. During covert sensitization the patient is asked to imagine himself engaging in the undesired behavior. When this is achieved he is asked to imagine at the same time a noxious scene, e.g. a pedophile might be asked to imagine himself masturbating a little boy who then proceeds to vomit all over both of them. The noxious scene need not be disgusting, but could instead be anxiety provoking. Kolvin (1967) described the treatment of a 14-year old boy who put his hand up women's skirts in the streets. This image was paired with sensations of falling out of bed while dreaming of falling from a great height. Other unconventional sexual images have been paired with anxiety-provoking ones such as a man brandishing a knife while threatening to castrate the subject unless he complied with homosexual demands, or the subject's wife looking in through a car window at the subject about to begin a homosexual encounter.

A pilot aversive method is *smell sensitization*, in which deviant stimuli are paired with real unpleasant smells like ammonia or ammonium sulfide or valeric acid. In the author's unit smell aversion has not been very successful. Another pilot technique is *shame aversion* in which the patient is required to perform the deviant act repeatedly in front of other people, the aversion coming from embarrassment. Staff are enlisted to act as observers. Shame can be effective quite unexpectedly. A prim and naive patient of the author's was asked to buy sadomasochistic pictures in the red-light district of London for use in his aversion. On return to hospital he expressed such shock at the atmosphere in which his perversion was practiced that he lost his deviant urges and required no further treatment.

A *rubber band worn around the wrist* can be held taut and snapped back suddenly to sting the skin as effectively as most electric shock apparatus.

It is simple, and the patient can use it as a "self-regulator" or "thought-stopper" as well as an aversive stimulus. In recent years electric aversion has been increasingly replaced by methods like covert sensitization or a rubber band on the wrist. These methods require no equipment, can be readily self-induced, and can be combined with other aspects of a self-management program. Electric aversion given by the therapist and/or self-administered by the patient may be reserved for those patients in whom the deviant urges are so strong that weaker aversive stimuli do not help the patient to control them.

Whatever form of aversion is chosen, ultimately the patient has to learn to exercise control of his unconventional sexual urges in tempting situations which are likely to trigger such urges. Treatment thus consists of sessions with a therapist in which the patient starts by practicing control of his deviant urges stimulated by fantasy or by slides and pictures or real stimuli by means of aversive methods such as electric shock, covert sensitization, or snapping a rubber band sharply on the wrist; as he acquires control over these urges he is then encouraged to carry out these maneuvers in increasingly tempting situations outside the treatment sessions (cue exposure). The patient then plans systematic cue exposure and practices these methods repeatedly between sessions until he is able to switch off deviant urges rapidly. He is then asked to slowly go first into mildly tempting situations while practicing these self-control methods. Once these are mastered he is then encouraged to enter more tempting situations and to practice these approaches further, until complete control is possible even in the most attractive (to him/her) situations, e.g. an exhibitionist might first only look at young girls in the distance and learn to dampen down his desires to expose by means of an aversive fantasy he finds effective such as imagining being arrested, or by means of the sharp sting of a rubber band snapped smartly on his wrist, or by giving himself a shock from a portable shockbox. Having achieved this successfully several times, he will then be asked to practice these maneuvers while waiting outside the gate of a girls' school at the end of the day when all the girls are leaving school.

Behavioral treatments of the kinds described generally achieve substantial amelioration of deviant desires (Marks et al., 1970; Marks, 1978). Failures are usually the result of noncompliance where patients feel they are entitled to their deviance, are coming purely because of social or legal pressure, and do not wish to change. In a few cases, however, despite excellent compliance the urges still cannot be brought under control. In such cases, as a last resort, hormones to reduce libido have been employed with varying success; mainly estrogens or "antiandrogens" have been used (Bancroft et al., 1974). Even such "chemical castration" may fail, as in a patient of the author's who, after cyproterone acetate was administered, merely changed from exposing with an erect penis to exposing with a flaccid penis.

TREATMENT CONTROVERSIES

It will be obvious from the foregoing that behavioral treatments (including aversion) cannot be forced on the patient because they must be used in a self-management context. The ethics of aversion are, in principle, no different from those of any other therapy, provided that it is given with discretion and compassion and with the patient's overall needs always in mind. For example, it may be easier to help a pedophile to become an adult homosexual rather than heterosexual. The strategy of treatment needs to be worked out by consensus with the patient, his partner (where available), and the therapist. Heterosexuality need not be the aim of treatment.

Most of the controlled studies for the efficacy of behavioral methods with unconventional sexual behaviors have examined electric aversion (which is no longer often used). Very little controlled outcome work has been done in this area in the last few years; most studies were done in the early 1970s.

Electric Aversion

Three forms of electric aversion were compared by McConaghy and Barr (1973). They randomly assigned 46 male homosexuals (mean age 25) to classical, avoidance, or backward electric aversive conditioning. Each subject was treated in 14 sessions as an inpatient for five days. During treatment 60 slides of male children, adolescents, and adults were shown for 10 seconds at a time. On some occasions following the removal of the slides showing males and cessation of shock, patients assigned to avoidance or backward conditioning were also shown 30 slides of nude or partially clothed young adult women. Follow-up, usually with booster shock, was at monthly intervals for six months and at one year.

Results showed no significant differences between these three forms of electric aversion. Patients who attended for six or more booster treatments during follow-up did best. At one-year follow-up, half the subjects reported decreased homosexual and half increased heterosexual feeling. A quarter showed increase in coital frequency and a quarter a decrease in homosexual relations, the correlation between these being significant.

There was no significant relationship between outcome and a measure of "appetitive conditionability"—erections to red circles preceding female movies and to green triangles preceding male movies. However, there was a significant correlation between outcome and a measure of "aversive conditioning"—the galvanic skin response to tones preceding shocks. That backward conditioning equalled the other two forms of aversion in efficacy suggested that aversion therapy does not act by setting up conditioned reflexes. Patients treated with aversion did not show arm withdrawal to the shocks or report anxiety if they viewed homosexual pictures after treatment. Instead they reported less sexual interest and showed fewer erections to these pictures. Patients under the age of 30 were more likely to commence heterosexual intercourse after treatment.

Feldman and MacCulloch (1971) treated 43 male homosexual patients (7 of these pedophiles) by electric shock given in an anticipatory avoidance paradigm with follow-up lasting a year or more. Shocks were given while the subject viewed slides of males on a screen. Slides of males could sometimes be turned off prior to receipt of shock. As soon as the slides of males left the screen, slides of females were introduced as relief stimuli, on a variable-ratio basis. Patients could request the return of a female slide at times, this request being met occasionally. About 24 stimulus presentations were given per 30-minute session on an inpatient basis, the average number of sessions being 18–20. Thirty-six of the 43 patients who began treatment completed it. Of these, 25 were significantly improved at the end of the year. Success was defined as cessation of homosexual behavior, the use of no more than occasional and mild homosexual fantasy and/or mild homosexual interest in directly observed males, together with strong heterosexual fantasy or behavior. Post-treatment measures were a structured clinical interview and a sexual orientation questionnaire. Within-treatment measures were of avoidance response latencies and changes in pulse rate to the male slides which were used as conditional stimuli. The two measures cohered in indicating change or not. Prognosis was best in patients with a prior history of pleasurable heterosexual behavior and without a "weak-willed or attention-seeking" personality. This relationship held even when controlled for age.

These workers also carried out a controlled trial in 30 more homosexuals who were assigned at random to treatment by anticipatory avoidance learning, classical conditioning, or "psychotherapy." Aversion treatment was given over 24 half-hour sessions, and "psychotherapy" over 12 one-hour sessions. Six aversion patients after 24 sessions were crossed over to the alternative form of aversion in a further 24 sessions while 7 psychotherapy patients who failed then received aversion. Bias against psychotherapy was not excluded from the design. Follow-up was an average of 44 weeks. Both aversion techniques were equally successful with most patients who had a prior heterosexual history. Of the 27 patients who finally had aversion, 17 showed successful change in sexual orientation at a mean of 46 weeks follow-up. Of the two patients who received psychotherapy only, one failed and one defaulted at follow-up. All three treatments were almost totally unsuccessful in patients without a history of prior heterosexuality.

An elegant controlled comparison of electric aversion with imaginal desensitization was made by Bancroft et al. (1974). He assigned 60 patients at random to treatment by desensitization in fantasy to fears of heterosexuality or to electric aversion. There were 30 treatment sessions each lasting an hour. In half the aversion sessions, patients were shocked when they developed erections to slides of males and in half patients were shocked on reporting the production of homosexual fantasies. Measures of change consisted of ratings of sexual behavior and attitude, and actual erections to slides. Immediately after treatment only aversion significantly reduced erections and attractions to males; erections and attraction to females increased significantly both with aversion and with desensitization. On no measure at the end of treatment did aversion differ significantly from desensitization. At six to nine months follow-up, only 5 of the 30 averted and 5 of the 30 desensitized patients were improved—results were not as good as those of Feldman and MacCulloch; erections were not measured, but there was a suggestion that desensitized patients showed more heterosexual behavior. Both aversion and desensitization reduced homosexual behavior; aversion decreased homosexual and desensitization increased heterosexual attitudes. Only one case showed persistent signs of conditioned anxiety. Desensitization resulted in more improvement among patients who had shown previous anxiety about heterosexuality. Aversion increased heterosexual erections more in younger and less in anxious patients.

The value of heterosexual arousal for favorable outcome was suggested by one finding. At the end of treatment, although homosexual erections decreased in many patients, more of those with *heterosexual* interest (attitudes and erections) subsequently did well at six months follow-up.

Bancroft made the important observation that changes often began in patients two months *before* treatment. This reviewer has also observed this at times. It suggests that factors like motivation are important.

Another careful comparison of electric aversion with a nonaversive (placebo) control was reported by Birk et al. (1971). Of 60 homosexual referrals, 18 were selected for treatment and 16 remained after two years' treatment. During these two years, they all received group psychotherapy with a male and female cotherapist team. At the end of the first year's group therapy, the sample was assigned at random to shock or placebo conditioning. This was followed immediately by 12 hours of individual treatment and another year of group psychotherapy. Twenty to twenty-five half-hour conditioning sessions were given over six weeks. Each patient selected his own male and female pictures for use in sessions. There were 25 pictures per session given at intervals of 20 seconds. Within each session several forms of electric aversion were given: avoidance trials with escape by a female slide, classical conditioning with inevitable shock, delayed escape, delayed avoidance and intertrial approach learning. Placebo conditioning controls received no shock but instead saw an amber light in the same program and were told that this was "associative conditioning."

After 12 sessions of conditioning 0/8 placebo and 5/8 aversion patients showed changed sexual feelings. One year after the end of conditioning two of the five improved aversion patients remained free of homosexuality and were active heterosexually. On the Kinsey ratings aversion was significantly better than placebo at the end of conditioning, but not at the end of follow-up. However, homosexual cruising, petting, and orgasm was significantly decreased at the end of follow-up in aversion patients compared to placebo conditioning subjects (Fig. 11-1). Really good results were obtained in only two out of eight patients with aversion and in none of those who received placebo conditioning.

Total treatment time was 79–140 hours, most of which was in group psychotherapy. The design of the experiment precludes accurate assessment of the contribution made by group psychotherapy to the changes,

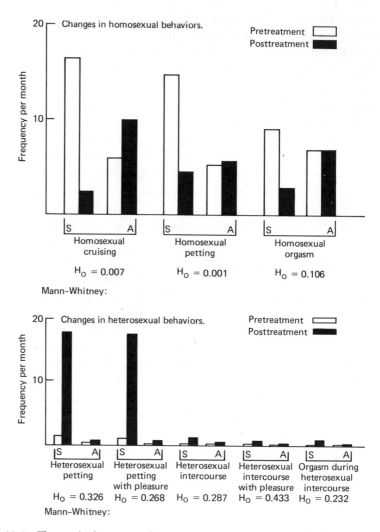

Fig. 11-1. Change in homosexuals one year after aversive or placebo conditioning. Patients in both conditions also had two years' group psychotherapy. S = aversion (shock); A = placebo (associative conditioning). (Redrawn from *Archives of General Psychiatry*, October 1971, Vol. 25, pp. 314–325. Copyright 1971, American Medical Association)

as it was balanced across aversive and placebo conditioning. However, the poor results in the psychotherapy and placebo group suggest that group psychotherapy was not very useful unless one posits a specific interaction between it and aversion. Overall results were not as good as those obtained by Feldman and MacCulloch, but the evidence did favor contingent shock over contingent light where both were given in the context of group psychotherapy.

Tanner (1974) compared male homosexuals in a wait list control group with those receiving electric shock aversion therapy. The latter showed significantly more erection and subjective arousal to *female* slides, and more sexual thoughts, socializing, and sex with females.

The controlled studies so far all concern homosexuality. One controlled comparison has also been made of aversion in exhibitionism (Rooth and Marks, 1973). Twelve persistent, chronic exposers were treated as inpatients, ten of whom had been convicted for exhibitionism. A parallel study with long-term follow-up was not practicable, so instead a design was adopted which examined changes in feelings and behavior three days after the end of each form of treatment. Three treatments were given, one form of treatment per week over three consecutive weeks, in a balanced incomplete Latin-square design. The treatments were aversion, self-regulation, and muscular relaxation chosen as a placebo control method unlikely to have a specific effect on the target problem. There were eight therapy sessions a week, each session lasting an hour. During aversion, patients were shocked either on reporting that they had produced an image of exposing or during their rehearsal and description of an exposure act in front of a mirror. Shocks were given on all trials, followed by the "aversion relief" of conversation with the therapist. There were about 15 trials per session. Shocks were given from a portable shock box to the subject's forearm. In the second half of the trial, patients were also required to shock their own exposure fantasies in their own rooms, and to administer self-aversion to their forearm with a portable shock box in potential exposure situations.

In self-regulation sessions, discussions would elucidate internal and external triggers of the exposure impulse–response chain, and a repertoire of alternative behaviors (e.g. smoking, mental arithmetic, reading) was selected for use in interrupting the early stage of sequences that might lead to exposure. To enhance awareness of deviant behavior patterns, prerecorded accounts of typical acts were repeatedly played back while the subject exposed to himself in the mirror and tried to express his

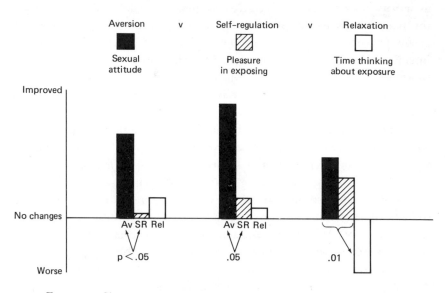

FIG. 11-2. Short-term outcome in 12 exhibitionists. (Redrawn from Rooth and Marks, In *Archives of Sexual Behavior* (ed. R Green), Vol. 3, pp. 227–248, 1974)

feelings about the situation. In the second half of the trial, patients spent an additional daily session on self-administered covert sensitization in their rooms, and were also required to rehearse self-regulation techniques in provocative situations. The aversive and self-regulation procedures overlapped to the extent that the self-administered aversion which patients carried out between sessions could be construed as a form of self-regulation, and also the covert sensitization which patients practiced during self-regulation could be regarded as a form of aversion.

Relaxation treatment consisted of Jacobson's method of progressive muscular relaxation. In the second half of the trial, the patients carried out daily relaxation sessions in their room. They also went into tempting situations each day, with the instruction that they should counteract incipient tension by attempting to generate feelings of mental and physical relaxation.

Results showed the order of efficacy of the three treatments to be aversion best and self-regulation second, with relaxation being last and ineffective. Measures of change were necessarily based mainly on self-reports. Aversion produced significant improvement on four measures, self-regulation on two and relaxation on none. Aversion was significantly superior to self-regulation and to relaxation on two measures (Fig. 11-2). Self-regulation was significantly superior to relaxation on only one measure. Aversion was most effective when given as the first treatment, while on one measure, self-regulation was potentiated when preceded by aversion. During follow-up, results could be attributed to any or all of the three treatments because of the crossover design. At 12–14 months follow-up, significant improvement continued despite the chronicity and severity of the disorder before treatment. However, of the 12 patients, 7 had reexposed at some stage and 4 had been reconvicted.

COVERT SENSITIZATION

A small, controlled study of covert sensitization (Barlow et al., 1972) examined the contribution of therapeutic instructions to the procedure. Four homosexuals were told that convert sensitization to a nauseating image would increase their sexual deviation and that simply visualizing deviant images repeatedly was therapeutic. They then received treatment in a repeated measures design which consisted of (1) repeated visualization of deviant images (no pairing); then (2) covert sensitization with negative instructions; then (3) no pairing (repeating no. 1); then (4) covert sensitization with more positive instructions. The number of sessions and pairings was matched across covert sensitization and the preceding condition on one occasion. Subjects were treated three to five times weekly, three as outpatients and one as inpatient, to a total of 28 to 42 sessions.

Results shortly after sessions showed that, regardless of instructions, erections to male slides were reduced significantly more after covert sensitization than after visualizing deviant images without the nauseating image (Fig. 11-3). One patient did improve during a no-pairing conditioning but there was a suggestion that he might have used covert sensitization himself at this stage. Only four subjects were used in this study, but results suggested that overall instructions and patient expectations play but a minor role in covert sensitization, as measured during the short time after treatment.

An attempted comparison of covert sensitization with electric aversion was reported by Callahan and Leitenberg (1973) in a study using six sexual deviants (three homosexuals, two exhibitionists, and one transves-

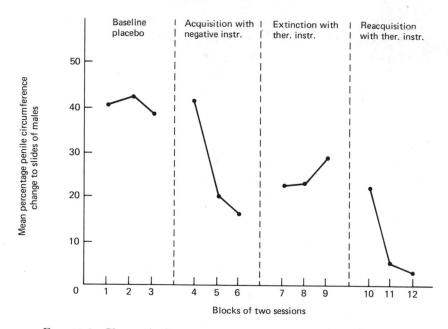

FIG. 11-3. Change in homosexuals using covert sensitization versus repeated imagery. (Redrawn from Barlow *et al.*, In *Behaviour Research and Therapy* (ed. S Rachman), Vol. 10, pp. 411–415, 1972)

tite transsexual). The two forms of aversion produced similar improvement in erections to deviant stimuli and frequency of deviant sexual behavior. Covert sensitization produced greater suppression of deviant urges than did shock. Unfortunately, the balance of design which the authors planned could not be attained, making adequate comparison of the two treatments impossible, and significance figures of difference were not reported.

The long-term effects of covert sensitization remain to be demonstrated in a controlled fashion. Since subjects learn to summon up their own noxious fantasies when they have deviant temptations, the method can be regarded as a form of self-regulation.

Shame Aversion

This has not yet been subjected to controlled study. Serber (1972) reported five male deviants who received shame aversion as the sole treatment; all showed some repetition of their deviance by six months follow-up. Ten other patients received shame aversion over two weeks, plus graduated retraining which included assertive training (the "stand up for yourself" type) and heterosexual social retraining with a female therapist. Further retraining was assisted by a full-length mirror and audio tape recorder for immediate feedback. The retraining included modeling, behavior rehearsal, and role playing, and was carried out once or twice a week over a three-month period.

Of the 10 patients who received shame aversion plus social retraining eight did not repeat their deviant behavior during a one-year follow-up. Two improved but continued some deviant behavior. Serber suggested that patients with marked heterosexual deficit might begin heterosexual retraining *before* applying aversion.

Shame aversion was called "provoked anxiety" by Jones and Frei (1977). They treated 15 male exhibitionists, who were required to undress completely in front of 5–12 male and female staff while describing past exhibitionist episodes. The fifth session was videotaped and the patient saw this videotape as the sixth session. The audience was detached in manner and asked the exhibitionist about his behavior and feelings. No measures were taken, but at 1–5 years follow-up, all were said to be heterosexual and 10 patients had stopped exposing.

GENERAL ISSUES IN AVERSION THERAPY

The unpleasantness of aversion therapy varies greatly depending on its mode of administration. There is no evidence that extreme unpleasantness is important. Just enough shock is given to overcome the pleasure which patients experience from deviant stimuli; the aim is not to produce suffering but to abolish pleasure (Marks et al., 1970). Electric aversion was rated by patients as less unpleasant than a dental visit (Hallam et al., 1972). Aversion can thus be given humanely in a manner which is acceptable to most patients. Obviously, however, if more pleasant treatments can be found which are equally effective, these should replace aversive methods.

Although aversion decreases deviance more than several other methods, the overall effects are not startlingly large even when significant. A favorable prognostic factor is the presence of some prior heterosexual interest which predicts more heterosexual behavior after treatment (Feldman and MacCulloch, 1971; Bancroft, 1974; Bancroft, 1970; Marks and Gelder, 1967; Rooth and Marks, 1973).

Evidence that aversion works mainly by leading to conditioned anxiety is unimpressive (McConaghy and Barr, 1973; Bancroft, 1974; Bancroft, 1970; Hallam and Rachman, 1972; Marks et al., 1970). Patients who improve after aversion usually report, not anxiety, but indifference to their formerly attractive stimuli (Bancroft, 1970; Marks et al., 1970; Marks et al., 1977; Hallam and Rachman, 1972). Aversion therapy produced changes which are neutralizing rather than aversive. In general, aversion seems to work best in patients with higher self-esteem and less anxiety before and during treatment (Marks et al., 1970; Bancroft, 1974; Bancroft, 1970; Morgenstern et al., 1965; Feldman and MacCulloch, 1971).

The importance of an *aversive* stimulus is suggested by the results of Birk et al. (1971) in which a placebo conditioning procedure produced inferior results. However, this does not argue for *conditioning* processes—only a noncontingent shock control could prove this, and has not yet been reported in sexual deviants. The fact that backward conditioning has produced as good results as forward conditioning argues against conventional conditioning mechanisms (McConaghy and Barr, 1973).

NONAVERSIVE METHODS

Fading
Here the deviant stimuli are gradually shifted toward a more conventional heterosexual content during periods of sexual arousal. The technique has been used by several authors (Bancroft, 1971; Beech et al., 1971; Gold and Neufeld, 1965; Barlow and Agras, 1973), but is still experimental.

Self-Regulation
With this method the precise conditions are defined under which self-control is deficient and the client is then trained to control his impulses by interrupting the response chain, e.g., by switching thoughts (Bergin, 1969). As this is one of the commonest behavioral approaches used now in paraphilia, some detail is appropriate.

The only controlled trial of self-regulation to date is the study of exhibitionism by Rooth and Marks (1973). Self-regulation had a significant short-term effect, but less so than aversion. The method required the patient and therapist to discuss the most recent exhibitionistic urges; data were obtained from a time sheet and daily self-regulation form. Choice points were identified and, where faced with alternative moves, the patient was instructed to take the action less likely to lead to exposure. Possible future situations were rehearsed and responded to, e.g. one patient would get resentful when he felt unfairly treated at work or at home and would then plan to expose over the next few days. He was instructed to challenge such resentful or other moods and to articulate the covert decision to expose which was made at this point. Many patients disguised their decision to expose by pretending they wanted to go out for a walk or to go fishing. During self-regulation they became more aware of their exposure plans and focused on choice points. As the patient moved towards a potential exposure situation, e.g. park or train, he had to become aware of the situation and its danger, and execute *alternative* behavior which would decrease the likelihood of exposure, e.g. walk away from young girls, or if he could not do so, look at a shop window or read a newspaper, or memorize verse, solve crossword puzzles, think of his family or look at a photograph of his children or think of a policeman coming. The latter is a form of covert sensitization.

On that measure which improved most with self-regulation, the effect was significantly greater when it was preceded by electric shock aversion. The possibility of treatment combining both methods thus arises. One patient said that he felt unable to apply self-regulation when exhibitionistic urges were very strong, but when their strength had been reduced by aversion he could bring self-regulatory maneuvers into play.

Canton-Dutari (1974) and Canton-Dutari (1976), working in Panama, trained young homosexuals to control their homosexual arousal by a combination of desensitization, aversion, and self-regulation by a breathing-contraction technique; thereafter they were asked to masturbate to heterosexual stimuli. The patient was taught to relax all his muscles, then shown how to diminish sexual arousal by alternately contracting and relaxing his thighs, meanwhile breathing with his abdominal muscles. Having mastered this technique, the patient was instructed to masturbate as his sole sexual outlet for three weeks, trying to prolong the erection as long as possible. During this time if he became homosexually aroused he was instructed to practice the control breathing-contraction technique. Then for three weeks he was given electric aversion while imagining homosexual fantasies and looking at homosexual slides and films. Thereafter the patient was instructed to masturbate in the presence of heterosexual stimuli, the aim being to prolong erections in the presence of such stimuli rather than to achieve orgasm. From the thirteenth week in treatment onward, the patient's relationship with his male therapist was analyzed and compared with other male relationships in actual social situations. Canton-Dutari treated 54 homosexuals who had a mean age of only 17 and found that 90% achieved worthwhile results in terms of changed sexual orientations up to four years follow-up. His homosexual sample was much younger than most reported in the literature, and therefore had a higher chance of achieving heterosexuality.

INCREASING HETEROSEXUAL BEHAVIOR

There are undoubtedly sexual deviants who have normal heterosexual skills without heterophobia, and in such patients it seems futile to concentrate on increasing heterosexual skills further rather than to reduce the deviant urges. In those deviants who do have heterosexual anxiety and deficits, it is moot how much decrease in deviance might result simply from production of a heterosexual repertoire. There are case reports of such instances in homosexuality (Kraft, 1967; Stevenson and Wolpe, 1960; Huff, 1970) and in exhibitionism (Bond and Hutchinson, 1960). Such reports give no reliable guide to practitioners who must decide when to opt for reducing heterophobia and increasing heterosexual skills, and when to reduce deviance. An optimal strategy might be a combination of techniques both to reduce deviance and to increase heterosexuality. The patient's history might serve as a guide.

There is no clear-cut relationship between the presence of deviance and heterosexuality; while in some the one seems reciprocal to the other, in others the two are independent. The author has known transvestites and exhibitionists who engage in repeated heterosexual intercourse to try to keep their deviant urges at bay, but in vain. The mainsprings of deviant behavior are thus many, and only one of these is heterosexual anxiety or deficit. In those subjects where this is clearly present, it would seem logical to try increasing heterosexual behavior. Several methods have been used in this endeavour.

Desensitization
Case reports of desensitization in homosexuality come from Kraft (1967), Bergin (1969a), Huff (1970), and LoPiccolo (1971). The most systematic

study to date is that of Bancroft described earlier. Only one of his 15 patients who were desensitized in fantasy lacked heterosexual anxiety and he dropped out of treatment. The result of imaginal desensitization was modest, only five of the fifteen showing marked improvement at follow-up of nine months. So far, Barlow's (1973) conclusion is valid: there is no experimental evidence that desensitization increases heterosexual responsiveness. Research in this area is badly needed in patients with clear heterophobia on history or examination.

Social Retraining

Assertive training, modeling, and behavior rehearsal might be used to increase heterosexual skills. Pilot studies of their use have been conducted (Serber, 1972; Hanson and Adesso, 1972; Blitch and Haynes, 1972; Stevenson and Wolpe, 1960; Cautela and Wisocki, 1969). The technology of social skills training is improving in this crucial field.

Pairing

Pairing of sexual arousal with heterosexual stimuli is another way of evoking heterosexual behavior (Moan and Heath, 1972; Herman et al., 1973). *Fading* and *shaping*, described earlier, are special variants of these. *"Orgasmic conditioning"* is the pairing of sexual arousal during masturbation with heterosexual stimuli and has been used in the treatment of homosexuality, sadomasochism, voyeurism, and heterosexual pedophilia (Barlow and Agras, 1973). Subjects usually masturbate to pictures or fantasies which progressively resemble the heterosexual target.

In *aversion relief*, a heterosexual stimulus is paired with cessation of a noxious stimulus. This might be classified as a form of aversion, since the effect of electric shock aversion given as backward conditioning is similar to that given as forward conditioning (McConaghy and Barr, 1973). In his review, Barlow concludes that evidence still fails to support the value of aversion relief in increasing heterosexual behavior in paraphilias.

Subcultural Considerations

An obvious factor complicating the treatment of homosexuals is the subculture to which they often belong. A homosexual wishing to make the transition to heterosexuality may need to break with his previous gay environment. The same applies to transvestites who belong to transvestite clubs.

DECISION TREE (Fig. 11-4)

The standard course of treatment is reduction of deviant desires through aversive-self-regulatory methods, plus reduction of any heterophobia (or homophobia if appropriate) which might be present.

SELECTION OF PATIENTS SUITABLE FOR TREATMENT

1. Patient must have repetitive deviant behavior triggered by particular external cues (e.g. sight of fetish objects), or internal cues (e.g. boredom).
2. The problem should be definable in precise, observable terms, e.g. "repeated urges to masturbate slim young boys under age 11" or "repeated desires to expose myself to women when I am bored."
3. Based on these problems the patient should define specific goals desired in treatment, e.g. "be able to see young boys under age 11 and resist any tempting thoughts" or "be able to be near young women without exposing myself and finding interesting things to do when bored."
4. Overcoming the patient's problem should make a difference to his life, e.g. to reduce formerly adverse consequences of deviant behavior such as marital friction, likelihood of arrest, or loss of job.
5. The patient should be willing to invest the time and effort necessary to overcome his problem by practicing self-regulatory, aversive, and other maneuvers; keeping a diary of his urges and behavior; and asking to see his therapist when the urges are in danger of escaping control.
6. Where sexual partners are present it is helpful if they are willing to participate as cotherapist in the treatment of the patient for the reduction of deviant behavior. For the reduction of heterophobia or sexual dysfunction this is critical.
7. The patient should not have suicidal depression, schizophrenia, or organic deficits.

STRATEGY FOR BEHAVIORAL TREATMENT

1. Is heterophobia or sexual dysfunction present? If no, treat deviance only: if yes, worth considering exposure and social skills train-

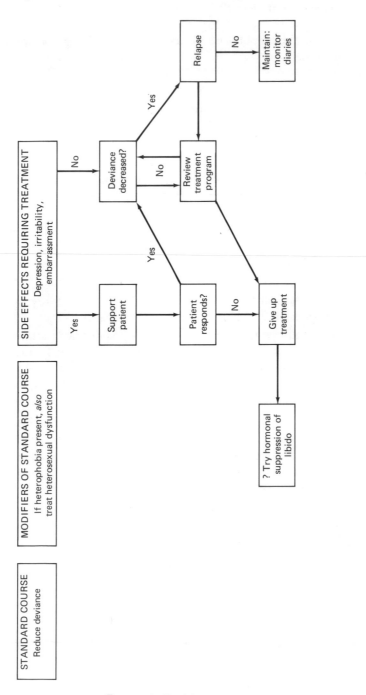

FIG. 11-4. Decision tree.

ing for heterophobia and sexual skills training for specific sexual dysfunctions (see Chap. 12). These can be given concurrently with measures to reduce deviant behavior.

2. Write down specific problems and goals to be worked on.

3. What are the sensations and behaviors when aroused? (e.g. searching for opportunities to engage in deviant behavior, prolonged deviant fantasies, tumescence).

4. Choose appropriate self-regulatory tactics to reduce sensations and behaviors (aversive fantasies of covert sensitization, sting from elastic band on wrist, self-shocking portable electric device, or bottle containing noxious smell).

5. If self-regulatory tactics are insufficient, give additional therapist-aided aversion with covert sensitizing images, shocks, or shame, aversion etc.

Modifiers of standard course: The main one is to treat any heterophobia which is present, as well as to reduce deviance.

Side effects requiring treatment: Common events during treatment are short-lived anxiety, depression, irritability, hostility, or embarrassment. For these the patient needs to be supported until the episode is over.

Adequate response in the treatment consists of reduction in strength and frequency of deviant sexual urges.

Relapse indicates the need for reanalysis of factors precipitating unconventional sexual behaviors. The therapist may need to deal with any depression, marital conflict, or interpersonal problems which might have generated relapse and perhaps administer additional therapist-aided aversion or self-regulatory maneuvers.

Maintenance requires adequate record keeping by the patient of diaries and rating scales of heterosexual and unconventional sexual behavior. The diaries are sent back to the therapist at intervals for monitoring.

SUMMARY

Patients usually ask for treatment of unconventional sexual behavior when it brings them into conflict with the law or their partner. Where such deviance is associated with heterosexual dysfunction, then treatment of that dysfunction by sexual and social skills training with a partner is appropriate, and can be combined with an aversion–self-regulation program to reduce the strength and frequency of deviant urges. Where there is normal heterosexuality, reduction of deviance alone is the aim. For this purpose, controlled studies have found aversion and self-regulation to be useful. Successful behavioral treatment requires that patients should have repetitive deviant behavior triggered by particular cues and be willing to have treatment and cooperate in an aversion–self-regulation program, including "homework" between sessions. This can include self-administered aversion, covert sensitization, and cue exposure initiated by the therapist and then practiced by the patient between sessions, with recording of details in daily diaries. If behavioral treatment fails, hormonal suppression of libido, which has been used with varying success, can be tried.

References

Bancroft JHJ: A comparative study of aversion and desensitization in the treatment of homosexuality. Chapter in: Behavior Therapy in the 1970's. Burns, LE and Worsley, JH (eds). Bristol, Wright. 1970.

Bancroft JHJ: The application of psychophysiological measures to the assessment and modification of sexual behaviour. Behav Res Ther. 9:119–130, 1971.

Bancroft JHJ: Deviant Sexual Behaviour. Oxford University Press, New York. 1974.

Bancroft JHJ, Tennent G, Lucas K, Cass C: Control of deviant sexual behaviour by drugs: behavioural changes following estrogens and antiandrogens. Brit J Psychiat. 125:310–315, 1974.

Barlow DH: Increasing heterosexual responsiveness in the treatment of sexual deviation. A review of the clinical and experimental evidence. Behav Ther. 4:655–671, 1973.

Barlow DH, Abel GG, Blanchard EB: Gender identity change in transsexuals: an exorcism. Arch Sex Behav. 6:387–395, 1977.

Barlow DH, Agras WS: Fading to increase heterosexual responsiveness in homosexuals. J Applied Behav Anal. 6:355–366, 1973.

Barlow DH, Agras WS, Leitenberg H, Callahan EJ, Moore RC: The contribution of therapeutic instruction to covert sensitization. Behav Res Ther. 10:411–415, 1972.

Beech HR, Watts F, Poole AD: Classical conditioning of sexual deviation: a preliminary role. Behav Ther. 2:400–402, 1971.

Bergin AE: A self regulation technique for impulse control disorders. Psychotherapy: Theory, Research and Practice. 6:113–118, 1969.

Bergin AE: A technique for improving desensitization via warmth, empathy and emotional reexperiencing of hierarchy events. Chapter in: Proceedings of the Association for Advancement of the Behavioural Therapies. Rubin, RD, Franks, CM, Lazarus, AA (ed). Academic Press. New York 1969a.

Birk L, Huddleston W, Miller E, Cohler B: Avoidance conditioning for homosexuality. Arch Gen Psychiat. 25:314–323, 1971.

Blitch JW, Haynes SN: Multiple behavioral techniques in a case of female homosexuality. J Behav Ther Exp Psychiat. 3:319–322, 1972.

Bond IK, Hutchinson HC: Application of reciprocal inhibition therapy to exhibitionism. Can Med Assoc J. 83:23–25, 1960.

Callahan EJ, Leitenberg H: Aversion therapy for sexual deviation: contingent shock and covert sensitization. J Abnorm Psychol. 81:60–73, 1973.

Canton-Dutari A: Combined intervention for controlling unwanted homosexual behavior. Arch Sex Behav. 3:367–371, 1974.

Cautela JR, Wisocki PA: The use of male and female therapies in the treatment of homosexual behavior. Chapter in: Advances in Behavior Therapy. Rubin, R and Franks, C (eds). Academic Press, New York 1969.

Feldman MP, MacCulloch MJ: Homosexual Behaviour: Therapy and Assessment. Pergamon, Oxford. 1971.

Gold S, Neufeld IL: A learning approach to the treatment of homosexuality. Behav Res Ther. 2:201–204, 1965.

Hallam R, Rachman S: Some effects of aversion therapy on patients with sexual disorders. Behav Res Ther. 10:171–180, 1972.

Hallam R, Rachman S, Falkowski W: Subjective, attitudinal and physiological effects of electrical aversion therapy. Behav Res Ther. 10:171–180, 1972.

Hanson RW, Adesso VJ: A multiple behavioral approach to male homosexual behavior: a case study. J Behav Ther Exp Psychiat. 3:323–325, 1972.

Herman SH, Barlow DH, Agras WS: An experimental analysis of classic conditioning as a method of increasing heterosexual arousal in homosexuals. Behav Ther. 5:33–47, 1973.

Huff FW: The desensitization of a homosexual. Behav Res Ther. 8:99–102, 1970.

Jones IH, Frei D: Provoked anxiety as a treatment of exhibitionism. Brit J Psychiat. 131:295–300, 1977.

Kolvin I: "Aversive imagery" treatment in adolescents. Behav Res Ther. 5:245–249, 1967.

Kraft T: A case of homosexuality treated by systematic desensitization. Am J Psychother. 21:815–821, 1967.

LoPiccolo J: Systematic desensitization of homosexuality. Behav Ther. 2:394–399, 1971.

Marks IM: Living with Fear. McGraw-Hill, New York. 1978.

Marks IM, Gelder MG: Transvestism and fetishism: clinical and psychological changes during faradic aversion. Brit J Psychiat. 113:711–739, 1967.

Marks IM, Gelder MG, Bancroft JHJ: Sexual deviants two years after aversion. Brit J Psychiat. 117:173–185, 1970.

Marks IM, Hallam RS, Connolly J, Philpott R: Nursing in Behavioral Psychotherapy. Royal College of Nursing Research Series. Henrietta Place, London W1. 1977.

McConaghy N, Barr RF: Classical, avoidance and backward conditioning treatments of homosexuality. Brit J Psychiat. 122:151–162, 1973.

Moan CE, Heath RG: Septal stimulation for the initiation of heterosexual behavior in a homosexual male. J Behav Ther Exp Psychiat. 3:23–30, 1972.

Morgenstern FS, Pearce JF, Rees WL: Predicting the outcome of behaviour therapy by psychological tests. Behav Res Ther. 2:191–200, 1965.

Rooth FG, Marks IM: Aversion, self-regulation and relaxation in the treatment of exhibitionism. Arch Sex Behav. 3:227–248, 1973.

Rosen I: Sexual Deviation. Oxford University Press, New York. 1979.

Ross MW, Stalstrom OW: Exorcism as psychiatric treatment: a homosexual case study. Arch Sex Behav. 8:379–383, 1979.

Serber M: Shame aversion therapy with and without heterosexual training. In: Advances in Behaviour Therapy. Academic Press, New York. pp. 115–119, 1972.

Stevenson I, Wolpe J: Recovery from sexual deviations through overcoming nonsexual neurotic responses. Am J Psychiat. 116:737–742, 1960.

Stravynski A, Shahar A: The treatment of social dysfunction in volunteer and nonpsychotic clinical populations: outcomes and related issues. Submitted for publication. 1980.

Tanner BA: A comparison of automated aversion conditioning in a waiting list control in the modification of homosexual behavior in males. Behav Ther. 5:29–32, 1974.

Ward NG: Successful lithium treatment of transvestism associated with manic-depression. J Nerv Ment Dis. 161:204–206, 1975.

12 | Psychosexual Dysfunctions

HELEN SINGER KAPLAN and
JAMES LAWRENCE MOODIE

Progress in the understanding and treatment of sexual disorders, though erratic, has been made throughout this century. Work in this area has been impeded mainly by a socially restrictive moral climate that associated reproductive functions with immorality. Nonetheless, major contributions were made by Freud, Kinsey, Masters and Johnson, and others, and current concepts of the physiology of sexual response, sexual pathology, and methods of treatment of sexual disorders have finally caught up with the rest of psychiatry and medicine.

Freud described the powerful natural urge within human beings to reproduce themselves, which in the context of repressive social attitudes becomes convoluted in its manifestations, but which nonetheless constitutes a compelling force that consciously and unconsciously influences many aspects of our lives. He discovered childhood sexuality and called our attention to infantile desires and the taboos that shape our adult sexual natures (Freud, 1953). As everyone knows, these ideas were controversial and further evidence was needed before the medical community and the public at large would begin to look rationally into sexual health and pathology.

Kinsey's survey helped to add empirical evidence that many common taboos had no scientific validity. He confirmed that men and women of all ages have sexual feelings and that masturbation and other frowned upon sexual practices were not only secretly common but seemed to produce no harmful effects (Kinsey, 1948; Kinsey, 1953).

The next breakthrough was Masters and Johnson's bold and impressively detailed scientific study of sexuality which described the physiology of male and female sexual excitement and orgasm. Their work also demonstrated that sexual dysfunctions, such as impotence or anorgasmia, were not invariably the product of serious psychopathology, but could often be traced to minor anxiety states which might be cured with relatively brief treatment methods—the now familiar sexual tasks and conjoint counseling of sex therapy. The goals of the Masters and Johnson approach were to educate, improve communication between sexual partners, and interrupt the milder forms of sexual anxiety (Masters and Johnson, 1970).

Since then, concepts of sexual physiology and psychopathology have been refined, sex therapy has become accepted in a much wider sense, and the methods have been modified and extended by clinicians of various disciplines. In 1974 Kaplan attempted to integrate various concepts of sexual disorders derived from physiology, psychoanalytic theory, "systems" formulation, and behavior therapy in modifying some sex therapy strategies. The psychosomatic sexual dysfunctions are ultimately the product of physiological concomitants of anxiety or defenses against anxiety. The object of treatment is to diminish the sexually related anxiety, thereby restoring genital functioning. This approach employs an amalgam of behavioral and psychodynamic techniques.

Kaplan described the sources of sexually disruptive anxiety in terms of multiple levels of causality. Examples of immediate causes are fear of failure, i.e. performance anxiety; inadequate stimulation; "spectatoring," i.e. obsessive self-observation; and poor communication. These immediate causes often are consciously perceived and readily reversed by brief sex therapy techniques.

In other patients, however, the sexual symptoms may be the product of a deeper or unconscious sexual conflict, as postulated by psychoanalytic theory and also by systems theory. These include serious intrapsychic conflicts and relationship difficulties. Some of these patients may also respond to brief treatment methods that integrate structured sexual interactions and psychotherapy if they are modified to give more emphasis to insight. A certain degree of insight into unconscious underlying conflict may be necessary to produce and maintain reversal of the immediate cause. This is often true when a person is troubled by conflict over competition, success, intimacy, or pleasure, which may derive from very early conflicts. Thus, traditional psychoanalytic concepts need not clash with behavioral strategies but can be used in an integrated manner to identify and address the multiple sources of anxiety that may result in sexual pathology.

Much of the recent success of sex therapy has come from distinguishing separate phases of the sexual response. In particular, separating the excitement phase (or vasocongestive phase leading to erection in men and lubrication and swelling in women) from the orgasm phase of males and females (or phase of genital muscle contraction) helped to explain many clinically observed differences and facilitated the development of specific treatment methods. More recently a third phase of sexual functioning, the desire phase, with its own physiology and potential disturbances, has been described. This phase, previously neglected by sex therapists, has helped to explain many of the failures seen with traditional sex therapy approaches which work best with excitement and orgasm phase disorders. Although modified techniques that focus more sharply on producing insight have been helpful with an increasing number of these problems of desire, more work needs to be done to clarify the etiology and develop effective treatments for these problems.

TREATMENT GOALS

In the treatment of sexual disorders the goals are typically quite specific, e.g. the relief of manifest symptoms such as low or inhibited sexual desire, absent or inadequate erection or lubrication, failure to achieve orgasm, lack of control over ejaculation, unconsummated marriage, or pain in either partner on intercourse. In order to reach these goals, the immediate causes or antecedents of the symptom must be modified. This typically involves the reduction of sexual anxiety, reduction of interpersonal anger and resentment, acquisition of sexual information and techniques, improvement in partner communication about sex, reduction in nonerotic obsessive thoughts, and for premature ejaculation focusing in on the level of arousal. In general, more extensive goals like personality change, resolution of deep conflict, and improvement in the couple's relationship are not pursued unless they are essential to progress toward the specific goal. Most often the simpler goals described above are attainable without personality change, intrapsychic exploration, or major changes in the marital system. Indeed, it became possible to establish symptom relief as a goal when clinical evidence began to show that most couples with sexual problems were able to obtain symptomatic relief and go on to enjoy sex without any adverse reactions.

CURRENTLY AVAILABLE TREATMENTS

The therapeutic goal in the treatment of sexual disorders is to reduce sexual anxiety and conflict to a point where sexual functioning is adequate and pleasurable. To achieve this fundamental goal it is necessary to modify the immediate antecedents of the sexual symptom. In order to accomplish this one must sometimes resolve the deeper intrapsychic and/or interactional conflicts which have given rise to the immediate causes. Currently several alternative therapeutic strategies are used to achieve these objectives.

1. *Individual insight therapy* may be helpful in reducing some of the basic intrapsychic causes of anxiety, anger, and conflict, although even when underlying conflicts are resolved, the sexual symptoms may persist. The purely verbal psychotherapies apparently often fail to modify directly the immediate and specific antecedents of sexual symptoms.

2. *Conjoint insight psychotherapy* is likely to be helpful in improving mutual understanding and communication and in reducing resentment and the kinds of anxiety that are evoked by marital conflict. Unless this approach is combined with specific structured sexual tasks that modify the immediate causes of the sexual symptom, however, it is unlikely to yield quick progress or to help resolve many of the immediate causes of sexual dysfunction like inadequate stimulation, performance anxiety, spectatoring, or a lack of awareness of arousal as in premature ejaculation. It appears that many mutually cooperative, well meaning partners do not instinctively know how to relax themselves or their partners or how to provide appropriate stimulation. Much of this must often be learned in a gradual, structured manner designed to minimize the anxiety which so frequently accompanies sexual interactions.

3. *Behavior therapy* can provide patients with specific tasks to reduce anxiety gradually, acquire new skills, and communicate assertively. It has been highly successful in some cases of sexual dysfunction associated with minor anxiety. It is less likely to be effective in cases where the roots of anxiety and anger are deeper and less consciously perceived, e.g. where issues of fear of competition, fear of success, or fear of intimacy may be involved. In addition, individual behavior therapy is not likely to deal adequately with the "systems" interactional components of many sexual problems.

4. *Sex therapy*, although practiced differently by different therapists, generally integrates the use of structured sexual tasks with psychotherapeutic exploration of resistances. This can be done by cotherapists or individual therapists, generally working in conjoint sessions with both members of a couple. The frequency of sessions can vary greatly. Masters and Johnson use daily sessions for two weeks; many other therapists prefer weekly sessions. A brief course of treatment is common. This

places emphasis on the efficient use of each therapeutic session, either to make progress with the structured tasks or to deal directly with resistances.

A group approach, used especially with anorgastic women and with men who have inadequate ejaculatory control, has also been effective when combined with regular structured tasks (Kaplan, 1974).

5. *Medication*. Psychoactive medication can be extremely useful in cases of dysfunction where phobic anxiety, depression, or psychotic thinking interferes with the ability of patients to make progress in therapy. In our experience, medication alone does not produce a remission of sexual avoidance or dysfunction, but rather reduces anxiety or disturbed thinking to a point where treatment can be effective. On the other hand, antidepressant medication, when it effectively reduces an underlying depression, may increase libido in the inhibited, sexually dysfunctioning patient without specific sexual therapy. In evaluating a patient for a sexual dysfunction, it should always be kept in mind that some cases simply will not progress at all or may be aggravated by sexual tasks attempted in the presence of an underlying psychiatric disorder unless the patient is effectively treated for that disorder.

CRITERIA FOR SEX THERAPY

Before beginning sex therapy, the clinician should determine whether the problem is potentially amenable to sex therapy. Some conditions should be excluded from sex therapy because they either do not warrant it or will not respond to this approach. Other conditions may be partially helped by sex therapy but are more appropriate for other forms of treatment. The evaluation should screen out patients whose sexual complaints are not true dysfunctions, sexual phobias, or psychogenic dyspareunias, those whose problems have an organic basis, and those cases of sexual difficulties that are secondary to major psychopathologic states or severe marital discord.

Conditions to be excluded are:

1. Normal persons who mistakenly seek sex therapy from ignorance or misunderstanding of sexual functions. These individuals generally need only reassurance and possibly sources of further information.

2. Obsessions. Many patients become obsessed with their sexual

functioning or the sexual response of their partners and erroneously believe they or their partners have a sexual disorder. These patients defend against other forms of anxiety by dwelling on their obsessions. They need to be reassured about their sexuality and referred for individual treatment for specific obsessive disorders (Salzman, 1968).

3. Gender disorders, including transsexualism, in general, do not respond to sex therapy. Such patients should be referred for further evaluation and treatment before consideration of approaches like hormonal or irreversible surgical sex reassignment.

4. Paraphilias and homosexuality. Paraphilias and some cases of homosexuality may be regarded as special instances of inhibition of desire in the heterosexual situation. Traditionally, it has been held that such patients, if indeed they desire a change, suffer from deep and profound conflict which requires lengthy insight therapy. Recent evidence suggests that some of these patients have developed their variant sexual response pattern on the basis of relatively minor anxieties that are amenable to brief, specific treatment procedures.

Conditions warranting specialized evaluation and treatment before sex therapy is considered or concurrent with it are:

1. Sexual dysfunctions associated with organic factors, e.g. impotence from diabetes, antihypertensive medication, or pelvic atherosclerosis; or low sex desire from testosterone deficiencies, hepatic disease, or renal disease.

2. Conditions secondary to major psychopathology; severe depression, severe anxiety, phobic states, and psychosis may be the primary cause of sexual disorders and will require specific treatment.

3. Sexual problems related to substance abuse, such as alcoholism or opiate dependence, will not respond unless the primary conditions are resolved.

4. Sexual problems consequent to severe marital problems requiring marital therapy before sex therapy.

5. Sexual problems secondary to severe stress of a nonsexual nature, e.g. job loss, separation, which must be resolved first.

SEX THERAPY TREATMENT—THE GENERAL APPROACH

Although the different sexual disorders respond to specific techniques, there is a general approach that applies to virtually all cases (Kaplan,

1979). Its essential characteristics are: (1) to focus on a sexual symptom, e.g. anorgasmia, impotence, premature ejaculation, etc.; and (2) to integrate behavioral and psychotherapeutic methods.

THE SESSIONS

In each sex therapy session the therapist follows a strategy somewhat analogous to that of crisis intervention and views the couple's interaction around the problem or assigned task as a "crisis." The therapist then attempts to balance support and confrontation to facilitate progress. Each session typically includes:

1. a review of the results of the last assigned task,
2. support and encouragement for behavioral and emotional progress,
3. careful confrontation of resistances to progress,
4. interpretation of possible unconscious intrapsychic or interactional conflicts causing resistances,
5. a new or modified assignment.

THE THERAPEUTIC TASKS

The tasks used by Masters and Johnson are similar for all the dysfunctions. Recent modifications (Kaplan, 1974; Kaplan, 1979) of sex therapy have retained some of these highly effective maneuvers, but have introduced additional interactions which are specifically tailored to each couple and to the particular syndrome. The goal is to select a task which will not create so much anxiety that it is avoided but which will advance progressively toward relief of the sexual symptom. The focus of the tasks is to modify the immediate antecedents of the anxiety or conflict that has inhibited normal sexual response in the past. In each individual these immediate antecedents are quite specific and must be identified by the therapist.

In the case of premature ejaculation, for instance, we hypothesize that the immediate cause is the man's failure to perceive the erotic sensations of the late excitement stage. This high level of excitement seems to evoke anxiety which is defended against by suppression, repression, or distraction. As the man loses touch with his arousal level he is unable to learn or effect ejaculatory control. The immediate cause is this perceptual failure. However, there may be numerous remote causes responsible for the anxiety he feels at high pleasure levels. Some men may have trained themselves to ejaculate quickly under pressured conditions, others may have performance anxiety, others may have guilt over pleasure, still others may harbor anger toward their partners. Although the remote causes are varied, the treatment tasks are chosen to reverse the immediate cause by teaching the man to maintain awareness of his sensations at high levels of sexual excitement just as a child needs to learn to recognize a full bladder to control urination. Treatment typically bypasses the more remote, "deeper" etiologies if, in fact, they exist in a particular case, unless resistance is significant and these issues must be addressed.

The following pages describe the specific tasks currently used by Kaplan and colleagues for each of the sexual disorders. Although most patients proceed through these steps, individual variation demands that the pace and ingredients of each stage of therapy be tailored to the needs of each patient.

PREMATURE EJACULATION (302.75)

ESSENTIAL FEATURES

Ejaculation occurs before the individual wishes it, because of recurrent and persistent absence of reasonably voluntary control of ejaculation and orgasm during sexual activity. The judgment of "reasonable control" is made by the clinician's taking into account factors that affect duration of the excitement phase, such as age, novelty of the sexual partner, and the frequency and duration of coitus.

TREATMENT

The aim of the treatment of premature ejaculation is to facilitate learning voluntary control over ejaculation by fostering the patient's awareness of, and increasing his tolerance for, the pleasurable genital sensations that accompany the intense sexual excitement which precedes orgasm.

Any method that encourages the man's concentration on preorgastic erotic sensations, including the "squeeze" and the "stop-start" methods, can be used to implement this goal. Our group use the following variation of the stop-start method:

The patient is advised to concentrate on his erotic sensations only and not to attempt to "hold back."

1. The partner stimulates the patient's penis manually, until he feels that he is near climax. He then asks her to stop. A few seconds later, when he feels the acute sensations diminish, he asks her to start again. He climaxes on the fourth period of stimulation.

2. The stop-start stimulation of the penis manually by the partner is repeated, this time using a lubricant, petroleum jelly. This simulates the sensations produced by the vaginal environment.

3. Stop-start stimulation is conducted intravaginally, in the female superior position. The woman straddles her partner with his erect penis inside her vagina. His hands are on her hips to guide her motion. She moves up and down until he feels he is near climax and motions her to stop. Then he signals her to start again. He climaxes on the third period of stimulation. At first he does not thrust during this exercise. After he attains control he proceeds to thrusting.

4. Stop-start intravaginally is conducted in the side-to-side position.

5. Stop-start intravaginally in the male superior position.

6. Stop-slow intravaginally. After the patient has learned control by stopping at a high plateau of excitement, if necessary he can improve his control by slowing rather than coming to a complete stop at high excitement levels. This "stop slow" sign may be employed when the man is having difficulty integrating his new ejaculatory control into his behavior.

ORGASM INHIBITION IN FEMALES AND MALES
(302.73, 302.74)

Essential Features

DSM-III defines *inhibited female orgasm* as: recurrent and persistent inhibition of the female orgasm as manifested by a delay in or absence of orgasm following a normal sexual excitement phase during sexual activity that is judged by the clinician to be adequate in focus, intensity, and duration.

Inhibited male orgasm is defined as: recurrent and persistent inhibition of the male orgasm as manifested by a delay in or absence of ejaculation following an adequate phase of sexual excitement.

TREATMENT

The aim in treating orgasm inhibition is to modify the patient's tendency to obsessively observe his/her preorgasmic sensations and to foster abandonment to erotic feelings, which is a necessary condition of orgastic release. These aims can be implemented by structuring the situation so that the patient receives effective penile or clitoral stimulation under the most tranquil conditions that can be arranged. At the same time, he/she is distracted from the obsessive self-observations. The usual means of distraction is fantasy, but external distractions such as reading or observing pictures or films may also be employed to circumvent the difficulties some patients have with fantasy.

Kaplan et al. use the following method unless the evaluation reveals reasons to modify the treatment plan.

TOTAL ANORGASMIA—FEMALES AND MALES

If the patient is totally anorgastic, the initial aim of treatment is to have the patient experience an orgasm while he or she is alone, as follows.

1. Self-stimulation of the penis or clitoris—this is first done manually. If manual stimulation is not sufficient to overcome the resistance to orgasm, the intensity of the stimulus is increased. Towards this end males employ a lubricant and females a vibrator.

2. Concomitant distraction by imagery. This may entail concentration on the person's favorite erotic fantasy, on reading erotic literature or viewing erotic pictures, or on a neutral, nonerotic image. The mental imagery occurs while the patient is stimulating himself or herself.

Anorgasmia with a Partner—Females and Males

After a patient can reach orgasm when alone, the next step is to learn to have an orgasm in the partner's presence. Since shared sex is usually far more anxiety provoking than solitary sexual activity, orgasm alone usually precedes shared orgasm unless there is profound resistance to masturbation.

The steps to shared orgasm are:

1. Self-stimulation to orgasm in the partner's presence. This should occur with a gradual increase in intimacy. First the partner turns away while the patient masturbates. Then the partner can hold the patient while he or she masturbates. The partner can masturbate to orgasm after the other has climaxed, but the patient should not attempt to reach orgasm during intercourse at this stage of the treatment.

2. Manual genital stimulation by the partner to orgasm, while the patient uses fantasy for distraction. (This is preceded by sensate focus I and II as needed. See p. 378)

Coital Anorgasmia

Treatment for this complaint essentially consists of progressive in vivo desensitization to orgastic release during vaginal containment. The treatment procedures for males and females are slightly different at this point.

Female Coital Anorgasmia

The aim of the treatment of female coital anorgasmia is to diminish any anxieties, if they exist, that are provoked by penetration; this will lower the woman's orgastic threshold. In addition, the patient is trained to maximize the relatively low level of clitoral stimulation provided by penetration and to accustom herself to have orgasms in this manner. Most women can learn to have orgasm on coitus with concomitant clitoral

stimulation with these techniques. But only a relatively few are successful in achieving coital orgasm without "clitoral assistance."

The method we employ for the treatment of coital anorgasmia has the
following sequence:

1. Self-stimulation with pelvic thrusting. Under usual circumstances, women reach orgasm during coitus by actively thrusting
the pelvis against the partner's pubic bone and not, as during masturbatory, manual, or oral stimulation, by passive reception of stimulation. Therefore, coitally anorgastic women are first taught to
stimulate themselves to orgasm by thrusting their pelvis down against
their stationary hand. This pattern of orgastic release improves the
probability of learning to reach orgasm during coitus.
2. The bridge maneuver. This consists of concomitant clitoral stimulation and vaginal intromission. While the penis is inserted, the
woman or her partner stimulates her clitoris until she reaches orgasm. This is most comfortable in the side-to-side or rear entry po-
sitions. Intromission is delayed until the woman is highly aroused
by foreplay.
3. Progressively earlier cessation of clitoral stimulation while the
penis is inserted in order to climax without "clitoral assistance."

Many apparently normal women do not learn to climax during intercourse without clitoral assistance, at least by these methods. Such couples are counseled to adapt their love-making to the woman's pattern of
climax, without considering this as "settling for second best."

RETARDED EJACULATION

1. Orgasm is reached by manual self-stimulation of genitals in the
presence of the partner. This is done progressively nearer to the
partner's vagina, until orgasm can comfortably be achieved near the
mouth of the vagina.
2. Orgasm is achieved by manual stimulation by the partner.
3. The partner stimulates the man's penis manually to a point close
to orgasm. Then the penis is inserted into the vagina at the moment
of orgasm.
4. The procedure is repeated but the penis is inserted into the va-

gina progressively earlier until the need for manual stimulation diminishes.

5. Concomitant manual and vaginal stimulation of the penis. The female stimulates the base of her partner's penis manually as he thrusts in and out of her vagina. This maneuver supplies additional stimulation. It is sometimes used to supplement the progressive desensitization described in steps 1 through 4.

PARTIAL EJACULATORY RETARDATION

The immediate antecedents of this syndrome are similar if not identical to the immediate causes of general retardation of the entire male ejaculatory reflex, and treatment follows the same tactics: relaxation and stimulation concomitant with distraction by fantasy.

INHIBITED SEXUAL EXCITEMENT (MALE AND FEMALE) (302.72)

ESSENTIAL FEATURES

Inhibited sexual excitement is characterized by: recurrent and persistent inhibition of sexual excitement during sexual activity, manifested by: in males, partial or complete failure to attain or maintain erection until completion of the sexual act, or in females, partial or complete failure to attain or maintain the lubrication—swelling response of sexual excitement until completion of the sexual act.

Furthermore, DSM-III requires that sexual activity be adequate in focus, intensity, and duration and that the disturbance not be caused exclusively by organic factors (such as physical disorders or medication).

MALE IMPOTENCE OR ERECTILE DYSFUNCTION

The performance anxiety which is so frequently associated with impotence can be diminished in many cases by structuring the sexual interactions so that they are nondemanding and reassuring. The patient is encouraged to substitute the nonpressuring goal of pleasure for the stress-producing goal of performance, and the sexual situation is arranged so that it is highly stimulating but has a low level of demand for performance or pressure. The basic Masters and Johnson method accomplishes these goals in a substantial number of patients.

1. Sensate focus I—This consists of taking turns caressing or "pleasuring" each other's bodies without genital stimulation.
2. Sensate focus II—This consists of taking turns body pleasuring and also includes gentle, nondemanding genital stimulation which may proceed to erection but not to orgasm.
3. Brief intromission without orgasm in the female superior position. The woman inserts her partner's penis into her vagina, thrusts a few times, and gets off before her partner feels anxiety or loses erection. The man reaches orgasm by manual stimulation, which is provided by himself or by his partner, depending on which is more comfortable for him.
4. Intromission to orgasm in the female superior position.
5. Intromission to orgasm in the male superior position.

This method is highly effective in those cases where the etiology is a simple fear of failure. However, many impotent men are basically afraid of sexual success and require a more flexible treatment approach which is designed to accommodate their specific needs. The following tasks may be used to circumvent or "bypass" sexual anxiety which is not primarily related to performance fears. They are designed to reduce the pressure on the man still further, and also to provide him with the tools to deal with anxiety if it arises.

1. The use of fantasy concomitant with genital stimulation, especially during anxious moments.
2. Having the partner learn to accept clitoral stimulation as an alternative to coitus, thus relieving the pressure on the man.
3. Teaching the couple the use of self-stimulation at times of tension.

PARTIAL IMPOTENCE

It may be speculated that males who, on a psychogenic basis, cannot ejaculate with a full erection have reinforced the incomplete erections by ejaculating in that state. This reinforcement sequence may be regarded as the immediate cause of the syndrome of partial impotence. Treatment is based on the rationale of extinguishing that response, and reinforcing full erection instead.

The man or his partner stimulates his penis. He is advised not to allow himself to climax unless he is fully erect. If he feels that he is near orgasm he stops until he is fully erect. Finally, when he has a full erection, he climaxes. This is a frustrating but effective treatment procedure.

INHIBITED SEXUAL EXCITEMENT—FEMALE

The aim of treatment of this rather uncommon disorder is to reduce the anxiety which is evoked during the excitement phase, and which inhibits its expression. The original Masters and Johnson method is effective, although there are advantages in being flexible enough to accommodate the patient's individual needs.

1. Sensate focus I—Taking turns at pleasuring or caressing each other's bodies without genital stimulation.
2. Sensate focus II—Taking turns at pleasuring each other's bodies with gentle, nondemanding genital stimulation which does not proceed to orgasm.
3. Slow, teasing genital stimulation by partner. The vulva, clitoris and vaginal entrance and the nipples are caressed. This is interrupted if the woman feels near orgasm, and then continued a little later, when arousal is diminished somewhat.
4. Coitus is withheld until the woman is well lubricated. To avoid frustration and to reduce pressure on the woman, the partner is advised to have extracoital orgasms during this phase of treatment.
5. Slow, teasing, nondemanding intromission in the female superior position under her control, for the purpose of focusing on her vaginal sensations.

When the patient's anxiety does not diminish sufficiently with these desensitizing exercises, we suggest "bypass" via distracting erotic imagery during stimulation, to give her a tool for managing her anxiety.

INHIBITED SEXUAL DESIRE (302.71)

ESSENTIAL FEATURES

Inhibited sexual desire is defined in DSM-III as follows: persistent and pervasive inhibition of sexual desire. The judgment of inhibition is made by the clinician's taking into account factors that affect sexual desire such as age, sex, health, intensity and frequency of sexual desire, and the context of the individual's life.

TREATMENT

The sexual exercises used to treat this persistent and pervasive inhibition are designed to confront patients with their activity, which consists of unconscious and involuntary avoidance of sexual feelings and activities and/or their tendency to focus on negative images and thoughts and to suppress sexual feelings which may emerge despite the patients' defenses against this.

As mentioned above, desire phase disorders also seem, with some exceptions, to be associated with more severe and tenacious underlying psychopathology than is typically found with the genital dysfunctions. Consequently, psychosexual treatment of these disorders often necessitates much more extensive psychotherapeutic intervention than does the treatment of orgasm and excitement phase disorders.

The structured sexual experiences are designed to reduce sexual anxiety and to promote sexual pleasure. At the same time, they play the role of a "probe" to rapidly ferret out and foster the emergence of deeper anxieties and resistances and make these available for psychotherapeutic exploration in the sessions. The blocks against sexual desire must be clearly identified and resolved or bypassed before sexual desire can return.

In these disorders the sequence of treatment is much more variable than with premature ejaculation or secondary impotence. The therapist decides on exercises according to the specific psychodynamic needs of the couple. In order to illuminate these dynamics, however, it is often useful to begin treatment with the "classical" Masters and Johnson therapeutic sequence which is employed in the excitement phase disorders:

1. Sensate focus I
2. Sensate focus II
3. Self-stimulation—If the woman is inhibited in her desire and also anorgastic, she first learns to have an orgasm by herself. When both partners are orgastic alone they masturbate together in each other's presence.
4. Exploring fantasies—In blocked patients the exploration of fantasies is often useful, both to increase desire and to reveal psychological blocks.
5. Sharing erotic fantasies with partner.
6. Sharing erotic material with partner.
7. Slow and nondemanding intromission.
8. Focus on the emotional interaction of the couple before lovemaking.

FUNCTIONAL VAGINISMUS (306.51)

Essential Features

According to DSM-III, the diagnostic criteria are: a history of recurrent and persistent involuntary spasm of the musculature of the outer third of the vagina that interferes with coitus. Also, the disturbance must not be caused exclusively by a physical disorder.

Treatment

The treatment of vaginismus is designed to extinguish the conditioned spasm of the muscles surrounding the vagina by means of systematic desensitization. Gradual dilation of the spastic introitus is the basic approach. We use the following sequence:

1. Inspection of vaginal opening by the patient using a mirror.
2. Daily insertion of one of her fingers into her vaginal opening until comfortable. A lubricant may be used in all the dilation exercises. Also, graduated dilators may be substituted for fingers.
3. Daily insertion of two fingers into vaginal opening until comfortable.
4. Daily insertion of three fingers into vaginal opening until comfortable.
5. Insertion of one or two fingers into vaginal opening by partner.
6. Insertion of penis without thrusting under patient's control. This is usually most comfortable in the female superior position.
7. Insertion with thrusting.

When vaginismus is mild enough to permit penetration, but severe enough to make intercourse painful, gradual dilation of the vagina is also highly effective. The use of a lubricant is helpful.

DISORDERS NOT LISTED IN DSM-III

There are a few clinically significant conditions which were not described in DSM-III but which we feel must be included in an up-to-date treatment manual. These include *ejaculatory pain due to muscle spasm* and *sexual phobias*. These are discussed below.

EJACULATORY PAIN DUE TO MUSCLE SPASM

DIAGNOSTIC CRITERIA

Although not described in DSM-III, a number of men clinically report a history of a recurrent, painful sensation in the proximal end of the penis immediately after ejaculation. It seems most likely that this is a consequence of muscle spasm.

The muscle spasm which occurs immediately after ejaculation, and which is the immediate cause of this syndrome, is treated by systematic desensitization. A variety of psychological anxiety-reducing methods, such as reassurance and explanation, may be employed, as well as procedures that relax muscles by physical means.

SEXUAL PHOBIAS

Although not specifically separated in DSM-III from *panic disorder* (300.01), we have found it clinically useful and important to emphasize that a significant number of patients have a history of acute anxiety and/or panic which is evoked by sexual feelings and/or activity. The anxiety attack typically prevents excitement and orgasm from occuring and reduces desire for sexual activity overall. This may be a part of a broader syndrome of multiple phobias.

TREATMENT

The immediate cause of sexual phobias and their attendant avoidance behavior is acute anxiety and/or panic which is evoked by sexual feelings and/or activities. Sexual phobias respond to the same treatment procedures as other kinds of phobias. Specifically, when the sexual phobia is part of a phobic anxiety syndrome, treatment is with gradual exposure (Klein, 1978; Wolpe, 1958) and additionally with antidepressant drugs if panic is present and unresponsive to exposure alone. Many sexually phobic patients can be helped by these drugs, which protect them against the panic attacks they experience in the phobic situation (Zitrin et al., 1978). The residual anticipatory anxieties can then be diminished with exposure in vivo by means of gradual sexual exercises and sometimes with systematic sexual assertiveness. In those cases where no medication is required, a combination of very gradual exposure and psychotherapeutic support and confrontation with resistances is often effective. It is not possible to construct a sequence of tasks that is appropriate for all phobic patients, because the anxiety patterns are highly individual.

The successful management of unconsummated marriage rests on the accurate diagnosis of the specific immediate causes of the problem. A couple may be unable to have intercourse for a variety of reasons. These include a sexual phobia on the part of either partner, ignorance, dyspareunia, or sexual dysfunction. Treatment will, of course, vary with the specific cause.

FUNCTIONAL DYSPAREUNIA (302.76)

ESSENTIAL FEATURES

According to DSM-III, this is coitus associated with recurrent and persistent genital pain in either the male or the female, which is not caused exclusively by a physical disorder and is not due to lack of lubrication, *functional vaginismus*, or another Axis I disorder.

TREATMENT

The treatment for either males or females with apparent functional discomfort would typically include a gradual approach toward intercourse. Sensate Focus I or II would be used as exploratory exercises to elicit contributing emotional factors that may be coalescing at the point of intercourse to create a negative experience. Concurrent psychodynamic exploration usually demonstrates the factors which must be resolved to allow intercourse to be experienced pleasurably. This is similar to the approach for *inhibited sexual desire*.

TREATMENT CONTROVERSIES

Debate in the field of sex therapy is predominantly about the theoretical framework that best conceptualizes and enables practitioners to treat the various sources of anxiety which contribute to sexual symptoms. Unfortunately, many clinicians who are committed to a particular theory have difficulty acknowledging the value of utilizing the techniques of alternative theoretical approaches. Thus, the strict behaviorists reject the notion of unconscious conflicts and the orthodox psychoanalysts do not accept or utilize the directive desensitization and assertive communication techniques. However, these are false dichotomies. The behavioral and psychodynamic models merely describe human behavior at different levels. The evidence for unconscious motivation is overwhelming, but unconscious wishes and fears are learned. They have been acquired and can be extinguished according to the laws of learning theory. Sex therapy employs a rational amalgam of behavioral strategies and intrapsychic exploration. The value of this integrated approach, however, will not be fully established until systematic outcome studies, comparing it with both "pure" insight and "pure" behavioral methods, are completed.

The use of medication is also controversial. Drugs are more likely to be administered by clinicians familiar with drug therapy of phobic anxiety, depression, and schizophrenic states.

The treatment of desire disorders is relatively new, poorly understood, and the least effective of sex therapies. Thus, these problems are most likely to be overlooked or handled according to the theoretical bias of the therapist.

Some controversy still exists regarding the need for meticulous evaluation of potentially organic sexual disorders. In our view such evaluation should not be neglected. New diagnostic tools, such as the nocturnal tumescence monitor, have increased our ability to detect subtle organic etiologies, and the widespread use of these techniques has called our attention to the unsuspectedly high prevalence of organic factors, especially in the aging male population.

References

Freud S: Three Essays in the Theory of Sexuality, Vol. 7 of Standard Edition of The Complete Psychological Works of Sigmund Freud. Hogarth Press, London. 1953.

Kaplan HS: The New Sex Therapy. Brunner/Mazel, New York. 1974.

Kaplan HS: Disorders of Sexual Desire. Brunner/Mazel, New York. 1979.

Kinsey AC: Sexual Behavior in the Human Male. Saunders, Philadelphia. 1948.

Kinsey AC: Sexual Behavior in the Human Female. Saunders, Philadelphia, 1953.

Klein DF: Antidepressants, Anxiety, Panic and Phobia. In: Psychopharmacology a Generation of Progress. Lipton M, DiMascio A, and Killian KF (eds). Raven Press, New York. 1978.

Masters W, Johnson V: Human Sexual Inadequacy. Little, Brown, Boston. 1970.

Salzman L: The Obsessive Personality. Aronson, New York, 1968.

Wolpe J: Psychotherapy by Reciprocal Inhibition. Stanford University Press, Stanford, 1958.

Zitrin CM, Klein DF, Woerner MG: Behavior therapy, supportive psychotherapy, imipramine and phobias. Arch Gen Psychiat. 35:307–316, 1978.

13 | Factitious Disorders

JAMES W. JEFFERSON and
HERBERT OCHITILL

FACTITIOUS DISORDER WITH PSYCHOLOGICAL SYMPTOMS (300.16)

Factitious disorder with psychological symptoms has been known as Ganser's syndrome since it was described by Ganser in 1898. Originally, the syndrome was considered to be a hysterical twilight state with the following essential features: (1) *Vorbeigehen* (approximate answers or near misses of the correct answer), (2) clouding of consciousness, (3) somatic conversion features, and (4) hallucinations (Enoch et al., 1967a). Since then, the syndrome has been subjected to a number of reviews (Weiner and Braiman, 1955; Enoch et al., 1967a; Whitlock, 1967) and over the years case reports, frequently approximating but not duplicating the original essential features, have been added to the literature (Goldin and MacDonald, 1955).

Diagnostic Criteria

The DSM-III diagnostic criteria for *factitious disorder with psychological symptoms* are quite different from Ganser's essential features and represent a redefinition of the disorder. These criteria are:

A. Psychological symptoms are apparently under voluntary control,

B. The symptoms are not explained by another mental disorder,

C. The individual's goal appears to be that of assuming the patient role and is not otherwise explained by his environmental circumstances.

While DSM-III states that patients with this disorder have no obvious reason for assuming the patient role, other authors have maintained that the syndrome ". . . is precipitated by a situation where the patient would derive benefit from a lessening of his responsibility" (Rieger and Billings, 1978).

The difficulty in determining the nature of the syndrome was concisely stated by Whitlock (1967): "Despite Ganser's designation of the condition as hysterical, controversy over its precise nosological status has persisted over the past sixty-odd years." The syndrome has been considered a form or result of the following:

1. hysterial dissociative state
2. malingering
3. schizophrenia (and other psychoses)
4. affective disorder
5. organic brain syndrome (dementia, head trauma, alcohol excess)
6. epilepsy

DSM-III states that the syndrome is "almost always superimposed on a severe Personality Disorder" and that an individual may engage in substance abuse to create a nonorganic appearing mental disorder. Furthermore, DSM-III emphasizes that distinguishing factitious disorder from other mental disorders is quite difficult (in fact, one wonders whether it actually exists as a free-standing entity).

TREATMENT

Given the long-standing diagnostic controversy and disagreement as to nosological status, coupled with the relative rarity of the disorder (well under 100 cases reported over the last 80 years), it is not surprising that there is *no* established treatment of choice for this disorder. There have been *no* controlled studies and it is unlikely that the disorder can ever be subjected to rigorous scientific study.

Several points should be emphasized.

1. Ganser's syndrome is usually short-lived and complete recovery is the rule rather than the exception. Case reports frequently describe the "spontaneous" resolution of symptoms over the course of hours to days, usually during a period of observation in the hospital (Weiner and Brai-

man, 1955; Enoch et al., 1967a; Whitlock, 1967; Tsoi, 1973). Hospitalization can also be considered a means of removing a person from a stressful situation and, in this sense, symptom resolution would not be considered spontaneous.

Since some authors contend that the disorder is often associated with a severe external stressor, efforts should be made to identify and deal with pertinent stressors. Some patients diagnosed as having Ganser's syndrome have been involved in compensation cases; criminal proceedings; or domestic, sexual, or financial difficulties.

2. Other disorders frequently, if not always, coexist with Ganser's syndrome. DSM-III diagnostic criterion B ["the symptoms produced are not explained by another mental disorder (although they may be superimposed on one)"] may be quite difficult to apply in clinical situations. It implies that if an associated disorder is identified and treated, and this is followed by resolution of the factitious symptoms, then the diagnostic criteria for factitious disorder would not have been met. Avoiding further diagnostic quibbles, suffice it to say that any patient appearing to have *factitious disorder with psychological symptoms* should be given a comprehensive diagnostic evaluation. One patient with features of Ganser's syndrome recovered after removal of a sagittal meningioma (Sim, 1974). Another patient with Ganser's syndrome superimposed on an involutional depression recovered completely following three modified electroconvulsive treatments (Goldin and MacDonald, 1955). Although Tyndel (1956) stated that "E.C.T. has proved beneficial not only in cases where depression was a prominent feature, but also for breaking the Ganser state as such," he provided no evidence to substantiate the claim.

3. DSM-III diagnostic criteria B and C would exclude many, if not most, of the cases reported in the literature as Ganser's syndrome. Since *factitious disorder with psychological symptoms* is a creation of DSM-III, it lacks a history on which one can base therapeutic recommendations. For the time being, generalizations made from a limited number of nonsystematized, anecdotal reports of Ganser's syndrome must be the tenuous framework for treatment recommendations. They are, in summary: (1) identify and remove stressors, (2) identify and treat associated disorders, and (3) anticipate spontaneous remission.

CHRONIC FACTITIOUS DISORDER WITH
PHYSICAL SYMPTOMS (301.51)

In 1951 Asher described a series of patients who wandered from hospital to hospital telling dramatic but plausible stories suggesting illness which resulted in extensive, sometimes dangerous medical evaluations or procedures. Negative evaluation coupled with disruptive, quarrelsome behavior aroused much staff frustration and hostility and hospitalization usually terminated in premature discharge against medical advice (Asher, 1951). Although various descriptive terms such as (1) the syndrome of hospital addiction, (2) hospital hoboes, (3) peregrinating problem patients, (4) pathologic malingering, (5) hospital vagrants, (6) Ahasuerus syndrome, and (7) Kopernickiades have been applied to these people, Asher's designation, Munchausen's syndrome, has been most widely accepted (Enoch, et al., 1967b; Berney, 1973; Justus et al., 1980).

Essential Features

The corresponding DSM-III disorder is *chronic factitious disorder with physical symptoms*, the essential feature of which is the individual's plausible presentation of factitious physical symptoms to such a degree that he or she is able to obtain and sustain multiple hospitalizations.

Although the disorder is accordingly defined as a discrete disorder, the boundaries between Munchausen's syndrome, malingering, somatoform disorder, and factitious illness in the absence of the Munchausen stereotype are often quite blurred (Cramer et al., 1971; Berney, 1973; Rumans and Vosti, 1978). For example, Aduan et al. (1979) describe Munchausen's syndrome as "a bizarre variant of chronic factitious illness." A similar disclaimer is made by Justus et al. (1980): "Admittedly, the exact interrelations between Munchausen's syndrome, self-induced factitious illnesses, malingering, hysteria, and the "polysurgery syndrome" are incompletely understood, and we make no claims that they are totally clear in our minds."

Diagnostic considerations become increasingly important when treatment is considered, since the presence of underlying or associated diagnostic entities may have a major modifying influence on outcome. Most reports (using pre-DSM-III terminology) emphasize the heterogeneity of underlying psychiatric conditions which include sociopathy, hysteria, schizophrenia, organicity, and drug addiction (Spiro, 1968; Berney, 1973; Mendel, 1974; Stern, 1980). More recently, the presence of borderline personality characteristics in many of these patients has been stressed (Stone, 1977; Aduan, 1979; Nadelson, 1979; Ries, 1980).

TREATMENT

Diagnostic uncertainties, the relative rarity of the condition (Spiro's 1968 review of Munchausen's syndrome was based on 38 cases), and lack of patient cooperation have precluded any organized effort to define and evaluate treatment. There have been no controlled or otherwise standardized studies of the treatment of this disorder. In fact, patients with *chronic factitious disorder with physical symptoms* are unlikely to even engage in any type of meaningful treatment program. As Cassem (1979) aptly states: "Even though the physician assumes that the patient needs help with emotional problems and confronts the patient very gently with the diagnosis and offers help the patient usually becomes outraged, denies the allegation and signs out of the hospital." The report of a single case successfully treated with a "dynamic behavior modification program" applied over a hospitalization period of *three years* (with two-year follow-up) must be viewed as exceptional (Yassa, 1978). More typical was Ford's experience with four patients with Munchausen's syndrome (1973): (1) after three months of psychiatric hospitalization no progress was made and the patient had to be "discharged against his wishes," (2) after two months of psychiatric hospitalization, "attempts at establishing a psychotherapeutic relationship were futile," (3) patient signed out against medical advice, (4) patient refused inpatient psychiatric referral.

Somatic Therapy
Unsuccessful treatments have included hypnosis, insulin coma, electroshock, and lobotomy (summarized in Ireland et al., 1967). No role has been established for the use of psychiatric drugs in treating this condition although their use could be justified in the presence of an associated or underlying psychiatric disorder that was potentially drug responsive. One would anticipate major compliance problems with any drug

treatment program and the potential for substance abuse in at least some of these patients.

Psychotherapy

Most authors have accepted some type of psychotherapy as the most appropriate therapeutic intervention. For example, O'Reilly and Aggeler (1976) state: "By establishing a therapeutic relationship the physician can help the patient recognize the psychological basis of his illness and the genuineness of his emotional disorder. Then, the physician can motivate the patient to desire a healthy mental state instead of an attractive 'sick role'." Fras (1978) adds: "In spite of enormous difficulties and frequent lack of success, psychiatric therapy is the only definitive treatment for factitial disease. Treatment consists of patient, often very supportive, cautious psychotherapy, with emphasis on maintaining the relationship with the patient."

Such approaches make intuitive sense, yet the fact remains that *there is no established successful treatment for chronic factitious disorder with physical symptoms.* Nadelson (1979) states this position more harshly: "Despite much that has been said about the potential for help in the form of psychotherapy, it would appear that such statements represent the reparative impulses of psychiatrists, and their consequent susceptibility to participation in the patient's sadomasochism, rather than any realistic possibility."

Other Suggestions

Unfortunately, the lack of effective treatment does not mean that clinicians will not have to cope with these patients. A number of somewhat fanciful treatment suggestions have been made:

1. Tattoo the diagnosis on the patient's abdomen to alert the *next* physician.
2. Publish a blacklist, central register, or International Rogues Gallery.
3. Imprison the patient as a penalty for unremitted hospital expenses.
4. Tell the patients they have Munchausen's syndrome with the hope that this will facilitate diagnosis by the *next* physician.
5. Encourage the patient to adopt "pseudo-factitious" behavior which hopefully would satisfy psychological needs while avoiding risky and

uncomfortable medical and surgical procedures. (The patient with "factitious Münchausen's syndrome" described by Gurwith and Langston (1980) had abdominal surgical "scars" which were readily removed with soap and water.)

Confrontation

Once the diagnosis is established (or at least strongly suspected), how to convey this to the patient becomes an issue. Most authors agree that forceful direct confrontation (especially if premature) is usually met with emphatic denial and departure from the medical setting. Stone (1977) takes exception stating: "My own feeling is that if anything positive is to happen, it will only come through timely, vigorous, and repeated confrontation about the true nature of the patient's illness and about his vengeful, exploitative, antisocial attitudes."

In discussing their approach to patients with factitious fever and self-induced infection, Aduan et al. (1979) stress the value of a team approach (including primary physician, attending physician, nursing staff, social worker, and psychiatrist) which permitted confrontation of the patient only after a social/psychiatric care plan had been arranged. Although confrontation was then made in a "straightforward, nonaccusational, and nonpunitive manner," patients usually responded with anger and rage directed at some team members. Continued support by others apparently allowed therapy to occur and many of the patients responded "very well." No information, however, was provided with regard to type of therapy, quality and magnitude of response, or duration of follow-up. An effective technique for confrontation and for shifting attention from the physical to the psychological aspects of the disorder has not yet been established, although a gentle, supportive approach makes intuitive sense.

Underlying Psychiatric Diagnoses

Although *chronic factitious disorder with physical symptoms* appears to be associated with a variety of underlying diagnoses, borderline personality features may be present in many patients (Nadelson, 1979, Aduan et al., 1979). It is possible that the application of current and emerging therapeutic approachs that are useful in the treatment of *borderline personality disorder* (see Chap. 17) may be useful for this particular subgroup of patients.

Underlying Physical Illness

Even if the diagnosis is well established, the physician must confront the ever present specter that the patient may ultimately develop a genuine, nonfactitious, serious medical or surgical condition. For this reason, refusing admission or neglecting to perform an adequate evaluation is ill advised. The physician, unfortunately, must sail a course between Scylla and Charybdis and do so without an accurate map.

Staff Management

Since these patients are so refractory to treatment and so aggravating and frustrating to those involved in their care, the psychiatrist can play a major role in consulting to the staff. As Nadelson (1979) states: "Perhaps the best help comes from promoting an understanding of the dynamics of the doctor–patient interaction—specifically, the issues of aggression, counter-transference, and splitting." It is important that the psychiatrist not become a vehicle for punitively conveying staff anger to the patient. Instead, the psychiatrist might best serve as organizer and director of a coordinated team approach to most effectively deal with the situation.

CONCLUSION

Although there is no established effective treatment for *chronic factitious disorder with physical symptoms*, the following suggestions may prove useful:

1. Once the diagnosis is established, carefully assess whether underlying or associated psychiatric disorders are present, since specific treatment may be available for these.
2. Adequately evaluate the possibility of true medical or surgical problems while minimizing the cost and risk of such procedures (easier said than done).
3. Confront the patient with the diagnosis in a nonpunitive, gentle fashion, attempting to redirect the focus from physical to psychological.
4. Evolve a coordinated team approach to the patient and deal with staff counter-transference issues.

5. Attempt to gather clinical data in a consistent, standardized fashion to facilitate further investigation and understanding of this disorder.

6. Set realistic expectations for dealing with this group, while remembering that while most patients are refractory to treatment, successful interventions may be possible with the exceptional patient.

REFERENCES

Aduan RP, Fauci AS, Dale DC, et al.: Factitious fever and self-induced infection. A report of 32 cases and review of the literature. Ann Intern Med. 90:230–242, 1979.

Asher R: Munchausen's syndrome. Lancet. 1:339–341, 1951.

Berney TP: A review of simulated illness. S Afr Med J. 47:1429–1434, 1973.

Cassem EH, In: case records of the Massachusetts General Hospital, weekly clinicopathological exercises. Case 35-1979. N Engl J Med. 301:488–496, 1979.

Cramer B, Gershberg MR, Stern M: Munchausen syndrome. Its relationship to malingering, hysteria, and the physician-patient relationship. Arch Gen Psychiat. 24:573–578, 1971.

Enoch MD, Trethowan WH, Barker JC: The Ganser syndrome. In: Some Uncommon Psychiatric Syndromes. Williams & Wilkins, Baltimore. pp. 41–55, 1967a.

Enoch MD, Trethowan WH, Barker JC: The Munchausen (or hospital addiction) syndrome. In: Some Uncommon Psychiatric Syndromes. Williams and Wilkins, Baltimore. pp. 71–84, 1967.

Ford CV: The Munchausen syndrome: a report of four new cases and a review of psychodynamic considerations. Psychiat in Med. 4:31–45, 1973.

Fras I: Factitial disease: an update. Psychosomatics. 19:119–122, 1978.

Goldin S, MacDonald JE: The Ganser state. J Ment Sci. 101:267–280, 1955.

Gurwith M, Langston C: Factitious Münchausen's syndrome. N Engl J Med. 302:1483–1484, 1980.

Ireland P, Sapira JD, Templeton B: Munchausen's syndrome. Review and report of an additional case. Am J Med. 43:579–592, 1967.

Justus PG, Kreutziger SS, Kitchens CS: Probing the dynamics of Munchausen's syndrome. Ann Intern Med. 93:120–127, 1980.

Mendel JG: Munchausen's syndrome: a syndrome of drug dependence. Comp Psychiat. 15:69–72, 1974.

Nadelson T: The Munchausen syndrome. Borderline character features. Gen Hosp Psychiat. 1:11–17, 1979.

O'Reilly RA, Aggeler PM: Covert anticoagulant ingestion: study of 25 patients and review of world literature. Medicine. 55:389–399, 1976.

Rieger W, Billings CK: Ganser's syndrome associated with litigation. Comp Psychiat. 19:371–375, 1978.

Ries RK: DSM-III differential diagnosis of Munchausen's syndrome. J Nerv Ment Dis. 168:629–632, 1980.

Rumans LW, Vosti KL: Factitious and fraudulent fever. Am J Med. 65:745–755, 1978.

Sim M: Guide to Psychiatry. Churchill Livingstone, Edinburgh. pp. 486–488, 1974.

Spiro HR: Chronic factitious illness. Munchausen's syndrome. Arch Gen Psychiat. 18:569–579, 1968.

Stern TA: Munchausen's syndrome revisited. Psychosomatics. 21:329–336, 1980.

Stone MH: Factitious illness. Psychological findings and treatment recommendations. Bull Menninger Clin. 41:239–254, 1977.

Tsoi WF: The Ganser syndrome in Singapore: a report on ten cases. Brit J Psychiat. 123:567–572, 1973.

Tyndel M: Some aspects of the Ganser state. J Ment Sci. 102:324–329, 1956.

Weiner H, Braiman A: The Ganser syndrome, a review and addition of some unusual cases. Am J Psychiat. 111:767–773, 1955.

Whitlock FA: The Ganser syndrome. Brit J Psychiat. 113:19–29, 1967.

Yassa R: Munchausen's syndrome: A successfully treated case. Psychosomatics. 19:242–243, 1978.

14 | Disorders of Impulse Control

(not elsewhere classified)

ROBERT KELLNER

Under the classification "Disorders of Impulse Control Not Elsewhere Classified," DSM-III lists the following: *pathological gambling* (312.31), *kleptomania* (312.32), *pyromania* (312.33), *intermittent explosive disorder* (312.34), *isolated explosive disorder* (312.35), and *atypical impulse control disorder* (312.39). This chapter will survey and evaluate treatments that have been used for these disorders and other treatments that might be beneficial.

PATHOLOGICAL GAMBLING (312.31)

ESSENTIAL FEATURES

The essential features are a chronic and progressive failure to resist impulses to gamble and gambling behavior that compromises, disrupts, or damages personal, family, or vocational pursuits.

PSYCHOTHERAPIES

Pathological gamblers have been treated with analytically oriented psychotherapy (Bergler, 1957), aversion therapy (Barker and Miller, 1968; Seager, 1970; Goorney, 1968), family or marital therapy (Bolen and Boyd, 1968; Tepperman, 1976), paradoxical intention (Victor and Krug, 1967), and covert contingency punishment (Guidry, 1975) as well as with combinations of techniques (Aubry, 1975; Colter, 1971; Moran, 1975). In addition they have been referred to Gamblers Anonymous, an organization modeled on Alcoholics Anonymous (Gamblers Anonymous, 1964). Here, gamblers who want to break this habit are provided the support of other pathological gamblers in their effort to establish a new lifestyle. Unfortunately, only 5–8% of gamblers who join Gamblers Anonymous refrain from gambling (Fighting the Odds, 1979). Their spouses may join a similar organization—Gam-Anon—for psychological support. At present (May, 1981), there are four inpatient programs in the United States for the treatment of compulsive gamblers; three are in Veterans' Administration medical centers (Custer, 1979) and a small unit is in Baltimore, Maryland.

The programs are highly structured; the program at the VA Medical Center, Breckville, Ohio, has the same program for gamblers as for alcoholics, and they found that mixing the two groups presents few problems and has advantages. The staff is consistent, firm, and accepting. The patients who are admitted usually have severe difficulties, both psychological and social, and the early stages of treatment consist of crisis management. Later, they appear able to accept support from other patients and are visited by volunteers from Gamblers Anonymous. There are many opportunities for education about gambling. The therapists play active roles and patients have an opportunity to interact with the therapists in many situations. Reasonable limits are set and the therapists expect cooperation and self-responsibility during treatment. After the initial crises are over and the patients recognize that gambling is the crucial problem, the therapist directs the patients to take control of their lives in a more mature and satisfactory manner (Glen et al., 1975). About one-half of the patients who complete these programs refrain from gambling on a follow-up lasting for about one year (Fighting the Odds, 1979) and about one third on follow-up lasting several years (Taber, 1981).

The treatment guidelines which follow are based on the psychopathology of gamblers, predominantly as described by Custer (1979) and on published reports describing treatment of pathological gamblers, predominantly those by Custer et al. (1975), Glen et al. (1975), Custer (1979), and Taber (1979) and on the principles of management of impulse control, which are discussed elsewhere in this chapter.

In pathological gambling, there is a progressive increase in the urge to gamble. The pathological gambler is unlikely to encounter a therapist in the early stages; he seeks treatment only when he is emotionally dependent on gambling and when he is in severe emotional crisis. He has debts, often has lost his job, and his family life is a shambles. He has spent his savings, cashed insurance policies, has borrowed large amounts of money legally, later from bookies, and later still from loansharks, and has perhaps misappropriated funds. He may be in danger of divorce, imprisonment, injury, and death. He has been bailed out many times by his spouse, parents, or in-laws, and these bail-outs appear to be particularly damaging in that they resemble "wins" and do not allow the pathological gambler to assume responsibility for his own behavior. His gambling has lately increased to a frenzied pace in the belief that one huge win would repair all these problems. Under this pressure, the once skilled gambler's expertise completely breaks down and he risks further illegal loans and nonviolent crime to obtain money for gambling. He rationalizes the illegal behavior on the ground that he intends to repay what he has borrowed or taken. By this time, gambling does not provide pleasure. Finally, the world comes crashing down; he is physically and psychologically exhausted, with a feeling of hopelessness and helplessness. Depression and suicidal thoughts and attempts are common at this time (Custer, 1979).

When the patient presents for treatment, the usual principles of crisis management apply (Kellner, 1971). The severity of the crisis must be assessed, suicide risk evaluated, and a decision made as to whether hospitalization is necessary. One initial task is recognition. The patient may present with emotional symptoms, but not admit to gambling, and the history may have to be obtained from the spouse. If the patient is a veteran, he may be referred to one of the VA medical centers which has a program for pathological gamblers. Otherwise, if the patient needs hospitalization and he does not appear to be a serious risk for suicide, an alcohol treatment program appears to be more suitable than an acute psychiatric inpatient unit (Glen et al., 1975).

A few days after admission, some of the patients have headaches, diarrhea, cold sweats, and nightmares which resemble a withdrawal reaction but which actually may be symptoms of exhaustion and sleep deprivation. Patients usually respond to sleep, regular diet, vigorous exercise, supportive therapy, and reassurance.

When the acute emotional crisis has abated, patients remain distressed facing a large number of social and family problems. The future seems hopeless, the problems appear to be insurmountable, submission to hospital discipline is required, and gambling is not permitted.

If the therapist has other gamblers as patients, group psychotherapy should be included in the treatment plan because these patients appear to benefit from group therapy. If there is a local chapter of Gamblers Anonymous, a member should be asked to get in touch with the patient. At some stage, family therapy may have to be added because family members need support and should be educated about the patient's condition; and family therapy appears to be important in helping repair the damage.

The therapist must remain accepting, empathetic, and warm while dealing firmly with a number of attitudes which are likely to impede treatment. Custer (1979) describes four such consistent beliefs and attitudes: (1) lack of money is *the* problem, (2) the patient expects an instant or miraculous cure, (3) he cannot conceive of life without gambling, (4) he sees complete restitution of debts or stolen money as desirable but impossible. In addition, some will admit during therapy to idiosyncratic beliefs or rationalizations which tend to perpetuate gambling. Later, particularly when the depression begins to lift, plans for the future are often unrealistic; these may include gambling as a method of getting money to repay the debts. Since the gambler will anticipate the therapist's disapproval, he may not be willing to admit to these plans.

Once a therapeutic relationship has been established, these erroneous beliefs and attitudes must be challenged; the patient must be persuaded that they are false and harmful and are likely to lead to another disaster. The techniques in persuasion might be similar to those in rational-emotive therapy (Ellis, 1973).

Taber (1979), however, warns that in the early stages, the therapist must resist the tendencies to be overly directive and confronting. In a group, gamblers are easy to work with, being themselves direct, confrontive, and talkative. A biography written by the patient is usually approached with trepidation and later remembered with positive feelings. Taber suggests the main topics for group psychotherapy (which also appear to be appropriate for individual therapy) are the social stigma, a profound sense of personal failure, denial and resistance, alienation and distrust, magical thinking, continuing overwhelming debt, return to responsible living, vocational problems and job failure, other disorders of impulse, compulsive lying, how to deal with relapse, resentment of

Gamblers' Anonymous and violent and abusive behavior. Dealing with these topics directly seems to be more effective than probing the past for neurotic distortions.

Vocational rehabilitation may be a major need for the recovering gambler (Kramer and Mascia, 1978). Gamblers often gamble while working at jobs which permit them considerable discretion about the use of time and resources. They tend not use work as a vehicle for self-actualization (Taber, 1979). For some gamblers, suitable employment may become a time and energy consuming activity which substitutes in part for their cravings for excitement and challenge. Apart from easing their financial pressures, it provides them with a sense of gaining control over their lives (Custer, 1979).

When a gambler is on trial for offenses connected with gambling, such as misappropriation of funds, the goal should be neither incarceration nor unqualified release (Taber, 1979). Instead, with the help of an understanding judge an effective living plan should be structured and enforced by prolonged periods of probation. This should include attention to family obligations, regular employment, total abstinence of all gambling, consistent attendance at Gamblers' Anonymous (if available), restitution within reason, and periodic full accountability. Imprisonment would remove all opportunity to learn through corrective living arrangement and would make restitution unlikely; it should be used only when the gambler refuses to follow the prescribed living plan.

When the patient recognizes that his life has to be drastically changed and when he regains hope, rehabilitation can be fairly rapid. The patients are often intelligent, industrious, have a great deal of energy, competitiveness, and desire for independence.

The treatment goals are life without gambling, full restitution of debts, and a lifestyle which provides some satisfaction, challenges, and some excitement. The therapist must be available during follow-up. Temptations recur and relapses are common (Taber, 1981). A few patients can manage with Gamblers Anonymous alone; others will need treatment by a therapist. Several of the principles described in the management of disorders of impulse control (see elsewhere in this chapter) can be incorporated in the treatment plan, because it seems likely that they will contribute to the effective treatment of pathological gambling. If these treatments are unsuccessful, other treatments which have been described in the literature can be tried. When gamblers are first encountered, the prospect of rehabilitation may seem hopeless both to patient and therapist. Treatment, however, may be a gratifying experience since prognosis (at least short term) is good in a large proportion of pathological gamblers.

SOMATIC THERAPIES

There have been no studies evaluating the effectiveness of drug treatment for pathological gambling. Antianxiety drugs might be considered for treating tension associated with the disorder or for the patient who claims that such a drug helps them in refraining from the unwanted behavior.

SUMMARY

While a variety of approaches have been used to treat pathological gambling, there is no clearly established treatment of choice. Gamblers Anonymous is economical but helpful to only a small proportion of patients. Some of the inpatient programs appear to be substantially more successful. Since successes have been reported in uncontrolled studies and case reports using diverse techniques and combinations of techniques and since no controlled studies have been done, no specific recommendations can be made. Tentative guidelines for treatment have been described. These should be read in conjunction with the guidelines for the other treatments in this chapter, because it seems likely that some of the principles of psychotherapy and behavior modification are similar in diverse disorders of impulse control, particularly those which give the patient pleasure or a release from tension.

KLEPTOMANIA (312.32)

ESSENTIAL FEATURES

The essential features are recurrent failure to resist impulses to steal objects that are not for immediate use or their monetary value: The objects taken are either given away, returned surreptitiously, or kept and hidden.

THERAPIES

Small, uncontrolled studies and single case reports characterize the literature on the psychotherapy of kleptomania. Among the treatments suggested are psychoanalysis (Castelnuovo-Tedesco, 1974; Zavitzianos, 1971), aversion therapy (Kellam, 1969), breath-holding aversion conditioning (Keutzer, 1972), systematic desensitization (Marzagao, 1972), and a combination of techniques (Robertson and Meyer, 1976; Stumphauzer, 1976). There are no published studies of psychotropic drug use in the treatment of kleptomania.

SUMMARY

There are no controlled studies of any type of treatment for kleptomania. A review of open studies and case reports indicates that symptom-directed treatments seem to be as effective as the more time-consuming, nondirective therapies. Since only a small number of treated cases have been published and since there is a tendency for only successful cases to be submitted for publication, it is not possible to estimate the proportion of patients with kleptomania that have been successfully treated. Treatment should include exploration of the patient's psychopathology. Strategies for impulse control, including stress inoculation, habit reversal, and aversive conditioning (preferably in imagery) should be planned. Since kleptomania tends to have a disruptive effect on the family (or may be a reflection of family psychopathology), family therapy has some logical appeal.

An investigation should be made for coexisting psychiatric disorders, the effective treatment of which may have a modulating effect on the kleptomanic behavior. The psychotherapy of kleptomania is discussed below together with that of pyromania.

PYROMANIA (312.33)

ESSENTIAL FEATURES

The essential features are a recurrent failure to resist impulses to set fires and intense fascination with setting fires and seeing them burn. Before setting the fire, the individual experiences a buildup of tension; and once the fire is underway, he or she experiences intense pleasure or release.

PSYCHOTHERAPIES

Suggested treatments for pyromania have been based on case reports and small, uncontrolled studies. They include psychoanalytically oriented individual therapy (Kaufman et al., 1961), aversive conditioning (Denholtz, 1972), and a combination of techniques (Awad and Harrison, 1976; Lewis and Yarnell, 1951).

Since there are no controlled studies of kleptomania and pyromania, no firm treatment recommendations can be made. Those that follow are tentative guidelines, based on case histories, on techniques that have been found effective in controlling unwanted impulses such as anger (described elsewhere in this chapter), and on treatments used for certain unwanted habits (Azrin et al., 1980).

An initial phase of nondirective therapy may be helpful in establishing a trustful relationship with the patient. During this phase the therapist should be empathetic and accepting, since these qualities have been associated with good outcome in studies with client-centered therapy and in studies with delinquents (Truax and Carkuff, 1967; Truax et al., 1966; Jesness, 1975). The next step is a detailed exploration of ideas, beliefs, emotions, impulses, and images which precede, accompany, and follow the act. Strategies may have to be designed to combat several of these experiences in the various stages of the chain.

It may be helpful to ask the patient to keep a diary of thoughts, preoccupations, impulses, and behaviors, both to evaluate the progress of treatment and to monitor whether new ideas or new impulses are occurring. The contents of the diary can serve as a topic for discussion with the patient in subsequent sessions and for the modification of strategies. Some patients may have irrational and self-damaging attitudes or beliefs which enhance the unwanted activity. For example, a patient with pyromania may have the vague belief that he is revenging himself, but the target of his retribution may be unrelated to owners of the property which he burned down; a kleptomaniac may have rationalized that it is right to steal because everybody does it, yet he is desperate, and genuinely appears to want to stop stealing. These beliefs should be challenged and attempts should be made to persuade the patient that they are false and self-damaging, perhaps by using a rational-emotive therapy approach (Ellis, 1973). The patient's self-statements are recorded (Meichenbaum, 1977) and coping strategies are devised to interrupt the chain in which these self-statements are a link.

For some patients in whom tension builds up before the impulse is acted upon, systematic desensitization combined with muscular relaxation (Wolpe, 1958) can be added to the program and the patient can practice at home. Covert sensitization (Cautela, 1967) or covert aversive contingency management (Guidry, 1975) appears to be preferable (at least as the first choice) to aversive conditioning with electric shocks. There is no evidence to suggest that the latter is more effective than the former in the treatment of these conditions, and aversive conditioning in imagery is more acceptable to patients. Moreover, it can be incorporated in the patient's daily life, can be frequently practiced by the patient at home, and can be modified by the patient in ways that are most effective for him.

The patient can be advised to change certain habits which are conducive to perpetuation of the unwanted impulse. For example, a female shoplifter who wears dresses under which she can hide stolen items or a man who wears a raincoat for the same purpose is advised to wear an attire which would make concealment difficult. A patient with pyromania who buys kerosene is advised to rid himself of plastic bottles and is helped in devising strategies which stop him from buying inflammable substances.

When the patient is in the exposed situation he should practice (at least initially) thoughts and behaviors which make the unwanted behavior more difficult and which change the chain of habits. For example, the shoplifter should approach only shelves where there is an attendant or another customer and at the same time imagine that a store detective is suspecting and watching him.

The principles of stress inoculation (Meichenbaum, 1977) are likely to be helpful in treatment. The patient rehearses with the therapist's guidance various coping strategies, his new chain of thinking, selftalk, and acting, and later the patient may practice the new thinking and behavior in situations where he is exposed to the temptation.

In treating disorders of impulse control which give pleasure or lead to a relief from tension, the therapist frequently needs patience and persistence because relapses tend to be common. In the author's experience, patients with these disorders who recovered relapsed a few times before they finally abstained. It may be that the patient needs the experience of a relapse to learn to resist the impulse. When the patient relapses, the treatments have to be repeated and he can be assured that this is a stage in his progress. Subsequent attempts at treatment appear to be more successful in that they can be shorter and lead to longer periods of abstinence before the patient finally desists altogether.

SOMATIC THERAPIES

There is no established role for psychiatric drugs in the treatment of pyromania. Antianxiety drugs may be considered for the treatment of tension which often occurs with this condition or for the patient who claims that the drug helps him or her to refrain from the unwanted behavior.

SUMMARY

Available evidence is too sparse to allow firm recommendations for the treatment of pyromania. Symptom-directed treatments seems as effective as the more time-consuming nondirective techniques. Tentative strategies for the treatment of pyromania and kleptomania are described above. The number of published cases is too small to form an opinion as to what proportion of patients with pyromania will desist from setting fires after treatment.

Should there be coexisting psychiatric disorders, their management should be included in the treatment plan (Tennent et al., 1971; Macht and Macht, 1968; Monkenmoeller, 1912).

Perhaps a combination of treatments such as habit reversal or those successful in anger control (see below) can be successfully applied to pyromania and kleptomania.

INTERMITTENT EXPLOSIVE DISORDER (312.34)

ESSENTIAL FEATURES

The essential features are several discrete episodes of loss of control of aggressive impulses that result in serious assault or destruction of property. For example, with no or little provocation the individual may suddenly start to hit strangers and throw furniture. The degree of aggressivity expressed during an episode is grossly out of proportion to any precipitating psychosocial stressor.

PSYCHOTHERAPIES

While there have been no controlled studies of the psychotherapy of intermittent explosive disorder, there have been two controlled studies on the control of anger, one of which included people who acted violently when angry.

Rimm et al. (1971) conducted a controlled study of systematic desensitization in male psychology students who became either uncomfortable or inappropriately angry while driving a car. Thirty students were randomly divided into a desensitization group, a placebo group who were only questioned about their experiences with anger, and an untreated control group. After treatment, the subjects who had desensitization treatment were found to have significantly lower self-rating scores of anger and a significantly greater reduction in the GSR (galvanic skin response) than those in the control groups. This difference was maintained on follow-up tests two weeks after the last session.

The study showed that self-reported anger and GSR decreased after desensitization when the subjects were exposed to imagined scenes of stress during driving; however, it did not indicate the extent to which these findings would apply in times of real provocation. In addition, the population studied cannot be considered analogous to people who would meet the diagnostic criteria for intermittent explosive disorder.

Novaco (1975) conducted a controlled study comparing self-instruction with relaxation ("combined treatment"), self-instruction alone, relaxation training alone, and an attention-control group. The last group had five sessions with a therapist who remained nondirective. These subjects were asked to keep a diary about anger and to explore factors which precipitated or ameliorated their anger. Assignment to the treatments was random. The eight or nine volunteers in each group were selected because they reported difficulty in coping with anger which, in some, had resulted in physical assault or property destruction.

The self-instruction method was derived, in part, from Meichenbaum's cognitive behavior modification and stress inoculation (1977). Participants were asked to record anger-related self-statements on the premise that anger is fomented and maintained by self-statements that are made when provocation occurs. Sets of other self-statements were offered as examples of ways to regulate anger, and the subjects were encouraged to develop their own self-instruction. They were taught how to deal with various stages of the provocation encounter. Beliefs which tended to aggravate their anger were challenged. Self-statements, attitudes, and acts which were incompatible with anger (such as cooperation and empathy) were trained and encouraged. Outcome measures which included blood pressure, GSR, anger diary, self-ratings, and behavior ratings were used to evaluate subjects in situations designed to provoke anger.

The most consistent differences were found between the combined treatment group and the control group; such differences were significant for almost all measures. The combined treatment resulted in a striking improvement in the ability to regulate and manage anger. "Relaxation alone" was significantly less effective than the combined treatment on several measures.

In this study, the combined treatment was statistically more effective than the other two. However, since all the subjects were motivated volunteers, it is not known how effective the technique would be in treating patients with the more severe intermittent explosive disorder.

SOMATIC THERAPIES

Drugs
There is one relatively small double blind, placebo controlled study (Lion, 1979) in which chlordiazepoxide (CDP) and oxazepam were compared in

patients with histories of temper outbursts, assaultive behavior, and belligerence (several had committed criminal acts). All were anxious, irritable, and hostile and described as having moderately severe character disorders with mixed explosive, antisocial, and passive-aggressive features. The study lasted four weeks. For the first two weeks, the patients received either CDP (100 mg daily), oxazepam (120 mg daily), or placebo in divided doses. During the last two weeks these doses were doubled. Forty-five patients completed the study. Physician ratings of target symptoms showed oxazepam significantly more effective than CDP and placebo in reducing anxiety, superior to placebo in reducing irritability, and more effective than CDP in reducing indirect hostility on the Buss-Durkee scale.

The number of patients who finished the study was too small for an adequate comparison of treatment effects. Many of the patients apparently had explosive traits, but it is not clear what proportion would be classified as having intermittent explosive disorder. Moreover, the outcome was evaluated by ratings and self-ratings and not by observed changes in explosiveness. The study is summarized here because it suggests that large doses of oxazepam tend to reduce irritability and hostility and might reduce the tendency for explosiveness.

A number of studies dealing with the drug treatment of irritability, impulsiveness, and aggression have been summarized in the chapter on personality disorders (Chap. 16). It seems likely that some of these drugs (antipsychotic agents, stimulants, and lithium) may be effective in the treatment of patients with intermittent explosive disorder. Since anticonvulsants have been recommended for the treatment of this disorder, and since they are not discussed in the personality disorder chapter, pertinent studies will now be surveyed.

Several of the many *uncontrolled* studies on the effects of phenytoin (DPH) on aggression, hostility, and impulsiveness suggest that the drug is effective in behavior disorders, particularly in controlling explosive and aggressive behavior both in children and adults (Bogoch and Dreyfus, 1970; Bogoch and Dreyfus, 1975). A small number of double-blind controlled studies have compared the effectiveness of DPH with placebo or another drug in the treatment of aggressive, hostile, and violent behavior. Stephens and Shaffer (1970) compared DPH 300 mg daily with DPH 15 mg daily in 30 patients suffering from anxiety neurosis. The smaller dose was used as a control in place of an inert placebo. Both physician ratings and self-ratings showed a significantly greater reduction of irritability, temper outbursts, quarrelsomeness, and impatience with the larger doses of DPH.

Conners et al. (1971), under double-blind conditions, compared DPH 200 mg daily with methylphenidate 20 mg daily and placebo over a two-weeks period in delinquent boys. There were no differences between the effects of the two drugs which, in turn, were no more effective than placebo.

Gottschalk et al. (1973) compared DPH 300 mg daily with DPH 24 mg daily over a six-month period in 44 inmates of an institution for emotionally disturbed criminal offenders. The outcome, which was evaluated by the Gottschalk-Gleser method of speech content analysis, showed no difference between the two doses with regard to hostile attitudes or verbal hostility. Lefkowitz (1969) compared 250 mg DPH daily with placebo in young delinquent boys who showed aggressive and destructive behavior. After 2½ months, there was no difference between DPH and placebo and some important items even favored placebo. This was a well-designed study in which DPH had no favorable effect on aggression, other unwanted behaviors, or psychopathology.

Carbamazepine differs from other anticonvulsants in that it is an iminostilbene derivative with a ring structure similar to that of imipramine. It is an effective anticonvulsant both in grand mal epilepsy and partial complex seizures. Studies in which changes in mood and behavior were reported had been reviewed (Dalby, 1975). Most uncontrolled studies with epileptic patients reported a decrease in irritability, hostility, and impulsiveness and improved social adjustment. However, in a few patients, especially those with brain atrophy and dementia, irritability increased and explosiveness was aggravated. Carbamazepine improved mood and behavior in a few studies when compared with other anticonvulsants but this was not observed when the drug was compared with placebo. Carbamazepine has not been used in a controlled study in patients with intermittent explosive disorder.

In several studies, anticonvulsants were combined with other drugs in the treatment of aggression and explosiveness. In an uncontrolled study, Monroe and Wise (1965) reported that some patients with episodic behavioral changes suggestive of an altered state of awareness benefited from the combination of primidone and a phenothiazine. Itil and Rizzo (1967) treated a group of adolescents who had explosive and aggressive traits with a combination of DPH and thioridazine. The outcome was compared to that of drug treatment of another group without anticonvulsants, but the authors did not mention whether the latter study was double-blind. Use of the drug combination was associated with an improvement in psychopathology which was highly correlated with a decrease of slow activity, a reduction of epilepticlike pattern, and an increase of alpha index on the electroencephalogram (EEG).

Boelhouwer et al. (1968) compared the effects of DPH and thioridazine in young adults and adolescents who had uncontrolled impulsive or antisocial behavior. The treatment compared thioridazine 300–600 mg daily and DPH 300 mg daily, given either alone or in combination in a modified Latin-square design. The authors compared the effects of the drugs in patients who showed 14 and 6 per second positive spiking on the EEG and those without positive spiking. The group with positive spiking showed a better response to the combination of thioridazine and DPH than to either drug alone, whereas the group without positive spiking showed the best response to DPH alone. The results of the study are congruent with the previous study in that they showed a correlation between EEG findings and response to psychotropic drugs.

In addition to the treatments thus far described in this chapter and in Chapter 16, tricyclic antidepressants have been recommended for the treatment of explosive personalities in adults who were hyperkinetic in childhood (Morrison and Minkoff, 1975). Those authors suggested imipramine or amitriptyline in doses of 150–300 mg/day but the recommendations were based on the treatment of only a few cases. In an uncontrolled study, Elliott (1977) treated seven patients with belligerent behavior following acute brain damage with propranolol (daily doses of 60–320 mg) and observed a conspicuous reduction of aggressive outbursts. At present, however, there are no controlled studies of the treatment of intermittent explosive disorder with either tricyclic antidepressants or propranolol.

Psychosurgery

There are no controlled studies of psychosurgery in patients with intermittent explosive disorder. In uncontrolled studies of patients with severe and dangerous explosiveness, improvement in a substantial proportion has been reported after amygdalotomy and other stereotactic procedures (Goldstein, 1974; Bridges and Bartlett, 1977). In the absence of potentially correctable organic brain pathology, the use of psychosurgery for this disorder is controversial. Psychosurgery should be offered only when the patient's rights are fully protected (National Commission for the Protection of Human Subjects of Biomedical and Behavioral Research, 1977), when all other reasonable treatments have failed, and when the dangers and suffering from the condition outweigh the risks and consequences of the surgical procedure.

SUMMARY

A combination of techniques (Novaco, 1975) and to a lesser extent, systematic desensitization in imagery (Rimm et al., 1971) were found effective in these two studies of the control of anger. The participants were motivated volunteers and the follow-up was short. It is not known whether these methods would be effective in patients with more severe intermittent explosive disorder. However, a combination of cognitive therapy, systematic desensitization, and stress inoculation may be a useful approach in patients with this disorder.

Although drug therapy of patients with strictly diagnosed intermittent explosive disorder has not been adequately studied, a large body of literature exists dealing with the treatment of anger, hostility, impulsiveness, and aggression and of entities such as "explosive personality," "emotional dyscontrol syndrome," and "episodic behavioral disorder" (Monroe, 1970). Much of this work has been discussed in the chapter on personality disorder (Chap. 16). In addition, treatment guidelines have been outlined by Elliott (1976) and Monroe (1975) and are incorporated into the recommendations which follow.

There is no specific drug or class of drugs that is preferred for all patients with explosive behavior. The appropriate drug or drug combination must be individually determined.

Unless there are specific indications for a particular drug, the benzodiazepines, because of their relative safety, should be tried first (see also Chap. 16).

If there is a history of seizures, anticonvulsants may be the initial treatment choice for intermittent explosive disorder. While phenytoin has been most extensively studied, its merits in controlling explosive behavior have not been firmly established. Nonetheless, especially if a seizure disorder appears to coexist, it is the logical first-choice anticonvulsant. Carbamazepine can alter both mood and behavior but it is not known whether it would be more effective than other anticonvulsants in the treatment of intermittent explosive behavior.

Should anticonvulsants alone prove ineffective in controlling explosive behavior, consideration should be given to combining the anticonvulsant with either a benzodiazepine anxiolytic or an antipsychotic drug such as thioridazine. While none of these treatment approaches is firmly established, studies suggest that they may be of merit in some patients.

Use of drugs such as lithium, stimulants, and antipsychotics is discussed in the Chapter 16 on personality disorder. While their effectiveness in the treatment of intermittent explosive disorder has not been established, the results of a few studies suggest that they may be of value in some patients.

Finally, in an uncontrolled study, the beta-adrenergic receptor antagonist propranolol has shown promise for controlling belligerent behavior associated with organic mental disorders (Elliott, 1977; Biological Therapies in Psychiatry, 1981).

There is some evidence to suggest that some patients benefit more from a combination of drugs than from any single drug. Combinations should be used only if individual trials with each constituent have been ineffective. In view of difficulties in evaluating the contribution of each drug and the increased risk of side-effects, combinations should be avoided unless the benefits are clearly superior to those afforded by the individual drugs. Even if a combination appears effective, efforts should be made every few months to taper and discontinue one of the constituents to determine if continued use of the combination is necessary.

In conclusion, the most appropriate treatment for intermittent explosive disorder has not been established. Available evidence suggests that drug therapies are more likely to be effective than psychotherapies, yet this issue cannot be resolved until controlled studies become available. Psychosurgery may be of value for a few severe, otherwise refractory patients, but only when several stringent conditions are fulfilled.

ISOLATED EXPLOSIVE DISORDER (312.35)

Since this disorder is defined in DSM-III as "a single, discrete episode in which failure to resist an impulse led to a single, violent, externally directed act that had a catastrophic impact on others" and since the criteria for the disorder also include "no signs of generalized impulsivity or aggressiveness prior to the episode," it is not likely that high-risk patients could be identified. Therefore, by definition, isolated explosive disorder must be considered a disorder for which there can be no treatment.

REFERENCES

Gamblers Anonymous. G.A. Publishing, Los Angeles. 1964.

National Commission for the Protection of Human Subjects of Biomedical and Behavioral Research: Report and Recommendations. Psychosurgery. Washington, D.C. U.S. Government Printing Office. 1977.

Aubry WE: Altering the gambler's maladaptive life goals. Int J Addictions. 10:29–33, 1975.

Awad GA, Harrison SI: A female fire-setter: a case report. J Nerv Ment Dis. 163:432–437, 1976.

Azrin NH, Nunn RG, Frantz SE: Treatment of hairpulling (trichotillomania): a comparative study of habit reversal and negative practice training. J Behav Ther Exp Psychiat. 11:13–20, 1980.

Barker JC: Miller M: Aversion therapy for compulsive gambling. J Nerv Ment Dis. 146:285–302, 1968.

Bergler E: The Psychology of Gambling. Hill & Wang, New York. 1957.

Boelhouwer C, Henry CE, Glueck BC: Positive spiking. A double blind control study on its significance in behavior disorders, both diagnostically and therapeutically. Am J Psychiat. 125:65–73, 1968.

Bogoch S, Dreyfus J: The Broad Range of Use of Diphenylhydantoin. Bibliography and Review. Dreyfus Med. Foundation, New York. 1970.

Bogoch S, Dreyfus J: DPH, 1975. A Supplement to the Broad Range of Use of Diphenylhydantoin, Vol. 2. Dreyfus Med. Foundation, New York. 1975.

Bolen DW, Boyd WH: Gambling and the gambler. Arch Gen Psychiat. 18:617–630, 1968.

Bridges PK, Bartlett JR: Psychosurgery: yesterday and today. Brit J Psychiat. 131:249–260, 1977.

Castelnuovo-Tedesco P: Stealing, revenge and the Monte Cristo Complex. Int J Psychoanalysis. 55:169–181, 1974.

Cautela J: Covert sensitization. Psychol Rep. 20:454–468, 1967.

Colter SB: The use of different behavioral techniques in treating a case of compulsive gambling. Behav Ther. 2:579–581, 1971.

Conners CK, Kramer R, Rothschild GH: Treatment of young delinquent boys with diphenylhydantoin sodium and methylphenidate. Arch Gen Psychiat. 24:156–160, 1971.

Custer RL: An overview of compulsive gambling. Presented at South Oaks Hospital, Amityville, NY. 1979.

Custer RL, Glen A, Burns R: Characteristics of compulsive gambling. Presented at Second Annual Conference on Gambling, Lake Tahoe, Nev. 1975.

Dalby MA: In: Advances in Neurology, Vol. 2, Chap. 18, Penry, JK Daly, DD (eds). Raven Press, New York. 1975.

Denholtz MS: "At home" aversion treatment of compulsive fire-setting behavior: case report. In: Advances in Behavior Therapy, Rubin, RD, Henderson, JD, Ullman, LP (eds). Proceedings of the Fourth Conference of the Association for Advancement of Behavior Therapy. p. 233, 1972.

Elliott FA: The neurology of explosive rage: the dyscontrol syndrome. Practitioner. 217:50–60, 1976.

Elliott FA: Propranolol for the control of belligerent behavior following acute brain damage. Ann Neurol. 1:489–491, 1977.

Ellis A: Humanistic Psychology: the Rational-Emotive Approach. Julian Press, New York. 1973.

Gelenberg AJ (ed): Biological Therapies in Psychiatry: The long arm of propranolol: extension to organic mental disorders. 4:13–14, 1981.

Glen A, Custer RL, Burns R: The inpatient treatment of compulsive gamblers. Presented at Second Annual Conference on Gambling, Lake Tahoe, Nevada. 1975.

Goldstein M: Brain research and violent behavior. Arch Neurol. 30:1–35, 1974.

Goorney AB: Treatment of a compulsive horse race gambler by aversion therapy. Brit J. Psychiat. 114:329–333, 1968.

Gottschalk LA, Covi L, Uliana R, Bates D: Effects of diphenylhydantoin on anxiety and hostility in institutionalized prisoners. Comp Psychiat. 14:503–511, 1973.

Guidry LS: Use of a covert punishing contingency in compulsive stealing. J Behav Ther Exp Psychiat. 6:169, 1975.

Itil TM, Rizzo AE: Behavior-disturbed adolescents. Electroencephalogr Clin Neurophysiol. 23:81, 1967.

Jesness CF: Comparative effectiveness of behavior modification and transactional analysis programs for delinquents. J Consult Clin Psychol. 43:758–779, 1975.

Kaufman I, Heims LW, Reiser DE: A re-evaluation of the psychodynamics of fire setting. Am J Orthopsychiat. 31:123–137, 1961.

Kellam AMP: Shoplifting treated by aversion to a film. Behav Res Ther. 7:125–127, 1969.

Kellner R: Outlines of management of common psychiatric crises and emergencies in the community. Psychosomatics. 12:191–199, 1971.

Keutzer CS: Kleptomania: a direct approach to treatment. Brit J Med Psychol. 45:159–163, 1972.

Kramer AS, Mascia GV: Ambulatory care: another approach to rehabilitation of the compulsive gambler. Presented at the Fourth Conference on Gambling, Reno, Nevada, December 1978.

Lefkowitz MM: Effects of diphenylhydantoin in disruptive behavior: study of male delinquents. Arch Gen Psychiat. 29:643–651, 1969.

Lewis N, Yarnell H: Pathological Firesetting (Pyromania). Nerv Ment Dis Monogr, New York. Vol. 32, 1951.

Lion JR: Benzodiazepines in the treatment of aggressive patients. J Clin Psychiat. 40:71–72, 1979.

Macht, LB, Macht JE: The firesetter syndrome. Psychiatry. 31:277–288, 1968.

Marzagao LR: Systematic desensitization treatment of kleptomania. J Behav Ther Exp Psychiat. 3:327–328, 1972.

Meichenbaum D: Cognitive-Behavior Modification. An Integrative Approach. Plenum Press, New York and London. 1977.

Monkenmoeller X: Zur Psychopathologie des Brandstifters. Hans Gross Archiv fur Kriminal-Anthropologie und Kriminalistik. 48:193–312, 1912.

Monroe RR: Episodic Behavioural Disorders. Harvard University Press, Cambridge, Mass. 1970.

Monroe RR: Anticonvulsants in the treatment of aggression. J Nerv Ment Dis. 160:119–126, 1975.

Monroe RR, Wise SP: Combined phenothiazine, chlordiazepoxide and primidone therapy for uncontrolled psychotic patients. Am J Psychiat. 122:694–698, 1965.

Moran E: Pathological gambling. Brit J Psychiat, Spec. No. 9. 9:416–428, 1975.

Morrison JR, Minkoff K: Explosive personality as a sequel to the hyperkinetic child. Comp Psychiat. 16:343–347, 1975.

Novaco RW: Anger Control: The Development and Evaluation of an Experimental Treatment. Heath Publishers, Lexington, Mass. 1975.

Rimm DC, DeGroot JC, Boord P: Systematic desensitization of an anger response. Behav Res Ther. 9:273–280, 1971.

Robertson J, Meyer V: Treatment of kleptomania. A case report. Scand J Behav Ther. 5:87–92, 1976.

Sanger S, Dunne JA: Fighting the odds: How to treat the compulsive gambler. Behav Med Aug. 12–15, 1979.

Seager CP: Treatment of compulsive gamblers by electrical aversion. Brit J Psychiat. 117:545–553, 1970.

Stephens JH, Shaffer JW: A controlled study of the effects of diphenylhydantoin on anxiety, irritability and anger in neurotic outpatients. Psychopharmacologia. 17:169–181, 1970.

Stumphauzer JS: Elimination of stealing by self-reinforcement of alternative behavior and family contracting. J Behav Ther Exp Psychiat. 7:265–268, 1976.

Taber J: Personal communication. 1981.

Taber JI: The Brecksville inpatient program for pathological gamblers: current directions. Presented at the American Psychological Association, New York, September 1979.

Tennent TG, McQuaid A, Loughnane T, Hands AJ: Female arsonists. Brit J Psychiat. 119:497–502, 1971.

Tepperman JH: The Effectiveness of Short Term Group Therapy Upon the Pathological Gambler and Wife. California School of Professional Psychology, Los Angeles. 1976.

Truax CB, Carkuff RR: Toward Effective Counseling and Psychotherapy: Training and Practice. Aldine, Chicago. 1967.

Truax CB, Wargo DG, Silber LD: effects of group psychotherapy with high accurate empathy and nonpossessive warmth upon female institutionalized delinquents. J Abnormal Psychol. 71:267–274, 1966.

Victor RG, Krug CM: "Paradoxical Intention" in the treatment of compulsive gambling. Am J Psychother. 21:808–814, 1967.

Wolpe J: Psychotherapy by Reciprocal Inhibition. Stanford University Press, Stanford, CA. 1958.

Zavitzianos G: Fetishism and exhibitionism in the female and their relationship to psychopathy and kleptomania. Int J Psychoanalysis. 52:297–305, 1971.

15 | Adjustment Disorders

JOHN H. GREIST

ESSENTIAL FEATURES

The essential feature of an *adjustment disorder* is a maladaptive reaction that occurs within three months after the onset of an identifiable psychological stressor. The maladaptive nature of the reaction is indicated by either impairment of social or occupational functioning or symptoms that are in excess of a normal and expected reaction to the stressor. The disturbance is not merely one instance in a pattern of overreaction to a stressor, nor is it an exacerbation of another mental disorder. Adjustment disorders are subclassified according to the following predominant characteristics: (1) *depressed mood* (309.00), (2) *anxious mood* (309.24), (3) *mixed emotional features* (309.28), (4) *disturbance of conduct* (309.30), (5) *mixed disturbance of emotions and conduct* (309.40), (6) *work (or academic) inhibition* (309.23), (7) *withdrawal* (309.83), and (8) *atypical features* (309.90).

A DISORDER IN EVOLUTION

Adolf Meyer's concept of the individual reacting or adjusting to stressors in maladaptive ways was broadly based to include all of the psychobiological stressors individuals encounter throughout their lives. It balanced the magnitude of stressors with the strength and resilience of the individual and an awareness of the importance of long-term psychological development as well as immediate, temporal factors. Meyer's concept of psychobiological reactions, however, included not only what we now label adjustment disorders, but all other psychopathology as well (Meyer, 1948).

In DSM-II (American Psychiatric Association, 1968), adjustment disorders were called "reactions" and were subsumed under the broad heading of "transient situational disturbance." A diagnosis of adjustment reaction required an acute onset in individuals without apparent psychopathology faced with an overwhelming stressor. Symptom descriptions were not provided and if symptoms persisted after removal of the stressor, another diagnosis was to be substituted for the adjustment reaction.

It soon became apparent that clinicians were making diagnoses of adjustment reaction or transient situational disturbance based on criteria other than those specified in DSM-II. Andreasen (1980) found that stressors were often chronic, need not be overwhelming, often occurred in individuals with other psychiatric disorders, and could persist for many months or years. In her study, the 402 adolescents and adults who received a DSM-II diagnosis of "transient situational disturbance" over a four-year period represented approximately 5% of inpatients admitted to the University of Iowa Hospital.

Stressors had been present for more than one year in 59% of adolescents and 36% of adults. Symptoms persisted for at least three months in 77% of adolescents and in 47% of adults. Behavioral manifestations including acting-out were noted in three-quarters of the adolescents but in only one-quarter of adults with this diagnosis. Such behavioral manifestations included school truancy and conduct leading to suspensions or expulsion; delinquency; running away more than once; persistent lying; early sexual behavior; early drinking; theft; vandalism; academic performance lower than expected; chronic rule violation; drinking to intoxication weekly; temper outbursts; running up debts/defaulting; illegal drug use; serious arrests more than twice; and poor occupational performance. Even behavior that would presumably be more common in adults, such as the last two items on this list, was more frequently reported in adolescents.

Adults had significantly more depressive symptoms ($p < .00001$) than adolescents; 87% of adults versus 64% of adolescents reported them. All depressive symptoms, with the exception of actual suicide attempts, were more common in adults.

The most common precipitants or stressors leading to diagnoses of adjustment disorder in adolescents were school problems (60%), parental rejection (27%), alcohol/drug problems (26%), parents separated/divorced (25%), girl friend/boyfriend problems (20%), and marital problems in parents (18%). Death of a loved one ranked as the ninth most frequent precipitant among adolescents (11.5%). The most common precipitants for adults were marital problems (25%), separation or divorce (23%), a move (17%), financial problems (14%), school problems (14%), and work problems (9%). Death of a loved one (only 3%) ranked thirteenth in this list.

Family histories were largely negative for known psychiatric illness with the exception that alcoholism in fathers was overrepresented in both adolescents (22%) and adults (12%).

The predominant treatment was psychotherapy, which 50% of adolescents and 62% of adults received. Family therapy was employed with 21% of adolescents but only 1.5% of adults. Behavior therapy was used in 9% of the adolescent cases and 2% of adult cases. Minor tranquilizers were prescribed for 3% of adolescents and 15% of adults, while major tranquilizers were given to 2% of both adolescents and adults. Six and a half percent of adolescents and 9.4% of adults received antidepressants. Despite the high frequency of marital problems in the adult population (25%), only 4% received marital counseling per se. Outcome data for the various therapies were not available. No treatment was prescribed for 36% of adolescents and 23% of adults, so that, "the diagnosis appears to be used in patients when the physician feels they are likely to recover with a minimum of treatment."

Wynne (1975), who was among the first to recognize the shortcomings of the classification of adjustment reactions in DSM-II, found that the classification was used in much the same way at the University of Rochester Hospitals. And he found again that depression was a prominent symptom among the patients given this diagnosis; 86% had "noteworthy depressive symptoms" and 22% had made suicide attempts. Twenty-two percent were described as having severe depression. In parallel with the behavioral or acting-out symptoms among Iowa patients, 35% of Wynne's Rochester patients were described as angry, hostile, and destructive.

Looney and Erickson (1978) reviewed the case histories of 2078 male Navy enlisted personnel who had been hospitalized with the diagnosis of transient situational disturbance during the period 1966 to 1969. The mean age was 24.6 years with a range from 17 to 48. Outcomes included separation from service at time of index hospitalization, return to military duty, and recurrence of symptoms as indicated by rehospitalization or impaired work effectiveness. Good work effectiveness was defined as "completion of six months on active duty after hospitalization and, if separated from the service after six months, completion of current enlistment with a favorable discharge and a positive recommendation for re-enlistment." Noneffectiveness was defined as rehospitalization for a psychiatric condition, receiving an unfavorable discharge "such as unsuitability or bad conduct," or receiving a negative recommendation about reenlistment because of substandard performance. The average length of follow-up was three and one half years. No details on treatment were provided.

Individuals with a diagnosis of transient situational disturbance had better outcomes than Navy personnel assigned other psychiatric diagnoses. Thus, 90% of the men given a diagnosis of transient situational disturbance returned to military duty compared with 66% of those with neuroses, 41% of those with personality disorders, and 27% of those with psychoses. Men with a diagnosis of transient situational disturbance who did not return to military duty were generally young and less skilled in their naval occupations. Length of hospitalization was relatively short for adjustment reaction patients (15 days), while neurotics (29 days) and psychotics (65 days) were hospitalized for significantly longer periods ($p < .01$).

Posthospital outcome for the 90% of patients who returned to military duty was generally good. During the three- to four-year follow-up period, 27% were rehospitalized for psychiatric reasons, 10% received early discharge, and 4% were not recommended for reenlistment because of poor work performance. Thus, 59% of the men who returned to duty at the index hospitalization performed in an effective manner as defined by not being rehospitalized for psychiatric reasons and satisfactorily completing their military enlistment.

Readmitted patients most frequently received a diagnosis of personality disorder (47%). Neurosis, including psychophysiologic disorders, was the next most frequent classification (25%), while 21% again received a diagnosis of transient situational disturbance and 7% were diagnosed as psychotic.

Andreasen and Hoenck (in press) have conducted a five-year follow-up of 100 adjustment disorder patients (52 adolescents and 48 adults) from the earlier sample of 402 psychiatric inpatients (Andreasen, 1980). Seventy-nine percent of the adults were well at follow-up but 8% of those had had some intervening psychiatric problem. Those adults who were ill at follow-up tended to suffer from either major depression or alcoholism. Fifty seven percent of the adolescents were well at follow-up but 13% of these "well" adolescents had had an intervening psychiatric problem. Diagnoses for adolescents who had not remained well after recovery from the adjustment disorder were more heterogeneous than those for adults and included schizophrenia, schizoaffective disorder, major depression, bipolar disorder, antisocial personality, alcoholism, and drug use. The most powerful predictors of poor outcome were chronicity of adjustment disorder, number of behavioral symptoms, and number of precipitants.

This study suggests that the DSM-II diagnosis of adjustment disorder has considerable predictive validity for adults since most individuals recover after the precipitating stressor disappears. Patients with several behavioral symptoms (falling into the DSM-III category of "disturbance of conduct") are most likely to have a poor outcome. Age and chronicity appear to be important predictors of subsequent outcome, as adolescents and those with long-standing adjustment disorders have relatively poor outcomes. Interestingly, the presence of depressive symptoms at the index hospitalization was not predictive of subsequent depression.

Although adjustment disorders usually have a benign outcome, one adolescent (retrospectively diagnosed as schizophrenic) and two adults (diagnoses unspecified) committed suicide during the five-year follow-up period. This suggests the need for careful evaluation and serious consideration of treatment for each individual given this diagnosis.

In summary, these studies show that adjustment disorders have been widely diagnosed under DSM-II, that depressive symptoms usually accompany these disorders in all age groups, and that behavioral manifestations (acting-out) are common among adolescents. Although adjustment disorders are usually short-lived, many patients receive some form of psychotherapy and a few receive drugs.

TREATMENT

There have been no controlled studies of the treatment of any type of adjustment disorder. Thus, treatment recommendations are based on empirical observations and common sense. Since spontaneous improvement appears to be the rule rather than the exception, the role of specific interventions is often difficult to evaluate.

Several general principles seem important in adjustment disorders whatever their symptomatic presentation. Primary mood, anxiety, and behavioral disorders (such as bipolar disorder-depressed, major depressions, cyclothymic disorder, and dysthymic disorder; phobias with and without panic attack, obsessive-compulsive disorder, and generalized anxiety disorder; and conduct disorders, antisocial personality, isolated childhood, adolescent or adult antisocial behavior, pathological gambling, kelptomania, pyromania, and explosive disorder) should be differentiated from those occurring in response to some indentifiable stressor. This separation of primary from adjustment disorders is somewhat artificial since stressors can almost always be found if diligently sought and may or may not play a precipitating role in the initiation of "primary" disorders (Andreasen, 1980; Lloyd, 1980; Lloyd, 1980a). Nevertheless, a decision about the weight to be accorded to etiologic factors in "primary" versus "adjustment" disorders is helpful in determining the course of treatment. Primary disorders should be promptly treated with the specific approaches described in other parts of this book. Adjustment disorders usually warrant a more conservative approach, particularly with regard to medications, since they are likely to remit spontaneously as the individual's basic recuperative powers assert themselves and/or as the stressors which presumably brought on the disorder diminish.

Treatment of adjustment disorders requires that attention be paid to the patient's symptoms; circumstances of living; and failures of adjustment (developmental arrest or regression to a less mature level) that play a role in precipitating or perpetuating the stressors which led to the adjustment disorder.

Most patients receive some form of psychotherapy, often crisis-oriented. Common sense elements of the crisis model include rapid reduction of stressors to relieve symptoms; restoration of functional capacity through support, reassurance and explanations of what has happened; and rapid return of the restored individual to the same setting after stressors have been reduced.

Symptom relief can usually be gained by temporarily separating the patient from the stressors that appear to be causing them. While hospitalization accomplishes this goal, it is generally best to maintain the patient in close proximity to his usual surroundings with a clear goal of returning him to adequate functioning in that setting as quickly as possible. Symptom relief may require nothing more complicated than transient removal from the stressful circumstances (i.e. a few days away from school, spouse, children, or work), regular and wholesome meals, and adequate sleep. While this simple treatment course is not always sufficient, the important general principles of making the minimum interventions required and allowing the individual's restorative powers to assert themselves and thereby reestablish him or her at the previous or a higher functional equilibrium should be applied before using more intrusive methods.

If sleep cannot be obtained without the use of hypnotics, they should be provided for a few days. Marked anxiety that does not diminish quickly suggests the short-term use of anxiolytic drugs such as the benzodiazepines.

After patients have been separated from the stressors thought to precipitate their adjustment disorder and have returned to a healthful pattern of eating and sleeping, they should be encouraged to discuss their perceptions of the causes of the disorder and to express whatever feelings they may wish to share. Supportive psychotherapy emphasizing the role of the stressor in producing their present symptoms and the strong likelihood that they will quickly regain their capacity to function is appropriate.

As soon as a patient's immediate health and symptom state have been stabilized, attention should be directed to the precipitating stressors with the goal of reducing or eliminating them. Since the most common precipitants often involve family problems or other social interactions, family members or significant others should usually take part in therapy. School problems are the most common precipitant among adolescents so that, with the permission of the adolescent and his family, it can be an advantage to have school counselors and teachers participate.

Given a respite from the stressors and symptoms they bring on, most individuals can quickly return to their previous level of functioning. It appears that some individuals with adjustment disorders can even reach a higher level of functioning through understanding of the relationships between stressors and the stress they experience and development of coping skills to avoid or decrease stressors and manage stress once it occurs. Some may become partially "immunized" against the stressors that have been troubling them by repeated exposure to and mastery of previously overwhelming stressors (Marks, 1981). It is appropriate to continue to see patients with an adjustment disorder for a period of a few months, and gradually decrease the frequency of visits; the therapist should also counsel family members, significant others, school counselors and teachers, etc. to ensure, as much as possible, that a new and healthier pattern of interaction has been established and can be maintained.

If the individual does not appear to be making a good recovery after four weeks of treatment as described above, further attention must be paid to whatever is maintaining the disorder. Since most patients receiving this diagnosis are outpatients (71% of adults and 58% of adolescents in the Andreasen and Hoenck study based on DSM-II diagnoses) and most complete treatment within four weeks (73% of adults and 76% of adolescents in Andreasen and Hoenck's study), it seems reasonable to expect that most patients will have made substantial gains and will have returned to their previous level of functioning within one month. Even among patients who are hospitalized, rapid recovery seems to be the pattern; 95% of adults and 69% of adolescents were discharged from the University of Iowa Hospital within four weeks.

When a patient does not recover in that period, one must reconsider whether a medical disorder or a different psychiatric disorder could be responsible for his or her symptoms. If an adjustment disorder with depressed mood does not respond to the above interventions, treatment with tricyclic or other antidepressant medications should be considered. If stressors have not subsided or seem impossible to reduce, a more complete and lasting separation from them may be necessary. It is also important to consider whether the individual has some stake (more or less conscious) in maintaining the symptoms, stressors, or relationship between them.

SUMMARY

Adjustment disorders appear to account for about 5% of all psychiatric diagnoses. They are viewed as a response to a stressor that exceeds an individual's adaptive capacity and produces symptoms which usually lead to the patient's disturbed reaction. It may be further conceptualized that anyone could develop an adjustment disorder given a stressor sufficiently in excess of their adaptive capacity. The stressor need not be a single overwhelming one, since the accumulation of seemingly small stressors may lead to the proverbial "straw that broke the camel's back."

Adjustment disorders may occur in individuals with or without apparent underlying mental disorders, may have an acute or gradual onset and, while usually shortlived, may become chronic. Major manifestations are depression, behavioral disturbance, and anxiety. Assuming that one has made a careful evaluation for the presence of underlying psychiatric or medical disorders requiring direct intervention, the treatment of adjustment disorders focuses on:

1. temporarily separating the person from the stressful environment
2. relieving symptoms through good nutrition, rest, and recreation
3. treating persistent anxiety and sleep disturbance for short periods with benzodiazepines
4. carefully assessing the individual's circumstances and lifestyle (not overemphasizing the immediate precipitant) to reduce, where possible, stressors that appear overwhelming
5. achieving early return to previous or higher level of functioning in less stressful circumstances
6. reevaluating symptoms, stressors, and possible underlying disorders in patients who have not improved within a month
7. evaluating possible secondary gains which may be involved in persistence of adjustment disorder beyond one month.

REFERENCES

American Psychiatric Association: Diagnostic and Statistical Manual of Mental Disorders, 2nd ed. (DSM-II) Washington, D.C. 1968.

Andreasen NC: Adjustment disorders in adolescents and adults. Arch Gen Psychiat. 37:1166–1170, 1980.

Andreasen NC, Hoenck PR: The predictive value of adjustment disorders: a follow-up study. In Press.

Lloyd C: Life events and depressive disorder reviewed. I. Events as predisposing factors. Arch Gen Psychiat. 37:529–535, 1980.

Lloyd C: Life events and depressive disorder reviewed. II. Events as precipitating factors. Arch Gen Psychiat. 37:541–548, 1980a.

Looney JG, Erickson EKE: Transient situational disturbances: course and outcome. Am J Psychiat. 135:660–663, 1978.

Marks I: Cure and Care of Neuroses. Wiley-Interscience, New York. 1981.

Meyer A: Collected Papers of Adolf Meyer, 4 Vols. Johns Hopkins Press, Baltimore. 1948.

Wynne LC: Adjustment reaction of adult life. In: Comprehensive Textbook of Psychiatry, 2nd ed, Freedman, AM, Kaplan, HI and Sadock, BJ (eds). Williams and Wilkins, Baltimore. pp. 1609–1618, 1975.

16 | Personality Disorders

ROBERT KELLNER

Personality disorders (coded on Axis II in DSM-III) are described as personality traits that are inflexible and maladaptive and cause either significant impairment in social or occupational functioning or subjective distress. These disorders refer to long-term, enduring patterns of functioning as opposed to discrete, time-limited periods of illness.

Although 12 personality disorders are classified in DSM-III (paranoid, schizoid, schizotypal, histrionic, narcissistic, antisocial, borderline, avoidant, dependent, compulsive, passive-aggressive, and atypical, mixed or other), a separate discussion of the treatment of each disorder is not practical. Some have not been defined clearly enough in pre-DSM-III nosology to provide adequate evidence about treatment outcome. Others which do have pre-DSM-III equivalents have not been studied with sufficient consistency to justify inclusion. Since many of the DSM-III personality disorders are not discussed in this chapter, a listing of essential features for each disorder has been omitted.

The chapter is divided into two sections: psychotherapies and somatic therapies. Treatment approaches are given within each section for disorders where there is sufficient knowledge to warrant inclusion.

PSYCHOTHERAPIES

Psychotherapy of personality disorders is considerably more difficult than that of many other conditions. These disorders have been present for a large part of a person's life and, regardless of etiology, are likely to be more resistant to change than are disorders of shorter duration. The efficacy of psychotherapy in the treatment of personality disorders has not been extensively evaluated and, at present, there are only a few controlled studies which indicate that one treatment is more effective than another.

429

It is unlikely that psychotherapy will be equally effective in different disorders or even in different individuals in the same diagnostic category. Characteristic traits may differ markedly from one disorder to the next and sometimes the most prominent trait in one disorder may be virtually absent in another. For example, a patient with antisocial personality disorder is likely to be impulsive and seek pleasure with little consideration of the consequences. Conversely, a patient with a compulsive disorder will prize work and productivity to the exclusion of pleasure; when pleasure is considered, it is something to be planned and worked for. A patient with an antisocial personality may, for various reasons, make decisions on the spur of the moment. His pursuit of pleasure may have an overriding insistence or his impulsively chosen course may appear flawless to him at the time. The compulsive individual, on the other hand, will avoid or postpone decisions because of his inordinate fear of making a mistake.

Some of the evidence supporting the use of different psychotherapeutic strategies for people with differing personality features is summarized in this chapter. For example, a person who suffers because of his conflicts with society because of poor impulse control or his inability to consider the future will be taught techniques of self control and postponement of gratification. In contrast, a person with overcontrolled and rigid behavior is aided in abandoning a distressing preoccupation with the future and encouraged to find some pleasure in pursuits which may not serve a purpose.

Because of the paucity of adequate research and differences in the orientation of psychotherapists, it is inappropriate to recommend psychotherapeutic strategies for most personality disorders; such recommendations would depend on this reviewer's interpretation of scant evidence. An exception is the treatment of antisocial personality about which a great deal of research has been published (studies dealing with the treatment of anger are discussed in Chap. 14—Disorders of Impulse Control).

ANTISOCIAL PERSONALITY DISORDER (301.70)

Most of the many studies dealing with the psychotherapy of patients with antisocial personalities have been uncontrolled series or case reports. The controlled studies, primarily of antisocial offenders or criminals, predate DSM-III and an undetermined number of subjects probably would not meet DSM-III criteria for antisocial personality disorder.

There are several surveys which include controlled studies of psychotherapy with delinquents and antisocial personalities (Akman et al., 1968; Mullen and Dumpson, 1972; Smith and Berlin, 1974; Goldstein and Stein, 1976; Suedfeld and Landon, 1978). The studies summarized below were chosen either because they were controlled or had features which may influence the choice of treatment. The recommendations for treatment at the end of the section are based on these studies. Throughout the chapter, "significant" is used as a statistical term and means results which were at or below the conventional probability of less than 5% chance occurrence.

The Cambridge-Somerville Youth Study is a well-known, outstanding experiment in the prevention of juvenile delinquency (Powers and Witmer, 1951). Six hundred fifty boys judged to be underprivileged and likely to become delinquent were divided into a treatment and control group. The counselors' method of choice for the treatment group emphasized "friendship" but many boys had formal psychotherapeutic interviews in accord with the principles of psychiatric social casework. There were some differences in outcome but the work of the counselors was, on the whole, no more effective than the usual forces in the community that prevented boys from committing delinquent acts.

Although the investigation revealed that the counseling program had not prevented juvenile delinquency, a follow-up study showed that some of the boys *may* have benefited from treatment. McCord and McCord (1959) found that while as many treated boys as controls had been convicted of crimes, boys who had intensive counselor contact at a younger age were somewhat less likely to commit crimes.

In an uncontrolled study of 650 prisoners at the California Medical Facility (most of whom were recidivists), Showstack (1956) evaluated the effectiveness of dynamically oriented permissive group psychotherapy. The aim of therapy was to resolve conflicts, to change attitudes, and to redirect energies. Parole revocation rates were compared with those from other institutions and there was a trend for the treated prisoners to violate parole less frequently.

These findings are difficult to evaluate. When comparing the outcome of treatment in two different institutions, biases such as deliberate or unintentional placement of certain offenders in one of the institutions may intrude. After excluding sex offenders (who were overrepresented in the treatment program), the differences between recidivism rates were small. It appears that prisoners exposed to group psychotherapy in the Medical Facility had a better outcome than those in an ordinary prison where there was no group psychotherapy, but the extent to which this was the effect of group therapy is not certain.

Grant and Grant (1959) and Grant (1963) evaluated different kinds of supervision for marines and sailors confined after court martial for various offenses. Three hundred and thirty-five offenders underwent group therapy and group living in closed groups for six to nine weeks. The criterion of adjustment was return to active service for six months without further offense. There was no untreated control group. Offenders were rated on an interpersonal maturity scale and supervisors were rated with regard to personality and behavior. While flexible and mature supervisors had the best results with relatively *mature* offenders, a rigid disciplinary approach by other supervisors apparently reduced the reconviction rate of *immature* offenders. This was the first study to show that the interaction between the personality of the offender and the characteristics of the supervisor substantially influenced treatment outcome.

Adams (1961) conducted a large, well designed counseling experiment with older juvenile offenders. Two-hundred prisoners described as bright, insightful, verbal, anxious, and with an apparent desire to change were judged to be *amenable* to counseling. Two hundred judged to be *nonamenable* lacked these qualities. Half of each group had once or twice weekly psychotherapy, mostly in groups, and the other half served as untreated controls. The best results were in the group of treated "amenables" who had significantly better outcome on most measures, including revocation of parole or reconviction, during the 33 month follow-up. Untreated "amenables" and untreated "nonamenables" performed approximately the same; therefore, having been judged to be amenable alone did not predict outcome. Treated "nonamenables" had a trend toward a worse outcome than the untreated control groups.

Shelley and Johnson (1961) examined the effect of counseling which focused on vocational and educational matters and problems of personal adjustment in felons under the age of 25. Fifty prisoners were matched with an untreated control group in another camp. Eighty hours of group and individual counseling over six months was offered and the prisoners also saw the counselors informally and briefly many times a day. The group that received counseling had significant decreases on antisocial scores of the Thematic Apperception Test (TAT) and significantly fewer returned to prison following revocation of parole. Generally, those who failed on parole had either unchanged or increased antisocial scores on the TAT. The findings suggest that counseling led to a better adjustment of the prisoners, although the authors did comment that staff attitudes may also have influenced outcome.

Weeks (1958) compared the performance of young delinquents treated in an experimental program ($n = 229$) with those in a traditional reformatory ($n = 116$). There were no locks and bars in the experimental program and the boys participated regularly in "guided group interaction sessions" (discussions in the presence of a group leader). The aim was to create an environment without punitive or aggressive measures in which the boys would feel free to discuss their behavior with adults and peers and try out new modes of more satisfactory and rewarding behavior. Although little change was noted on psychological tests, the experimental group had significantly fewer reconvictions (the difference was found largely in black boys). It is difficult to determine the role played by group psychotherapy in the treatment outcome, since the favorable results in the experimental group may also have been influenced by factors such as subject selection, staff quality and attitude, and more pleasant physical environment.

Among young male delinquents in a psychiatric hospital, Craft et al. (1964) compared the effect of an intensive group psychotherapy program in a relatively permissive residential setting ($n = 25$) with an authoritarian program ($n = 25$) in which there was moderate punishment for breaches of discipline and only brief superficial psychotherapy. Virtually all outcome criteria favored the authoritarian unit. Fourteen months after discharge, the boys from the authoritarian program had committed significantly fewer offenses after release, were rated to be in a better clinical state, and showed significantly greater improvement on several psychological tests including a significant improvement in their IQ. The authors concluded that work training alone in a friendly but disciplined residential setting is probably better than work training combined with group psychotherapy in a relatively permissive residential setting. They comment that negativism in delinquents often results from exposure to a permissive and friendly environment and, perhaps, these short-term attempts to change personality merely leave the patients in a confused and bewildered state.

Persons (1965) treated 12 sociopaths in a federal reformatory with 20 sessions of eclectic counseling while 40 sociopathic prisoners were randomly allocated to a control group. After treatment, the counseled prisoners showed a significantly greater improvement on a variety of psychological tests. Only one disciplinary report was issued to a member of the therapy group, whereas there were 38 reports to members of the control group.

In an uncontrolled study, Glasser (1965) treated institutionalized older adolescent girls with "reality therapy." This technique emphasized individual responsibility and focused on present behavior, issues of right and wrong, and the morality of behavior. Close involvement of the therapist with the patient was also emphasized. The author noted that while 90% of girls institutionalized for delinquency violate their parole and are reinstitutionalized, fewer than 12% of the treated girls returned to the institution during the three years of the treatment program.

Although the study was uncontrolled, patient selection may have been biased, and it is not certain whether the duration of follow-up was the same for both groups; the treated girls had all been recidivists and many had not been helped by previous outpatient psychotherapy. The outcome appeared to be unusually good compared to that of girls from other institutions.

In a state reformatory, Persons (1966, 1967) evaluated a combination of group and individual therapy (60 sessions over a 20-week period) in 41 delinquent adolescent boys who were matched with untreated controls. Initially, the therapists attempted to develop a warm, interpersonal relationship with their patients and teach them to behave in less self-defeating ways. Later they used interpretations, negative reinforcement of inappropriate behavior, approval of appropriate behavior, and role playing. They attempted to teach the boys to discriminate between acceptable and unacceptable behavior. The Taylor Manifest Anxiety Scale, the Delinquency Scale and several scales of the MMPI significantly favored the treated group. In addition, the treated boys received passes sooner, had fewer disciplinary reports, and their academic functioning improved significantly more than the controls. Fewer were reinstitutionalized and significantly more were employed.

Truax et al. (1966) compared 40 institutionalized delinquent adolescent girls treated with 24 sessions of time-limited, client-centered group psychotherapy with 30 untreated controls (random assignment). The two therapists who conducted the group sessions were selected on the basis of high rankings in empathy and nonpossessive warmth. At the end of treatment there were significantly greater improvements on psychological tests in the treated group, and at one-year follow-up the treated girls had spent a significantly shorter time in institutions.

Truax and Wargo (1967) examined how therapists' behavior related to results in juvenile delinquents. Outcome was evaluated by a combined score (Z score) which included time spent outside institutions during follow-up. Therapists who were rated as warm, empathetic, and genuine had significantly more success than therapists who did not possess these qualities.

In another study, adolescent antisocial boys with a history of truancy, aggression, and delinquency were contacted at a time of crisis (immediately after dropping out or being expelled from school). Ten were treated for 10 months with psychotherapy and ten were randomly assigned to a control group. The therapists focused on practical issues, including relationships with others, and helped the boys find jobs and adjust to work after they left school (Massimo and Shore, 1963; Massimo and Shore, 1967; Shore and Massimo, 1966). At two- to three-year follow-up, outcome was decidedly better in the treated group. The boys who received psychotherapy continued to improve and all but one had an above average employment record. On the other hand, three of the untreated boys were incarcerated for major crimes and four were unemployed. Most of the untreated boys showed deterioration in all areas of functioning.

Meyer et al. (1965) evaluated the outcome of casework with adolescent girls who were judged to be predelinquent. The girls were randomly assigned either to casework ($n = 139$) or to a control group ($n = 132$). Those in the latter group continued at school and had no additional treatment. Casework was carried out predominantly in homogeneous groups to make it easier to deal with girls who had similar personalities and similar problems. The duration of treatment and the number of sessions varied; over one-third had 20 or more sessions. The duration of follow-up also varied. Outcome was evaluated on several measures, including the number graduating from high school, suspensions from school, conduct, grades, and rating by staff. At the end of treatment and follow-up there were no significant differences on several outcome measures including suspensions, academic failures, and conduct grades between the treated group and the control group. This is in contrast with the study by Massimo and Shore (described above) in which intensive involvement with boys who had dropped out of school led to a markedly better outcome than in boys who were in an untreated control group.

It is not certain why there were such striking differences between these studies. It may be that because the boys in the Massimo and Shore study were contacted immediately after leaving school, when they appeared to be in a crisis, and the therapist managed to establish an unusual relationship with them and could guide them through the initial difficulties of looking for jobs and help them to adjust to work. The treatment in the Cambridge-Somerville and the Meyer studies may have been largely ineffective because of the different circumstances. The youngsters were not in a crisis when approached and were not at a particular turning point in their lives. Also, they may not have felt the same need of guidance and emotional support and may not have established the same kind of bond with the therapist. Perhaps the therapist in the Massimo and Shore study was unusually capable.

Schwitzgebel and Kolb (1964) studied delinquent adolescent boys who had spent some time in a reformatory or prison. Twenty delinquents in their experimental group were matched with another twenty who had no contact with the experimenters. The treated group was offered part-time employment and told they were participating in research. Their task was to talk into a tape recorder. The kind of topics discussed during these sessions depended on the orientation of the different therapists. Timely attendance was reinforced by rewards. After three years' follow-up, the mean number of arrests and the mean number of months incarcerated were significantly smaller in the treated boys and there was a nonsignificant trend for the number of prison sentences to be smaller. The authors attributed the favorable treatment outcome to successful shaping of behavior by rewards and to the good relationship between the delinquent and experimenter, a relationship which apparently generalized to other older and educated persons such as employers.

Sarason (1968) compared two treatment methods in a reception center for juvenile offenders. One was modeling in which acceptable behaviors in various situations (such as job interviews) were demonstrated and the second was a role playing situation in which the boys themselves chose the scripts. When compared to a control group, both treatment groups' behavior improved; modeling was apparently more effective than role playing. There was no follow-up outside the institution.

Jesness (1975) compared the effects of transactional analysis and behavior modification in a large study of institutionalized juvenile delinquents. More than 900 delinquents randomly assigned to two institutions participated in the study for periods of seven months to two years. All had fairly extensive criminal records. In the behavior modification program a contingent point system was used; each boy had to accumulate a predetermined number of behavior change units. The transactional analysis consisted of mutually agreed upon verbal contracts; the boys described how they wanted to be different and the staff agreed to work only toward socially desirable goals. Group therapy was held twice a week.

The boys from both programs showed considerable improvement in rated behavior. Though there was no difference in subsequent conviction rates between the two groups, some treatment effects were specific to each program. Those in the behavioral program achieved greater gains in observer ratings of behavior, whereas those in transactional analysis showed greater gains in attitudes on self-reports. The boys' positive regard for the staff appeared to contribute as much to outcome as the type of treatment. The outcome on parole for these two programs was significantly better than that of similar programs which did not include psychotherapy or behavior modification. However, the improvement appeared transitory in most of the boys since after two years only 23% had no further arrests.

The Community Treatment Project of the California Youth Authority is the largest experiment on the treatment of juvenile delinquents in the community (Palmer, 1971; Palmer, 1971a; Palmer, 1971b; Rubenfeld, 1967; Warren, 1969; Warren et al., 1966). Over 1000 young first-time offenders were randomly assigned either to the experimental group or to a group that was confined in prisons or other institutions. In the experimental group, parole officers counseled and helped the offenders, intervened in family disputes, and helped with school and employment difficulties. Among the various experiments, there was an attempt to match offenders with therapists who had behavior and personality characteristics suited to that particular type of delinquent. Classification of offenders was based on Sullivan's theory of interpersonal maturity (Sullivan et al., 1957).

Outcome was evaluated on many measures including reconviction rates and time spent in institutions. Several of the authors who conducted the study concluded that the offenders had been helped by treatment in the community and that matching the maturity level of the offender with a therapist with suitable personality traits made the treatment more effective.

The interpretations of these findings have been criticized by several authors. For example, Beker and Heyman (1972) asserted that the theory of interpersonal maturity had not been adequately validated and apparently does not apply to black offenders. Another criticism has been that both detection and punishment of offenses were biased so that the criteria of revocation of parole and time spent in institutions were unsuitable outcome measures. Nevertheless, the beneficial effect of matching offender and therapist has been found in another study (Jesness, 1968), and the findings of Grant and Grant (1959) suggest that matching might enhance efficacy of treatment. Treating the offenders in the community appeared to be at least as effective (and far less expensive) in preventing reconvictions as traditional punishment.

COMMENTS

There are too few adequate studies to recommend a specific psychotherapeutic technique for most of the personality disorders. The exceptions are psychotherapy of the antisocial personality disorder and psychotherapy of anger and hostile behavior, traits which occur in several of the personality disorders. The treatment of anger is described in Chapter 14 (Disorders of Impulse Control).

The studies of psychotherapy for antisocial behavior suggest that psychotherapy may be effective in some patients with antisocial personality disorder. It is not possible to make definite treatment recommendations because there are too few studies which compare specific techniques and some results appear to be in conflict. A few trends, however, do emerge from the available controlled studies. It appears that nondirective methods are, on the whole, less effective with antisocial patients than with neurotic patients. Some patients with antisocial personalities appear to respond differently to therapies which appear to be effective in neurotics (Kellner, 1967). It appears that effective treatment of antisocial personalities includes involvement by the therapist, acceptance of the patient, and the establishment of a trustful relationship. Yet, in delinquents who are immature, a rigid, disciplinarian approach appears to be more effective than a permissive, flexible therapeutic milieu in achieving adjustment during a short-term follow-up after release from an institution.

There is some evidence to suggest that matching of delinquents and therapists leads to somewhat better outcome than random assignment to therapists. Effective treatments appears to include counseling and guidance, the teaching of social skills, and the reinforcement of appropriate behavior. Coaching on practical matters such as how to cope with employment and how to differentiate between right and wrong is also effective. Most of the successful treatments were carried out either with young people or with patients who appeared to have had an incentive to cooperate with treatment.

There are no controlled studies available of adults who had antisocial personalities and who were treated as outpatients; clinical experience suggests that short-term outcome in this group is generally poor. However, the findings of the controlled studies suggest that psychotherapy is likely to be helpful for at least a few of these patients. It appears that, even in outpatients, an attempt should be made to use psychotherapy if the patient can be so persuaded. If the patient's attendance is irregular and he does not want to pursue treatment, the therapist may still try to establish a bond and remain available to resume the therapeutic relationship when the patient returns. The patient may accept guidance about the use of medication, sometimes accept counsel or advice on other matters, and may, albeit imperceptibly, benefit from the treatment and the relationship with the therapist. Long-term studies suggest that even in the absence of treatment, a substantial proportion of patients with antisocial personalities become more mature and more law abiding as they get older (Craft, 1969; Weiss, 1973).

SOMATIC THERAPIES

Drugs

The drug treatment of personality disorders is more difficult than that of other disorders for several reasons. Compared to schizophrenia and affective disorders, far less research has been carried out on the effects of drug therapy. In many studies of personality disorders, diagnostic criteria have not been adequately described and it is uncertain how diagnoses can be related to DSM-III. The ongoing difficulty of diagnosing personality disorders has only been partly alleviated with the introduction of DSM-III. The use of the new classification system has substantially increased agreement among diagnosticians because the conditions have been more clearly defined. However, agreement on a descriptive label does not necessarily mean agreement on a pathological entity. To choose a simple analogy, two observers who are using an old medical nomenclature might agree that an individual suffers from the syndrome of "colic" (colicky abdominal pain, nausea, and anorexia) which is merely a label but this does not necessarily mean that they agree on the pathological state—the diagnosis—responsible for the syndrome.

Sometimes the same underlying disorder can produce differing clinical presentations. It is common to see patients who, over time, have been diagnosed as having several types of schizophrenia, which suggests that the same pathology manifested itself as different clinical syndromes. Conversely, different psychopathologies can lead to similar syndromes. For example, the syndrome of persistent law-breaking, inability to learn from experience, and apparent disregard for group standards can stem in one person from the sociopathic traits of callousness, excessive egocentricity, and the absence of guilt; in another from impulsiveness and inadequate self control; and in still another from emotional inadequacy (which prevents coping in a competitive society, and contributes to a guilt-ridden and fearful descent into crime). The difficulty in choosing an appropriate drug treatment for conditions which have only been labeled descriptively has been decribed more fully elsewhere (Kellner and Rada, 1979).

Drug treatment of personality disorders is symptomatic. Only a few studies suggest that the label describing the condition predicts which drug treatment will be most effective. For the most part, treatment is directed at the most troublesome symptom or the most conspicuous disturbance of behavior. The choices of treatment discussed below are based on a survey of studies dealing with personality disorders and with symptoms such as hostility, irritability, and mood swings that are commonly associated with them (Kellner, 1979). The main emphasis is on double-blind, controlled drug trials; however, several open studies are reviewed, mainly where a drug was reported to be effective but few controlled studies had been published.

Hostility, Impulsiveness, and Aggression

Hostility, anger, and aggression are manifested in several personality disorders and are sometimes the most conspicuous or troublesome feature for the patient or for others. It is practical to evaluate the drug treatment of these traits together, in part because they often coexist in the same individual, and in part because they have often been evaluated together.

Antianxiety agents (minor tranquilizers). Antianxiety drugs have been compared with placebo or with each other in several studies. Most have dealt with the effect of benzodiazepines on hostility, either in neurotic patients or in normal volunteers.

There appears to be a complex interaction of the effects of minor tranquilizers on anxiety, depression, and hostility. Unexpected outbursts of rage have been reported in patients taking chlordiazepoxide and diazepam, but they are very rare in individuals who have not shown these tendencies before taking the drug. An increase in self-rated hostility was found with chlordiazepoxide in normal subjects (Gardos et al., 1968; DiMascio et al., 1969); and in depressed female outpatients, diazepam increased hostile mood but apparently did not increase impulses to be overtly aggressive (Covi et al., 1977). In neurotic outpatients, chlordiazepoxide reduced hostility and irritability and may have increased healthy assertiveness (Rickels and Downing, 1967). The effects of different benzodiazepines on hostility and anger may depend, in part, on personality factors; in one study with female volunteers in which a single dose of diazepam (10 mg) was used, "action oriented" subjects reported an increase in hostility whereas "nonaction oriented" subjects reported a decrease (McDonald, 1967).

There is no evidence, at present, that oxazepam increases hostility and there is some evidence that in neurotic patients it leads to a greater reduction in hostility than other benzodiazepines (Feldman, 1967). In clinical practice it is rare for a patient who complains of excessive hostility to get a satisfactory result with oxazepam when the older benzodiazepines have failed; nonetheless, oxazepam is a rational choice in anxious and hostile patients, particularly if the hostility appears to have been enhanced by diazepam or chlordiazepoxide.

The extent to which the findings in neurotics and normals who are hostile can be replicated in patients who have personality disorders is not certain, although a single dose of chlordiazepoxide reduced observer-rated hostility in juvenile delinquents in one study (Gleser et al., 1965). Most studies have examined changes in verbal hostility as measured by self-rating or rating scales but not changes in hostile or aggressive behavior. There is no adequate evidence from controlled studies to show that minor tranquilizers are effective in the treatment of hostility and anger in patients with personality disorders such as antisocial personality.

Studies of meprobamate (McNair et al., 1965; Lorr et al., 1961) in anxious patients, some of whom had personality disorders, showed either that the drug was no more effective than placebo in reducing hostility or that it increased hostile mood or verbal hostility. In view of these results and also because of the greater risk of toxic effects and addiction, meprobamate should not be prescribed to hostile or impulsive patients.

The results of a few controlled studies suggest that some patients who are anxious, irritable, and angry benefit from treatment with benzodiazepines; however, such studies have been conducted principally with neurotic patients. The recommendations which follow are based on these studies and on clinical impressions; they have not been adequately confirmed in controlled studies with personality disorders. Based on both overall effectiveness and safety, the benzodiazepines are the antianxiety drugs of choice in treating these disorders.

Clinical experience suggests that some patients with personality disorders need larger doses of benzodiazepines than are generally prescribed for neurotic patients, particularly if there is a history of alcoholism. This poses difficult problems because (1) there is inadequate research support for larger doses, (2) there is no research evidence that large doses have beneficial effects if given for a long time, and (3) some patients, particularly former alcoholics, may abuse benzodiazepines. Yet a patient may be severely distressed and in need of treatment; a decision has to be made as to the most beneficial and safest drug. The studies in which benzodiazepines have been used in unusually large doses in patients with severe neuroses and personality disorders have been largely uncontrolled. Solomon (1978) reviewed the literature of uncontrolled studies and reported on the treatment of a few patients who had not responded to other treatments. Kellner et al. (1979) used chlordiazepoxide in higher doses than customary in a short, double-blind study with depressed and anxious neurotics. Lion (1979) has used large doses of benzodiazepines in patients with personality disorders who were explosive and hostile (that study is summarized in Chap. 15). Patients should be observed, in part, because chlordiazepoxide and diazepam may occasionally increase hostile feelings and be associated with aggressive acts. Oxazepam apparently does not have this tendency. Patients who have been on large doses of any benzodiazepine should not stop the drug suddenly because of the risk of withdrawal symptoms. Dose reduction should be periodically attempted with the goal of discontinuing the drug or maintaining the patient on the smallest dose which gives adequate symptom relief.

Although it is rare to get a satisfactory result with oxazepam if chlordiazepoxide or diazepam has failed to reduce anger and hostility, oxazepam should be tried if the response to the previous benzodiazepine was inadequate. As with the other benzodiazepines, the highest recommended dose of oxazepam (120 mg daily) may be inadequate to control a patient's symptoms (Lion, 1979). If the recommended dosage for any benzodiazepine is exceeded, it is advisable to document the rationale for using the high dose and obtain informed consent from the patient.

Some patients with personality disorders, especially those who get relief from severe, chronic anxiety, or those who have a history of substance abuse, have a tendency to self-medicate with excessive amounts of benzodiazepines. These patients are poor candidates for long-term treatment with these drugs.

Antipsychotic agents (major tranquilizers). Several controlled studies have shown that hostility and aggression are reduced in acute and chronic schizophrenics who are treated with antipsychotic drugs. In only three controlled studies have antipsychotic drugs been used to treat patients with personality disorders. In two, the findings were inconclusive (Klein et al., 1973; Molling et al., 1962), whereas in a small study by Barnes (1977) with adolescents who had various personality disorders, mesoridazine was significantly more effective than placebo in reducing the severity of several symptoms.

There are many uncontrolled studies in which clinicians apparently have effectively treated personality disorders with neuroleptics. Some of the studies summarized in Chapter 15 (Disorders of Impulse Control) suggest that neuroleptics may be effective in some nonpsychotic patients. If at all possible, the long-term use of neuroleptics should be avoided in nonpsychotic patients because of the risk of tardive dyskinesia. For patients with personality disorders, neuroleptics should be reserved only for those who have the following characteristics: (1) need of drug treatment, (2) hostile, aggressive, or anxious behavior, (3) contraindications to the use of other drugs, such as a history of drug abuse or dependence, (4) inadequate response to treatment with other drugs, and (5) apparent benefit from a trial of neuroleptics.

If a neuroleptic is used, it is prudent to use the smallest possible effective dose and to prescribe it for short periods. There is no firm evidence favoring the use of a particular neuroleptic. Individuals vary in their response to these drugs and in the types of side effects they experience. Occasionally, explosive behavior may actually be aggravated by neuroleptic treatment. Because of a low evidence of extrapyramidal side effects and some evidence of efficacy in anxiety and nonendogenous depression, thioridazine may have some advantages and there is some evidence that mesoridazine may be effective in adolescents with personality disorders.

Stimulants. Many years ago two uncontrolled studies of adult psychopaths suggested that some of these patients benefited temporarily from amphetamines (Hill, 1947; Shovron, 1947). In two other studies (Korey, 1944; Eisenberg et al., 1963) the aggressive behavior of young male delinquents improved significantly with stimulants and the boys reported that they were feeling better. Conners et al. (1971) did not find such an effect but their two-week trial may have been too short to show measurable differences between drug and placebo.

There have been several reports that adults diagnosed in childhood as suffering from minimal brain dysfunction (MBD) have persistent psychiatric abnormalities in adult life which include personality disorders (Weiss et al., 1979; Milman, 1979). A few uncontrolled studies suggest that in some of these patients stimulants are beneficial not only in childhood but in adult life as well. Wood et al. (1976) carried out a double-blind crossover study with methylphenidate (up to 60 mg daily) and placebo, with each phase lasting two weeks. The patients' most prominent symptoms were impulsivity, irritability, inattentiveness, and emotional lability. They had been diagnosed as having a variety of nonpsychotic disorders including antisocial disorder, drug or alcohol abuse, and anxiety disorder. Four out of five self-rating scales favored methylphenidate over placebo. Self-ratings on a scale which included the extremes of happiness and sadness did not discriminate between the treatments, suggesting that the improvement was not primarily due to the euphoriant effects of the drug. During the study no patient abused methylphenidate and two women who had a prior tendency to abuse drugs stopped doing so when their irritability and anger diminished during the study. Some of the patients were also apparently treated successfully with either pemoline or a tricyclic antidepressant, both of which have been used in children with MBD.

Since adults with persisting symptoms of childhood MBD may either be misdiagnosed as having a personality disorder or have a coexisting personality disorder, accurate diagnosis is essential. With careful patient selection and proper attention to possible abuse of these drugs, a trial of stimulant drug therapy may prove beneficial. There is a need for well designed, controlled, long-term studies to determine the role of stimulants in treating hyperkinetic adults.

Lithium. Sheard (1971) treated 12 male inmates of a maximum-security state prison with lithium or placebo in a single blind study lasting three months. Lithium and placebo were given in alternating four-week periods with initial allocation to drug or placebo done in random fashion. Subjects were selected on the basis of (1) preprison history of three or more episodes of violent assaultive crime; (2) prison behavior characterized by continuing verbal and physical aggressive behavior; (3) no overt psychosis or brain damage; (4) no renal or cardiovascular diseases; (5) high scores on aggression items of MMPI and Buss rating scale for aggression; and (6) IQ over 85 on group Stanford-Binet Test.

As contrasted to placebo periods, the lithium periods (serum lithium 0.6–1.5 mEq/l) were associated with a significant reduction in physical or verbal aggressive episodes (as measured by number of "tickets" given by staff) and aggressive affect (as measured by self ratings). In those individuals who experienced anxiety along with their aggressive acts, reduced aggression was not associated with increased depression or anxiety. When aggression was reduced in individuals whose aggression was not usually accompanied by anxiety, an increase in anxious and depressive affect was noted.

Tupin et al. (1973), in an open study, evaluated the effects of lithium in 27 prisoners who had shown recurring violence and who had reacted rapidly to slight provocations with anger and violent behavior. The patients had a variety of diagnoses, including personality disorders. There was a significant decrease in the number of disciplinary actions for violent behavior during lithium treatment as compared to the same time period before lithium. The prisoners reported that they had experienced a greater capacity to reflect on the consequences of their actions, a greater ability to control angry feelings when provoked, and a diminished intensity of angry affect. The dosage of lithium tended to be higher than necessary for the maintenance treatment of manic depressive illness.

Sheard et al. (1976) carried out a three-month double blind study of lithium administered to delinquents with severe personality disorders who had committed serious aggressive crimes such as murder, manslaughter, or rape and had a history of either long-standing assaultive behavior or impulsive antisocial behavior. Sixty-six delinquents completed the study. There was a significantly greater decrease in infractions in the lithium group, and "major infractions" (that is, acts of violence) decreased month by month until at the end of the study it had reached zero. The number of infractions increased again after lithium was withdrawn.

Maintenance therapy with lithium is a promising development in the management of individuals with impulsive, violent, and explosive traits.

446 | Treatment of Mental Disorders

The effective serum level appears to be similar or, perhaps, somewhat higher than that required to prevent affective episodes in patients with affective disorders. The characteristics of persons suitable for this treatment have been described by various authors; however, a good response in any individual cannot be accurately predicted.

Patients with personality disorders who show serious unpremeditated aggression and damaging impulsiveness should have a trial with lithium, particularly if the effects of other treatments have been inadequate. Unfortunately, drug side effects are often poorly tolerated by impulsive and emotionally unstable individuals and many lack the self-discipline to take drugs regularly in the prescribed dosage and to adhere to the regular testing of serum levels.

If lithium is used, the initial aim should be a blood level in the therapeutic range with careful observation of the results. If there is a gradual improvement, lithium should be continued for up to four months since there is evidence to suggest that it can take that long before the maximum therapeutic effect is achieved. If after two months there is no improvement and the patient has tolerated his current blood level, the dosage should be increased toward a blood level approaching 1.5 mEq/l; again, this level should be tried for two months or longer. Blood levels over 1.5 mEq/l can be dangerous and should be tried only if the patient can be closely observed for toxicity, if all other treatments have failed and if treatment with a lower blood level appears to have been partially successful.

Some of these patients show evidence of brain damage or epilepsy. If lithium is given to patients who have epilepsy, it should be used with caution. Tupin's study, however, suggests that a history of brain damage or an abnormal EEG without seizures is not a contraindication to treatment with lithium.

Anticonvulsants. There are no controlled studies showing anticonvulsants to be effective in the symptomatic treatment of patients with personality disorders. The use of anticonvulsants in treating impulsive and uncontrollable aggression is discussed in Chapter 14 under heading "Intermittent Explosive Disorders" (p. 410).

Mood Swings in Personality Disorders

Mood swings are common in histrionic, narcissistic, antisocial, and borderline disorders and may also occur in other personality disorders. The affective disturbance that prompts the patient to seek treatment is usually depression, predominantly with exogenous features and often presenting as an adjustment reaction with depressed mood. Sometimes periodic mood swings appear to have an endogenous quality and may be a manifestation of a cyclothymic disorder without conspicuous hypomanic episodes. If this condition coexists with a personality disorder, treating the cyclothymic disorder should be considered.

Rifkin et al. (1972) carried out a double-blind crossover study with lithium and placebo in hospitalized young patients who had emotionally unstable character disorders. These patients were characterized by mood swings not usually reactive to environmental or interpersonal events, poor acceptance of authority, maladaptive behavior patterns, poor work record, manipulativeness, frequent sexual promiscuity, and abuse of drugs. They shared some of the traits of the histrionic personality and borderline personality. Lithium was markedly more effective than placebo in reducing the severity of the mood swings, although many patients complied poorly with treatment after leaving the hospital. In a previous open study Klein et al. (1973) were apparently successful in using chlorpromazine to treat such patients.

Although there is inadequate research evidence on the treatment of mood swings in patients with other personality disorders, lithium seems to be a logical choice if the disturbance is severe. If it appears that the affective changes are predominantly adjustment disturbances, treatment with antianxiety agents may be tried. It is not certain whether these drugs have a direct antidepressant effect; it seems more likely that the antidepressant effect is secondary to relief of anxiety (Kellner et al., 1979; Schatzberg and Cole, 1978). There is no firm evidence that tricyclic antidepressants are effective but they may be tried if other methods are unsuccessful.

Borderline Disorders

In a study of "chronic borderline" patients who had symptoms of anxiety, depression, and insomnia, diazepam proved to be more effective than a small dose of trifluoperazine (Vilkin, 1964). Klein (1967) found imipramine more effective than placebo in patients described as pseudoneurotic schizophrenics. Hedberg et al. (1971) found that pseudoneurotic schizophrenics had less pathology while treated with tranylcypromine than with a small dose of trifluoperazine or with a fixed dose combination of the two drugs. Brinkley et al. (1979) reviewed the literature on drug treatment of borderline patients and presented five uncontrolled case histories describing the effective use of low-dose neuroleptics. These studies have not been replicated and it is not certain from the descriptions given how the disorders would be classified using the DSM-III nomenclature. Carroll et al. (1981) found that it can be difficult to diagnose melancholia if it occurs in patients with a borderline disorder and these patients may benefit from antidepressants.

On the whole, response to drug treatment is poor. When target symptoms are treated, a few patients appear to benefit from treatment with antianxiety, antidepressant, or antipsychotic drugs. At present, no consistent drug treatment can be recommended in the treatment of borderline personality disorder.

Other Personality Disorders
There have been no controlled studies of drug treatment of patients with personality disorders such as paranoid, schizotypal, narcissistic, or dependent. Symptomatic treatment of a coexisting disorder is likely to make them less distressed and, perhaps, enable them to cope more adequately with their difficulties. Lifelong character traits are unlikely to change as a consequence of drug treatment, but the distress of intercurrent psychiatric disturbances may be highly amenable to drug therapy.

ELECTROCONVULSIVE THERAPY (ECT)

There is no systematic evidence from authoritative reviews (Fink, 1979; American Psychiatric Association, 1978) that ECT has any role in the management of personality disorders. Case reports of beneficial effects of ECT in patients with personality disorders probably describe the response to a coexisting disorder.

PSYCHOSURGERY

At present there is no place for psychosurgery in the treatment of personality disorders unless the patient also has another psychiatric disorder. Some patients suffer chronically from severe or incapacitating depression or anxiety that appears to be either consequent to or an integral part of their personality disorder. These patients may have an extremely poor prognosis; some have made multiple suicide attempts and others destroy themselves by abusing drugs or alcohol in an attempt to relieve their distress.

No controlled studies of psychosurgery for personality disorders have been conducted, and if this treatment is considered it should be used with the fullest safeguards for the patients' rights (DHEW Publ. No. (05) 77-0001, 1977). Uncontrolled studies with careful psychological assessment suggest that stereotactic psychosurgery, such as cingulotomy, relieves distress and improves social functioning in a substantial proportion of patients with severe chronic anxiety or severe depression (DHEW Publ. No. (05) 77-0001, 1977; Mitchell-Heggs et al., 1976; Bridges and Bartlett, 1977; Hitchcock et al., 1979). Psychosurgery should be considered only when other treatments have failed, when there is little or no hope for spontaneous recovery, and when the patient's suffering is extreme.

REFERENCES

Reports and Recommendations—Psychosurgery, National Commission for the Protection of Human Subjects of Biomedical and Behavioral Research. U.S. Govt. Printing Office. DHEW Publ. No. (OS) 77-0001, Washington, D.C. 1977.

American Psychiatric Association. Task Force Report 14. Electroconvulsive Therapy, Washington, D.C. 1978.

Adams S: Interaction between individual interview therapy and treatment amenability in older youth authority wards. Monogr. No. 2, Board of Corrections, State of California. 1961.

Akman DD, Normandeau A, Wolfgang ME: The group treatment literature in correctional institutions: an international bibliography, 1945–67. J Crim Law, Criminology & Police Sci. 59:41–51, 1968.

Barnes RJ: Mesoridazine (serentil) in personality disorders. A controlled trial in adolescent patients. Dis Nerv Syst. 38:258–264, 1977.

Beker J, Heyman DS: A critical appraisal of the California differential treatment typology of adolescent offenders. Criminology, 10:3–59, 1972.

Bridges PK, Bartlett JR: Psychosurgery: yesterday and today. Brit J Psychiat. 131:249–260, 1977.

Brinkley JR, Beitman BD, Friedel RO: Low-dose neuroleptic regimens in the treatment of borderline patients. Arch Gen Psychiat. 36:319–326, 1979.

Carroll BJ, Greden JF, Feinberg, M: Neuroendocrine evaluation of depression in borderline patients. Psychiat Clin North Am. 4:89–99, 1981.

Conners CK, Kramer R, Rothschild GH: Treatment of young delinquent boys with diphenylhydantoin sodium and methylphenidate. Arch Gen Psychiat. 24:156–160, 1971.

Covi L, Lipman RS, Smith VK: Diazepam induced hostility in depression. Paper presented at the Annual Meeting of the American Psychiatric Association, Toronto, Canada, May 2–6. 1977.

Craft M: The natural history of psychopathic disorder. Brit J Psychiat. 115:39–44, 1969.

Craft M, Stephenson G, Granger C: A controlled trial of authoritarian and self-governing regimes with adolescent psychopaths. Am J Orthopsychiat. 34:543–554, 1964.

DiMascio A, Shader RI, Harmatz J: Psychotropic drugs and induced hostility. Psychosomatics. 10:46–47, 1969.

Eisenberg L, Lachman R, Molling PA: A psychopharmacologic experiment in a training school for delinquent boys: methods, problems, findings. Am J Orthopsychiat. 33:431–447, 1963.

Feldman PE: Current Views on Antianxiety Agents. Pamphlet from a scientific exhibit presented at the Annual Meeting of the American Medical Association, Houston, Texas, November. 1967.

Fink M: Convulsive Therapy: Theory and Practice. Raven Press, New York. pp. 39, 218. 1979.

Gardos G, DiMascio A, Salzman C: Differential actions of chlordiazepoxide and oxazepam on hostility. Arch Gen Psychiat. 18:757–760, 1968.

Glasser W: Reality Therapy. A New Approach to Psychiatry. Harper and Row, New York. 1965.

Gleser GC, Gottschalk LA, Fox R: Immediate changes in affect with chlordiazepoxide. Arch Gen Psychiat. 13:291–295, 1965.

Goldstein AP, Stein N: Prescriptive Psychotherapies. Pergamon Press, Elmsford, NY. 1976.

Grant DJ: Current trends of individual and interpersonal approaches to rehabilitation of the offender. Conference: Mobilizing resources toward rehabilitation of the offender. New York, April. 1963.

Grant JD, Grant MQ: A group dynamic approach to the treatment of nonconformists in the navy. Ann Am Acad Pol Soc Sci. 322:126–135, 1959.

Hedberg DL, Houch JH, Glueck BC: Tranylcypromine-trifluoperazine combination in the treatment of schizophrenia. Am J Psychiat. 127:1141–1146, 1971.

Hill D: Amphetamine in psychopathic states. Brit J Addiction. 44:50, 1947.

Hitchcock ER, Ballantine HT, Meyerson BA: Modern Concepts in Psychiatric Surgery. Elsevier/North Holland Biomedical Press, New York. 1979.

Jesness CF: The Preston Typology Study. Sacramento, California, Institute for the Study of Crime and Delinquency. 1968.

Jesness CF: Comparative effectiveness of behavior modification and transactional analysis programs for delinquents. J Consult Clin Psychol. 43:758–779, 1975.

Kellner R: The evidence in favour of psychotherapy. Brit J Med Psychol. 40:341–358, 1967.

Kellner R: Drug treatment of personality disorders and delinquents In: The Psychopath, A Comprehensive Study of Antisocial Disorders and Behaviors. Reid WH (ed). Brunner/Mazel, New York. pp. 29–63, 1979.

Kellner R, Rada RT: Pharmacotherapy of personality disorders. In: Psychopharmacology Update: New and Neglected Areas. Davis JM and Greenblatt D (eds). Grune & Stratton, New York. pp. 29–63, 1979.

Kellner R, Rada RT, Andersen T, Pathak D: The effects of chlordiazepoxide on self-rated depression, anxiety, and well-being. Psychopharmacology. 64:185–191, 1979.

Klein DF: Importance of psychiatric diagnosis in prediction of clinical drug effects. Arch Gen Psychiat. 16:118–126, 1967.

Klein DF, Honigfeld G, Feldman S: Prediction of drug effect in personality disorders. J Nerv Ment Dis. 152:183–198, 1973.

Korey SR: The effects of benzedrine sulfate on the behavior of psychopathic and neurotic juvenile delinquents. Psych Quart. 18:127–137, 1944.

Lion JR: Benzodiazepines in the treatment of aggressive patients. J Clin Psychiat. 40:71–72, 1979.

Lorr M, McNair DM, Weinstein GJ: Meprobamate and chlorpromazine in psychotherapy. Arch Gen Psychiat. 4:75–83, 1961.

Massimo JL, Shore MF: The effectiveness of a comprehensive, vocationally-oriented psychotherapeutic program for adolescent delinquent boys. Am J Orthopsychiat. 33:634–642, 1963.

Massimo JL, Shore MF: Comprehensive vocationally oriented psychotherapy: a new treatment technique for lower class adolescent boys. Psychiatry. 30:229–236, 1967.

McCord J, McCord W: A follow-up report on the Cambridge-Somerville Youth Study. Ann Am Acad Pol Soc Sci. 322:90–96, 1959.

McDonald RL: The effects of personality type on drug response. Arch Gen Psychiat. 17:680–686, 1967.

McNair DM, Goldstein AP, Lorr M: Some effects of chlordiazepoxide and meprobamate with psychiatric outpatients. Psychopharmacologia. 7:256–265, 1965.

Meyer HJ, Borgatta EF, Jones WC: Girls at Vocational High: An Experiment in Social Work Intervention. Russell Sage Foundation, New York. 1965.

Milman DH: Minimal brain dysfunction in childhood: outcome in late adolescence and early adult years. J Clin Psychiat. 40:371–380, 1979.

Mitchell-Heggs N, Kelly D, Richardson A: Stereotactic limbic leucotomy: a follow-up at 16 months. Brit J Psychiat. 128:226–240, 1976.

Molling PA, Lockner AW, Sauls RJ: Committed delinquent boys. Arch Gen Psychiat. 7:96–102, 1962.

Mullen EJ, Dumpson JR: Evaluation of Social Intervention. Jossey-Bass, San Francisco. 1972.

Palmer TB: California's community treatment program for delinquent adolescents. J Res Crime and Delinquency. 8:74–92, 1971.

Palmer TB: Patterns of adjustment among delinquent adolescent conformists (six subgroupings of middle maturity, immature conformists). CTP Report Series 1, California Youth Authority. 1971a.

Palmer TB: California's Community Treatment Project: the Phase I, II and III experiments: developments and progress, CTP Research Report 10, California Youth Authority. 1971b.

Persons RW: Psychotherapy with sociopathic offenders: an empirical evaluation. J Clin Psychol. 21:204–207, 1965.

Persons RW: Psychological and behavioral change in delinquents following psychotherapy. J Clin Psychol. 22:337–340, 1966.

Persons RW: Relationship between psychotherapy with institutionalized boys and subsequent community adjustment. J. Consult Psychol. 31:137–141, 1967.

Powers E, Witmer HL: An Experiment in the Prevention of Delinquency. The Cambridge-Somerville Youth Study. Columbia University Press, New York. 1951.

Rickels K, Downing RW: Chlordiazepoxide and hostility in anxious outpatients produced by chlordiazepoxide therapy. J Nerv Ment Dis. 145:154–157, 1967.

Rifkin A, Quitkin F, Carrillo C: Lithium carbonate in emotionally unstable character disorder. Arch Gen Psychiat. 27:519–523, 1972.

Rubenfeld S: Typological approaches and delinquency control: a status report. U.S. Public Health Service Publication 1627. 1967.

Sarason IG: Verbal learning, modeling, and juvenile delinquency. Am Psychologist. 23:254–266, 1968.

Schatzberg AF, Cole JO: Benzodiazepines in depressive disorders. Arch Gen Psychiat. 35:1359–1365, 1978.

Schwitzgebel R, Kolb DA: Inducing behavior change in adolescent delinquents. Behav Res Ther. 1:297–304, 1964.

Sheard MH: Effect of lithium on human aggression. Nature. 230:113–114, 1971.

Sheard MH, Marini JL, Bridges CI: The effect of lithium on impulsive aggressive behavior in man. Am J Psychiat. 133:1409–1413, 1976.

Shelley ELV, Johnson WF: Evaluating an organized counseling service for youthful offenders. J Counsel Psychol. 8:351–354, 1961.

Shore MF, Massimo JL: Comprehensive vocationally oriented psychotherapy for adolescent delinquent boys: a follow-up study. Am J Orthopsychiat. 36:609–615, 1966.

Shovron JJ: Benzedrine in psychopathy and behavior disorders. Brit J Addiction. 44:58, 1947.

Showstack N: Preliminary report on the psychiatric treatment of prisoners at the California Medical Facility. Am J Psychiat. 112:821–824, 1956.

Smith AB, Berlin L: Treating the Criminal Offender. Issues and Problems. Oceana Publications, Dobbs Ferry, New York. p. 303, 1974.

Solomon K: High-dose benzodiazepines in the treatment of severe neurotic anxiety. J Clin Psychiatry. 39:610–613, 1978.

Suedfeld P, Landon PB: Approaches to treatment. In: Psychopathic Behavior: Approaches to Research, Hare RD and Schalling D (eds). Wiley, New York. pp. 347–377, 1978.

Sullivan C, Grant MQ, Grant JD: The development of interpersonal maturity: applications to delinquency. Psychiatry. 20:373–385, 1957.

Truax CB, Wargo DG: Antecedents to outcome in group psychotherapy with juvenile delinquents: effects of therapeutic conditions, alternate sessions, vicarious therapy pre-training and client self-exploration. Unpublished manuscript, Arkansas Rehabilitation Research and Training Center, University of Arkansas. 1967.

Truax CB, Wargo DG, Silber LD: Effects of group psychotherapy with high accurate empathy and nonpossessive warmth upon female institutionalized delinquents. J Abnorm Psychol. 71:267–274, 1966.

Tupin JP, Smith DB, Clanon TL: The long-term use of lithium in aggressive prisoners. Comp Psychiat. 14:311–317, 1973.

Vilkin MI: Comparative chemotherapeutic trial in treatment of chronic borderline patients. Am J Psychiat. 130:1004, 1964.

Warren MQ: The case for differential treatment of delinquents. Ann Am Acad Pol Soc Sci. 381:47–59, 1969.

Warren MQ, Neto VT, Palmer TB, Turner JK: Community Treatment Project-Fifth Progress Report: An Evaluation of Community Treatment for Delinquents. CTP Research Report 7, California Youth Authority. 1966.

Weeks HA: Youthful Offenders at Highlands. An evaluation of the Effects of the Short-Term Treatment of Delinquent Boys. Ann Arbor Paperbooks. Univ. of Michigan Press. 1958.

Weiss G, Hechtman L, Perlman T, Hopkins J, Wener A: Hyperactives as young adults. A controlled prospective ten-year follow-up of 75 children. Arch Gen Psychiat. 36:675–681, 1979.

Weiss JMA: The natural history of antisocial attitudes. What happens to psychopaths? J Geriat Psychiat. 6:236–242, 1973.

Wood DR, Reimherr FW, Wender PH, Johnson GE: Diagnosis and treatment of minimal brain dysfunction in adults. Arch Gen Psychiat. 33:1453–1460, 1976.

17 | V Codes for Conditions not Attributable to a Mental Disorder that are a Focus of Treatment

CARL J. GETTO

V codes have been adapted from ICD-9-CM to describe those conditions that are a focus of treatment but are not attributable to any other mental disorder. V codes would apply to instances where no other mental disorder is found, or when the diagnostic evaluation has not been adequate to determine the presence or absence of a mental disorder, but there is need to note the reason for contact with the mental health care system. They also apply to those cases where a mental disorder is present, but the focus of attention or treatment is on a condition that is not due to the mental disorder.

This chapter focuses on three of the conditions listed in DSM-III—malingering, marital and family disorders, and uncomplicated bereavement. These were chosen because of the frequency with which they present to psychiatrists either directly or in consultation with other health professionals.

MALINGERING (V65.20)

ESSENTIAL FEATURES

The essential feature of *malingering* is the voluntary production and presentation of false or grossly exaggerated physical or psychological symptoms. The symptoms are produced in pursuit of a goal that is obviously recognizable with an understanding of the individual's circumstances rather than of his or her individual psychology. Examples of such obviously understandable goals include: to avoid military conscription or duty, to avoid work, to obtain financial compensation, to evade criminal prosecution, or to obtain drugs.

TREATMENT GOALS

1. To provide a thorough medical, social, and psychiatric evaluation leading to the diagnosis.
2. To inform the patient of the diagnosis and to make this information available to legal, health, and social agencies with which the patient may have contact.
3. To facilitate appropriate medical, psychiatric, or social treatment for the patient.
4. To minimize overutilization of the health-care system.

TREATMENTS

The most frequent scenario of the malingerer is the "gotcha" syndrome. Initially, the personal charm of the malingerer and curiosity about his presenting symptom entices the physician into providing the malingerer with some gain (a place to stay, escape from legal difficulties, or drugs). In effect, the malingerer says "gotcha" to the physician. Within a short period of time, however, the diagnostic work-up is completed and it becomes apparent that the symptom was intentionally feigned. The physician confronts the malingerer with the diagnosis (usually in an angry or moralistic manner), and terminates treatment. It is now the physician's turn to say "gotcha." This may then be repeated with other physicians or social agencies, and, in fact, may reinforce the problem.

An alternative treatment is illustrated in Figure 17-1. The first step in the treatment process involves viewing the patient's symptoms as legitimate until a thorough diagnostic evaluation is completed. Although this is not radically different from the treatment illustrated above, it is only the first step in the process rather than the termination.

The diagnostic evaluation should include thorough, although not necessarily extensive, evaluations of the patient's physical, social, and psychiatric status. In addition to the usual psychiatric diagnostic interview, an amytal interview (Naples and Hackett, 1978; Skoichet, 1978) or hypnosis (Walberg, 1975) may provide useful information.

When the diagnosis of malingering has been established, it is important to inform the patient in a manner which would allow for further psychiatric treatment if indicated, or to provide an alternative approach for the patient to achieve his purpose. Hackett (1978) illustrates how a patient can be so informed in a creative and "face-saving" way without embarrassing the patient or the physician. In essence, he advocates the following:

1. Explaining the results of the work-up to the patient
2. Offering a benign diagnosis for the patient's symptom
3. Emphasizing that the patient's symptom has a good prognosis
4. Advising the patient that the symptom will improve with time and conservative treatment.

Once informed of the diagnosis, the patient may choose to leave treatment. If this is the case, the physician may be asked to share his information with other agencies. Most frequently these include local emergency rooms, social services such as public assistance, or agents of the court.

Instead of leaving treatment, the patient may not accept the diagnosis, and request that he see a consultant or specialist for a "second opinion." The primary physician is in a position to facilitate such a consultation, without requiring the patient to repeat his charade before another unknowing doctor. In fact, many facilities such as the Veterans Administration have such consultations built into their evaluation process.

The psychiatrist can provide more specific treatment if the patient's

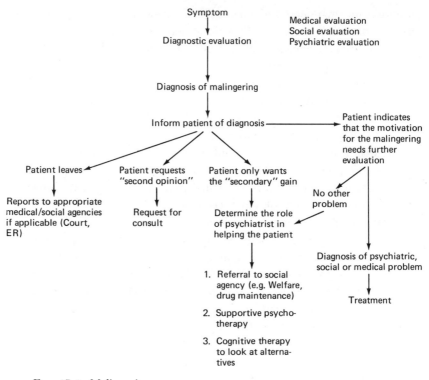

FIG. 17-1. Malingering.

evaluation suggests an underlying primary psychiatric problem, or if the patient requests psychiatric help in obtaining the desired gain by more direct and appropriate means. Referral to appropriate agencies (legal aid, public assistance) may provide the patient with at least a partial solution to his problem. Supportive psychotherapy can be quite beneficial while the patient is attempting to deal with a legal or social problem, and cognitive psychotherapy may offer insights into alternative ways of coping with specific environmental stresses. Each of these therapeutic approaches offers more efficient and less expensive ways of dealing with the malingerer than by sending him away to further strain limited health-care resources.

The most important component in the treatment of the malingerer is the definition of a therapeutic goal that is mutually acceptable to the patient and the physician. It is difficult for treatment to succeed if therapy becomes an adversarial process. A careful diagnosis allows for the clarification of the patient's goals, and therapy can then focus on alternative strategies for attaining them.

UNCOMPLICATED BEREAVEMENT (V62.82)

ESSENTIAL FEATURES

The essential feature of *uncomplicated bereavement* is a normal or expected reaction to the death of a loved one. The full depressive syndrome may be present, however morbid preoccupation with worthlessness, prolonged and marked functional impairment, and marked psychomotor retardation are uncommon and suggest that the bereavement is complicated by the development of a major depression.

TREATMENT GOALS

1. To encourage, guide, and support the bereaved person through the process of grieving.
2. To prevent pathological grief reactions.
3. To provide consultation to clergymen, physicians, and other professionals who work with the bereaved.

In his classic description of the grief process and its treatment, Lindemann (1944) describes "grief work" as encompassing the following goals: "The emancipation of the bereaved from bondage to the deceased, readjustment to the environment from which the deceased is missing, and the formation of new relationships."

Parkes (1972) elaborates the task of the psychiatrist (or other "helping person") as:

(1) Helping the bereaved recognize their loss and the changes associated with that loss.
(2) Validating the feelings of the bereaved, demonstrating that these are not to be feared, and allowing them to emerge into consciousness.

(3) Emphasizing the fact that grief cannot be avoided.

(4) Empathically supporting the bereaved in their pain.

(5) Providing reassurance that the grief process is normal, time-limited, and not a symptom of mental illness.

(6) Approving the changes in feelings, attitudes, and behaviors that are turning points in the course of bereavement.

(7) Approving the expression of negative feelings toward the deceased.

(8) Encouraging emotional attachments to other individuals.

Most bereaved persons never enter a psychiatrist's office. Studies of the natural history of bereavement, reviewed by Clayton (1979), indicate that the vast majority of widows and widowers experience a significant increase in depressive symptoms (depressed mood, crying, sleep problems, loss of appetite, fatigue, difficulty concentrating, guilt, hopelessness, and hallucinatory experiences) shortly after the death of a spouse. However, during the first year of bereavement, most deal with the loss "with minimal morbidity and mortality." The only exceptions to this are (1) younger widows and widowers (under age 45) who have more symptoms of physical distress and may take more drugs, and (2) older widowers (over 65 years of age) who have a slight increase in mortality during the first six months of bereavement.

It appears then that bereavement is quite adequately treated by the social milieu of the bereaved. Friends, relatives, clergymen, and general physicians seem capable of supporting the bereaved without the intervention of psychiatrists or the mental health system. This is borne out by Vachon (1980) who compared the postbereavement adaptation of widows with a "widow-contact" (another widow who provided emotional support and assistance) with a matched control group without intervention. They found that the course of adaptation was the same in both groups, the only significant difference being that the group with "widow-contact" achieved adaptation more rapidly than the control group.

Polack's (1979) study of crisis intervention in bereavement offers a similar perspective. He found that many families refused mental health crisis intervention. These families felt that they were capable of dealing with the crises themselves, and regarded the mental health professional as an unwelcome "intruder" who did not fit into the family's concept of mourning.

Furthermore, the group that accepted treatment showed a poorer adjustment six months after the death than the untreated group. By the end of the eighteenth month follow-up period, there were no significant differences between the groups. Polack attributes this difference to the therapeutic technique which encourages emotional release, and discourages repression and denial. In fact, successful mourning may require a degree of repression and denial which is incompatible with this type of therapeutic intervention, and bereaved persons may do better without treatment.

Even though contemporary research tends to regard grief as a normal consequence of living, which is self-limited, without serious morbidity and not requiring treatment, several questions remain.

1. *Is there a significant mortality associated with bereavement?*
Clayton (1979) reviewed the literature on the subject of mortality during bereavement, including her own prospective study of 109 widows and widowers (Clayton, 1974). She concluded that there is no appreciable increase in mortality in bereaved persons. Furthermore, she has found no significant increase in morbidity (from physical illness) in the bereaved. These findings are quite different from those of Parkes (1969) and Rees and Lutkins (1967) who found significantly higher rates of mortality and morbidity in the bereaved when compared with the general population matched for sex and age. Furthermore the studies of Engel (1968) and Holmes (1978) have implicated bereavement as a significant factor in illness onset. It is difficult to totally dismiss the impact of the death of a significant loved-one, such as a spouse, and yet it seems that correlations with mortality may not be justified by the data currently available.

2. *Which persons are at higher risk for having problems with grief?*
All of the studies previously cited indicate that there is a subpopulation of bereaved persons who suffer significant psychiatric dysfunction as a result of bereavement. Clayton (1979) and Parkes (1972) have identified the abuse of alcohol as having negative effects on the outcome of bereavement. Polack (1979) felt that families with a past history of unstable functioning prior to the death were at risk for having more difficulty in mourning. All the authors point to the importance of social contact during bereavement; conversely, social isolation may adversely effect the process of grief. Finally, the tendency of younger widows and widowers

to abuse medications (tranquilizers and sedatives) has been noted. This too would predict a person who might have more-than-usual difficulty during bereavement.

3. *What is the role of the psychiatrist in the treatment of uncomplicated bereavement?*

This discussion has focused on studies which tend to indicate that uncomplicated grief is a self-limiting condition which ordinarily does not require the attention of a psychiatrist. However, for those patients who do come to a psychiatrist's attention, either directly or in consultation with other health professionals (i.e. physicians, nurses, clergymen), the psychiatrist has a very specific role.

First, he may need to establish the diagnosis, separating it from other depressive disorders. This problem becomes especially important when the grief concerns the loss of a person other than a spouse (i.e. children). The second function of the psychiatrist is to directly treat those "high-risk" patients noted above, or those patients whose grief is complicated by other mental or physical illness. Such treatment follows the same outline already discussed and does not differ significantly depending on the person lost. Finally, it is the function of the psychiatrist to serve as an educational and referral source to those professionals working directly with the bereaved.

MARITAL AND FAMILY PROBLEMS

Essential Features

The category *marital problems* (V61.10) can be used when a focus of attention or treatment is a marital problem that is apparently not due to a mental disorder. An example is marital conflict related to estrangement or divorce.

The category *other specified family circumstances* (V61.80) can be used when a focus of attention or treatment is a family circumstance that is apparently not due to a mental disorder and is not a *parent-child problem* (V61.20) or a *marital problem*. Examples are interpersonal difficulties with an aged in-law, or sibling rivalry.

Treatment Goals

1. Diagnose areas of conflict.
2. Reduce symptoms of conflict.
3. Facilitate communication between family members.
4. Mediate problem areas, encouraging the family to negotiate mutually acceptable decisions.
5. Help all members of the family maximize their own potential within the relationship.
6. Facilitate the dissolution of the relationship when indicated.

From a clinical standpoint, the treatment of marital and family problems is very similar. Such problems usually represent difficulties in the relationship between the members of the family rather than a defect intrinsic to any individual. Many of the therapeutic strategies originally developed for exclusive use with either couples or families have been successfully applied to both. Furthermore, many of the research studies evaluating treatment outcome do not distinguish between marital and family therapy. It is, therefore, appropriate to consider these collectively.

There are, in general, three major theoretical orientations toward the practice of marital and family therapy; psychodynamic, interactional, and behavioral. Within each of these theoretical constructs there are many "schools" or models of practice which translate the general theory into specific treatment approaches. It is beyond the scope of this brief chapter to detail the intricacies of all these specific approaches, and the reader is referred to more comprehensive references such as Gurman and Kniskern (1981), Martin (1976) and Paolino and McCrady (1978).

Psychodynamic Approaches

Psychodynamic approaches are based on the principles of psychoanalysis and object relations theory. Marriages and families are viewed as intimate relationships between individuals. As such, each individual brings to the relationship a set of needs and expectations (conscious and unconscious) which have been derived from personal, genetic, developmental, and environmental influences. The partners in such a relationship have a defensive need to maintain their own internal self-image by supporting the image of the other through the defensive process of *projective identification*. The personal development of each individual takes place within the context of the relationship's development. As such, the relationship has a developmental history which demands that certain tasks—separation from families of origin, raising children, allowing one's children to separate—be accomplished in a sequential fashion.

Difficulties in a relationship are seen to arise from the failure of one partner to have his or her needs or expectations satisfied by the other members. Frequently, the symptomatic expression is seen in more than one family member. A complementary view conceives of difficulties as arising from the family's difficulty in accomplishing a certain developmental task.

Treatment focuses on making conscious the developmental (individual and relationship) needs and expectations of the members of the couple or family. This is done by increasing communication between the family members. Expression of emotions is encouraged as a way of facilitating communication and uncovering unconscious material. The therapist attempts to clarify and interpret the material in a way that allows the family to understand it. Insight is viewed as a goal of treatment, as well as a tool which can aid the family in altering patterns of behavior. Transference toward the therapist and between the members of the family is used to foster insight. Change is measured in terms of increased comfort on the part of the family members, decreased symptomatology (anxiety, depression, acting-out behavior, etc.), and formation of new, more adaptive behaviors.

BEHAVIORAL APPROACHES

Behavioral marital/family therapy consists of the clinical application of social learning theory. Relationships are formed and maintained by reciprocal positive reinforcement in the form of observable behaviors. Problems in a relationship arise when there is a reduction in positive reinforcement, or an increase in the partner's aversive attempts to modify the other's behavior. Such a change in the behavior of any member will elicit like changes from the other members. This results in some behavioral symptoms of dysfunction, which can be described by the couple or family.

The treatment of dysfunction is basically a structural, cognitive approach in which:

1. The members of the couple or family specify and concisely describe problem behaviors, as behaviors to be changed.
2. Each problem behavior is then approached by the couple or family in a problem solving way. Alternative positive behaviors are suggested.
3. The members then contract in a *quid pro quo* way, whereby the desired behavior of one member is reciprocated by a positive behavior by another.
4. The contracts may be written.
5. The couple or family is instructed to practice the behaviors contracted.
6. This process continues with each identified problem behavior.

Within this approach, the therapist acts to teach skills, directs and structures the therapy, models new interpersonal behavior, clarifies communications, and provides rationale for difficulties encountered and treatment offered. The therapist is a consultant to the patients and imparts to them the sense that they *can change* others behavior in a mutually satisfactory way.

INTERACTIONAL APPROACHES

General systems theory forms the conceptual basis for interactional approaches to marital and family therapy. The couple or family is viewed as a system in which the members are constantly interacting with each other, and redefining their relationships.

Conflict is defined in terms of present interactions. They are conceptualized as struggles for power or control in the relationship, or as a manifestation of contradictory (double-bind) messages from another member. The individual is seen as being expressed through relationships; individual symptoms can be understood as ways of defining and controlling a relationship.

Therapy consists of determining: (1) *What* is occurring in the interactional system; (2) *how* such interactions are *maintained*, and (3) *how* they can be *altered*. Problems are defined by the therapist as "paradoxes" (or double-binds). The response to this by the family results in symptomatic change in one member, which then causes change in the system. In such therapy, the *process* of interacting is viewed as more important than the *content* of interactions. Furthermore, the therapist becomes an active part of the system and it is through his/her interactions that change occurs. Another important task of the interactional therapist is to provide the couple/family with some understanding of how change is effected in treatment, in order to help the couple/family continue to change outside of formal therapy.

GENERAL PRINCIPLES

While these theoretical orientations may appear to define unique, specific approaches to the therapy of marital/family dysfunction, and while many of the charismatic leaders of various therapeutic schools advocate the rigid application of specific principles and techniques, it is clear that most clinicians are fairly eclectic in actual practice. Different families may require different approaches, and techniques from one orientation frequently complement those of another. In fact, Gurman and Kniskern (1978) have reported that in general, therapists from all three orientations tend to share the following process goals in their treatments:

1. specification of problems
2. clarification of each member's individual desires and needs
3. redefining the nature of difficulties
4. encouraging each partner's recognition of his/her mutual contribution to the marital discord
5. recognition and modification of communication patterns, "rules," and interactional patterns
6. increasing reciprocity
7. decreasing the use of coercion and blaming
8. increasing cooperative problem solving
9. modification of individual needs
10. increasing each member's ability to express his or her feelings clearly and to "hear" the other members

11. the preferred treatment approach is conjoint; that is meeting with all members of a couple/family

Furthermore, the therapist's tasks are described as:

1. Directing and structuring the therapy sessions, and sequencing treatment goals.
2. Challenging the assumptions, beliefs, and attitudes of the couple or family about the nature of marriage and families, and providing alternative views.
3. Clarifying communication.
4. Providing homework.

In addition to the general treatment of marital and family dysfunction, therapists have developed strategies for preventing dysfunction and for interviewing in specific relationship disorders. In particular, the development of "marital enrichment programs," divorce counseling, and the treatment of family violence is noteworthy.

Marital enrichment or skill-training programs have been developed as a *functional* way of helping couples and families increase their adjustment, satisfaction, and relationship skills, as well as preventing subclinical dysfunction from becoming symptomatic or disruptive to the relationship. For the most part, these programs are brief, ranging from six one-hour sessions to a weekend retreat. Rather than work with a single couple or family, these programs are designed to deal with groups of 3 to 20 units. They are highly structured relative to usual therapeutic approaches and combine elements of the following:

1. *Education* regarding the conceptual nature of relationships.
2. *Skill-training* in various techniques (i.e. speaking for self, expressing feelings, making interpretations, paraphrasing).
3. Practicing *problem-solving* techniques, such as negotiating.
4. Anticipating problem areas in the relationship.
5. Assertiveness training.
6. Learning to deal with anger and aggression in a constructive way ("fair-fighting").

Divorce therapy consists of the application of the principles of marital and family therapy to the emotional, behavioral, and interpersonal difficulties surrounding separation and divorce. Most of the therapeutic strategies are based on the recognition that divorce proceeds through distinct stages and concomitant feelings and tasks. Kaslow (1981) suggests the following progression in Table 17-1:

Feelings	Tasks
Predivorce	
Disillusionment	Confronting partner
Deliberation period	
Dissatisfaction	Seeking therapy
Ambivalence	Negotiating alternatives
Dread	Physical and emotional withdrawal
Emptiness	
Low self-esteem	
During divorce: Litigation	
Depressed	Separating physically
Detached	Filing for legal divorce
Angry	Considering economic arrangements
Hopeless	Considering custody arrangements
Confusion	Grieving and mourning
Sadness	Telling relatives and friends
Loneliness	
Relief	
Postdivorce: Reequilibration	
Resignation	Finalizing divorce
Regret	Forming new friendships
Acceptance	Undertaking new activities
Self-confidence	Stabilizing new life schedule
Curiosity	Resynthesis of identity
Independence	Seeking new love object
	Completing "psychic divorce"
	Helping children accept divorce and form new relationship with both parents

Most authors prefer to work with the couple or family conjointly until the divorce has been completed. Treatment of couples in groups has also been advocated. Treatment approaches tend to be similar to those outlined for general marital and family therapy. However, an alternative approach termed *structured mediation* has been advocated by Coogler (1978). Under this approach, the mediator is a trained, neutral "third-party" who aids the divorcing couple resolve the following types of issues: property division, terminating dependence on the relationship, and deciding the continuing responsibility for children. The partners must agree to follow specific mediation rules. Within the process of mediation, issues are clearly defined, all options for settlement are examined, consequences of decisions are examined, and impasses are resolved by arbitration. This model, which is a highly structured, cognitive approach to a difficult problem, appears to provide a viable alternative to other traditional models.

Domestic violence is a marital/family problem quite different from the others considered in this chapter. Rather than a symptom of mild to moderate dysfunction, it represents a major problem which demands immediate attention. Various programs have been developed by police and mental health agencies to try to treat the abuser and the members of the family who are the victims of the violence. The first step in the treatment involves separating the parties. "Safe houses" and shelters have been formed where a battered spouse (usually the wife) can be protected from the abuser. Information regarding legal rights, employment opportunities, divorce procedures, and therapeutic intervention is provided by peers (usually women who have been victims of abuse). If the battered spouse decides to terminate the relationship, emotional, social, and legal support is provided.

For those spouses who choose to stay together, therapy consists of treatment of the abused spouse and children, the abuser, and the couple or family as a unit. Most often, treatment is provided in groups, which can offer support and practical advice. Therapy focuses on the relationship, rather than the individual. In particular, the antecedants to violence are identified (i.e. alcohol), alternatives to physical violence (i.e. verbal fighting, relaxation techniques) are provided, a therapeutic contact (such as a 24-hour hotline) is made available to couples, new ways of "fighting" which do not include violence are taught, ways for the couples to increase each other's self-esteem are explored, practical problem solving (especially around financial problems) is offered, and the couple/family is encouraged to explore mutually satisfying goals for themselves.

CONTROVERSIES

There are many ongoing areas of dispute in marital/family therapy, many of which deal with specific techniques, such as the merit of including several generations in the therapy, or the optimal number and length of treatment sessions, or differences in effectiveness of the different approaches. I would, however, like to examine several questions which have relevance to general psychiatric practice.

1. *What are the indications for individual treatment (one spouse or family member) in marital or family problems?*

Gurman and Kniskern (1978a) indicate that individual therapy for marital problems is less effective and appears to have more negative effects than conjoint treatment. However, the literature on the treatment of spouse abuse (Moore, 1979) and divorce (Kaslow, 1981) suggests that individual treatment may at times be the treatment of choice for these conditions. In addition, conjoint therapy becomes impossible when one member persistently refuses to attend therapy or when one member deteriorates during conjoint therapy.

2. *Are skill-training and divorce therapy clinically effective?*

The researchers who have developed these programs indicate that these are effective strategies for increasing family functioning and reducing psychiatric morbidity. Empiric evidence, however, does not support those claims. In spite of this, large numbers of families are approaching such therapy (especially marital enrichment) to enhance their own growth.

3. *To what extent should the practicing psychiatrist be involved in the treatment of marital/family problems?*

The debate over this question has been raging for as long as marital and family therapy has been advocated. The spectrum of opinion ranges from the approach that psychiatrists as medical specialists should deal with severe disturbances and that "relationship problems" should be dealt with by those who are better trained (i.e. social workers, psychologists). In fact, many psychiatry residencies reflect this bias in providing little experience and even less clinical supervision in working with couples and families.

At the other end of the spectrum are those who would argue that the growth of marital and family therapy demands that psychiatrists have basic knowledge and skills in the field. For example, the treatment of many psychiatric disorders (alcoholism, drug abuse, sexual problems, child and adolescent problems) requires the assessment and treatment of the family. Furthermore, growing evidence indicates that certain types of marital/family treatment may be the treatment of choice for disorders such as anorexia nervosa or sexual dysfunction. Finally, can a psychiatrist really act as a consultant to other mental health or medical professionals if he is devoid of knowledge in this basic and burgeoning area of mental health treatment?

REFERENCES

Clayton PJ: Mortality and morbidity in the first year of widowhood. Arch Gen Psychiat. 30:747–750, 1974.

Clayton PJ: The sequelae and nonsequelae of conjugal bereavement. Am J Psychiat. 136:1530–1534, 1979.

Coogler GJ: Structured Mediation in Divorce Settlement. Lexington Books, Lexington, Mass. 1978.

Engel GL: A life setting conducive to illness. Ann Internal Med. 69:293–300, 1968.

Gurman AS, Kniskern DP: Research on marital and family therapy: progress, perspective, and prospect. In: Handbook of Psychotherapy and Behavior Change. Garfield SL and Bergin DE (eds). Wiley, New York, pp. 817–901, 1978.

Gurman AS, Kniskern DP: Contemporary Marital Therapies: A Critique and Comparative Analysis of Psychoanalytic, Behavioral and Systems Theory Approaches. In: Marriage and Marital Therapy. Paolino TJ and McCrady BS (eds). Brunder/Mazel, New York. pp. 445–566, 1978a.

Gurman AS, Kniskern DP: Handbook of Family Therapy. Bruner/Mazel, New York, 1981.

Hackett TP: The Malingerer. In: Massachusett's General Hospital Handbook of General Hospital Psychiatry. Hackett, TP and Cassem, NH (eds). C. V. Mosby, St. Louis. pp. 238–240, 1978.

Holmes TH: Life situations, emotions and disease. Psychosomatics. 19:747–754, 1978.

Kaslow FW: Divorce and divorce therapy. In: Handbook of Family Therapy. Gurman AS and Kniskern DP (eds). Bruner/Mazel, New York. pp. 662–696, 1981.

Lindemann E: Symptomatology and management of acute grief. Am J Psychiat. 101:141–149, 1944.

Martin PA: A Marital Therapy Manual. Bruner/Mazel, New York. 1976.

Moore DM: Battered women. Sage publications, Beverly Hills, Calif. 1979.

Naples M. Hackett TP: The amytal interview: history and current uses. Psychosomatics. 19:98–105, 1978.

Paolino TJ, McCrady BS: Marriage and Marital Therapy. Bruner/Mazel, New York. 1978.

Parkes CM: Broken heart: a statistical study of increased mortality among widowers. Brit Med J. 1:740–743, 1969.

Parkes CM: Helping the bereaved. In: Bereavement: Studies of Grief in Adult Life. International University Press, New York. pp. 149–181, 1972.

Polack RP: Follow-up research in primary prevention: a model of adjustment in acute grief. J Clin Psychol. 35:35–45, 1979.

Rees WD, Lutkins SG: Mortality of bereavement. Brit Med J. 4:13–16, 1967.

Skoichet RP: Sodium amytal in the diagnosis of chronic pain. Can Psychiat Assoc J. 23:219–228, 1978.

Vachon MLS: A controlled study of self-help intervention for widows. Am J Psychiat. 137:1380–1384, 1980.

Walberg LR: Hypnotherapy. In: American Handbook of Psychiatry, Vol. 5. Arieti, S. (ed). Basic Books, New York. pp. 235–253, 1975.

18 | Diagnosis and Treatment of Sleep Disorders

JOYCE D. KALES,
CONSTANTIN R. SOLDATOS,
and ANTHONY KALES

We were unable to base our discussion of sleep disorders on the diagnostic classification of sleep disorders proposed by the Association of Sleep Disorders Centers (ASDC) (1979) because of its general lack of usefulness for clinical practice. Thus, we propose an alternative diagnostic classification and will describe in detail the treatment of sleep disorders based on this classification.

The ASDC classification was not incorporated into DSM-III and instead appears in Appendix E of that manual (1980). This unofficial classification of sleep disorders is not compatible with the DSM-III format and is not practical for clinical use since it is overly complicated, too specific, and misleading; it includes a multitude of diagnoses for sleep disorders, many of which are not adequately substantiated.

The ASDC classification is incompatible with the DSM-III format for a number of reasons. Many of the individual ASDC diagnoses constitute an artificial fusing of a general sleep disorder with another distinct medical or psychiatric condition. Such a fusing fails to meet the DSM-III requirement for separately diagnosing each disorder according to a multiaxial model. Furthermore, a single diagnosis referring to two separate conditions implies a cause-and-effect relationship when there may not be one. For example, the diagnosis of "persistent insomnia associated with chronic alcoholism" implies that insomnia and chronic alcoholism are related etiologically, whereas the two conditions may or may not be directly related to each other and, in fact, may both be caused by an underlying personality disorder. Finally, the ASDC coding system requires six digits (1979) whereas DSM-III and the *International Classification of*

Diseases, 9th Revision, Clinical Modification (ICD-9-CM) do not allow for more than five digits (1980; 1978).

The ASDC classification (1979; 1980) is unnecessarily complex, listing about 70 specific diagnoses that refer to only six to eight general conditions of disturbed sleep or, if these are divided into organic and nonorganic diagnoses, to no more than about 15 conditions. The individual diagnoses, although very specific, are not adequately substantiated in the scientific literature. Many of the diagnoses lack clinical relevance and some refer to neurophysiological disturbances that are hypothetical. For example, at least four diagnoses ("insomnia with repeated REM sleep interruptions," "insomnia with atypical polysomnographic features," "insomnia with sleep-related (nocturnal) myoclonus," and "asymptomatic polysomnographic findings") not only are poorly substantiated, but also imply that certain electrophysiological findings have clinical significance, even though there is not adequate proof that such claims are warranted. Finally, a number of diagnoses are based on anecdotal information or on preliminary, unpublished, or insufficient data. One example is "childhood-onset insomnia." There is no evidence that this condition is any different than insomnia beginning at any other age. Similarly, the diagnoses of "delayed sleep phase syndrome," "short sleeper," "long sleeper," "subjective insomnia without objective findings," and "subjective disorder of excessive sleep without objective findings" are based primarily on anecdotal information and insufficient data.

The sleep disorder diagnoses of the ICD-9-CM (1978) are practical, and their format is compatible with DSM-III. Thus, we recommend the use of ICD-9-CM for diagnosing sleep disorders and DSM-III for diagnosing the psychiatric disorders frequently associated with sleep disturbances. The ICD-9-CM diagnoses divide sleep disturbances into nonorganic (307.40–307.49) and organic (780.50–780.59) disorders, whereas conditions that may occur in sleep and/or wakefulness are listed separately, e.g. enuresis (307.6), bruxism (306.8), and head-banging (307.3). Narcolepsy (347) is classified with the disorders of the central nervous system. The ICD-9-CM "specific disorders of sleep of nonorganic origin" are listed in Table 18-1 (terms in parentheses are ours).

This classification (1978) is acceptable with minor modifications such as retaining well-established and widely used terms such as insomnia and hypersomnia, and excluding the diagnosis of "repetitive intrusions of sleep" since it is unsubstantiated and lacks clinical relevance. The part of the ICD-9-CM dealing with sleep disturbances of organic origin (780.50–780.59) could be altered to mirror the classification of the non-

TABLE 18-1.
ICD-9-CM SLEEP DISORDERS CLASSIFICATION

307.40	Nonorganic sleep disorder, unspecified
307.41	Transient disorder of initiating or maintaining sleep (transient insomnia)
307.42	Persistent disorder of initiating or maintaining sleep (persistent insomnia)
307.43	Transient disorder of initiating or maintaining wakefulness (transient hypersomnia)
307.44	Persistent disorder of initiating or maintaining wakefulness (persistent hypersomnia)
307.45	Phase-shift disruption of 24-hour sleep-wake cycle
307.46	Somnambulism or night terrors
307.47	Other dysfunctions of sleep stages or arousal from sleep
307.48	Repetitive intrusions of sleep
307.49	Other

organic sleep disorders (307.40–307.49). This would greatly facilitate the physician's decision-making process and would be more clinically meaningful. The ICD-9-CM classification would be further improved by including a separate diagnosis for sleep apnea among the sleep disturbances of organic origin. Sleep apnea is a condition that is often most associated with hypersomnia and rarely with insomnia. In any event, its presence warrants a separate diagnosis.

Based on the considerations just discussed, we envision an improved classification of sleep disorders, as listed in Table 18-2.

Other disorders occurring in sleep and/or wakefulness, as well as narcolepsy, would continue to be classified separately, as in the current ICD-9-CM.

INSOMNIA

Analysis of the personality patterns of patients with chronic insomnia strongly suggests that these patients characteristically internalize their emotions instead of expressing them outwardly (Kales et al., 1976; Marks

TABLE 18-2.
PROPOSED SLEEP DISORDERS CLASSIFICATION

SPECIFIC DISORDERS OF SLEEP OF NONORGANIC ORIGIN	SPECIFIC DISORDERS OF SLEEP OF ORGANIC ORIGIN
Nonorganic sleep disorder, unspecified	Organic sleep disorder, unspecified
Transient insomnia	Transient insomnia
Persistent insomnia	Persistent insomnia
Transient hypersomnia	Transient hypersomnia
Persistent hypersomnia	Persistent hypersomnia
Phase-shift disruption of 24-hour sleep-wake cycle	Sleep apnea
Somnambulism or night terrors	Somnambulism or night terrors
Other dysfunctions of sleep	Other dysfunctions of sleep

and Monroe, 1976). The internalization of psychological conflicts may lead to chronic emotional arousal, which in turn results in physiological arousal and, consequently, insomnia (Kales et al., 1976b). The fact that poor sleepers have high levels of daytime anxiety (Coursey et al., 1975) and higher levels of physiological arousal during sleep (Monroe, 1967) supports this hypothesis. During the day, the insomniac typically tries to deny and repress conflicts. At night, however, when there is less external stimulation and distraction, the patient's attention is focused internally, he relaxes, and regression occurs. Anger, aggression, and sadness threaten to break through into consciousness, and as the insomniac struggles against the emergence of negative feelings, sleeplessness worsens (Kales et al., 1981). Thus, in addition to the psychological conflicts that typically underlie the complaint of insomnia, a fear of sleeplessness that is independent of the primary psychological causes soon develops in patients with insomnia. Also, a chronic pattern of disturbed sleep eventually conditions the patient to expect insomnia. The ultimate result is a vicious circle of continued sleep disturbance, with an escalation of emotional arousal, physiological arousal, sleeplessness, fear of sleeplessness, further arousal, and still further sleeplessness (Kales et al., 1976b).

In transient insomnia, a similar mechanism can be hypothesized. The individual experiencing a major life-stress situation mobilizes his coping mechanisms, which may or may not be adequate. This mobilization may lead to emotional arousal, which in turn leads to physiological arousal and sleeplessness. If the life-stress situation does not subside or the coping mechanisms are not successful, then a fear of sleeplessness may subsequently develop, possibly leading to the same vicious circle that develops in chronic insomnia.

Thus, in the overall therapy of insomnia, the psychiatrist attempts to treat not only the underlying psychological conflicts, the impaired ability to cope with life stress, or any medical factors, but also the consequences of insomnia itself (Kales et al., 1981; Soldatos et al., 1979b).

A number of general measures involving personal health habits and lifestyle patterns may be helpful in most cases of insomnia, whether transient or chronic (Kales et al., 1981; Soldatos et al., 1979b; Kales et al., 1974b). The patient is encouraged to increase physical activity and exercise during the day, but not close to bedtime since exercise at that time may raise the level of physiological arousal. Complex mental activity, such as studying too late in the evening, may aggravate an insomniac condition; thus, patients are instructed to avoid mentally stimulating situations and engage instead in relaxing mental activities before bedtime. In addition, patients should regulate their daily schedules and establish a regular bedtime hour, although some flexibility of the patient's sleep schedule is desirable so that he does not become obsessive about the schedule itself. The insomniac should go to bed only when he is sleepy. If he is unable to sleep, he should get up, leave the bedroom, and engage in a relaxing activity. In this way, he learns to associate the bedroom with sleep rather than with obsessive thoughts and concerns. Naps during the day should be discouraged. Finally, smoking cigarettes (Soldatos et al., 1980) and drinking beverages containing caffeine (Karacan et al., 1976) should also be discouraged, particularly close to bedtime.

TRANSIENT INSOMNIA

Since transient insomnia is often a reaction to psychological or physical stress, it usually subsides when the individual has adapted to the situation through his own coping mechanisms. If elimination of the stress-generating situation is impossible or impractical, the main therapeutic role of the physician should be directed toward strengthening the patient's ego defenses and other psychological as well as physical adaptive mechanisms (Kales et al., 1981). Depending on the nature of the patient's problem, the psychiatrist selects a form of brief psychotherapy using supportive or insight-oriented techniques or a method combining both approaches. Both supportive and insight-oriented approaches assist the patient in understanding and resolving psychological conflicts, and thereby help him to reduce his emotional and physiological arousal at night. In addition, reassuring the patient that his condition is treatable helps to minimize a fear of sleeplessness, which in itself may be a factor in the development of chronic insomnia (Kales et al., 1976b; Kales et al., 1981; Soldatos et al., 1979b).

When transient insomnia appears to be secondary to neurotic anxiety states, prescribing anxiolytic medication for a short period of time may be helpful. The use of benzodiazepine anxiolytics (e.g. chlorazepate, chlordiazepoxide, diazepam, or lorazepam) is indicated both for the daytime anxiety and, in an increased bedtime dose, for the sleep difficulty (Soldatos et al., 1979b).

In some cases, it may be necessary to prescribe a hypnotic drug as an adjunct to the overall management of transient insomnia (Soldatos et al., 1979b). The use of hypnotic medication may be effective for short-term reduction of physiological and emotional arousal (Kales et al., 1981). There is a risk, however, that the patient may develop the fear that he will not be able to sleep without his sleeping pill.

Barbiturates are not recommended because of a number of shortcomings. They interact with anticoagulants (Greenblatt and Shader, 1975), and they have a high potential for inducing drug-withdrawal insomnia (Kales et al., 1974a) and drug dependence. Most important, barbiturate overdoses are highly lethal. Benzodiazepines, on the other hand, have a very wide therapeutic window and can be used with relative safety. Most of them are effective for a period of one to two weeks (Kales et al., 1977a), which is the usual length of treatment for transient insomnia. Nevertheless, not all benzodiazepines are alike. Those with shorter half lives have been shown to produce rebound insomnia even after they have been given in single nightly doses at therapeutic levels for short periods of time (Kales et al., 1978). Long-acting benzodiazepine hypnotics, however, may impair performance during the day following their bedtime administration (Oswald et al., 1979; Church and Johnson, 1979); short-acting drugs, however, have not been systematically evaluated for this side effect. Certain benzodiazepines may also induce anterograde amnesia (Bixler et al., 1979; Kales et al., 1976c) and others have simply not proven to be very efficacious, even with short-term administration (Bixler et al., 1978).

The clinician needs to be aware of the side effects of benzodiazepines, and he should instruct his patients accordingly (Kales et al., 1981). When shorter-acting benzodiazepines are prescribed, tapering the dosage before complete withdrawal should minimize the difficulty with rebound insomnia. Impairment of memory or daytime performance will be avoided if patients are made aware of their potential occurrence with certain benzodiazepines and know that they should avoid tasks that require heightened memory or performance capabilities.

Over-the-counter hypnotics are not a satisfactory alternative to prescribed hypnotic drugs. Claims that they effectively induce or maintain sleep have not been verified in the sleep laboratory (Kales et al., 1971; Soldatos et al., 1978). Moreover, those containing scopolamine not only lack proven effectiveness, but also can be hazardous since even in the recommended dose range they may precipitate acute glaucoma, especially in elderly patients who have a narrow corneal-iris angle. Higher than recommended doses of these compounds have, at times, produced transient disorientation and hallucinations (Bernstein and Leff, 1967).

On occasion, other drugs may be used for transient insomnia. For example, antidepressants may be prescribed when symptoms of depression are clearly present. The use of other drugs for the treatment of insomnia, however, usually applies to the treatment of persistent rather than of transient insomnia.

PERSISTENT INSOMNIA

The successful treatment of persistent insomnia is a difficult task. The chronic insomniac who presents to the family physician often appears to have a monosymptomatic problem that consists solely of insomnia. The patient gives this impression because of his strong denial of underlying psychological conflicts, and because he has incorporated his insomnia problem into his lifestyle, which usually provides considerable secondary gain. For these reasons, the patient's efforts at helping himself not only fail to alleviate his sleeplessness, but actually aggravate the condition. The more the patient tries to "help" himself, the more disappointed and upset he becomes by not being able to solve his problem. Also, when he seeks medical assistance, he does so in a way that almost always precludes a successful treatment outcome. Thus, more anxiety is generated, which in turn intensifies the insomnia.

In treating chronic insomnia, then, the psychiatrist keeps in mind the disorder's multidimensional nature: any approach that treats only one of the factors involved will usually be unsuccessful. In general, the most effective treatment combines the following elements: (1) general measures for improving personal health habits, (2) supportive, insight-oriented, and/or behavioral psychotherapies, and (3) appropriate, adjunctive use of pharmacotherapy (antidepressant or hypnotic medication) (Kales et al., 1981; Soldatos et al., 1979b; Kales et al., 1974b).

In treating the psychological aspects of chronic insomnia, the psychiatrist needs to be active and direct in exploring conflict areas rather than using a gradual, uncovering approach (Soldatos et al., 1979b; Kales et al., 1974b). Insomniacs tend to reject the reality that psychological conflicts underlie their sleep disorder. Instead, they focus on the somatic aspects of their problem and are mainly interested in symptomatic relief. These patients are more likely to become actively involved in therapy if areas of psychological conflict are delineated early in treatment.

Insight-oriented psychotherapeutic techniques may help to delineate and resolve the conflicts that frequently underlie insomnia and its development (Soldatos et al., 1979b; Kales et al., 1974b). A chronic insomniac may fear going to bed because of suppressed memories of traumatic events and experiences in childhood that were associated with sleep or bedtime. Also, insomniacs often have difficulty expressing and controlling their aggressive feelings. Going to sleep may represent a loss of control, and insomnia is a defense against this fear. Psychodynamic therapy provides a means for dealing with the unexpressed psychological conflicts and emotions that predispose the patient to emotional and physiological arousal at night (Kales et al., 1981). Getting the depressed person in touch with anger, and restoring the balance of outwardly expressed versus self-restrained aggression during the day, can be important tasks of treatment that will reduce nighttime emotional release and the resulting arousal at bedtime.

When insomnia becomes chronic, the patient's lifestyle, particularly his interaction with those close to him, usually changes significantly through the course of illness. These problems with interpersonal relations, although partly a result of the insomnia itself, are closely interwoven with the patient's unresolved psychological conflicts, and in this way are intimately tied to both the development and persistence of chronic insomnia.

For example, insomniac patients may experience sexual difficulties, such as avoidance of sexual relations or unsatisfying attempts at sexual intercourse. These problems may relate to a fear of aggressive impulses, or they could represent an attempt to control or manipulate the spouse through the insomnia, i.e. the patient is "too tired to have sex." In these cases, conjoint marital therapy along with sexual counseling is indicated (Soldatos et al., 1979b; Kales et al., 1974b).

Behavioral treatment can be beneficial, particularly in patients with difficulty falling asleep. Relaxation training combined with suggested pleasant imagery has a therapeutic effect since it focuses the thoughts of the insomniac patient on a positive or neutral theme (Montgomery et al., 1975). This helps the patient to avoid rumination by shifting his attention from the internal to the external. Thus, patterned thinking replaces the ruminative concerns that maintain the insomniac's high levels of cognitive arousal. Another advantage of behavioral therapy is the individual's active participation in achieving relaxation, which gives him a sense of mastery and reduces his feelings of passivity and helplessness.

Whenever hypnotic medication is considered for the treatment of chronic insomnia, it is always an adjunct to the main therapeutic endeavors (Soldatos et al., 1979b; Kales et al., 1974b; Kales et al., 1980a). The guidelines for using hypnotic medication in transient insomnia also apply to the treatment of chronic insomnia. An additional consideration is whether the hypnotic drug to be used continues to be effective beyond short-term administration (Kales et al., 1977a).

Only two hypnotics, nitrazepam (Adam et al., 1976) and flurazepam (Kales et al., 1976a; Kales et al., 1975b) to date have been reported to be effective beyond a two-week period. (Nitrazepam is not available in the United States.) In most patients, treatment should be initiated with a dose of 15 mg of flurazepam at bedtime. If the 15 mg dose does not sufficiently improve sleep after one to two weeks, the dose can be increased to 30 mg (Soldatos et al., 1979b; Kales et al., 1974b). Increasing the dose in older people as well as in people who are known to have impaired drug metabolism should be avoided or cautiously implemented, since accumulation of active drug metabolites is more likely in these individuals (Kales et al., 1980a; Salzman et al., 1975). In general, patients taking flurazepam should be alerted to possible decrements in their daytime performance (Oswald et al., 1979; Church and Johnson, 1979; Kales et al., 1980a).

On the first and second nights following withdrawal of flurazepam, sleep is still significantly improved (Kales et al., 1976a), whereas the withdrawal of most hypnotic drugs leads to an immediate return of sleep difficulty to predrug levels, or in some cases, to rebound insomnia (Kales et al., 1978). This carryover effectiveness of flurazepam facilitates withdrawal from the drug.

The proper use of anxiolytics or antidepressants is effective in relieving the anxiety or depression underlying insomnia, and their sedative side effects help to ameliorate the sleeplessness itself (Kales et al., 1981; Soldatos et al., 1979b; Kales et al., 1974b). When insomnia is secondary to anxiety states, anxiolytic benzodiazepine drugs (e.g. clorazepate, chlordiazepoxide, diazepam, or lorazepam) are indicated both for the daytime anxiety and, in an increased bedtime dose, for the sleep difficulty. Insomnia associated with agitated depression should be treated with an antidepressant that has a sedative side effect (e.g. amitriptyline or doxepin). Administration of most or even all of the daily dose of the sedative antidepressant at bedtime not only alleviates sleeplessness, but also reduces the likelihood of daytime sleepiness.

Antidepressant medication can be most effective in treating insomnia if the following shortcomings are avoided: failing to attain a sufficient dose level, producing undesired daytime sedation, and inducing impairment of daytime performance. A major problem with the tricyclic antidepressants that have sedating side effects is that many patients are given too much of their medication during the day rather than at bedtime (Kales et al., 1975a). The tricyclic antidepressants have immediate sedative side effects, while the antidepressant effect is more likely to occur after about two weeks. Confusing the side effects of these drugs with their basic action may account for undesired daytime sedation, difficulty in attaining a sufficient total daily dose, and inappropriate adjustment of the daytime-to-bedtime dose ratio. While a large initial dose of a sedative tricyclic antidepressant is usually desirable, the nightly dose should be increased gradually. This prevents the development of severe decrements in performance the following day, as is often the case when a sedative tricyclic is initiated in a bedtime dose of 50–100 mg (Kales et al., 1981). Unless the patient has previously tolerated high doses of such medication, initiation of the antidepressant with a 25 mg dose followed by 25 mg increments is usually best tolerated.

For the treatment of insomnia associated with schizophrenic psychosis or the manic phase of manic-depressive psychosis, neuroleptics with sedative properties, such as chlorpromazine, are preferable (Kales et al., 1981; Soldatos et al., 1979b; Kales et al., 1974b). A larger bedtime dose is usually effective in controlling the patient's sleeplessness and avoids the need for hypnotics. Nevertheless, it should be noted that even when a nonsedative neuroleptic is administered, sleep that is disordered by psychosis often returns to normal with remission of the psychosis.

Certain drugs may contribute to the development and persistence of insomnia. The amphetamines and methylphenidate generally cause sleeplessness, as do other CNS stimulants that are used to suppress appetite, control narcolepsy, or for other purposes. When taken chronically, these drugs lose their therapeutic effectiveness, and larger doses are required to preserve the same treatment outcome. Some patients take extremely high daily doses of CNS stimulants and/or take their medication too close to bedtime. These patients are more likely to develop insomnia (Kales et al., 1981; Soldatos et al., 1979b). If treatment with stimulants is necessary, the starting dose should be as low as possible and increases should be avoided. Also, the patient should be instructed to take the last dose before 5:00 p.m. In patients taking large doses of CNS stimulants that are ineffective, withdrawal should be gradual and very carefully supervised.

Drugs other than those known as classic CNS stimulants also have stimulant properties (Kales et al., 1981; Soldatos et al., 1979b). These include steroid preparations, beta adrenergic blockers, and bronchodilating drugs, as well as substances used for nonmedical purposes, such as coffee (Karacan et al., 1976), colas, and cigarettes (Soldatos et al., 1980). Also, tranylcypromine, an MAO inhibitor, is structurally quite similar to amphetamine and can cause insomnia if given too close to bedtime. Minimizing the daily dose of any of these drugs or substances and avoiding them close to bedtime will be very helpful.

NARCOLEPSY

The disorders of excessive sleepiness are narcolepsy and the various hypersomnias, including those associated with sleep apnea. The narcoleptic tetrad includes sleep attacks and the three auxiliary symptoms of cataplectic attacks, sleep paralysis and hypnagogic hallucinations (Yoss and

Daly, 1957; Zarcone, 1973; Daly and Yoss, 1974; Dement et al., 1976; Roth, 1976; Soldatos et al., 1979a). For the treatment of excessive sleepiness and sleep attacks, stimulants are indicated. Methylphenidate is recommended because of its prompt action and the relatively low incidence of side effects (Yoss and Daly, 1957; Daly and Yoss, 1974). The initial dose should be 5 mg t.i.d., with the last dose given at about 5:00 p.m.; depending on the outcome, the dose may be increased. Some narcoleptic patients respond more favorably to the amphetamines. The best tolerated of the amphetamines, and one with few sympathomimetic side effects, is methamphetamine (Daly and Yoss, 1974). Patients taking methamphetamine are initially given 10 mg upon arising in the morning; this dose is then gradually increased until the appropriate level is reached.

Patients with mild narcolepsy may avoid using stimulant medication by scheduling therapeutic naps and arranging their daily activities around these naps (Soldatos et al., 1979a). This is particularly practical for the patient who is not employed. In other patients, even limited use of naps may decrease the required total daily dose of stimulant drug. The psychiatrist needs to be aware, however, that the prolonged use of amphetamines may induce severe irritability, paranoid tendencies, or even frank psychosis (Soldatos et al., 1979a; Segal and Janowsky, 1978).

For the auxiliary symptoms of narcolepsy, the medication of choice is a tricyclic antidepressant; imipramine is most frequently used (Zarcone, 1973; Solatos et al., 1979a; Akimoto et al., 1960; Hishikawa et al., 1966; Rechtschaffen and Dement, 1969). In controlling cataplexy, the most common auxiliary symptom, imipramine has a much more rapid onset of action and is effective at lower doses compared with its use in treating depression. While the drug is quite effective in controlling cataplexy, it does not usually reduce sleep attacks.

When a patient complains of both sleep attacks and auxiliary symptoms, treatment with a stimulant and imipramine may be combined. This combination may produce serious side effects such as hypertension. Therefore, drug administration must be carefully titrated and monitored (Soldatos et al., 1979a).

Supportive psychotherapy is helpful as an adjunct to the basic pharmacologic treatment of narcolepsy since its overall management is facilitated by alleviation of the serious psychosocial consequences of the disorder. Narcoleptics often are considered by their family, friends, fellow employees, and employers as being lazy, malingering, or psychologically disturbed (Soldatos et al., 1979a; Rechtschaffen and Dement, 1969). The physician must inform the patient and the individuals who are central to his family, social, and occupational lives that the sleep attacks and other symptoms are irresistible and beyond the patient's control.

The patient should be aware of the potential risks of long-distance driving or other activities that would expose him to danger if a sleep attack or cataplectic episode were to occur (Yoss and Daly, 1957; Soldatos et al., 1979a). Nevertheless, the psychiatrist should not be overly restrictive of the patient's activities. Warnings should not exceed those warranted by the clinical course of the illness before, and especially after, treatment. Finally, side effects of the prescribed medication should be thoroughly covered with the patient and his family.

HYPERSOMNIA AND SLEEP APNEA

The hypersomnias or disorders of excessive daytime sleepiness include transient hypersomnia and persistent hypersomnia. Excessive daytime sleepiness, or hypersomnolence, is also a prominent symptom in sleep apnea. Therefore, sleep apnea is also discussed in this section although the presence of this condition would warrant a separate diagnosis.

TRANSIENT HYPERSOMNIA

It is not known why some individuals react to an environmental change or to a stressful situation with excessive daytime somnolence while others develop insomnia. In some cases, daytime somnolence is the result of inadequate sleep at night. Thus, a condition that causes insomnia may indirectly cause daytime sleepiness as well, although insomniacs more frequently experience a sense of fatigue.

Most often, no special treatment is required for transient hypersomnia. It usually subsides when adaptation to the environmental change is achieved or when the stressful situation is overcome. The psychiatrist should therefore try to strengthen the patient's coping mechanisms if the stress-generating situation cannot be eliminated. Depending on the individual's psychological difficulties, some form of psychotherapy may be used. For example, helping the patient to become more assertive can alleviate a problem of hypersomnia that is secondary to an avoidance of life stresses. On the other hand, psychological difficulties stemming from the patient's family relations would require family therapy.

In general, symptomatic treatment using stimulant drugs should be avoided. If it is necessary for the patient to be fully alert throughout the day, however, a daily dose of 10 mg methylphenidate can be given for a period of only a few days or on a p.r.n. basis. Increasing the dose should be avoided to minimize the potential for dependence and other consequences of the chronic administration of methylphenidate. Stimulants should not be taken close to bedtime because they may lead to disturbed nocturnal sleep, which will further complicate the problem of daytime somnolence.

PERSISTENT HYPERSOMNIA

Persistent hypersomnia may be idiopathic, psychogenic, periodic, or secondary to organic conditions (Zarcone, 1973; Roth, 1976; Rechtschaffen and Dement, 1969; Broughton, 1971; Sours, 1963). Psychogenic hypersomnia is usually related to a depressive disorder (Detre et al., 1972; Kupfer et al., 1972). The Kleine-Levin syndrome, the best-known type of periodic hypersomnia, is associated with excessive appetite and is most often seen in adolescent males (Critchley and Hoffman, 1942). Excessive sleepiness related to sleep apnea is a type of hypersomnia secondary to an organic condition (Lugaresi et al., 1972; Dement et al., 1978; Guilleminault et al., 1978). Other types of organic hypersomnia are related to brain dysfunction due to tumors, vascular lesions, infections, or toxic encephalopathies, endocrine conditions, and metabolic disorders (Broughton, 1971).

It is essential to differentiate between persistent hypersomnia of the idiopathic type and narcolepsy. The periods of excessive daytime sleepiness and sleep attacks of idiopathic hypersomnia are usually longer than those associated with narcolepsy; they may last up to one or more hours (Zarcone, 1973; Dement et al., 1976; Roth, 1976; Soldatos et al., 1979a; Rechtschaffen and Dement, 1969; Broughton, 1971). Also, hypersomniacs' nocturnal sleep is often prolonged, but otherwise it is not disturbed. Another occasional but striking symptom of persistent idiopathic hypersomnia is sleep drunkenness, a condition of difficulty in fully awakening in the morning that lasts from 15 minutes to about an hour (Roth et al., 1972).

The psychiatrist should educate the hypersomniac patient and his family regarding the symptomatology of hypersomnia and clarify any misconceptions they may have about the disorder. Supportive, and less frequently, insight-oriented psychotherapy may be helpful for certain patients with hypersomnia.

Stimulant drugs are indicated for treating the excessive daytime sleepiness, prolonged nocturnal sleep, and sleep drunkenness of idiopathic hypersomnia (Rechtschaffen and Dement, 1969; Roth et al., 1972). They may also be used during the phases of excessive sleep in periodic hypersomnia. Methylphenidate is the drug of choice, primarily because of its prompt action and few side effects. For sleep drunkenness, a family member awakens the patient and gives the dose about an hour before the desired time of arising. For excessive daytime sleepiness, drug administration is scheduled according to the patient's needs for heightened vigilance.

In psychogenic hypersomnia, when endogenous or characterological depression is considered the primary difficulty, nonsedating tricyclic antidepressants, such as imipramine or protriptyline, are indicated (Kales and Soldatos, in press). Lithium can be used to treat the hypersomniac patient in a depressive phase of a bipolar disorder, whereas the patient with an "atypical" depression may respond more favorably to an MAO inhibitor. The sedating tricyclics are generally contraindicated.

Hypersomnia Associated with Sleep Apnea

In treating sleep apnea, the total syndrome is addressed rather than simply treating the specific symptom of daytime hypersomnolence. Sleep apnea has been classified into three types: central, peripheral, and mixed. Because the characteristic presentation of sleep apnea often includes sleepiness and sleep attacks, this disorder is confused with narcolepsy unless a careful history and appropriate sleep laboratory examination are obtained. Questioning the spouse, parent, or other family members for the presence of snoring with interrupted nocturnal breathing is important in diagnosing sleep apnea. The physician determines if there are frequent periods of interrupted nocturnal breathing associated with snoring, gasping, gurgling, choking, periodic loud snorting, or morning headache. Other associated symptoms that should alert the physician to the possibility of sleep apnea are: essential hypertension, loss of libido, sexual impotence, and secondary enuresis (Guilleminault et al., 1978)

The snoring associated with sleep apnea is unique: periods of suspended respiration of more than ten seconds are followed by very loud and abrupt snorting sounds that are two to four seconds in duration. The common type of snoring in nonapneic individuals is not as loud; it fluctuates in intensity and is continuous, without any gaps of appreciable duration (Lugaresi et al., 1975).

When sleep apnea occurs in overweight patients, weight reduction as a first means of treatment, although helpful is some cases, must not replace treatment for the life-threatening aspect of this disorder (i.e., intermittent nocturnal hypoxia and cardiac arrhythmias). Tracheostomy is in most cases of severe obstructive sleep apnea the treatment of choice. The results obtained from a modified tracheostomy (i.e., open during sleep and closed during wakefulness) are almost invariably effective in treating the sleep apnea and excessive daytime sleepiness (Coccagna et al., 1972; Lugaresi et al., 1973; Tilkian et al., 1976).

Both before and after tracheostomy, the psychiatrist needs to be aware that the obstructive sleep apnea itself and its ultimate treatment, tracheostomy, can have profound psychosocial consequences for the patient and can significantly alter his postoperative lifestyle and level of functioning. During the illness, these patients and their families are appropriately concerned about the life-threatening consequences of the disorder as well as the severe disability it causes in daily functioning. Thus, the family needs reassurance and support in the decision-making process that leads to effective treatment. After treatment with tracheostomy, which often produces striking improvement, the physician needs to encourage the patient to resume a normal level of functioning, and should support him and his family so that a smooth transition will be made in an appropriate period of time.

As yet, an effective treatment for central sleep apnea has not been well established. Imipramine, and particularly chlorimipramine (not available in the United States), may be somewhat effective (Guilleminault et al., 1978). Medroxyprogesterone acetate may also be somewhat effective (Strohl et al., 1981). Diaphragmatic pacing has also been studied but may lead to degenerative lesions of the phrenic nerve.

DISORDERS OF THE SLEEP-WAKE SCHEDULE

Rapid changes between time zones ("jet lag") and shifts in customary sleep-wake schedules upset internal biological rhythms and cause a transient syndrome of insomnia, excessive daytime somnolence, psychomotor impairment, anxiety, depression, and various somatic complaints (Siegel et al., 1969; Weitzman et al., 1970). This syndrome lasts a few days while the internal biological rhythms adjust to the new environment and/or to the new sleep-wake schedule.

Special treatment is seldom required for transient disruption of sleep-wake patterns. Simply educating and reassuring the patient will be helpful. The patient may be informed that adhering to the new time zone schedules can accelerate the adaptation process, although napping when sleepy for a few days is both sensible and comfortable. When aberration of the sleep-wakefulness schedule is chronic, resynchronization to a consistent, 24-hour, rest-activity schedule should be advised by the clinician.

SLEEPWALKING AND NIGHT TERRORS

These two conditions have many similar etiological, clinical, and physiological characteristics (Kales et al., 1980b; Kales et al., 1980c; Kales et al., 1980d). Both sleepwalking and night terrors begin in childhood and are usually outgrown before adulthood (Kales et al., 1980c; Kales et al., 1980d), and the episodes of both disorders occur out of slow-wave sleep (Gastaut and Broughton, 1964; Jacobson et al., 1965; Kales et al., 1966; Fisher et al., 1973a; Fisher et al., 1974) and are typically associated with impaired arousal (Broughton, 1968). Further, development of these disorders in childhood and adolescence is related to a maturational/developmental lag (Kales et al., 1980c; Kales et al., 1980d; Kales et al., 1966), but when they persist or begin in adulthood, psychological factors are more prominent (Kales et al., 1980c; Kales et al., 1980d). Finally, the same patient may present with both conditions or may initially have somnambulism and later develop or change to having night terrors. Thus, the two conditions have been considered as two different manifestations of the same pathophysiological substrate, with sleepwalking being the more frequent and less severe condition (Kales et al., 1980b; Kales et al., 1980c; Kales et al., 1980d). From a practical point of view, management of sleepwalking and night terrors is similar.

Safety measures are essential for patients with night terrors as well as for sleepwalkers (Kales et al., 1980c; Kales et al., 1980d; Kales and Kales, 1970; Kales and Kales, 1974). Safety measures include latches for outside doors, accommodations for sleeping on the ground floor, and special locks or bolts for bedroom windows. Episodes of either condition should not be interrupted if previous interference has caused more confusion and fright.

Parents need to be reassured that their children will probably outgrow the condition and are not psychologically disturbed (Kales et al., 1980c; Kales et al., 1980d; Kales and Kales, 1970; Kales and Kales, 1974). On the other hand, underlying psychopathology is suggested when the conditions begin after age 10–12, when they occur frequently over a lengthy period of time, when there is a negative family history of either disorder, or when the onset of the conditions appears to be related to major life-stress events (Kales et al., 1980c; Kales et al., 1980d). Although adults who sleepwalk or have night terrors may also have had a delay in CNS maturation, psychological factors appear to be more important in the condition's development, and particularly in the persistence of sleepwalking and night terrors in adults.

MMPI profiles of sleepwalkers are consistent with active, outwardly directed, aggressive behavioral patterns (Kales et al., 1980c). Patients who have similar profiles commonly struggle to deal with life's frustrations and become extremely angry when frustrated. Excessive anger in response to frustration, failure, or loss of self-esteem is directed outward rather than at the self, as is the case in depression. Sleepwalkers typically cope in an externally directed manner rather than struggling internally with distress.

Insight-oriented psychotherapy may be beneficial for these patients. The psychological profiles of these patients suggest an approach in which the psychiatrist assists the patient in developing more constructive reactions to frustration (Kales et al., 1981). The psychiatrist helps the patient learn to identify and appropriately discharge feelings of frustration and anger so that he no longer needs to respond with aggression. The sleepwalker can be taught to think of a sleepwalking episode as a cue or indication that he is not dealing with an important, current frustration. In

essence, he tries to identify disturbing issues that may provoke an episode and are so troublesome and distressing that he avoids dealing with
them. It should be noted that controlled studies are needed to demonstrate the efficacy of insight-oriented psychotherapy for patients with
sleepwalking.

Psychological factors also contribute considerably to the development
and persistence of night terrors in adulthood (Kales et al., 1980d). Unlike
sleepwalkers, however, adults with night terrors tend to inhibit outward
expression of aggression, and their personality patterns are dominated
by anxiety, depression, phobic tendencies, and a secondary "schizoid"
self-negativity in the absence of overt psychoticism. Night terror patients' inability to express aggression may lead to the aggression being
directed inward, thereby precipitating night terror events that consist of
extreme defensiveness and fighting behavior that further frightens the
patients.

Since the adult with night terrors is conditioned to react to stress with
fear and apprehension, insight-oriented psychotherapy may be beneficial. Our clinical experience suggests that positive results may be gained
by using such psychotherapeutic approaches as actively exploring fears
of failure and hostility as well as apprehension of the night terror event
itself (Kales et. al., 1981). Furthermore, strengthening the patient's self-
assertiveness may help to counteract fears of hostility and anxieties over
how others will react if the patient experiences failures in life. Assuming
that night terrors discharge accumulated anxiety and fear, the patient
should appreciate the advantage of dealing with the anxiety, however
distressing, in psychotherapy, rather than discharging it during sleep.
Finally, if the fear is phobic, then desensitization and direct, implosive
exaggeration of the phobia may be useful. It should be noted, however,
that no controlled research evidence is yet available to document the
effectiveness of these techniques in treating night terrors.

Although benzodiazepine drugs that suppress slow-wave sleep, such
as diazepam (Kales et al., 1969), are effective in reducing the frequency
of night terror events (Fisher et al., 1973b), withdrawal usually leads to
a relapse. It is not clear whether diazepam's effectiveness in reducing
night terror events is related to its suppression of stage 4 sleep or to its
general anxiolytic properties (Fisher et al., 1973b).

Imipramine's effectiveness in reducing the frequency of sleepwalking
or night terror episodes has not been clearly established (Pesikoff and
Davis, 1971; Tec, 1974). The mechanism of a potential effect would not

be related to the drug's antidepressant action, nor would it be related to slow-wave sleep suppression, since imipramine does not significantly change slow-wave sleep. Any effectiveness of imipramine would probably relate to the fact that it increases wakefulness during the night, thus minimizing the potential for an arousal disorder that ordinarily occurs out of stages 3 and 4 sleep (Kales et al., 1977b).

Drug treatment, especially in children, should be used only when a reduction in the frequency of night terrors or sleepwalking is absolutely necessary. With children, the psychiatrist needs to prescribe medication cautiously and for very limited periods, since the long-term effects of psychotropic drugs on children's development is not known.

OTHER DYSFUNCTIONS OF SLEEP OR AROUSAL FROM SLEEP

NIGHTMARES

Nightmares are nocturnal episodes of intense anxiety and fear associated with a vivid and emotionally charged dream experience. They are a serious source of sleep disruption since spontaneous awakenings from nightmares often are associated with prolonged wakefulness. Nightmares, which occur in REM sleep, should be differentiated from night terrors, which occur in slow-wave sleep (stage 3 and 4). The night terror episode, in comparison with the nightmare, is accompanied by much more anxiety, vocalization, motility, and autonomic discharge, and there is much less recall (Gastaut and Broughton, 1964; Fisher et al., 1973a; Fisher et al., 1974; Broughton, 1968; Kales and Kales, 1974; Kanner, 1972).

Psychological factors play a major role in the development and maintenance of nightmares (Kales et al., 1980e). Adults who have nightmares show high levels of psychopathology; they are distrustful, alienated, and have chronically schizoid patterns of adjustment, but are usually not psychotic or paranoid. Chronic nightmares can be considered secondary to long-term schizoid adjustments in which the patient is consistently unable to deal with interpersonal hostility and resentment. When the excessive hostility resulting from intensely neurotic object relations is not entirely discharged in everyday life, it may be carried over and released in the nightmare. The nightmare is a vehicle not only for discharging unreleased hostility, but also for the extinction of unexpressed anger and generally negative emotionality. When this emotionality is finally expressed in the nightmare, it provokes anxiety.

Quite often, hypnotic drug withdrawal is associated with intense dreaming. If this is the case, the patient should understand the nature of his nightmares and should be instructed how to gradually withdraw from the medication (Kales et al., 1974a).

In childhood no psychiatric treatment is necessary, since nightmares are a common manifestation of emotional maturation and simply reflect the child's temporary difficulty in distinguishing reality from fantasy. Chronic nightmares in adulthood require psychiatric therapy, however, since there is usually considerable psychopathology (Kales et al., 1980e). Since monosymptomatic conditions, such as chronic fears and phobias, are seldom responsible for nightmares, behavioral treatment is applied infrequently. Based on our clinical experience, insight-oriented psychotherapies are more likely to be effective in the majority of cases.

A sound therapeutic relationship should be developed as early as possible in therapy, because distrustfulness and alienation are often present in the nightmare patient and the likelihood of his suddenly terminating treatment is very high (Kales et al., 1981). A subsequent therapeutic task is to have the patient achieve a better understanding of his emotions, particularly his anger. This would enable him to more efficiently cope with his emotions, rather than becoming excessively frustrated and discharging incompletely expressed resentments in his nightmares.

Although there is a schizoid adjustment in the nightmare sufferer's lifestyle, schizophrenic psychosis is rarely present (Kales et al., 1980e). When overt psychosis is associated with the presence of nightmares, however, the physician should proceed with the indicated antipsychotic treatment. Finally, the physician should be alert for the presence of depression, especially in men who have nightmares (Hartmann and Russ, 1979), since the nightmare patient tends to avoid professional help and thus a suicidal potential may go unnoticed (Kales et al., 1980e).

ENURESIS

The term "enuresis" refers to bedwetting that occurs after control of urinary bladder should have been acquired. In primary enuresis, the child has never been dry for more than one or two weeks. In secondary enuresis, he may be dry for several weeks, months, or years before enuresis begins.

In primary enuresis, genetic (Hallgren, 1960; Bakwin, 1971) and developmental/maturational (Starfield, 1967; Experanca and Gerrard, 1969), factors underlie the disorder, while in secondary enuresis, psychological factors are usually causative (Kanner, 1972). From a developmental standpoint, children with primary enuresis have a smaller functional bladder capacity (Starfield, 1967; Experanca and Gerrard, 1969). Psychological factors related to secondary enuresis may reflect a need to regress or a need for excessive attention, for example, at the time of birth of a new sibling. It also should be noted that bed-wetting may be a symptom of diabetes mellitus, diabetes insipidus, nocturnal epilepsy, or severe mental retardation (Starfield, 1972).

The psychiatrist should acquaint the parents of children who have primary enuresis with the need for tolerance, patience, and understanding of their child's disorder (Kales and Kales, 1974). Parental mishandling of the situation can result in guilt and anxiety being imposed on the child, and psychological problems may be created.

Since the functional bladder capacity of children with primary enuresis is small, bladder training exercises are often used to increase the bladder's capacity (Starfield, 1967; Starfield, 1972). The child drinks as much fluid as he can during the day and tries to keep from urinating as long as possible. This exercise gives the child a feeling of mastery and, by stretching the bladder, increases its capacity. Besides being useful in young children, bladder training exercises can help adolescents and adults to achieve mastery of bladder functioning. Subsequently, insight-oriented psychotherapy may help these patients to attain permanent dryness.

The management of secondary enuresis usually involves the use of various psychotherapies that are determined by the psychological basis of the problem. Family therapy, individual therapy for the parents and child, behavioral therapy, or simply educating and instructing the parents, are each helpful if appropriately applied by the psychiatrist. In adults secondary enuresis that is unrelated to any organic factors is treated with insight-oriented psychotherapy by most psychiatrists.

Imipramine has been shown to significantly reduce the frequency of enuretic events (Pouissaint and Ditman, 1965; Miller et al., 1968; Shaffer et al., 1968). While enuretic frequency is markedly reduced with medication, the relapse rate is high after withdrawal (Miller et al., 1968; Shaffer et al., 1968). Use of the drug is recommended only in older children, adolescents, or adults, and then for only limited periods of time and in special situations. It has not been established whether the drug is more effective for primary or secondary enuresis.

The FDA-approved dose for treating enuresis is 1.0 to 2.5 mg/kg per day, or 25–75 mg daily (Hayes et al., 1975). Treatment with imipramine is initiated with a dose of 25 mg one or two hours before bedtime, and this dose is then gradually increased to a therapeutic level. Imipramine should not be prescribed on a long-term basis since the effects of long-term administration of psychotropic medications in children have not been determined.

CONCLUSION

Most sleep disorders can be diagnosed and treated by physicians in the office setting. When cases of chronic or intractable sleep problems are referred to the psychiatrist, they can most often be evaluated and treated through the use of basic psychiatric and medical skills supplemented by a thorough knowledge of the various types of sleep difficulty. The use of expensive and time-consuming sleep laboratory procedures is only rarely helpful. In general, patients should be evaluated with electrophysiological recordings only when (1) sleep apnea is suspected, (2) narcolepsy is suspected but auxiliary symptoms, especially cataplexy, are not present, or (3) organic impotence needs to be differentiated from psychogenic sexual difficulty.

The physician is equipped with the basic skills and can acquire the knowledge needed to diagnose and treat sleep disorders, but cannot be a fully effective practitioner without a succinct and practical diagnostic classification. In this chapter, we propose such a classification of sleep disorders and discuss their treatment in a way that should aid the physician in providing effective management of patients with sleep disturbances.

REFERENCES

International Classification of Diseases, 9th Revision, Clinical Modification (ICD-9-CM). WHO Center for Classification of Diseases for North America. National Center for Health Statistics. Edwards Brothers Inc., Ann Arbor, Michigan, 1978.

Diagnostic Classification of Sleep and Arousal Disorders, Association of Sleep Disorders Centers. Sleep. 2:1–137, 1979.

Adam K, Adamson L, Brezinova V, Hunter WM, Oswald I: Nitrazepam: lastingly effective but trouble on withdrawal. Brit Med J. 1:1558–1560, 1976.

Akimoto H, Honda Y, Takahashi Y: Pharmacotherapy in narcolepsy. Dis Nerv Syst. 21:704–706, 1960.

Bakwin H: Enuresis in twins. Am J Dis Child. 121:222–225, 1971.

Bernstein S, Leff R: Toxic psychosis from sleeping medicine containing scopolamine. N Engl J Med. 277:638–639, 1967.

Bixler EO, Kales A, Soldatos CR, Scharf MB, Kales JD: Effectiveness of temazepam with short-, intermediate-, and long-term use: sleep laboratory evaluation. J Clin Pharmacol. 2&3: 110–118, 1978.

Bixler EO, Scharf MB, Soldatos CR, Mitsky DJ, Kales A: Effects of hypnotic drugs on memory. Life Sci. 25:1379–1388, 1979.

Broughton R: Neurology and sleep research. Can Psychiat Assoc J. 16:283–293, 1971.

Broughton RJ: Sleep disorders: disorders of arousal? Science. 159:1070–1078, 1968.

Church MW, Johnson LC: Mood and performance of poor sleepers during repeated use of flurazepam. Psychopharmacology. 61:309–316, 1979.

Coccagna G, Mantovani M, Brignani F, Parchi C, Lugaresi E: Tracheostomy in hypersomnia with periodic breathing. Bull Physiopathol Respir. 8:1217–1227, 1972.

Coursey RD, Buchsbaum M, Frankel BL: Personality measures and evoked responses in chronic insomniacs. J Abnorm Psychol. 84:239–249, 1975.

Critchley M, Hoffman HL: The syndrome of periodic somnolence and morbid hunger (Kleine-Levin Syndrome). Brit Med J (suppl), pp. 137–139, 1942.

Daly DD, Yoss RE: Narcolepsy. In: Handbook of Clinical Neurology, Vol. 15, The Epilepsies. Vinken PJ, Bruyn GW (eds). Volume edited by Magnus O, Lorentz De Haas AM. North-Holland, Amsterdam. pp. 836–852, 1974.

Dement WC, Carskadon MA, Guilleminault C, Zarcone VP: Narcolepsy: diagnosis and treatment. Primary Care. 3:609–623, 1976.

Dement WC, Carskadon MA, Richardson G: Excessive daytime sleepiness in the sleep apnea syndrome. In: Sleep Apnea Syndromes. Guilleminault C, Dement WC (eds). Alan R. Liss, New York. pp. 23–46, 1978.

Detre T, Himmelhoch J, Swartzburg M, Anderson CM, Byck R, Kupfer DJ: Hypersomnia and manic-depressive disease. Am J Psychiat. 128:123–125, 1972.

Experanca M, Gerrard JW: Nocturnal enuresis: studies in bladder function in normal children and enuretics. Can Med Assoc J. 101:324–327, 1969.

496

Fisher C, Kahn E, Edwards A, Davis D: A psychophysiological study of nightmares and night terrors I. Physiological aspects of the stage 4 night terror. J Nerv Ment Dis. 157:75–98, 1973a.

Fisher C, Kahn E, Edwards A, Davis D: A psychophysiological study of nightmares and night terrors: the suppression of stage 4 night terrors with diazepam. Arch Gen Psychiat. 28:252–259, 1973b.

Fisher C, Kahn E, Edwards A, Davis D: A psychophysiological study of nightmares and night terrors. Psychoanalysis and Contemporary Science. 3:317–398, 1974.

Gastaut H, Broughton R: A clinical and polygraphic study of episodic phenomena during sleep. Recent Advances in Biological Psychiatry. 7:197–220, 1964.

Greenblatt DJ, Shader RI: Drug interactions in psychopharmacology. In: Manual of Psychiatric Therapeutics. Shader, RI (ed). Little, Brown, Boston. pp. 269–279, 1975.

Guilleminault C, Van den Hoed J, Mitler MM: Clinical overview of the sleep apnea syndromes. In: Sleep Apnea Syndromes. Guilleminault C, Dement WC (eds). Alan R. Liss, New York. pp. 1–12, 1978.

Hallgren B: Nocturnal enuresis in twins. Acta Psychiat Scand (Suppl). 35:73–90, 1960.

Hartmann E, Russ D: Frequent nightmares and the vulnerability to schizophrenia: the personality of the nightmare sufferer. Psychol Bull. 15:10–12, 1979.

Hayes TA, Panitch ML, Barker E: Imipramine dosage in children: a comment on imipramine and electrocardiographic abnormalities in hyperactive children. Am J Psychiat. 132:546–547, 1975.

Hishikawa Y, Ida H, Nakai K, Kaneko Z: Treatment of narcolepsy with imipramine (Tofranil) and desmethylimipramine (Pertofran). J Neurol Sci. 3:453–461, 1966.

Jacobson A, Kales A, Lehmann D, Zweizig JR: Somnambulism: all night electroencephalographic studies. Science. 148:975–977, 1965.

Kales A, Kales JD: Evaluation, diagnosis and treatment of clinical conditions related to sleep. JAMA. 213:2229–2235, 1970.

Kales A, Kales JD: Sleep disorders: recent findings in the diagnosis and treatment of disturbed sleep. N Engl J Med. 290:487–499, 1974.

Kales A, Soldatos CR: Sleep disorders: description, assessment and treatment. In: Manual of Psychiatric Therapeutics. Shader RI (ed). Little, Brown, Boston (in press).

Kales A, Jacobson A, Paulson MJ, Kales JD, Walter RD: Somnambulism: Psychophysiological correlates I. All-night EEG studies. Arch Gen Psychiat. 14:586–594, 1966.

Kales A, Malmstrom EJ, Scharf MB, Rubin RT: Psychophysiological and biochemical changes following use and withdrawal of hypnotics. In: Sleep: Physiology and Pathology. Kales A (ed). Lippincott, Philadelphia. pp. 331–343, 1969.

Kales JD, Tan TL, Swearingen C, Kales A: Are over-the-counter sleep medications effective? All night EEG studies. Curr Ther Res. 13:143–151, 1971.

Kales A, Bixler EO, Tan TL, Scharf MB, Kales JD: Chronic hypnotic use:

ineffectiveness, drug withdrawal insomnia, and dependence. JAMA. 227:513–517, 1974a.

Kales A, Kales JD, Bixler EO: Insomnia: an approach to management and treatment. Psychiat Annals. 4:28–44, 1974b.

Kales A, Kales JD, Bixler EO, Martin E: Common shortcomings in the evaluation and treatment of insomnia. In: Hypnotics: Methods of Development and Evaluation. Kagan F, Harwood T, Rickels K, Rudzik A, Sorer H (eds). Spectrum, New York. pp. 29–40, 1975a.

Kales A, Kales JD, Bixler EO, Scharf MB: Effectiveness of hypnotic drugs with prolonged use: flurazepam and pentobarbital. Clin Pharmacol Ther. 18:356–363, 1975b.

Kales A, Bixler EO, Scharf MB, Kales JD: Sleep laboratory studies of flurazepam: a model for evaluating hypnotic drugs. Clin Pharmacol Ther. 19:576–583, 1976a.

Kales A, Caldwell AB, Preston TA, Healey S: Personality patterns in insomnia: theoretical implications. Arch Gen Psychiat. 33:1128–1134, 1976b.

Kales A, Kales JD, Bixler EO, Scharf MB, Russek E: Hypnotic efficacy of triazolam: sleep laboratory evaluation of intermediate-term effectiveness. J Clin Pharmacol. 8&9:399–406, 1976c.

Kales A, Bixler EO, Kales JD, Scharf MB: Comparative effectiveness of nine hypnotic drugs: sleep laboratory studies. J Clin Pharmacol. 17:207–213, 1977a.

Kales A, Kales JD, Jacobson A, Humphrey FJ, Soldatos CR: Effects of imipramine on enuretic frequency and sleep stages. Pediatrics. 60:431–436, 1977b.

Kales A, Scharf MB, Kales JD: Rebound insomnia: a new clinical syndrome. Science. 201:1039–1041, 1978.

Kales A, Kales JD, Scharf MB, Soldatos CR: Hypnotic drugs. In: Frequently Prescribed and Abused Drugs: Their Indications, Efficacy, and Rational Prescribing. Buchwald C, Cohen S, Katz D, Salmon J (eds). National Training System. Medical Monograph Series, Vol. II, No. 1. pp. 57–72, 1980a.

Kales A, Soldatos CR, Bixler EO, et al.: Hereditary factors in sleepwalking and night terrors. Brit J Psychiat. 137:111–118, 1980b.

Kales A, Soldatos CR, Caldwell AB, et al.: Somnambulism: clinical characteristics and personality patterns. Arch Gen Psychiat. 37:1406–1410, 1980c.

Kales JD, Kales A, Soldatos CR, Caldwell AB, Charney DS, Martin ED: Night terrors: clinical characteristics and personality patterns. Arch Gen Psychiat. 37:1413–1417, 1980d.

Kales A, Soldatos CR, Caldwell AB, et al.: Nightmares: clinical characteristics and personality patterns. Am J Psychiat. 137:1197–1201, 1980e.

Kales A, Soldatos CR, Kales J: Sleep disorders: office evaluation and management. In: American Handbook of Psychiatry, Vol. VII, 2nd ed. Arieti S, Brodie AKH (ed). Basic Books, New York. pp. 423–454, 1981.

Kanner L: Child Psychiatry, 4th ed. CC. Thomas, Springfield, Ill. 1972.

Karacan I, Thornby JI, Anch AM, Booth GH, Williams RL, Salis PJ: Dose related sleep disturbances induced by coffee and caffeine. Clin Pharmacol Ther. 20:682–689, 1976.

Kupfer DJ, Himmelhoch JM, Swartzburg M, Anderson C, Byck R, Detre TP: Hypersomnia in manic-depressive disease. Dis Nerv Syst. 33:720–724, 1972.

Lugaresi E, Coccagna G, Mantovani M, Cirignotta F, Ambrosetto G, Baturic P: Hypersomnia with periodic breathing: periodic apneas and alveolar hypoventilation during sleep. Bull Physiopathol Respir. 8:1103–1113, 1972.

Lugaresi E, Coccagna G, Mantovani M, Brignani F: Effects of tracheostomy in two cases of hypersomnia with periodic breathing. J Neurol Neurosurg Psychiat. 36:15–26, 1973.

Lugaresi E, Coccagna G, Farneti P, Manatovani M, Cirignotta F: Snoring. Electroencephalogr Clin Neurophysiol. 39:59–64, 1975.

Marks PA, Monroe LJ: Correlates of adolescent poor sleepers. J Abnorm Psychol. 85:243–246, 1976.

Miller PR, Campelli JW, Dinello FA: Imipramine in the treatment of enuretic schoolchildren. Am J Dis Child. 115:17–20, 1968.

Monroe LJ: Psychological and physiological differences between good and poor sleepers. J Abnorm Psychol. 72:255–264, 1967.

Montgomery I, Perkin G, Wise D: A review of behavioral treatments for insomnia. J Behav Ther Exp Psychiat. 6';93–100, 1975.

Oswald I, Adam K, Borrow S, Idzikowski C: The effects of two hypnotics on sleep, subjective feelings, and skilled performance. In: Pharmacology of the States of Alertness. Passouant P, Oswald I (eds). Pergamon Press, New York. pp. 51–63, 1979.

Pesikoff R, Davis P: Treatment of pavor nocturnus and somnambulism in children. Am J Psychiat. 128:134–137, 1971.

Pouissaint AF, Ditman KS: A controlled study of imipramine (Tofranil) in the treatment of childhood enuresis. J Pediatr. 67:283–290, 1965.

Rechtschaffen A, Dement WC: Narcolepsy and hypersomnia. In: Sleep: Physiology and Pathology. Kales A (ed). Lippincott, Philadelphia. pp. 119–130, 1969.

Roth B: Narcolepsy and hypersomnia: review and classification of 642 personally observed cases. Archives Suisses de Neurologie, Neurochirurgie et de Psychiatric. 119:31–41, 1976.

Roth B, Nevsimalova S, Rechtschaffen A: Hypersomnia with "sleep drunkenness." Arch Gen Psychiat. 26:456–462, 1972.

Salzman C, Van der Kolk B, Shader RI: Psychopharmacology and the geriatric patient. In: Manual of Psychiatric Therapeutics. Shader RI (ed). Little, Brown, Boston. pp. 171–184, 1975.

Segal DS, Janowsky DS: Psychostimulant-induced behavioral effects: possible models of schizophrenia. In: Psychopharmacology: A Generation of Progress. Lipton MA, DiMascio A, Killam KF (eds). Raven Press, New York. pp. 1113–1123, 1978.

Shaffer D, Costello AJ, Hill ID: Control of enuresis with imipramine. Arch Dis Child. 43:665–671, 1968.

Siegel PV, Gerathewohl SJ, Mohler SR: Time-zone effects. Science. 164:1249–1255, 1969.

Soldatos CR, Kales A, Bixler EO, Scharf MB, Kales JD: Hypnotic effectiveness of sodium salicylamide with short-term use: sleep laboratory studies. Pharmacology. 16:193–198, 1978.

Soldatos CR, Kales A, Caldieux R: Narcolepsy: evaluation and treatment. In: Amphetamine Use, Misuse, and Abuse. Smith DE, Wesson DR, Buxton ME, Seymour RB, Ungerleider JT, Morgan JP, Mandell AJ, Gail J (eds). G K. Hall, Boston. pp. 128–140, 1979a.

Soldatos CR, Kales A, Kales JD: Management of insomnia. Ann Rev Med. 30:301–312, 1979b.

Soldatos CR, Kales JD, Scharf MB, Bixler EO, Kales A: Cigarette smoking associated with sleep difficulty. Science. 207:551–553, 1980.

Sours JA: Narcolepsy and other disturbances in the sleep-waking rhythm: a study of 115 cases with review of the literature. J Nerv Ment Dis. 137:525–542, 1963.

Starfield B: Functional bladder capacity in enuretic and nonenuretic children. J Pediatr. 70:777–781, 1967.

Starfield B: Enuresis: its pathogenesis and management. Clin Pediatr. 11:343–350, 1972.

Strohl KP, Hensley MJ, Saunders NA, Scharf S, Brown R, Ingram RH: Progesterone administration and progressive sleep apneas. JAMA. 245:1230–1232, 1981.

Tec L: Imipramine for nightmares. JAMA. 228:978, 1974.

Tilkian AG, Guilleminault C, Schroeder JS, Lehrman KL, Simmons FB, Dement WC: Hemodynamics in sleep-induced apnea. Ann Intern Med. 85:714–719, 1976.

Weitzman E, Kripke D, Goldmacher D, McGregor P, Nogeire C: Acute reversal of the sleep-waking cycle in man. Arch Neurol. 22:483–489, 1970.

Yoss RE, Daly DD: Criteria for the diagnosis of the narcoleptic syndrome. Proceedings of the Staff Meetings of the Mayo Clinic. 32:320–328, 1957.

Zarcone V: Narcolepsy. N Engl J Med. 288:1156–1166, 1973.

19 | Treatment Compliance

BARRY BLACKWELL

Now that there are treatments of proven effectiveness for some psychiatric disorders, it is both alarming and annoying when patients with responsive disorders fail to comply with prescribed treatment. Clinicians often make pejorative statements about patients who comply poorly and fail to improve, while patients feel they have ample reason to blame their physicians for their lack of progress. This chapter reviews what is known about the role of compliance in the treatment of psychiatric disorders and recommends ways of improving patients' cooperation. It updates an earlier review (Blackwell, 1976) of the literature on this subject that was available before 1975.

Information on treatment compliance in general is rapidly expanding. The most recent annotated bibliography (Haynes, 1979) lists 853 articles written by 1978 compared with only 246 listed in a previous review (Sackett and Haynes, 1976). The former includes 96 references to psychiatric populations compared with the 55 reviewed by Blackwell (1976).

Despite this information explosion, there is scant agreement on even the essential parameters of the field. The authors of a recent major review found little relationship between disease state and noncompliance but noted as an exception that "psychiatric patients, particularly those with schizophrenia, paranoia or personality disorders tend to be low compliers" (Haynes, 1979). Yet another careful analysis of the data refutes this statement (Barofsky and Bulson, 1980). Findings in psychiatric patients were very similar to those in other populations requiring chronic medication, such as patients with hypertension, tuberculosis, and epilepsy. Hypertensive patients with minimal social support were the most noncompliant group and they overlapped in degree of noncompliance with chronic schizophrenic patients receiving phenothiazines. Only two studies compared the behavior of psychiatric and nonpsychiatric patients taking the same drugs. One reported that schizophrenic patients with tuberculosis were less compliant in taking isoniazid than nonschizophrenics (Ferebee, 1964); but the other study found that psychiatric and nonpsychiatric epileptics were equally noncompliant in taking anticonvulsant medication (Barofsky and Bulson, 1980). An extensive critical review of studies of various medical and psychiatric conditions found stable predictors of dropout, regardless of the type of treatment. These included social isolation, symptom relief, motivation, and family attitudes (Baekeland and Lundwall, 1975).

A recent editorial (1979) epitomized the confusion in this area with the rhetorical caption: "Noncompliance; does it matter?" The author pointed out that "in the case of much treatment with antibiotics and psychotropic drugs we know virtually nothing—not the optimum dose, nor the frequency, nor the duration of treatment . . . Do we know that low compliance interferes with the clinical goals of treatment? And is it established that treatment would do more good than harm in those who do not comply?"

SCHIZOPHRENIA

The reasons for this scepticism about the role of poor compliance in clinical outcome are well illustrated in the management of schizophrenia. The unequivocal efficacy of antipsychotic drugs in treating schizophrenia paved the way for deinstitutionalization, and a plethora of studies demonstrated that relapse and readmission were more frequent in placebo treated than in drug-treated patients. By the end of one year, over 70% of patients relapse on placebo compared to 33% on active drug and after two years the figures are 80% and 48%, respectively (Goldberg et al., 1977). Equally consistent are the findings that approximately one-fifth of schizophrenic inpatients and one half of schizophrenic outpatients fail to take medication regularly (Johnson and Freeman, 1972). These two observations have been linked to the twin assumptions that the major contribution to reinstitutionalization is poor compliance and that this can be effectively combated by using long-acting parenteral (depot) phenothiazines.

Both these assumptions are oversimplifications and may be erroneous. Previous reports on the benefit of depot phenothiazines have suffered from a variety of design defects. The use of cohort or "mirror image" designs in which patients serve as their own historical control has tended to confound the specific effects of medication with other aspects of an energetic treatment regimen, including intensive follow-up of patients who fail to attend for injections (Johnson and Freeman, 1972). Patients who dropped out of therapy were sometimes excluded from the analysis and have represented up to 43% of patients treated for prolonged periods (Carney and Sheffield, 1976). A definitive, prospective, double-blind study has now compared the effects of injectable and oral fluphenazine in preventing relapse in 214 schizophrenic patients followed up for one year after hospital admission (Schooler et al., 1980). The curves indicating readmission for both treatment regimens were virtually identical and at the end of the year 24% of patients on the injectable drug had been rehospitalized as opposed to 33% on oral drug—not a statistically significant difference. This study reminds us that many schizophrenic patients relapse despite known compliance in taking medication. One of the earliest studies of treatment adherence (Mason et al., 1963) found that 38% of schizophrenic patients were still taking their medication as prescribed at the time of readmission. The earlier enthusiastic claims for injectable phenothiazines tended to overlook this fact; in one study there were 57 readmissions in one year among 126 patients (45%) receiving these drugs (Johnson and Freeman, 1972).

Both recent studies and reanalysis of old data indicate that approximately 20% of schizophrenics remain well either on placebo or without drugs, that 40% relapse regardless of treatment, and that in about 40% medication prevents relapse. The characteristics of this latter group are important in understanding the compliance problem and in finding ways to improve prognosis. Patients with good premorbid adjustment (Goldstein, 1970) or those who live alone are likely to do relatively well without drugs, and in this group compliance does not contribute to outcome. At the other extreme, patients who live in frequent face-to-face contact with critical relatives may relapse despite the fact that they take the medication (Vaughn and Leff, 1976). The most sophisticated analysis of the roles of drug and social therapy in preventing relapse in schizophrenia is found in research conducted by the Psychopharmacology Research Branch of NIMH (Goldberg et al., 1977), which compares the effects of chlorpromazine, placebo, major role therapy (social casework and vocational rehabilitation), and a combination of drugs and role therapy. Five factors predicted good drug response: autism, family distress, patient's role satisfaction, compliance, and hours employed. Within these categories the greatest difference between drug and placebo groups occurred in the least withdrawn patients whose families were least distressed. Major role therapy provoked more rapid relapse in the less well adjusted patients but benefited those with fewer symptoms, suggesting that drugs and sociotherapy could interact beneficially in sequence.

Taken together, the results of both British and American research suggest that compliance is likely to be a significant factor when drugs help a less severely disturbed patient cope with a modestly stressful environment. If the family is critical of the patient or unsupportive toward therapy, there will be a predictable and interactive reduction in both drug response and compliance.

The possibility that it is the less sick patients who benefit most from drugs and are more compliant is also supported by a comparison between two extreme groups of habitual drug refusers and identified drug compliers (VanPutten, 1976). Drug refusers were sicker at discharge and relapsed into severe, grandiose psychoses while compliers experienced decompensation with anxiety, depression, and preservation of insight. Insight may be crucial not only to compliance but to strategies that improve it.

An elegant but overlooked study by hospital pharmacists (Nelson et al., 1975) divided male schizophrenic patients into two groups according to whether they accepted or resisted the premise that they were disturbed. The discrimination was based on responses to the Rorschach test (Weiner's criteria). Twenty-four patients from each group were then randomly assigned to a treatment condition in which they had control of their own medication before discharge or were administered drugs in the traditional manner. Compliance was measured by urine tests both before and after discharge at outpatient visits. Patients who accepted their illness and were trained to self-medicate showed 80% compliance before and after discharge. Patients who denied their illness or who were not trained to self-medicate showed only 50% compliance after discharge. The results indicate that those schizophrenics who retain insight can benefit considerably from self-medication training while those who reject their illness do not.

This same study also analyzed other variables and found that high compliance was associated with good physician–patient relationships and living within an intact family, while poor compliance was correlated with severity of side effects. The influence of side effects on compliance in schizophrenia is further supported by a two-year study of 85 outpatients. A highly significant relationship was found between reluctance to take drugs and subtler forms of akathisia and akinesia which mimic anxiety and depression and are especially distressing to the less disturbed patients (VanPutten, 1978).

Attention has been given to simplifying drug administration schedules in an effort to reduce the complexity, cost, and unwanted side effects of treatment (DiMascio and Shader, 1969). Chronic female schizophrenic patients taking phenothiazines who had been switched to a once-a-day schedule showed no deterioration in ward behavior compared to a matched control group that continued taking multiple daily doses (Callahan et al., 1975).

Another interesting approach has been the use of "coffee groups" to facilitate compliance by discussing medication in general, individual problems in particular, as well as renewing prescriptions. Masnik and his co-workers (1980) reported a nine-year follow-up study of 76 chronically ill psychiatric outpatients who attended coffee and cookie group sessions once or twice a month. In a subgroup of 18 schizophrenic patients taking neuroleptics, there was a statistically significant drop in hospitalization from nine days a year before the groups began to three and one-half days after their initiation.

The influence of medication cost on compliance has been studied by randomly assigning outpatient schizophrenics to medication either at traditional cost ($N=46$), or at a nominal charge ($N=44$) (Cody and Robinson, 1977). The unanticipated finding was that 34% of the low-cost group was readmitted compared to 15% of the full-cost group. Since the former figure is consistent with the relapse rates in the general literature and with the clinic's previous experience, the authors concluded that monetary investment on the patient's part may be an important ingredient in successful drug maintenance.

Taken together, these recent findings about schizophrenic patients suggest that previous definitions of the compliance problem and attempts to deal with it have been unduly simplistic. Only modest conclusions about the role of compliance can be drawn, namely that poor compliance plays a limited role in a restricted group of patients. The principles for effective management of this group are apparently similar to the techniques employed in any patient who has relatively intact insight. Our expectations about the effects of drugs, the significance of compliance, and our ability to influence either in schizophrenics should probably be more modest.

AFFECTIVE DISORDERS

More attention is being paid to problems of compliance in patients with affective disorders for two reasons; first, because of an increasing interest in long-term "prophylactic" or maintenance therapy and second, because we now have methods for monitoring the plasma levels of lithium and the tricyclic antidepressants.

DEPRESSIVE DISORDERS

There is no reason to suppose that depressed patients are unusually prone to poor compliance. In a study of 36 lower-class depressed female outpatients, Deykin and his colleagues (1975) found excellent attendance patterns and a very low dropout rate (5 patients or 17%) over an eight-month course of psychotherapy. The authors speculated that the strong superegos of depressed individuals, reflected in this punctuality and sense of obligation and responsibility toward the therapist, contributed to this pattern.

In an early, controlled study of antidepressant drug therapy, on the other hand, Glick (1965) found that 16 of 35 patients dropped out before the end of four weeks' treatment with either a monoamine oxidase inhibitor or a placebo. Seventy five percent of the dropouts occurred within the first ten days of treatment and those who dropped out tended to be less severely depressed and to have experienced significant improvement. Since the commonest reason for dropping out was complaints of side effects (7 out of 16 patients), the pattern of noncompliance in this study appears quite similar to that reported in studies of the failure to complete a course of antibiotics where recovery from the symptoms of infection leads to early discontinuation of treatment which sometimes results in relapse.

This supposition receives support from a more recent study in which a psychiatrist interviewed and followed up 73 patients treated for depression by family practitioners (Johnson, 1973). Ninety two percent of these patients were treated with antidepressants, two-thirds with less than full therapeutic doses. Sixteen percent stopped taking drugs within a week, 41% within two weeks, 59% by three weeks, and 68% at the end of a month. The most frequent reasons for stopping medication were recovery (26%), end of the initial prescription (21%), disbelief in drugs (21%), and side effects (7%). Any adverse consequences of this noncompliance are not described. In any event the rapidity of recovery, the low dosages of drugs used, and the fact that there was the same pattern of noncompliance as in the placebo-treated patients studied by Glick suggests that the findings cannot be generalized to the short-term management of severe depression, in which improvement is attributable to the specific pharmacologic action of adequate drug treatment. In fact, the more severely depressed patients in the study by Glick continued to comply despite the absence of benefit and occurrence of side effects. The findings from these studies do suggest that compliance problems may be encountered with long-term maintenance therapy in which patients are asked to continue medication despite feeling relief of depressive symptoms while still experiencing side effects.

Nevertheless, the problem of noncompliance with long-term therapy for depression might be less severe than the results above would indicate. In a recent study by Coppen et al. (1978), 32 patients who responded to amitriptyline were randomly allocated to either placebo ($N=16$) or active drug ($N=16$) (150 mg daily) and then followed up for one year. Five patients on placebo and three on amitriptyline relapsed. The noncompliance rate (19% for the drug treatment group) was almost identical to the dropout rate of 17% reported for psychotherapy alone over a comparable time period (Deykin et al., 1975). Furthermore, although relapse was attributed to a loss of pharmacologic effect, there was no correlation between plasma levels of amitriptyline and clinical response. Also, the compliance rates are not reported for the placebo patients who relapsed.

The results to date do not provide convincing evidence that noncompliance in depressed patients treated either acutely or prophylactically leads to relapse as a result of loss of the specific pharmacologic action of drugs. One reason may be the complexity of issues involved.

A particularly interesting study is the recent comparison of symptom reduction by drugs and short-term interpersonal psychotherapy in acute depression (DiMascio et al., 1979). Two compliance measures were used: acceptance of treatment and successful completion of 16 weeks of therapy. Treatment was rejected by only 9% of those placed in a control group which scheduled no regular therapy (but offered treatment on demand) and 4% of those offered both psychotherapy (one hour weekly) and drugs (amitriptyline 100 to 200 mg daily). By contrast, 17% of those offered only drugs and 32% of those offered only psychotherapy declined to participate. Following entry into treatment 61% of the control patients terminated prematurely compared to 20% on psychotherapy alone, 50% on drugs alone, and 29% of those receiving combined therapy. These data demonstrate the complexity of the issues involved in compliance and the importance of distinguishing between entry into and continuation with specific treatments. The overall completion rates for active therapy were highest for combined therapy (67% of those entering) and lowest for drugs alone (33%). These results may reflect the fact that clear additive benefits are gained from the differential effects of psychotherapy and drug treatment. It may be that patients who enter treatment are particularly influenced by preexisting beliefs about the appropriateness of what is offered while those who remain in treatment are more influenced by the actual benefits obtained.

The widespread assumption that noncompliance is causally related to relapse has resulted in the promulgation of strategies to detect and deal with the problem. Now that the technology for measurement of plasma levels of tricyclic antidepressants is more widely available, their routine use has been recommended as a means of monitoring compliance. In a study of 150 outpatients, Biggs and his colleagues (1976) found that 17% of patients had plasma levels of tricyclic antidepressants below what is generally regarded as therapeutic. However, they did not report any systematic relationship between compliance, plasma levels of drug, and clinical relapse.

Routine monitoring of plasma levels may be impractical for reasons other than the obvious one of expense and inconvenience. Hollister (1978) has published a report on the use of a tricyclic plasma level measuring service offered to psychiatrists. Out of 61 patients referred, poor compliance was detected in five (8%) and had already been suspected clinically in four of these patients. In 22 out of the 61 patients adequate plasma levels were correlated with good clinical response.

One common strategy to facilitate compliance in depressed patients has been the use of once-daily dosages made possible by the long plasma half-lives of tricyclic antidepressants. The widespread popularity of this practice is underlined by a mail survey that generated 481 responses from a representative sample of U.S. psychiatrists (Ayd, 1974). Fifty-one percent considered once-daily therapy effective for initial management and

87% for maintenance therapy. However, a review of the literature for all medications relating complexity of the regimen to compliance (Blackwell, 1979) indicated that negative influence was far stronger for multiple medications than for multiple dosages of the same medication. Only when the regimen reached more than three dosages daily was there clear evidence that multiple daily doses had an effect on compliance. Despite the absence of compelling scientific evidence, in general it is conceptually appealing to recommend once-daily medication as a strategy to improve compliance in depressed patients. Single-dose once-daily medication has one clear advantage—the possibility of prescribing lower cost, large-dose tablets or capsules. Efficacy is evidently maintained with once-daily medication and some side effects may be masked by sleep.

Because the side effects of tricyclic antidepressants are frequent and often precede therapeutic benefit, they are often thought to cause noncompliance. Myers and Calvert (1976) studied 100 outpatients taking dothiepin who were either forewarned about side effects or not. Two-thirds of the patients experienced side effects. Among those who were not forewarned, 41% discontinued medication (9 out of 22 patients) compared to 15% of those who were told (5 out of 33 patients). These differences are clinically meaningful but not statistically significant due to the small numbers involved. In a subsequent study, the same investigators found that providing patients with both written and verbal warnings significantly reduced the dropout rate in those who experienced side effects (Myers and Calvert, 1978). This strategy of forewarning patients has been more fully explored in depressed outpatients (Ley et al., 1976). Eighty patients were randomly assigned to four treatment groups, one serving as control and the others receiving written information about the medication and its side effects at three different levels of reading complexity. In the control group, 16% made medication errors (discrepancies between pills taken and prescribed). This compared with 3, 8, and 15% for written instructions at the three levels of increasing complexity.

Overall, studies of the management of depression by drug therapy indicate that noncompliance is very common in mildly to moderately depressed outpatients, but that the consequences have been inadequately defined and are not clearly linked to loss of a specific pharmacologic effect. Little practical value has been demonstrated for monitoring plasma levels, but once-daily medication and warnings about side effects (particularly in writing) may be useful.

MANIC DISORDERS

In an earlier report (VanPutten, 1975) it was suggested that patients' refusal to take lithium was associated with the denial of illness and lack of awareness of personal feelings and their relationships to treatment. These suggestions are amplified by a report of experience with 149 patients given lithium during a five-year period in a German clinic (Werner, 1973). Among these patients, 59% took medication continuously, 11% intermittently, and 30% stopped entirely. Demographic characteristics and features of illness were unrelated to compliance. However, the totally noncompliant group had been less well informed about the effects of lithium prophylaxis. The physician spent less time explaining treatment, including side effects, and the relationship of blood levels to outcome. In addition, the compliant patients more often were given written instructions and held clearer views of the risk–benefit ratio of the drug. Patients were much more likely to be compliant if regular blood level checks were accompanied by conversation with the physician. These findings underline a feature of the compliance literature in general: factors found to influence compliance tend to be interactional and interpersonal rather than fixed and statistical (such as demographic data and illness variables). This is seen, for instance, in a recent study of the influence of group psychotherapy on compliance with lithium therapy in manic patients (Shakir et al., 1979). Fifteen patients attended regular group meetings for an average of 51 weeks; these patients had fewer hospitalizations, briefer periods in hospital, and higher mean plasma lithium levels during this period than in the two years before group therapy began. In addition, the patients were reported to have more satisfactory work, social, and interpersonal adjustments.

A more mundane aspect of treatment reported to influence compliance is the bitter aspirinlike taste of lithium carbonate tablets. This can be avoided by the use of capsules that mask the taste.

ANXIETY DISORDERS

Minor tranquilizers are now the most widely used drugs in America, although only 18% are prescribed by psychiatrists (FDA, 1980). While it is today's conventional wisdom that the American population is overmedicated with these drugs, Halberstam (1978) found that 22 out of 50 patients questioned in office practice expressed negative views toward minor tranquilizers and another 9 were indifferent. When diazepam was made freely available to psychiatric inpatients, their requests for it were surprisingly infrequent (Winstead et al., 1974). Since anxiety is an episodic and often only mildly disruptive experience for most people, it would seem reasonable to expect that noncompliance might be prevalent but its consequences not serious. It can be argued that the unique circumstances of an individual's distress make it appropriate to take minor tranquilizers only when the individual feels acutely anxious rather than on a regular schedule. This may be another example of what Charney (1975) has described as the gap between precision and compliance that has protected the public in the past from such excessive therapeutic practices as cupping, bleeding, and purging. An attempt to conduct a controlled trial of antianxiety medications and placebo in 77 anxious outpatients supports this viewpoint (Stone et al., 1975). After two and a half weeks had passed, a third of the patients had stopped medication and when the treatment period ended after six weeks fewer than a quarter were still taking medication, although 80% recovered. Only 6% of the patients attributed a major part of the beneficial outcome to drugs, while 74% thought that most benefit could be attributed to talking. In an earlier study, Lipman and his colleagues (1965) found that almost half of 254 anxious outpatients prescribed meprobamate deviated from drug treatment procedures. The less compliant patients were characterized as more distressed and less motivated to make psychological readjustment or participate in psychotherapy, and were judged by the treating physician to have a poor prognosis. Another study of compliance with drug treatment, among 142 anxious male VA outpatients, also showed significant dose deviation in over half of the population (52%) during an eight-week treatment period (Michaux, 1961).

Until the principles for the rational use of minor tranquilizers are better understood and applied (Blackwell, 1975) and the effects of alternative coping strategies have been more clearly defined, the implications of noncompliance will be difficult to establish.

COMPLIANCE AND DSM-III

The upsurge of interest in compliance is a reflection of changing public and professional expectations. The consumer and patients' rights movements have led to greater involvement of patients in health care and to skepticism concerning overly simplistic technical solutions to inherently complex and incompletely understood problems. This has coincided with the development of a biopsychosocial model of health and health care that reaches beyond the purely biological aspects of treatment to incorporate psychological and social dimensions. These trends are reflected in the compliance literature by a movement away from simplistic assumptions to the recognition of multiple determinants and to a less reductionistic analysis of the problems surrounding patient cooperation in taking medication. It is timely that this shift has paralleled the development of DSM-III. The multiaxial format is intended to broaden the scope of clinical analysis. Axis IV (level of psychosocial stressors) and Axis V (adaptive functioning) may prove especially valuable in understanding the causes and consequences of poor compliance at the same time that discussions on treatment are linked to more rigorous clinical criteria under Axes I and II. Research along these lines is still in its infancy, so the suggestions that follow are plausible but not yet documented by systematic studies.

MANAGEMENT SUGGESTIONS

Management of compliance can be thought of as a three-stage process: *comprehension* (without which compliance cannot occur), *supervision* (often a necessary but not always a sufficient factor), and *independence* (a seldom achieved but ideal outcome).

Comprehension
The principles of adult education are only beginning to be applied to physician–patient transactions. Anxiety impairs learning, increases vulnerability, and enhances the tendency to deny illness. This helps explain the frequently poor retention or rapid denial of doctors' instructions about taking drugs, particularly when they are accompanied by dire admonitions about the consequences of poor compliance. Treatment instructions are more likely to be retained when delivered in a calm atmosphere with an optimistic discussion of the likely benefit.

It helps, of course, if the patient understands the goals of treatment and the role of medication in achieving them. In the case of psychotropic drugs this requires translation of drug effects into specific, easily grouped behavioral endpoints. Neuroleptics buffer the schizophrenic from intrusive relatives; they banish voices and repel alien influences. Lithium slows thoughts and controls impulses. Antidepressants elevate mood, abolish depressive ruminations, and reactivate the retarded patient. Antianxiety agents lessen the adverse consequences of social interaction by attenuating approach–avoidance conflicts. Such informal explanations of drug effects on behavior need to be couched in terms that are readily understandable to each individual in relation to his other life circumstances.

Instructions and explanation should be given in both verbal and written form to enhance retention. Repetition and reinforcement by nursing staff, pharmacists, and family also seem useful.

The only certain check of patients' understanding is to invite feedback from them about the details of management. This (and not the writing of the prescription) should mark the end of the interview.

Supervision
Understanding is a necessary beginning; once it is established, there are several strategies for motivating patients toward sustained compliance.

Lack of practice makes for imperfect performance. The patient is often propelled into the outside world without an attempt to observe, correct, or reinforce procedures for taking medication. Some patients cannot tell the time or easily fit medication taking into their daily activities. They become baffled by the complexity of the regimen or discouraged by unwanted effects on their social, sexual, or occupational lives. Some of these problems can be avoided by allowing patients to self-medicate before discharge from hospital and by encouraging outpatients to keep diaries to report and help resolve their difficulties. Simplifying the regimen, particularly reducing the number of different medications that need to be taken may well be helpful.

Even more important, patients should be given a clear sense of confidence in the reliability of the cause-and-effect relation between drug taking and personal behavior. This heightens the patient's belief in the value of treatment, reduces his sense of personal vulnerability, and diminishes the tendency to denial.

Efforts should also be made to incorporate partial rewards for compliance ranging from simple recognition of success expressed by the physician to feedback and encouragement from the patient's peer group or family. This can be accomplished through patient and family groups in which cookies, coffee, and an informal atmosphere help take the edge off social interaction and compliance monitoring.

Independence

Because some psychiatric patients lose insight during the early stages of relapse and become psychotic at variable rates, it is important in such instances to substitute some form of observation, if possible by friends or family.

Patients with some insight differ in the degree to which they can get along without supervision. Those with a strong sense of vulnerability may more readily adopt the sick role to avoid fears or facing up to their lack of the skills needed for independent existence. Such individuals value caretaking more than chemicals. Physicians also differ in their ability or willingness to satisfy the needs for nurturing of different patients; some tolerate dependency needs well while others feel uncomfortable when confronted with them and may be irritated by the apparent inconsistency of patients who fail to take medication but continue to seek help. The best resolution lies in a deliberate attempt to foster independence through graduated transfer of responsibility for aspects of care the patient can control. Patients are also reluctant or unable to relinquish the sick role unless they are given training in the occupational or social skills required for healthy existence and unless the rewards of sickness behavior are replaced by rewards and support from the family. Many patients or their families are unable to make this transition; the physician becomes a surrogate for the family and noncompliance may become a means of seeking asylum from the world.

REFERENCES

Editorial: Non-compliance: does it matter. Brit Med J. 2:1168, 1979.
Ayd F: Once-a-day dosage tricyclic antidepressant drug therapy: a survey. Dis Nerv Syst. 35:475–480, 1974.
Baekeland F, Lundwall L: Dropping out of treatment: a critical review. Psychol Bull. 82:738–783, 1975.
Barofsky I, Bulson RD: In: The Chronic Psychiatric Patient in the Community: Principles of Treatment. Spectrum Publications, Jamaica, NY. 1980.
Biggs JT, Chang SS, Sherman WR, Holland WH. Measurement of tricyclic antidepressent levels in an outpatient clinic. J Nerv Ment Dis. 162:46–51, 1976.
Blackwell B: Rational drug use in the management of anxiety. Rational Drug Therapy. 9:1, 1975.
Blackwell B: Treatment adherence. Brit J Psychiat. 129:513–531, 1976.
Blackwell B: The drug regimen and treatment compliance. In: Compliance in Health Care. Johns Hopkins Press, Baltimore. pp. 144–156, 1979.
Callahan EJ, Alevizos PN, Teigen JR, Newman H, Campbell MD: Behavioral effects of reducing the daily frequency of phenothiazine administration. Arch Gen Psychiat. 32:1285–1290, 1975.
Carney MWP, Sheffield BF: Comparison of antipsychotic depot injection in the maintenance treatment of schizophrenia. Brit J Psychiat. 129:476–481, 1976.
Charney E. Compliance and prescribance. Am J Dis Child. 129:1009–1010, 1975.
Cody J, Robinson AM: The effect of low-cost maintenance medication on the re-hospitalization of schizophrenic outpatients. Am J Psychiat. 134:73–76, 1977.
Coppen A, Ghose K, Montgomery S, Rama Rao VA, Bailey J, Jorgensen A: Continuation therapy with amitriptine in depression. Brit J Psychiat. 133:28–33, 1978.
Deykin E, Weissman M, Tanner J, Prusoff B: Participation in therapy. J Nerv Ment Dis. 160:42–48, 1975.
DiMascio A, Shader RI: Drug administration schedules. Am J Psychiat. 126:796–801, 1969.
DiMascio A, Weissman MM, Pousoff BA, Nen C, Zwilling M, Klerman G: Differential symptom reduction by drugs and psychotherapy in acute depression. Arch Gen Psychiat. 36:1450–1456, 1979.
FDA DB: Prescribing of minor tranquilizers. FDA Drug Bulletin. 10:2–3, 1980.
Ferebee SH: The schizophrenic and oral medication. Lancet. 2:147, 1964.
Glick BS: Dropout in an outpatient, double-blind drug study. Psychosomatics. 6:44–48, 1965.
Goldberg SC, Schooler NR, Hogarth GW, Roper M: Prediction of relapse in schizophrenic outpatients treated by drug and sociotherapy. Arch Gen Psychiat. 34:171–184, 1977.
Goldstein MJ: Premorbid adjustment, paranoid status and patterns of response to phenothiazines in acute schizophrenia. Schizophrenia Bull. 3:24–37, 1970.
Halberstam M: An office study of patient attitudes toward tranquilizing medication. Southern Med J. 2:15–17, 1978.
Haynes RB: Determinants of compliance: The disease and the mechanics of

treatment. In: Compliance in Health Care, Haynes, RB, Taylor, DW, Sackett, DL (eds). Johns Hopkins U Press, Baltimore. pp. 49–62, 1979.

Hollister LE: Monitoring plasma concentrations of tricyclics. Am J Psychiat. 135:618, 1978.

Johnson DAW: Treatment of depression in general practice. Brit Med J. 2:18–20, 1973.

Johnson DAW, Freeman H: Long acting tranquilizers. Practitioner. 208:395–400, 1972.

Ley P, Jain VK, Skilbeck A: A method of decreasing patient's medication errors. Psychol Med. 6:599–601, 1976.

Lipman RS, Rickels K, Uhlenhuth EH, Park LC, Fisher S: Neurotics who fail to take their drugs. Brit J Psychiat. 111, 1043–1049, 1965.

Masnik R., Olarte SW, Rosen A: "Coffee Groups": A Nine-Year Follow up Study. Am J Psychiat. 137:191–93, 1980.

Mason AS, Forrest IS, Forrest FM, Butler H: Adherence to maintenance therapy and rehospitalization. Dis Nerv Syst. 24:103–104, 1963.

Michaux WW: Side effects, resistance and dosage deviations in psychiatric outpatients treated with tranquilizers. J Nerv Ment Dis. 133:203–212, 1961.

Myers ED, Calvert EJ: The effect of forewarning on the occurrence of side effects and discontinuation of medication in patients on dothiepin. J Int Med Res. 4:237–240, 1976.

Myers ED, Calvert EJ: Knowledge of side effects and perseverance with medication. Brit J Psychiat. 132:527–577, 1978.

Nelson AA, Gold BH, Hutchinson RA, Benezra E: Drug default among schizophrenic patients. Am J Hosp Pharm. 32:1237–1242, 1975.

Sackett DL, Haynes RB: Compliance with Therapeutic Regimens. Johns Hopkins U Press, Baltimore. 1976.

Schooler NR, Levine J, Severe JB, et al.: Prevention of relapse in schizophrenia. Arch Gen Psychiat. 37:16–24, 1980.

Shakir SA, Volkmar FR, Bacon S, Pfefferbaum A: Group psychotherapy as an adjunct to lithium maintenance. Am J Psychiat. 136:455–456, 1979.

Stone WN, Green BL, Glaser GC, Whitman RM, Foster BB: Impact of psychosocial factors on the conduct of combined drug and psychotherapy research. Brit J Psychiat. 127:432–439, 1975.

VanPutten T: Why do patients with manic-depressive illness stop lithium?. Compr Psychiat. 16:179–183, 1975.

VanPutten T: Drug refusal in schizophrenia and the wish to be crazy. Arch Gen Psychiat. 33:1443–1446, 1976.

VanPutten T: Drug refusal in schizophrenia. Hospital and Community Psychiat. 29:110–112, 1978.

Vaughn CE, Leff JP: The influence of family and social factors on the course of psychiatric illness. Brit J Psychiat. 129:125–137, 1976.

Werner W: "Technical failures" in lithium prophylaxis. In: Psychopharmacology, Sexual Disorders and Drug Abuse, Ban TA et al. (eds). North Holland, Amsterdam. pp. 329–334, 1973.

Winstead D, Blackwell B, Anderson A, Eilers MK: Diazepam on demand: drug seeking behavior in anxious in-patients. Arch Gen Psychiat. 30:349–353, 1974.

Subject Index

Abreaction, in post-traumatic stress disorder, 260
Abused substances, pharmacological classification, 82
Acidification of urine, psychostimulant intoxication, 97
Activated charcoal, for polydrug abuse, 84
Acute paranoid disorder, 175–76
  antipsychotic, 176
  essential features, 176
  in migrants, 176
  psychotherapy, 176
  signs, 176
Adjustment disorders, 419, 421–28
  antianxiety drugs, 425
  antidepressants, 426
  behavioral manifestations, 420
  behavior therapy, 421
  classification, 419
  depression, 420, 421
  drug therapy, 421
  essential features, 419
  family history, 421
  family therapy, 421
  hypnotics, 425
  prognosis, 422, 423
  psychotherapy, 421, 424
  signs, 419
  stressors, 420, 423–26
  symptoms, 419
  treatment, 423
Affective disorders, 184–233
  bipolar disorder—depressed, 193
  bipolar disorder—manic, 192. *See also*
    Mania
  compliance, 506
  mania, 187
  treatment goals, 185
Aggression, drug therapy, 440–46
Aging, pharmacokinetics, 22

Agoraphobia, essential features, 234
Ahasuerus syndrome, 390
Alcohol
  obsessive-compulsive disorder, 254
  phobias, 254
Alcohol disorders, 44–61
Alcohol hallucinosis, 49
Alcohol idiosyncratic intoxication, 47
Alcohol intoxication, 44
  aspiration, 46
  chlordiazepoxide, 46
  death, 46
  differential diagnosis, 46
  essential features, 44
  gastric lavage, 46
  glucose, 46
  idiosyncratic, 47
  lethal level, 45
  physical restraint, 45
  short-term treatment, 44
  signs, 44
  suicide, 45
  treatment, 45
  unconsciousness, 45
  vomiting, 46
Alcohol withdrawal, 47–51
  antipsychotics, 49
  benzodiazepines, 49
  delirium, 49
  epilepsy, 49
  essential features, 47
  hypoglycemia, 51
  magnesium sulfate, 51
  phenytoin, 49
  seizures, 49
  short-term treatment, 49
  signs, 49
  symptoms, 47
Alcohol withdrawal delirium
  assaultiveness, 49

517

Alcohol withdrawal delirium *cont*.
  chlordiazepoxide, 50
  specific treatment, 50
  vitamins, 50
Alcoholics anonymous, 54, 399
Alcoholism, 51
  antidepressants, 53
  aversion: apomorphine, 53; electrical, 53;
    emetine, 53; succinylcholine, 53
  controlled drinking, 52, 57
  dependency, 58
  differential diagnosis, 51
  etiology, 58
  lithium, 54
  LSD, 53
  psychotherapy, 53
  role of fear, 58
  specific treatment, 54–59
  treatment goals, 52
Alexithymia, 278
Alkalinization of urine, sedative intoxication,
  66
Alzheimer's disease, 13
Amanita muscaria, 114
Amitriptyline
  compliance, 507
  dementia, 22
  depression—single episode, 203
  insomnia, 482
  intermittent explosive disorder, 412
Ammonium chloride, for psychostimulant
  intoxication, 97
Amnesia, 310
Amnestic syndrome, 25
  precipitating factors, 25; bilateral posterior
    cerebral arterial occlusions, 26; ECT,
    26; encephalitis, 26; seizures, 26; tem-
    poral lobe excision, 26
  short-term treatment, 25
  thiamine deficiency, 25
Amotivational syndrome, 117
Amphetamines, 93
  cause of insomnia, 483
  dementia, 23
  history, 93
  narcolepsy, 484
  patterns of use, 94
  personality disorders, 444
Amytal interview, 311
Anacin, 131
Anamnesis, associative, 312, 316

Androgen, 322
Androgyny, 330
Anger, 408–409, 413
Anorgasmia, 374
Antabuse, 53
Antabuse reaction, treatment, 46
Antiandrogens, 344
Antianxiety drugs, 403, 407, 421, 440–443,
  447
  adjustment disorders, 425
  borderline personality disorder, 448
  compliance, 511
  depression—bipolar, 194
  hypochondriasis, 300
  insomnia, 478, 482
  intermittent explosive disorder, 409–10,
    413
Anticholinergic intoxication syndrome, 107
Anticholinergics, 105–11
  alkalinization of blood, 111
  apple of Peru, 105
  Artane, 105
  cardiac complications, 109
  coma, 107
  devil's apple, 105
  devil's trumpet, 105
  diazepam, 110
  glucose, 111
  history, 106, 111
  intravenous fluids, 111
  jimsonweed, 105
  lidocaine, 111
  locoweed, 105
  management, 109
  naloxone, 111
  patterns of use, 106
  phenytoin, 111
  physical restraints, 110
  physostigmine, 110
  propranolol, 111
  scopolamine, 106
  stink weed, 105
  stramonium, 106
  support, 111
  symptoms, 107
  thorn apple, 105
Anticonvulsants, 446
  aggression, 413
  intermittent explosive disorder, 412
  organic hallucinosis, 32
  personality disorders, 446

Antidepressant drugs, 421–509
  adjustment disorders, 426
  alcoholism, 53
  borderline personality disorder, 448
  compliance, depression, 506
  depression—recurrent, 211
  dysthymic disorder, 213
  hypochondriasis, 300
  insomnia treatment, 479
  maintenance for depression, 210
  monoamine oxidase inhibitors as cause of
    insomnia, 483
  obsessive-compulsive disorder, 250
  phobias, 250
  psychogenic pain disorder, 285
  psychosexual dysfunctions, 369
  tricyclics, 340, 482
Antidepressants, tricyclic
  hypersomnia, 487
  intermittent explosive disorder, 412
  narcolepsy, 484
  personality disorders, 444
Antiparkinsonian agents, 159
  list of, 159
Antipsychotic drugs, 505
  acute paranoid disorder, 176
  alcohol withdrawal, 49
  borderline, 448
  compliance in schizophrenia, 502, 505
  delirium, 11
  depression—bipolar, 194
  depression—single episode, 207
  hallucinogen intoxication, 118
  hypochondriasis, 300
  insomnia, 483
  intermittent explosive disorder, 410, 411
  list of, 154
  maintenance for bipolar disorder, 197
  mania, 189
  psychogenic pain disorder, 284
  rapid tranquilization, 155
  route of administration, 11
  side effects, 158–60
  single dose, 158
  test dose, 155
Antisocial personality disorder, 429
Anxiety
  dementia, 20
  hypochondriasis, 288
Anxiety disorders, 234–58, 288
  caffeine, 133

  compliance in, 510
  dementia, 20
  leucotomy, 260
  psychosurgery, 260
  summary, 262
  treatment goals, 235
Anxiety management training, 259
Anxiety states, 258–62
  benzodiazepines, 260
  psychotherapy, 260
  summary, 261
  treatment controversies, 261
  treatment goals, 259
Apomorphine aversion
  alcoholism, 53
  polydrug abuse, 84
Aspiration, alcohol intoxication, 46
Association of Sleep Disorders Centers, 473
Asthma, 297
Atypical disorders
  bipolar, 226
  depression, 227
  dissociative, 309
  personality, 429
  somatoform, 286
Aversion conditioning, transsexualism, 325
Aversion relief, 357
Aversion therapy, 340, 406
  apomorphine, 53
  covert sensitization, 342; homosexuality,
    ego-dystonic, 351
  electrical, 342, 343, 344–51, 353, 355
  ethics, 344
  exhibitionism, 349
  general issues, 353–54
  homosexuality, ego-dystonic, 341, 344
  hormones, 343
  paraphilias, 341
  rubber band, 342
  shame, 342, 352–53
  transvestism, 333, 334
Avoidant personality disorder, 429

Barbitol, 62
Barbiturate assisted interview, 311, 316, 457
  multiple personality, 315
Barbiturate challenge test, 71, 73
Barbiturates, 478
  long acting, 62
  short acting, 62
Bedwetting. See Enuresis

Behavior therapy, 325
  adjustment disorders, 421
  chronic factitious disorder with physical symptoms, 391
  conversion disorder, 274
  depression, 219
  dissociative disorders, 313
  dysthymic disorder, 219
  gender identity disorder of childhood, 328, 330
  homosexuality, ego-dystonic, 360
  insomnia, 481
  kleptomania, 404, 406
  marital and family problems, 464
  obsessive-compulsive disorder, 235
  paraphilias, 344
  pathological gambling, 399
  phobias, 235
  psychogenic pain disorder, 281
  psychosexual dysfunctions, 368
  schizophrenia, 169
  somatization disorder, 268
  transsexualism, 325
  transvestism, 333
Benzodiazepines, 491
  alcohol withdrawal, 49
  alcoholism, 53
  anxiety states, 260
  delirium, 11
  dementia, 21
  insomnia, 478, 482
  night terrors, 491
  obsessive-compulsive disorder, 250
  phobias, 250
  route of administration, 10
Bereavement—uncomplicated, 459–62
  alcohol abuse, 462
  associated mortality, 462
  essential features, 459
  natural history, 459
  psychiatrist's role, 462
  symptoms, 459
  treatment, 459
  treatment goals, 459
Beta blockers, 163, 483
  intermittent explosive disorder, 414
  obsessive-compulsive disorder, 250
  phobias, 250
  schizophrenia, 163
Biofeedback
  obsessive-compulsive disorder, 246
  phobias, 246

Biopsychosocial model
  compliance issues, 512
Bipolar disorder. See also Mania
  maintenance treatment: antipsychotics, 197; carbamazepine, 199; controlled studies, 198; cost-benefit, 195; family role, 197; imipramine, 198; lithium, 198; monoamine oxidase inhibitors, 198; precipitation of mania, 198; psychotherapy, 200; summary, 200; tricyclic antidepressants, 198
Borderline personality disorder, 391, 429. See also Personality disorders
  antianxiety drugs, 448
  antidepressant drugs, 448
  antipsychotic drugs, 448
  diazepam, 447
  imipramine, 447
  tranylcypromine, 447
  trifluoperazine, 447
Brain damage, inhalants, 103
Briquet's syndrome, 266
Bromoquinine, 131
Buprenorphine, 136

Caffeine, 127–33
  anxiety disorders, 133
  essential features, 133
  history, 133
  intoxication, 132
  panic attacks, 133
  patterns of use, 129–30
  withdrawal, 132
Cannabis, 111, 114–20
  amotivational syndrome, 117
  history, 111–14, 120
  intoxication, 116, 117
  patterns of use, 114
  symptoms, 114, 117
Carbamazepine
  intermittent explosive disorder, 411, 413
  maintenance treatment, bipolar disorder, 199
  organic personality syndrome, 40
Carbon dioxide phobias, 250
Cardiac complications, anticholinergics, 107, 109
Cataplexy, 483, 484
Chen, K. K., 92
Chlomipramine, obsessive-compulsive disorder, 251

Chloral hydrate, 62
  dementia, 23
Chlordiazepoxide
  alcohol intoxication, 46
  alcohol withdrawal delirium, 50
  delirium, 10
  dementia, 21
  insomnia, 478, 482
  intermittent explosive disorder, 410
  personality disorders, 441, 442
Chlorimipramine, 488
  sleep apnea, 488
Chlorpromazine
  compliance, 503
  dementia, 23
  insomnia, 483
  mania, 190
  psychostimulant intoxication, 98
  rapid tranquilization, 156
  schizophrenia, 170
Choline dementia, 24
Cholinergic crisis, 110
Chronic factitious disorder with physical
    symptoms, 390–95
  behavior therapy, 391
  confrontation, 393
  essential features, 390
  fanciful suggestions, 392
  psychotherapy, 392
  somatic therapy, 391
  staff management, 394
  symptoms, 390
  team approach, 393
  underlying physical illness, 394
  underlying psychiatric conditions, 391,
    393
Clorazepate, insomnia, 478, 482
Cocaine, 93
  "free basing", 94
  history of, 91
  patterns of use, 93
Cocoa, 130
Coffee, 130
  insomnia, 483
Coffee groups, 505
Cognitive rehearsal, 238
Cognitive therapy
  depression, 220
  obsessive-compulsive disorder, 245
  phobias, 245
Coital anorgasmia. See Orgasm inhibition
Cola drinks, 129

Coma, anticholinergics, 107
Community treatment project, 437
Compliance, 501–14
  affective disorders, 510
  amitriptyline, 507
  anxiety disorders, 511
  chlorpromazine, 503
  coffee groups, 505
  comprehension, 514
  cost of drugs, 505
  depression disorders, 508, 509
  does it matter, 502
  drug side effects, 509
  DSM-III, 511
  fluphenazine, 503
  independence, 514
  lithium, 510
  management suggestions, 512
  manic disorders, 510
  meprobamate, 511
  plasma level monitoring, 508
  relapse, 508
  schizophrenia, 502, 505
  single daily dosage, 508
  supervision, 513
Complications
  hallucinogen intoxication, 119
  inhalants, 105
  phencyclidine intoxication, 102
Compulsive hoarding, 241
Compulsive personality disorder, 429
Compulsive slowness, 241
Confrontation, substance abuse, 134
Conjoint insight psychotherapy psychosex-
    ual dysfunctions, 368
Controlled drinking, 52, 57
Conversion disorder, 277
  behavior therapy, 274
  ECT, 275
  essential features, 271
  family therapy, 274
  hypnosis, 275
  individual psychotherapy, 272
  psychoanalysis, 272
  somatic therapy, 275
  supportive psychotherapy, 273
  symptoms, 272
  treatment goals, 272
Cope, 131
Countertransference
  depression, 215
  dysthymic disorder, 215

Couples therapy, depression, 225
Crisis intervention bereavement—uncomplicated, 462
Crisis management, pathological gambling, 400
Cross-dressing, 321
  see transvestism, 332
Cyclothymic disorder, 212–13, 447
Cyroterone acetate, 344

Day care
  schizophrenia, 152
Death
  alcohol intoxication, 46
  hallucinogen intoxication, 116, 117
  inhalants, 103
  opioid intoxication, 86
  psychostimulant intoxication, 95
  sedative withdrawal, 62
  sedatives, 65
Delirium, 4–12
  alcohol withdrawal, 47, 49
  antipsychotics, 11
  benzodiazepines, 10–11
  chlordiazepoxide, 10
  diazepam, 10
  environmental management, 8
  essential features, 4
  etiology: anemia, 7; anticholinergics, 9; arrhythmias, 7; carbon monoxide, 7; cataract surgery, 9; hyperthermia, 7; hypoglycemia, 6; hypoxia, 6; myocardial infarction, 7; oxygen, 7; prevention, 9–10; pulmonary disease, 7; steroids, 9; thiamine deficiency, 7; transfusions, 7; ventilatory assistance, 7; ventilatory impairment, 7
  glucose, 6
  hypnotics, 10
  medical support, 8–9
  medications, 9–11
  outcome, 11
  oxazepam, 10
  prevention, 9–10; benzodiazepines, 9; lithium, 9; thiamine, 10
  secondary, 5
  sedative withdrawal, 70, 72
  symptoms, 4
  thiamine—intravenous, 7
  treatment, 4, 11
Delinquency, juvenile, 431–38

Dementia, 12–24
  ambulation, 19
  amitriptyline, 22
  amphetamine, 23
  anxiety, 20
  benzodiazepines, 21
  chloralhydrate, 23
  chlordiazepoxide, 21
  chlorpromazine, 23
  choline, 24
  depression, 20, 22
  diazepam, 21
  differential diagnosis, 12–15
  doxepin, 22
  drug treatment, 20
  essential features, 12
  etiology, 12–14
  exercise, 19
  Gerovital-H3, 23
  haloperidol, 23
  hydergine, 23
  imipramine, 22
  insomnia, 20, 23
  lecithin, 24
  lorazepam, 21
  mania, 20
  medical care, 18
  need for treatment, 16
  nutrition, 18
  orientation, 19
  oxazepam, 23
  papaverine, 23
  paranoid symptoms, 23
  pentalenetetrazol, 23
  physician's role, 16–18
  promethazine, 23
  psychosis, 20
  psychotherapy, 20
  stimulation, 20
  stress, 19
  symptoms, 12
  thioridazine, 23
  treatment, 12–24
  treatment goals, 18; reduction of need for lost functions, 19; restitution of lost functions, 18–19; utilization of residual functions, 20
  treatment plan, 18
  vasodilators, 23
Dependent personality disorders, 429
Depersonalization disorder, 309

Depression, 193–212
  antidepressants, 211
  behavior therapy, 219
  cognitive therapy, 220
  combination treatment, 209
  compliance, 509
  countertransference, 215
  couples therapy, 225
  dementia, 20, 22
  essential features, 211
  family therapy, 223
  group psychotherapy, 222
  hallucinogen intoxication, 119
  insomnia, 482
  lithium, 212
  maintenance therapy, 209; antidepressants, 210; ECT, 211; lithium, 211; psychotherapy, 211; treatment goals, 210
  nortriptyline, 22
  obsessive-compulsive disorder, 252
  phobias, 252
  psychogenic pain disorder, 284
  psychostimulant intoxication, 98
  psychotherapy, 225
  psychotic, 202; electroconvulsive therapy, 203
  self-control techniques, 220
  self-evaluation, 220
  self-monitoring, 220
  self-reinforcement, 220
  short-term psychotherapy, 218
  social skills training, 219
  supportive therapy, 221
  symptoms, 211
Depression—bipolar, 195
  antianxiety, 194
  antipsychotics, 194
  ECT, 194
  essential features, 195
  lithium, 194
  monoamine oxidase inhibitors, 194
  psychotherapy, 194
  summary, 195
  symptoms, 195
  treatment goals, 193
  tricyclic antidepressants, 194
Depression—single episode, 200–211
  amitriptyline, 203
  antipsychotics, 207
  desipramine, 203

doxepine, 203
  electroconvulsive therapy, 207
  essential features, 211
  imipramine, 203
  isocarboxazid, 206
  lithium, 207
  monoamine oxidase inhibitors, 205
  nortriptyline, 203
  phenelzine, 206
  protriptyline, 203
  psychotherapy, 208
  stimulants, 207
  suicide risk, 201
  symptoms, 211
  tranylcypromine, 206
  treatment goals, 201
  tricyclic antidepressants, 202
Desenistization, 237
  ego-dystonic homosexuality, 357
  intermittent explosive disorder, 408
Desipramine, 203
Detoxification, 137
Dialysis, schizophrenia, 164
Diaphragmatic pacing, sleep apnea, 488
Diazepam, 511
  anticholinergics, 110
  borderline, 447
  delirium, 10
  dementia, 21
  hallucinogen intoxication, 118
  inhalants, 105
  insomnia, 478, 482
  night terrors, 491
  opioid withdrawal, 90
  personality disorders, 441, 442
  phencyclidine intoxication, 101
  psychostimulant intoxication, 98
Diazoxide, 101
Dimethyltryptamine, 116
Diphenylhydantoin, 410
Disease phobia, 298
Disorders of impulse control, 398–418
Dissociative disorders, 309–19
  acute, 315
  behavior therapy, 313
  chronic, 311, 315
  essential features, 309
  hypnosis, 313, 317
  legal issues, 315
  psychotherapy, 311
  somatic therapy, 311

Dissociative disorders *cont.*
  specific treatment, 315
  stimulant drugs, 311
  symptoms, 309
  treatment goals, 310
Disulfiram, 53
Disulfiram reaction, 46
Diuresis, 66
Divorce therapy, 467
DMT, 116
DOM, 116
Domestic violence, 469
Double-bind, 464
Doxepin
  dementia, 22
  depression—single episode, 203
  insomnia, 482
Dristan, 131
Drug abuse controversies, 79
Drug-free outpatient treatment, 136
Drug screening, 66
Drug therapy
  adjustment disorders, 421
  aggression, 440
  dementia, 20
  enuresis, 494
  hostility, 440
  hypersomnia, 485, 487
  impulsiveness, 440
  insomnia, 480
  night terrors, 491
  obsessive-compulsive disorder, 250
  phobias, 250
  sleep apnea, 488
  sleepwalking, 492
Drugs
  adjustment disorders, 425
  intermittent explosive disorder, 412
Dry side effects, 509
Dyspareunia, 384
Dysthymic disorder, 213–26
  antidepressants, 213
  behavioral therapy, 219
  countertransference, 215
  essential features, 213
  interpersonal psychotherapy, 218
  lithium, 213
  psychoanalysis, 217
  short-term psychotherapy, 218
  symptoms, 213
  women, 215
Dystonic reactions, 156

ECT, 389, 391
  conversion disorder, 275
  depression—bipolar, 194
  depression—single episode, 207
  depression—unipolar, 207
  dysthymic disorder, 213
  factitious disorder with psychological
    symptoms, 389
  maintenance, 211
  mania, 192
  personality disorders, 448
  psychogenic pain disorder, 284
  psychotic depression, 203
  schizophrenia, 160
  somatization disorder, 270
Efficacy, tricyclics, 202
Ego-dystonic homosexuality, 344
Ejaculation, retarded, 376
Ejaculatory pain due to muscle spasm,
    382–83
  diagnostic criteria, 382
  treatment, 383
Electric aversion
  alcoholism, 53
  ego-dystonic homosexuality, 344
  paraphilias, 344
Electroconvulsive therapy, 389
Electrosleep, 270
Emetine aversion, 53
Emotionally unstable character disorders,
    447
Enuresis, 493–96
  bladder training, 494
  drug treatment, 494
  imipramine, 495
  primary, 494
  psychotherapy, 494
  secondary, 494
Episodic dyscontrol syndrome, 413
Erectile dysfunction, 377
Essential features
  acute paranoid disorder, 176
  adjustment disorders, 419
  agoraphobia, 234
  alochol intoxication, 44
  alcohol withdrawal, 49
  amnestic syndrome, 25
  bereavement—uncomplicated, 459
  caffeine, 133
  chronic factitious disorder with physical
    symptoms, 390
  conversion disorder, 271

delirium, 4
dementia, 12
depression—bipolar, 195
depression—recurrent, 211
depression—single episode, 211
dissociative disorders, 309
dysthymic disorder, 213
functional dyspareunia, 384
functional vaginismus, 381
gender identity disorder of childhood, 326
generalized anxiety disorder, 258
homosexuality, ego-dystonic, 338
hypochondriasis, 286
inhibited sexual desire, 380
inhibited sexual excitement, 377
intermittent explosive disorder, 408
kleptomania, 403
malingering, 459
mania, 192
marital and family problems, 462
obsessive-compulsive disorder, 234
opioid intoxication, 86
opioid withdrawal, 91
organic affective syndrome, 34
organic delusional syndrome, 27
organic hallucinosis, 30
organic personality syndrome, 37
panic disorder, 258
paranoia, 174
paraphilias, 338
pathological gambling, 403
personality disorders, 429
post-traumatic stress disorder, 258
premature ejaculation, 372
psychogenic pain disorder, 277
pyromania, 405
schizophrenic disorder, 173
schizophreniform disorder, 173
sedative abuse, 64
sedative dependence, 64
sedative intoxication, 64
shared paranoid disorder, 175
signs, 338
social phobia, 234
somatization disorder, 266
transsexualism, 320
transvestism, 332
Estrogen, 322, 335, 344
Excedrin, 131
Exercise, dementia, 19
Exhibitionism, 338, 340, 353, 354, 356
  aversion therapy, 349

relaxation, 349
self-regulation, 349
Exorcism, 341
Explosive personality, 413
Exposure therapy, 235
  anxiety during, 247
  avoidance, 244
  booster treatment, 258
  controversies, 243
  cotherapists, 240
  duration, 242
  efficacy, 246
  group therapy, 243
  homework, 240
  interpersonal conflict, 246
  nightmares, 256
  outcome, 246
  reassurance, 240
  relaxation, 247
  satiation, 242
  self help, 244
  therapist assisted, 240
  therapy failure, 237

Factitious disorder with psychological
    symptoms, 387–89
  coexisting disorders, 389
  diagnostic controversy, 388
  diagnostic criteria, 387
  ECT, 389
  related disorders, 388
  spontaneous resolution, 388
  stressors, 389
  symptoms, 387
  treatment, 388–89
Fading homosexuality, ego-dystonic, 354
Family problems, 462
Family role, maintenance treatment—bipolar
    disorder, 197
Family therapy, adjustment disorders, 421
  conversion disorder, 274
  depression, 223
  family intensity, 169
  pathological gambling, 401
  schizophrenia, 167
  somatization disorder, 269
Fetishism, 338
Flashbacks, 119
Flooding, 237
Fluphenazine
  compliance, 503
  schizophrenia, 169

Flurazepam, for opioid withdrawal, 90
Frigidity, 379
Functional dyspareunia, 384
Functional vaginismus, 381

Gamblers Anonymous, 399
Ganser's syndrome, 387
Gastric lavage, 84
Gender identity disorder of childhood,
    326–32
  behavior therapy, 328, 330
  essential features, 326
  females, 327
  group therapy, 328
  Indian Guides Program, 329
  parental bonds, 331
  psychodynamics, 328
  psychotherapy, 328
  role modeling, 328
  symptoms, 326
  treatment, 328–29
  treatment controversies, 329–31
  treatment goals, 328; males, 327
Gender identity disorders, 320–32, 370
Gerovital-H3, for dementia, 23
Gestalt therapy, for substance abuse, 134
Glucose
  alcohol intoxication, 46
  anticholinergics, 111
  delirium, 6
  opioid intoxication, 88
  polydrug abuse, 83
  sedative intoxication, 66
Gotcha syndrome, 459
Grief, 459
Group therapy
  depression, 222
  exposure therapy, 243
  gender identity disorder of childhood, 328
  homosexuality, ego-dystonic, 347
  pathological gambling, 401
  psychogenic pain disorder, 281
  schizophrenia, 167
  somatization disorder, 268
  substance abuse, 134

Hallucinations, hypnagogic, 483
Hallucinogen intoxication
  antipsychotics, 118
  bad trips, 118

complications, 119
death, 117
depression, 119
diazepam, 118
flashbacks, 119
hospitalization, 119
management, 117
symptoms, 115
talk down, 118
Hallucinogens, 111–20
  death, 116
  history, 114
  patterns of use, 114
Haloperidol, 11
  dementia, 23
  mania, 189
  organic delusional syndrome, 28
  phencyclidine intoxication, 101
  psychostimulant intoxication, 98
  rapid tranquilization, 156
  schizophrenia, 170
Harrison Narcotic Act, 85
Hashish, 117
Hemodialysis
  schizophrenia, 164
  sedative intoxication, 66
Heterophobia, 341
Heterosexual behavior,
  increased, 356; desensitization, 357; pair-
    ing, 357; social retraining, 357; subcul-
    tural considerations, 357
Histrionic personality disorder, 429
Hoarding, 241
Home care,
  schizophrenia, 152
Homework
  obsessive-compulsive disorder, 238
  phobias, 238
Homosexuality, ego-dystonic, 320, 322, 324,
    330, 331, 333, 344, 370
  aversion therapy, 342
  behavioral strategies, 358
  desensitization, 356
  electric aversion, 344
  essential features, 338
  group therapy, 347
  increasing heterosexuality, 356
  patient selection, 358
  symptoms, 338
  treatment, 340–44
  treatment controversies, 344
  treatment goals, 339

Hormones
    aversion therapy, 344
    transsexualism, 322
    transvestism, 335
Hospitalization
    hallucinogen intoxication, 119
    mania, 188
    obsessive-compulsive disorder, 242
    phobias, 242
    psychostimulant intoxication, 98
    schizophrenia, 148–51
Hostility, drug therapy, 440–46
Huntington's chorea, 13, 30
Hydergine, for dementia, 23
Hydralazine, for phencyclidine intoxication,
    101
Hydration, psychostimulant intoxication,
    97
Hypercalcemia
    organic personality syndrome, 40
Hyperpyrexia
    psychostimulant intoxication, 97
Hypersexuality, 40
Hypersomnia, 485–88
    antidepressants, tricyclic, 487
    imipramine, 487
    lithium, 487
    methylphenidate, 486, 487
    persistent: drug therapy, 487; idiopathic,
        486–87; psychotherapy, 487
    protriptyline, 487
    sleep apnea, 487
    stimulant drugs, 486, 487
    transient, 485
    types, 486
Hypertension
    phencyclidine intoxication, 101
    psychostimulant intoxication, 97
Hypnosis, 275, 298
    conversion disorder, 275
    dissociative disorders, 313, 317
    multiple personality, 314
Hypnotics, 62
    adjustment disorders, 425
    delirium, 10
Hypochondriasis, 286–303
    antianxiety drugs, 300
    antidepressants, 300
    antipsychotics, 300
    anxiety, 288; treatment, 294
    beta-receptor blocking drugs, 300
    depression, 288

    essential features, 286
    iatrogenic factors, 289
    MMPI, 288
    physical examination, 295
    precipitating factors, 289
    prognosis, 301
    propranolol, 300
    psychopathology, 287
    psychotherapy, 290–300
    somatic symptoms, 287
    somatic therapy, 300
    symptoms, 286
    versus disease phobia, 297
Hypoglycemia alcohol withdrawal, 51
Hypoparathyroidism, organic personality
    syndrome, 41
Hysterical neurosis, 271

Illness phobia, 240
    treatment, 298
Imipramine, 484
    borderline personality disorder, 447
    dementia, 22
    depression—single episode, 203
    enuresis, 494
    hypersomnia, 487
    intermittent explosive disorder, 412
    maintenance treatment, bipolar disorder,
        198
    phobias, 252
    sleep apnea, 488
    sleepwalking, 491
    tricyclics, 203
Implosion, 237
Impotence, 377
Impulsiveness, drug therapy, 440–46
Increasing heterosexuality, paraphilias, 357
Individual psychotherapy
    conversion disorder, 272
    psychogenic pain disorder, 279
    psychosexual dysfunctions, 368
    somatization disorder, 267
    substance abuse, 134
Inhalants, 102–5
    brain damage, 103
    complications, 105
    death, 103
    diazepam, 105
    history, 105
    isobutyl nitrite, 103
    management, 104
    patterns of use, 104, 105

Inhalants *cont.*
  physical restraints, 105
  symptoms, 103
  types, 104
Inhibited female orgasm, 375
Inhibited male orgasm, 376
Inhibited sexual desire
  essential features, 380
  sensate focus I, 381
  sensate focus II, 381
  symptoms, 380
  treatment, 380
Inhibited sexual excitement, 334
  essential features, 377
  female: sensate focus I, 379; sensate focus
    II, 379; treatment, 379
  male: partial impotence, 379; sensate
    focus I, 378; sensate focus II, 378;
    treatment, 378
Insomnia, 69, 475–79, 482–83
  amitriptyline, 482
  antianxiety drugs, 482
  behavioral therapy, 481
  benzodiazepines, 478
  caffeine, 477
  chlordiazepoxide, 478, 482
  chlorpromazine, 483
  chronic, 475, 480, 481; drug-induced, 483;
    sexual difficulties, 481
  clorazepate, 478, 482
  coffee, 483
  dementia, 20, 23
  depression, 482
  diazepam, 478, 482
  doxepine, 482
  drug therapy, 480, 481
  drug treatment, 478
  flurazepam, 481
  general measures, 477
  general treatment measures, 480
  life stress, 477
  lorazepam, 478, 482
  nitrazepam, 481
  personality patterns, 475
  psychotherapy, 477, 480
  rebound, 479, 482
  scopolamine, 479
  sedative hypnotic drugs, 481
  transient, 477
  tranylcypromine, 483
  treatment, 477
Intensive outpatient care, schizophrenia, 152

Intermittent explosive disorder, 408–14
  amitriptyline, 412
  antianxiety drugs, 409, 413
  anticonvulsants, 410, 413
  antidepressants, tricyclic, 412
  antipsychotic drugs, 410, 411
  beta-blockers, 414
  carbamazepine, 411, 413
  chlordiazepoxide, 409
  desensitization, 408
  drugs, 409
  essential features, 408
  imipramine, 412
  lithium, 410
  methylphenidate, 411
  oxazepam, 409
  phenytoin, 410, 413
  propranolol, 412, 414
  psychosurgery, 412
  psychotherapy, 408
  somatic therapies, 409–13
  stimulants, 410
  symptoms, 408
  thioridazine, 411, 412
Interpersonal psychotherapy, dysthymic disorder, 218
Ipecac
  polydrug abuse, 84
  sedative intoxication, 66
Isocarboxazid depression—single episode, 206
Isolated explosive disorder, 414

Jet lag, 489
Jimsonweed, 106
Jorgensen, Christine, 323
Juvenile delinquency, 431

Kleine-Levin syndrome, 486
  sleep apnea, 488
Kleptomania, 333, 403–4
  behavior therapy, 404, 406
  essential features, 403
  psychotherapy, 404, 405
  somatic therapy, 404
  symptoms, 403
  treatment, 404
Korsakoff's syndrome, 12, 13, 26

Laboratory studies, delirium, 5
Lecithin, dementia, 24

Lethal dose
  opioid intoxication, 86
  sedatives, 65
Leucotomy anxiety disorders, 260
Lidocaine, anticholinergics, 111
Lithium, 275, 340, 447
  alcoholism, 54
  compliance, 510
  depression—bipolar, 194
  depression—recurrent, 212
  depression—single episode, 207
  dysthymic disorder, 213
  hypersomnia, 487
  intermittent explosive disorder, 410
  maintenance depression, 211
  maintenance therapy—bipolar disorder,
    198
  mania, 191
  organic affective syndrome, 36
  use in aggression, impulsiveness, 445–46
Living with Fear, 238
Locoweed, 106
Lorazepam: dementia, 21; insomnia, 478,
  482
LSD, 112
  alcoholism, 53

Magnesium sulfate, alcohol withdrawal, 51
Maintenance
  bipolar disorder, 195
  depression, 209
Major depression, single episode, 211
Major tranquilizers, 443
Malingering, 390, 456–59
  essential features, 459
  treatment goals, 459
Mania, 187–92
  antipsychotics, 189
  chlorpromazine, 190
  commitment, 188
  compliance, 510
  dementia, 20
  electroconvulsive therapy, 192
  essential features, 192
  haloperidol, 189
  hospitalization, 188
  lithium, 191
  psychotherapy, 192
  symptoms, 192
  thioridazine, 190
  treatment goals, 192
Mannitol, sedative intoxication, 66

Marijuana, 116
Marital and family problems, 462–70
  behavior therapy, 464
  divorce counseling, 467, 470
  divorce therapy, 467
  domestic violence, 469
  double-bind, 464
  essential features, 462
  interactional treatment approaches, 464
  marital enrichment programs, 467
  psychodynamic treatment approaches,
    463
  symptoms, 462
  treatment controversies, 469
  treatment goals, 462, 464
Marital enrichment programs, 467
MDA, 116
Medroxyprogesterone, sleep apnea, 488
Meprobamate
  compliance, 511
  personality disorders, 441
Mescaline, 113
Mesoridazine, personality disorders, 444
Methadone
  opioid withdrawal, 90
  opioids, 135
  substance abuse, 135
Methylphenidate. *See also* Stimulants
  cause of insomnia, 483
  hypersomnia, 486, 487
  intermittent explosive disorder, 411
  narcolepsy, 484
  personality disorders, 444
Meyer A., 419
Milieu treatment
  and medications, 151
  brief hospital care, 153
  day care, 152
  effectiveness, 150
  home care, 152
  inpatient, 153
  intensive outpatient care, 152
  outcome, 150
  outpatient after care, 153
  principles, 150
  studies of, 150
  toxicity, 151
  treatment resistance, 149
Minimal brain dysfunction, 444
Minor tranquilizers, 443
Mixed personality disorder, 429
MMPI, hypochondriasis, 288

Modeling, 237
Monoamine oxidase inhibitors
    atypical depression, 206
    depression—bipolar, 194
    depression—single episode, 205
    maintenance, bipolar disorder, 198
Morning glory seeds, 112
Motivation,
    organic personality syndrome, 38
    tobacco use, 126
Multiinfarct dementia, 13
Multiple personality, 309, 310, 314, 316
    barbiturate-assisted interview, 315
    hypnosis, 314
    treatment, 317
Munchausen's syndrome. See Chronic fac-
    titious disorder with physical symptoms
Myoclonus, nocturnal, 474

Naloxone, 136
    anticholinergics, 111
    polydrug abuse, 83
    sedative intoxication, 66
Naltrexone, 136
Narcan
    polydrug abuse, 83
    sedative intoxication, 66
Narcissistic personality disorder, 429
Narcolepsy, 474, 483, 484–85
    psychotherapy, 484
    scheduled naps, 484
    stimulants, 484
    tetrad, 483
    tricyclic antidepressants, 484
    vs. idiopathic hypersomnia, 486
    vs. sleep apnea, 487
Newborn, opioid withdrawal, 90
Night terrors, 489–92
    benzodiazepines, 491
    diazepam, 491
    drug therapy, 491
    psychotherapy, 491
    safety measures, 490
Nightmares, 492–93
    depression associated, 493
    drug withdrawal, 493
    exposure therapy, 256
    psychological factors, 492–93
    psychotherapy, 493
Nitrazepam, insomnia, 481
No Doz, 131

Normal-pressure hydrocephalus, 13
Nortriptyline
    depression, 22
    depression—single episode, 203
Nutrition
    dementia, 18
    sedative abuse, 65

Obsessive ruminations, 241
Obsessive-compulsive disorder, 258
    alcohol, 254
    antidepressants, 250
    behavior therapy, 235
    benzodiazepines, 250
    beta-blockers, 250
    biofeedback, 246
    clomipramine, 251
    cognitive therapy, 245
    controversies, 243
    depression, 252
    drug treatment, 250
    essential features, 234
    hospitalization, 242
    medical disorders, 254
    patient selection, 237, 253
    response prevention, 246
    specific treatment, 255
    symptom substitution, 242
    symptoms, 234
    treatment goals, 235
Operant conditioning, 237
Opioid abuse, medical disorders, 91
Opioid antagonists
    buprenorphine, 136
    cyclazocine, 136
    naloxone, 136
    naltrexone, 136
Opioid intoxication, 89
    death, 86
    essential features, 86
    glucose, 88
    lethal dose, 86
    management, 89
    naloxone, 88
    observation, 89
    physical restraint, 89
    street treatment, 89
    symptoms, 87
Opioid withdrawal, 89–91
    cheating, 90
    conning, 90

diazepam, 90
essential features, 91
evaluation, 90
flurazepam, 90
jacuzzi baths, 90
massage, 90
methadone, 90
newborn, 90
symptoms, 91
Opioids, 84–92
history, 92
methadone maintenance, 135
opioid antagonists, 135
patterns of use, 86
Organic affective syndrome, 34
adrenalectomy, 35
essential features, 34
lithium, 35, 36
precipitating factors, 34, 35; alphamethyldopa, 34; Cushing's syndrome, 35;
drugs, 37; epilepsy, 37; Huntington's
chorea, 34; hyperthyroidism, 37;
hypothyroidism, 36; metabolic disturbances, 37; propranolol, 34; reserpine,
34; steroids—exogenous, 36; viral infections, 37
short-term treatment, 34
signs, 34
tricyclic antidepressants, 36
Organic delusional syndrome, 27
essential features, 27
etiology: amphetamines, 27; folate deficiency, 29; temporal lobe epilepsy, 28;
vitamin B_{12} deficiency, 29
flashbacks, 28
haloperidol, 28
psychostimulant intoxication, 95
short-term treatment, 27
signs, 27
treatment, 28
Organic hallucinosis, 30
anticonvulsants, 32
essential features, 30
precipitating factors, 30; alcohol, 33; lesions of sensory structures, 32; sensory
deprivation, 32
short-term treatment, 30
signs, 30
treatment, 33
Organic mental disorders, 3–43
affective syndrome, 34

amnestic syndrome, 25
delusional syndrome, 27
diagnosis, 4
etiology, 4
hallucinosis, 30
personality syndrome, 37
Organic personality syndrome, 37–41
carbamazepine, 40
essential features, 37
etiology: brain injuries, 38; frontal lobe
trauma, 39; hypercalcemia, 40; hypoparathyroidism, 41; temporal lobe lesions, 40; Wilson's disease, 40
flexibility, 39
hypercalcemia, 40
hypersexuality, 40
hypoparathyroidism, 41
motivation, 38
precipitating factors, 38
propranolol, 38
sexual interest, 40
short-term treatment, 37
signs, 37
stress, 39
treatment, 38
Orgasm inhibition
anorgasmia, total, 374–75
essential features: females, 373; males, 374
females and males, 373–77
treatment, 374, 375; anorgasmia, female
coital, 375; retarded ejaculation, 376
treatment goals, 374
Orgasmic conditioning, 357
Orientation, dementia, 19
Osler, William, 78
Outcome
delirium, 11
electroconvulsive therapy, schizophrenia,
161
exposure therapy, 246
maintenance treatment, schizophrenia,
158
milieu treatment, 150
psychotherapy, schizophrenia, 166
substance abuse, 137
tricyclics, 202
Oxazepam
delirium, 10
dementia, 21, 23
intermittent explosive disorder, 410
personality disorders, 441–43

Pain, 277
Panic attacks, 383
Panic disorder, 383
　caffeine, 133
　essential features, 258
Papaverine, dementia, 23
Paranoia, 173–74
　early treatment, 174
　essential features, 174
　symptoms, 174
Paranoid personality disorder, 429
Paranoid symptoms, dementia, 23
Paraphilias, 338, 364, 370
　atypical, 338
　aversion therapy, 342
　behavior therapy, 341
　electric aversion, 344
　essential features, 338
　homosexuality, ego-dystonic, 338, 361
　increasing heterosexuality, 356
　patient selection, 358
　psychotherapy, 340
　treatment, 340–44
　treatment controversies, 344
　treatment failures, 340
　treatment goals, 339
Parental bonds, gender identity disorder of
　childhood, 331
Passive-aggressive personality disorder, 429
Pathological gambling, 398–403
　behavior therapy, 399
　clinical course, 399–400
　crisis management, 400
　essential features, 403
　family therapy, 401
　Gamblers Anonymous, 399
　group therapy, 401
　inpatient programs, 399
　psychotherapy, 398–403
　somatic therapies, 403
　symptoms, 403
　vocational rehabilitation, 402
Pathological intoxication, 47
Patterns of use
　amphetamine, 94
　anticholinergics, 106
　cannabis, 114
　cocaine, 93
　hallucinogens, 114
　inhalants, 105
　opioids, 86
　phencyclidine, 99

PCP, 98
Pedophilia, 338, 344, 345
Pemoline, personality disorders, 444
Pentalenetetrazol, dementia, 23
Personality disorders, 429–54
　amphetamines, 444
　antidepressants, tricyclic, 444
　antisocial, 429; behavior therapy, 436;
　　psychotherapy, 430–39; transactional
　　analysis, 436, 437
　atypical, 429
　avoidant, 429
　borderline, 429; drug therapy, 447–48
　chlordiazepoxide, 441, 442
　classification, 429
　compulsive, 429
　dependent, 429; drug therapy, 448
　diazepam, 441, 442
　ECT, 448
　essential features, 429
　histrionic, 429
　meprobamate, 441
　mesoridazine, 444
　methylphenidate, 444
　mixed, 429
　mood swings, 446–47
　narcissistic, 429; drug therapy, 448
　oxazepam, 441, 442, 443
　paranoid, 429; drug therapy, 448
　passive-aggressive, 429
　pemoline, 444
　psychosurgery, 448–49
　psychotherapy, 429–30
　schizoid, 429
　schizotypal, 429; drug therapy, 448
　somatic therapies, 439–48; antianxiety
　　drugs, 440–43
　somatic therapy
　antianxiety drugs, 447
　anticonvulsants, 446
　lithium, 444–46, 447
　stimulants, 444
　substance abuse, 134
　symptoms, 429
　thioridazine, 443
Peyotl cactus, 114
Pharmacokinetics, aging, 22
Pharmacological classification
　abused substances, 82
　amphetamine, 80
　anticholinergics, 81
　caffeine, 81

cannabis, 81
cocaine, 80
hallucinogens, 81
inhalants, 80
opioids, 80
PCP, 80
substance abuse, 82
tobacco, 81
Phencyclidine, 98, 102
history, 98
patterns of use, 99
Phencyclidine intoxication, 100
acidification of urine, 101
complications, 102
death, 101
diazepam, 101
diazoxide, 101
haloperidol, 101
hydralazine, 101
hypertension, 101
management, 101
physical restraints, 101
symptoms, 100
Phenelzine, depression—single episode, 206
Phenobarbital, 62
Phentolamine, psychostimulant intoxication, 97
Phenytoin
alcohol withdrawal, 49
anticholinergics, 111
intermittent explosive disorder, 410, 413
polydrug abuse, 84
Phobias, 234–58
alcohol, 254
antidepressants, 250
behavior therapy, 235
benzodiazepines, 250
beta-blockers, 250
biofeedback, 246
carbon dioxide, 250
cognitive therapy, 245
controversies, 243
depression, 252
drug treatment, 250
dysmorphophobia, 299
homework, 238
hospitalization, 242
illness, 289, 297
imipramine, 252
medical disorders, 254
patient selection, 237, 253
specific treatment, 255

symptom substitution, 242
therapy instructions, 239
treatment goals, 235
Phobias—sexual, 383–84
Physical restraints, 84
alcohol intoxication, 45
anticholinergics, 110
inhalants, 103, 105
opioid intoxication, 89
phencyclidine intoxication, 101
psychostimulant intoxication, 98
sedative intoxication, 66
Physostigmine
contraindications, 110
Polydrug abuse, 84
activated charcoal, 84
apomorphine, 84
diagnosis, 83
gastric lavage, 84
glucose, 83
ipecac, 84
naloxone, 83
narcan, 83
phenytoin, 84
sodium sulfate, 84
sorbitol, 84
treatment, 82
withdrawal, 84
Polysurgery syndrome, 390
Post-traumatic stress disorder
abreaction, 260
essential features, 258
summary, 261
Premature ejaculation, 371, 372–73
essential features, 372
squeeze method, 373
stop-start method, 373
treatment, 372–73
Promethazine, dementia, 23
Propranolol, 413
anticholinergics, 111
hypochondriasis, 300
intermittent explosive disorder, 412, 414
organic personality syndrome, 38
schizophrenia, 163
Protriptyline, 487
depression—single episode, 203
hypersomnia, 487
Pseudodementia, 13
Psilicybe mexicana, 113
Psychoanalytic therapy
conversion disorder, 272

Psychoanalytic therapy *cont.*
dysthymic disorder, 217
psychosexual dysfunctions, 366
transsexualism, 326
transvestisim, 333
Psychobiological reactions, 419
Psychogenic amnesia, 309
Psychogenic fugue, 309
Psychogenic pain disorder, 277–86
antidepressant drugs, 284, 285
antipsychotics, 284
behavior therapy, 281
depression, 284
diabetic neuropathy, 284
ECT, 284
essential features, 277
group therapy, 281
individual psychotherapy, 279
inpatient treatment units, 281
multidisciplinary approach, 279
somatic treatment, 284
treatment, 279–85
treatment goals, 282
tricyclics, 284
Psychosexual dysfunctions, 365–86
antidepressant drugs, 369
behavior therapy, 368
causes, 366
conjoint insight psychotherapy, 368
individual insight therapy, 368
medications, 369
psychoanalytic therapy, 366
sex therapy, 368
treatment, 367–69; drugs, 385
treatment controversies, 385
treatment goals, 367
Psychosis, dementia, 20
Psychostimulant intoxication, 95–98
acidification urine, 97
ammonium chloride, 97
aspirin, 97
CPZ, 98
death, 95
depression, 98
diagnosis, 98
diazepam, 98
essential features, 95
haloperidol, 98
hospitalization, 98
hydration, 97
hyperpyrexia, 97

hypertension, 97
long-term therapy, 98
organic delusional syndrome, 95
phentolamine, 97
physical restraints, 98
tricyclic antidepressants, 98
Psychosurgery, 412–13
anxiety disorders, 260
intermittent explosive disorder, 413
personality disorders, 448–49
Psychotherapy, 405
adjustment disorders, 421–24
alcoholism, 53
anxiety states, 260
chronic factitious disorder with physical
symptoms, 392
dementia, 20
depression, 214, 226
depression—bipolar, 194
depression—single episode, 208
dissociative disorders, 311
dysthymic disorder, 213
enuresis, 494
gender identity disorder of childhood, 328
hypersomnia, 485
hypochondriasis, 290
insomnia, 480
intermittent explosive disorder, 409
kleptomania, 404–7
maintenance, depression, 211
mania, 192
narcolepsy, 484
night terrors, 491
nightmares, 493
paraphilias, 340
persistent hypersomnia, 487
personality disorders, 429
pyromania, 407
schizophrenia, 164
sleepwalking, 491
somatization disorder, 267
transsexualism, 322
treatment, sleep apnea, 488
Psychotic depression, 202
Pyromania, 405–8
behavior therapy, 406
essential features, 405
somatic therapies, 407

Rapid tranquilization, 155–57
chlorpromazine, 156

choice of drug, 156
dosage, 156
dystonic reactions, 156
haloperidol, 156
thiothixene, 156
Real life test, 321, 323, 324
Regressive electroconvulsive therapy, 162
Relaxation, exposure therapy, 247
Response prevention, obsessive-compulsive
disorder, 246
Rivea corymbose, 113

Satiation, exposure therapy, 242
Schizoaffective disorder, 227
Schizoid personality disorder, 429
Schizophrenia, 146–73
antipsychotics, 153–60; acute episodes,
154; introduction, 153; plasma levels,
170; side effects, 158; treatment failures,
170
behavior therapy, 169
beta-blockers, 163
brief hospital care, 153
chlorpromazine, 170
combined treatment, 167, 173
compliance, 170, 502, 505
controversies, 145
cost-benefit, 144
day care, 152
design-relevance scale, 146
diagnosis, 146
dialysis, 164
drug-free interval, 154
electroconvulsive therapy, 160; combined
with antipsychotics, 161; controlled
studies, 162; efficacy, 161
essential features, 173
extrapyramidal side effects, 170
family treatment, 167; intensity, 169
fluphenazine, 169
goals, 145
group treatment, 167
haloperidol, 170
home care, 152
inpatient milieu treatment, 153
intensive outpatient care, 152
maintenance treatment, 157–58; discontinuation, 158; efficacy, 158
milieu treatment, 148–51
negative symptoms, 173
observation, 146

ongoing evaluation, 144
optimal treatment, 145
outpatient after care, 153
positive symptoms, 173
propranolol, 163
psychotherapy, 164–69; effectiveness,
165; efficacy, 166; indications, 166; individual psychotherapy, 164; timing,
166
rapid tranquilization, 155
regressive electroconvulsive therapy, 162
relapse, 158
research and DSM-III, 145
signs, 173
sociotherapy, 166
summary of treatment plan, 170
symptoms, 173
treatment approach, 145
vitamins, 163
Schizophrenia, pseudoneurotic, 447–48
Schizophreniform disorder, 173; essential
features, 173
Schizotypal personality disorder, 429
Scopolamine, 106
insomnia, 479
Sedative abuse, 64
epidemiology, 64
essential features, 64
nutrition, 65
rehabilitation, 73; education evaluation,
74; group therapy, 74; medical evaluation, 74; other treatments, 74; psychiatric evaluation, 74; psychotherapy, 75;
self help groups, 74
Sedative dependence, essential features, 64
Sedative hypnotic drugs
insomnia, 481; transient, 478
Sedative intoxication, 64, 65, 66–67
alkalinization of urine, 66
death, 65
diuresis, 66
drug screen, 66
essential features, 64
glucose, 66
hemodialysis, 66
ipecac, 66
lethal dose, 65
mannitol, 66
naloxone, 66
narcan, 66
physical restraints, 66

Sedative intoxication *cont.*
sedative withdrawal, 66
short-term treatment, 64
signs, 64, 65
sorbitol, 66
stimulants, 66
transfusions, 66
treatment, 66
vasopressors, 66
ventilatory assistance, 66
Sedative withdrawal
barbiturate challenge test, 73
death, 62
delirium, 70; treatment, 72
precipitating factors, 69
symptoms, 68, 69
time course, 70
treatment, 70–73
Sedative-hypnotic drugs, 311; over the counter, 479
Sedatives, 65
history of, 62
nonbarbiturate: benzodiazepines, 63; chlordiazepoxide, 63; diazepam, 63; ethchlorvynol, 63; ethinamate, 63; glutethimide, 63; lorazepam, 63; meprobamate, 63; methaqualone, 63; methyprylon, 63; oxazepam, 63; pharmacology, 62
Seizures, alcohol withdrawal, 49
Selective perception, 290, 293
Self-control techniques, depression, 220
Self help, exposure therapy, 244
Self-regulation, 238, 354–56
homosexuality, ego-dystonic, 354
paraphilias, 354
Sensate focus, 375
Sensate focus I and II
functional dyspareunia, 384
inhibited sexual desire, 381
inhibited sexual excitement: female, 379; male, 378
Sensitization, covert, 342
Sex reassignment surgery, 321, 323–26
Sex role stereotyping, 327
Sex therapy, 366, 368–86
criteria for, 369–70
general approach, 370–72
psychosexual dysfunctions, 368
therapeutic tasks, 371–72
treatment controversies, 384–85

Sexual behaviors, unconventional, 339
Sexual desire, inhibited, 380
Sexual dysfunction, 339, 481
organic, 370
Sexual masochism, 338
Sexual phobias, 383
Sexual response, phases, 366
Sexual sadism, 338, 340
Shaping, 238
Shared paranoid disorder, 174–75
Short-term psychotherapy
depression, 218
dysthymic disorder, 218
Short-term treatment, alcohol intoxication, 44
alcohol withdrawal, 49
amnestic syndrome, 25
organic affective syndrome, 34
organic delusional treatment, 27
organic hallucinosis, 30
sedative abuse, 64
sedative intoxication, 64
Signs
acute paranoid disorder, 176
adjustment disorders, 419
agoraphobia, 234
alcohol intoxication, 44
alcohol withdrawal, 49
anticholinergics, 107
bereavement—uncomplicated, 459
caffeine intoxication, 133
caffeine withdrawal, 132
cannabis, 117
chronic factitious disorder with physical symptoms, 390
conversion disorder, 272
delirium, 4
depression—bipolar, 195
depression—single episode, 200
dissociative disorders, 309
dysthymic disorder, 213
factitious disorder with psychological symptoms, 387
functional dyspareunia, 384
functional vaginismus, 381
gender identity disorder of childhood, 326
generalized anxiety disorder, 258
hallucinogens, 115
homosexuality, ego-dystonic, 338
hypochondriasis, 286
inhibited sexual desire, 380

intermittent explosive disorder, 408
kleptomania, 403
malingering, 459
mania, 192
marital and family problems, 462
obsessive-compulsive disorder, 234
opioid intoxication, 87
opioid withdrawal, 91
organic affective syndrome, 34
organic delusional syndrome, 27
organic hallucinosis, 30
orgasm inhibition, 374
panic disorder, 258
pathological gambling, 403
personality disorders, 429
phencyclidine intoxication, 100
post-traumatic stress disorder, 258
premature ejaculation, 372
psychogenic pain disorder, 277
psychostimulant intoxication, 95
pyromania, 405
schizophrenic disorder, 173
schizophreniform disorder, 173
sedative abuse, 64
sedative intoxication, 64, 65
sedative withdrawal, 68, 69
shared paranoid disorder, 175
social phobia, 234
somatization disorder, 266
transsexualism, 320
transvestism, 332
Sinarest, 131
Sleep apnea, 475, 486, 487–88
chlorimipramine, 488
diaphragmatic pacing, 488
drug therapy, 488
imipramine, 488
medroxyprogesterone, 488
psychotherapy, 488
tracheostomy, 488
types, 487
vs. narcolepsy, 487
weight reduction, 488
Sleep attacks, 483
Sleep disorders, 475
classification, 473
enuresis, 493
hypersomnia, 485
insomnia, 475
narcolepsy, 474, 483
night terrors, 489

nightmares, 492
Sleep drunkenness, 486
Sleep paralysis, 483
Sleep–wake schedule disorders, 489
Sleepiness, excessive daytime, 485
Sleepwalking, 489–92
drug therapy, 491
imipramine, 492
personality profile, 490
psychotherapy, 490
safety measures, 490
Snoring, 488
Social phobia
essential features, 234
symptoms, 234
Social skills training, 341
depression, 219
substance abuse, 134
Sociopathic personality, 433
Sociotherapy, schizophrenia, 166
Sodium sulfate, polydrug abuse, 84
Somatic therapy
chronic factitious disorder with physical
symptoms, 391
conversion disorder, 275
dissociative disorders, 311
hypochondriasis, 300
kleptomania, 404
pathological gambling, 403
personality disorders, 440
psychogenic pain disorder, 284
pyromania, 407
somatization disorder, 270
Somatization disorder, 266
behavioral therapy, 268
ECT, 270
electrosleep, 270
essential features, 266
family therapy, 269
group therapy, 268
psychotherapy, 267
somatic therapy, 270
summary, 271
treatment controversies, 270
treatment goals, 266
Somatoform disorders, 266–308, 390
Somnambulism, 489
Sorbitol
polydrug abuse, 84
sedative intoxication, 66
Spouse beating, 469

Squeeze method, premature ejaculation, 373
Stimulant drugs
    cause of insomnia, 483
    dissociative disorders, 311
    hypersomnia, 486, 487
Stimulant intoxication, 95
Stimulants
    depression—single episode, 207
    intermittent explosive disorder, 410
    narcolepsy, 484
    sedative intoxication, 66
Stimulation, dementia, 19, 20
Stink weed, 106
Stop-start method, premature ejaculation, 373
STP, 116
Stramonium, 106
Stress
    dementia, 19
    organic personality syndrome, 39
Stress inoculation, 407, 409
Stressors, 420, 424–426
Substance abuse
    confrontation, 134
    detoxification, 137
    diagnosis, 134
    drug-free outpatient treatment, 136
    Gestalt therapy, 134
    group psychotherapy, 134
    individual psychotherapy, 134
    long-term treatment, 134
    methadone maintenance, 135
    opioid antagonists, 135
    outcome, 137
    personality disorders, 134
    pharmacological classification, 82
    social skills training, 134
    therapeutic communities, 136
    vocational training, 134
Substance disorders other than alcohol and
    barbiturates, 78–142
Succinylcholine, alcohol aversion, 53
Suicide risk, 201
Sullivan, theory of interpersonal maturity,
    437
Supportive psychotherapy
    anticholinergics, 111
    conversion disorder, 273
    depression, 221
Surgery, transsexualism, 322
Symptom substitution

obsessive-compulsive disorder, 242
    phobias, 242
Symptoms. *See* Signs; *individual disorders*
Systematic desensitization, 237

Tardive dyskinesia, 23, 158, 159, 443
Team approach, chronic factitious disorder
    with physical symptoms, 393
Teonanacatl mushroom, 113
Tetrahydrocannabinol, 117
Theobromine, 130
Theophylline, 130
Therapeutic communities, substance abuse,
    136
Therapy failures, exposure therapy, 237
Therapy instructions, phobias, 239
Thiamine, alcohol withdrawal delirium, 50
Thiamine deficiency, amnestic syndrome, 25
Thiamine—intravenous, delirium, 7
Thioridazine
    dementia, 23
    intermittent explosive disorder, 411, 412
    mania, 190
    personality disorders, 443
Thiothixene, rapid tranquilization, 156
Thought stopping, 241, 298
Tobacco, 120–127
    addiction, 123
    history, 127
    lobeline, 126
    management, 124
    medical risks, 123
    motivation, 126
    patterns of use, 121–22
    physician smoking, 127
    physiologic effects, 122
    psychological effects, 122
    therapies for stopping smoking, 125
    toxicity, 125
    treatment failures, 126
    withdrawal syndrome, 124
Transactional analysis, 436
Transfusions
    delirium, 7
    sedative intoxication, 66
Transient insomnia, 477
Transient situational disturbance, 420
Transsexualism, 320–26, 327, 341, 370
    aversion conditioning, 325
    behavioral, 325
    diagnosis, 320

essential features, 320
follow up, 324
hormones, 322
psychoanalytic therapy, 326
psychodynamics, 325–26
psychotherapy, 322
surgery, 322
surgical, 323
treatment, 321–23
treatment controversies, 323, 326
treatment goals, 320
Transvestism, 322, 324, 332–35, 340
aversion therapy, 333, 334
behavior therapy, 333
essential features, 332
females, 334
hormones, 335
inhibited sexual excitement, 334
psychoanalytic therapy, 333
social organizations, 333
symptoms, 332
treatment controversies, 334
treatment goals, 332
Tranylcypromine
borderline personality disorder, 447
depression—single episode, 206
insomnia, 483
Treatment compliance, 501
Treatment controversies
anxiety states, 261
gender identity disorder of childhood, 329
homosexuality, ego-dystonic, 356
paraphilias, 356
somatization disorder, 270
transsexualism, 326
transvestism, 334
Treatment goals
affective disorders, 185
anxiety disorders, 235
anxiety states, 259
conversion disorder, 272
depression—bipolar, 193
depression—single episode, 201
dissociation disorders, 310
homosexuality, ego-dystonic, 339
malingering, 459
mania, 192
marital and family problems, 464
obsessive-compulsive disorder, 235
orgasm inhibition, 374
paraphilias, 339

phobias, 235
psychogenic pain disorder, 282
psychosexual dysfunctions, 367
somatization disorder, 266
transsexualism, 320
transvestism, 332
Tricyclic antidepressants
depression—bipolar, 194
depression—single episode, 202
maintenance treatment, bipolar disorder, 198
organic affective syndrome, 36
psychostimulant intoxication, 98
Tricyclics
antidepressant drugs, 482
choice of drug, 203
dosage, 204
efficacy, 202
imipramine, 203
mechanism of action, 203
outcome, 202
plasma levels, 203
psychogenic pain disorder, 284
Trifluoperazine, borderline, 447
Tybamate, 276

Uncomplicated bereavement, 459

Vaginismus, 381
Vasodilators, dementia, 23
Vasopressors, sedative intoxication, 66
Ventilatory assistance, sedative intoxication, 66
Violence, domestic, 469
Vitamins, alcohol withdrawal delirium, 50
schizophrenia, 163
Vivarin, 131
Vocational rehabilitation, pathological gambling, 402
Vocational training, substance abuse, 134
Vorbeigehen, 387
Voyeurism, 338

Weight reduction, sleep apnea, 488
Wernicke-Korsakoff syndrome, 7, 26, 50
Wife beating, 469
Wilson's disease, 40
Women
affective disorder, 215–217
dysthymic disorder, 215

Zoophilia, 338

Author Index

Abeles, M., 310, 314
Abrams, G. M., 148
Abrams, R., 161
Adam, G., 290
Adam, K., 481
Adams, I. H., 161
Adams, R. D., 47, 48, 49
Adams, S., 432
Adesso, V. J., 357
Aduan, R. P., 390, 391, 393
Aggeler, P. M., 392
Agras, W. S., 354, 357
Akil, H., 85
Akimoto, H., 484
Akiskal, H. S., 213, 226
Akman, D. D., 431
Alban, J., 275
Allison, B., 314
Anderson, W., 74
Andreasen, N.C., 420, 422, 424, 426
Appley, J., 291
Arky, R. A., 51
Asberg, M., 204
Asher, R., 390
Atsmon, A., 163
Aubry, W. E., 399
Awad, G. A., 405
Ayd, F. J., 92, 93, 112–14, 508
Azrin, N. H., 405

Baekeland, F., 502
Baker, A. A., 160, 161, 162
Bakwin, H., 494
Baldessarini, R. J., 192
Ballenger, J. C., 199
Ban, T. A., 163
Bancroft, J. H. J., 344, 346, 354
Baptiste, S., 281
Barber, T. X., 295
Barker, J. C., 398

Barlow, D., 325
Barlow, D. H., 341, 351, 354, 357
Barnes, R. J., 443
Barofsky, I., 501, 502
Barr, R. F., 344, 354, 357
Bartlett, J. R., 412, 449
Baughn, C., 167
Beal, E. W., 313
Bear, D. M., 40
Beck, A. T., 292, 298
Beech, H. R., 354
Beels, C., 223
Beker, J., 438
Bellak, L., 166, 275
Benjamin, H., 323
Benjamin, L. B., 185, 247
Benjamin, S., 247
Benson, D. F., 25, 39
Bentler, P., 332
Benvenuto, J. A., 66, 67
Berger, P. A., 78, 111–42
Bergin, A. E., 354, 356
Bergler, E., 398
Berlin, L., 431
Berney, T. P., 390, 391
Bernstein, S., 479
Bespalec, D. A., 125, 126
Bianchi, G. N., 288
Bibb, R. C., 270
Bick, E. C., 130, 131, 132
Biggs, J. T., 22, 508
Billings, C. K., 388
Bini, L., 160
Birk, L., 347, 354
Bishop, M. P., 146, 150
Bixler, E. O., 479
Blackwell, B., 92, 93, 112–14, 501–16
Blaine, J. D., 135
Bleuler, M., 165
Blitch, J. W., 357

Blum, E. M., 53
Blum, I., 163
Blum, R. H., 53
Blumenthal, R., 153
Blumer, D., 28, 39, 40, 279, 280
Boelhouwer, C., 412
Bogoch, S., 410
Bolen, D. W., 398
Bond, D. D., 260
Bond, I. K., 356
Bothwell, S., 225
Bowers, M. B., 203
Bowers, M. K., 313, 314, 317
Boyd, D. A., 284
Boyd, W. H., 398
Bracha, S., 161
Braiman, A., 387, 388
Branconnier, R., 24
Brandsma, J. M., 314
Bratfos, O., 276
Brecher, E. M., 85, 92, 120, 124, 128, 130–32
Brehm, M. L., 102–5
Brenner, I., 37
Bridges, P. K., 412, 449
Brill, N. O., 162
Brinkley, J. R., 447
Brody, S., 268, 269
Bronzo, A., 288
Brougham, L., 243
Broughton, R., 486, 489, 492
Broverman, I. K., 217
Brown, F., 301
Brown, G. W., 152, 167, 169
Brown, W. A., 35
Brust, J. C. M., 32
Budzynski, T. H., 299
Buie, D. H., 215
Bulson, R. D., 501, 502
Burns, B. H., 287, 295

Cade, R., 164
Caffey, E. M., 151, 153
Callahan, E. J., 351, 505
Calvert, E. J., 509
Canton-Dutari, A., 355
Carkuff, R. R., 293, 405
Carney, M. W. P., 503
Carroll, B. J., 35, 202, 448
Carroll, R. S., 150
Carter, A. B., 272, 274
Cassem, E. H., 391

Cassidy, W. L., 52
Castelnuovo-Tesesco, P., 404
Caudill, W. A., 148
Cautela, J. R., 357, 406
Centerwell, B. S., 10, 26
Cerletti, U., 160
Chappell, M. N., 291
Charney, E., 511
Chaudhary, N. A., 287
Chesler, P., 216
Childers, R. T., 161
Church, M. W., 478, 482
Claghorn, J. L., 168
Clancy, J., 53
Clark, M. L., 150
Clayton, P. J., 460, 461
Cliffe, M. J., 170
Cobb, J., 246
Cody, J., 505
Cohen, S., 82, 94, 99, 101–5, 114, 120, 121, 123, 126
Cohen, S. I., 35
Cole, J. O., 24, 154, 163, 202, 300, 447
Collins, W. F., 284
Colter, S. B., 399
Combs, G., 309–19
Connelly, F. H., 300
Conners, C. K., 411, 444
Coogler, G. J., 468
Cooper, T. B., 172
Cope, R. L., 295
Coppen, A., 203, 210, 507
Coursey, R. D., 476
Covi, L., 223, 441
Craft, M., 433, 439
Cramer, B., 390
Criqui, J. H., 10, 26
Critchley, M., 486
Cumming, E., 148
Cumming, J., 148
Custer, R. L., 399, 400–2

Dalby, M. A., 411
Daly, D. D., 484, 485
Danziger, L., 160
Davenport, Y., 200
Davis, J. M., 66, 67, 154, 157, 187, 190, 198, 212
Davis, P., 491
Dement, W. C., 484, 485, 486, 487
Denholtz, M. S., 405

Denko, J. D., 41
DesLauriers, A., 166
Detre, T. P., 3, 486
Deykin, E., 506, 507
Dickes, R. A., 274
DiMascio, A., 209, 218, 441, 505, 507
Ditman, K. S., 53, 494
Donlon, P. T., 155
Downing, R. W., 441
Drapsa, L. J., 291
Dreyfus, J., 410
Dumpson, J. R., 431
Duncan, G. W., 5, 26
Dunn, M. J., 78–142
Dupont, R. L., 88, 89
Duthie, A. M., 284
Dysken, M. W., 315

Eisenberg, L., 444
Ellinwood, E. H., 95–98
Elliott, F. A., 412–14
Ellis, A., 401, 406
Emmelkamp, P. G., 243, 246
Enelow, A. J., 218
Engel, G. L., 279, 461
Enoch, M. D., 387, 389, 390
Entwistle, C., 187, 190
Erickson, E. K. E., 421
Essig, C. F., 72
Evans, P. R., 288
Exner, J. E., 162
Experanca, M., 494

Fairweather, G. W., 151
Falk, W. E., 9, 36
Fedeo, P., 40
Feer, H., 164
Feldman, M. P., 345, 349, 353, 354
Feldman, P. E., 441
Fenichel, O., 272, 273
Ferber, A., 223
Ferebee, S. H., 502
Fieve, R., 191
Fink, M., 161, 192, 208, 448
Fisher, C., 489, 491, 492
Flemenbaum, A., 213
Fleming, M., 325
Fogelson, D. L., 164
Ford, C. V., 391
Fordyce, W. E., 281, 283
Foster, M. W., 161

Frankel, F. H., 275
Franz, D. N., 67
Fras, I., 392
Fraser, H. F., 68, 69, 73
Freedman, N., 149
Freeman, H., 502, 503
Freeman, T., 150
Frei, D., 353
Freinkel, N., 51
Freud, S., 92, 365
Friedman, M. J., 148
Fuchs, C. Z., 220
Fuller, M., 328

Gaitz, Z. M., 161
Gall, C., 312, 314, 315
Gallant, D. M., 146, 150, 227
Gallemore, J. L., 213
Gardos, G., 441
Gastaut, H., 489, 492
Gayle, R. F., 161
Gelder, M., 333, 354
Gerard, D. L., 54, 58
Gerbino, L., 191, 194, 198, 199
Gerrard, J. W., 494
Getto, C. J., 277–86, 455–72
Gibson, J. G., 287
Ginsberg, G., 192
Gipson, M., 300
Glasman, D. H., 202
Glasser, W., 434
Glatt, M. M., 52
Glen, A., 399, 400
Gleser, G. C., 441
Glick, B. S., 506, 507
Glick, I. D., 151
Glithero, E., 272
Glueck, B. C., 162
Gold, S., 354
Goldberg, A., 148
Goldberg, S. C., 148, 153, 166, 502, 503
Goldfrank, L., 106, 107, 109, 110, 111
Goldin, S., 387, 389
Goldstein, A. P., 431
Goldstein, M. J., 168, 412, 503
Goodwin, D. W., 44, 45, 52, 59–61, 203, 267
Goorney, A. B., 398
Gottlieb, J. S., 162
Gottschalk, L. A., 411
Gough, H. G., 288
Grad, J., 152

Graham, D. M., 129, 130, 132
Granacher, R. P., 107, 109–111
Grant, D. J., 432
Grant, J. D., 432, 438
Grant, M. Q., 432, 438
Greden, J. F., 133
Green, A. I., 135
Green, R., 320–37
Greenblatt, D. J., 11, 21, 63, 65, 73, 84, 88, 89, 117, 118, 478
Greenblatt, M., 151, 161, 162, 165, 166
Greene, M. H., 88, 89
Greenson, R., 328
Greist, J. H., 191, 192, 198, 201, 203, 205, 207, 244, 419–28
Greist, T. H., 201, 205, 207
Grinspoon, L., 161
Gritz, E. R., 120, 122, 123, 125
Groen, J. J., 297
Gruenwald, D., 313, 314
Guidry, L. S., 399, 406
Guillenminault, C., 486, 488
Gurman, A. S., 186, 216, 224, 463, 466, 470
Guze, S. B., 52, 267, 270

Haase, H. J., 170
Hackett, T. P., 457
Hadley, S. W., 260
Hafner, J., 247
Hahn, K. W., 295
Halberstam, M., 511
Hale, B., 291
Hallam, R., 353
Hallgren, B., 494
Hamilton, M., 151
Hanback, J. W., 290
Hanlon, T., 208
Hanson, R. W., 357
Harris, L. S., 115–117
Harrison, S. I., 405
Hartmann, E., 493
Harvey, S. C., 62, 65, 73
Haskell, D. S., 202
Hay, G. G., 300
Hayes, S. N., 357
Hayes, T. A., 495
Haynes, R. B., 501
Heath, R. G., 357
Hedberg, D. L., 447
Hellman, R., 321
Henderson, J. G., 29

Hendler, N., 281
Herman, E., 281
Herz, M. I., 151, 152
Hes, J. P., 161
Heyman, D. S., 438
Hilgard, E. R., 295
Hill, D., 444
Himmelhoch, J. M., 194
Hishikawa, Y., 484
Hitchcock, E. R., 449
Hoenck, P. R., 422, 426
Hoffman, H. L., 486
Hofmann, F. G., 63, 65, 70
Hogan, B. K., 223
Hogan, P., 223
Hogarty, G. E., 153, 166, 167
Hollister, L. E., 69, 72, 101, 114, 115, 156, 205, 508
Hollon, S. D., 219, 220
Holmes, T. H., 461
Holzman, P. S., 215, 218
Hope, J. M., 48
Huff, F. W., 356
Hunt, W. A., 125, 126
Hunter, R., 3
Huston, P. E., 162
Hutchinson, H. C., 356

Ifabumuyi, O. I., 31, 32
Ireland, P., 391
Isbell, H., 48, 68
Itil, T. M., 411

Jacobson, A., 184–233, 489
Jaffee, J. H., 121–26
James, W., 57
Jamieson, R. C., 22
Jannoun, L., 244–46
Janowsky, D. S., 484
Jarecki, H. G., 3
Jarvik, M. E., 120–26
Jasinski, D. R., 136
Jefferson, J. W., 191, 192, 198, 203, 207, 387–97
Jeffries, J. J., 31, 32
Jesness, C. F., 405, 436, 438
Johnson, D. A. W., 502, 503, 506
Johnson, F. N., 191, 192
Johnson, L. C., 478, 482
Johnson, V., 366
Johnson, W. F., 432

Johnston, D. W., 243
Jones, E., 236
Jones, H. G., 169, 170
Jones, I. H., 353
Jones, M. C., 52, 169
Justus, P. G., 390

Kaelbing, R., 41
Kales, A., 473–500
Kales, J. D., 473–500
Kalinowski, L. B., 160–62
Kanner, L., 492, 494
Kantor, S. J., 202
Kaplan, H. S., 365–86
Karacan, I., 477, 483
Kaslow, F. W., 468, 470
Kass, D. J., 268
Kaufman, I., 405
Kellam, A. M. P., 404
Kellner, R., 286–88, 291, 294, 295–303, 398, 400–18, 429–54
Kendwall, J. A., 160
Kennedy, A., 310–14
Kenyon, F. E., 287, 301
Kessler, K., 202, 204
Keutzer, C. S., 404
Khantziam, E. J., 72
Kiersch, T. A., 310, 314, 315
King, P., 161
Kino, F. F., 161
Kinsey, A. C., 365
Kissin, B., 135
Klein, D. F., 148, 160, 227, 253, 383, 443, 447
Klein, M. H., 185, 186, 216, 217
Klein, R. F., 280
Klerman, G. L., 37, 198, 199, 202, 210, 212
Kline, N. S., 54
Klotz, U., 21
Kniskern, D. P., 224, 463, 466, 470
Kolb, D. A., 436
Kolvin, I., 342
Korey, S. R., 444
Kornblith, S. J., 219
Kraft, T., 356
Kramer, A. S., 402
Krauthammer, C., 37
Krieger, D. T., 35
Krug, C. M., 398
Kuipers, A. C. M., 243

Kumar, K., 298
Kupfer, D. J., 486

Lacey, J. I., 290, 292
Ladee, G. A., 287, 301
Lader, M., 260
Landon, P. B., 431
Langsley, D. G., 161
Laub, D., 323, 324
Lazarus, A. A., 274
Leff, J. P., 167, 169, 503
Leff, R., 479
Lefkowitz, M. M., 411
Lehmann, H. E., 163
Leigh, D., 38
Leitenberg, H., 351
Lentz, R. J., 149, 169
Letermendia, F. J. J., 150
Levenson, H. S., 130, 131, 132
Levine, B., 222
Lewinsohn, P. M., 219
Lewis, N., 405
Ley, P., 292, 509
Lezak, M. D., 40
Liebowitz, M. R., 227
Liebson, I., 274
Lindemann, E., 459
Lindsay, P. G., 284
Lindstrom, H. H., 163
Ling, W., 135, 163
Linn, M. W., 152, 153
Lion, J. R., 409, 442, 443
Lipman, R. S., 511
Lipowski, Z. J., 11
Liskow, B., 62–77
Ljunberg, L., 272
Lloyd, C., 424
Looney, J. G., 421
LoPiccolo, J., 356
Lorr, M., 441
Lovaas, O., 328
Ludwig, A. M., 151, 309–19
Lugaresi, E., 486, 488
Lundwall, L., 502
Lutkins, S. G., 461

MacCulloch, M. J., 345, 349, 353, 354
MacDonald, J. E., 387, 389
Mace, J., 133
Macht, J. E., 407
Macht, L. B., 407

Mahender, R. A., 91
Main, T. F., 148
Malan, D. H., 218, 219
Maltsberger, A. T., 215
Malyou, A. K., 281
Mandel, 202
Mandel, M. R., 202, 203
Marks, I. M., 192, 298, 333, 338–64, 425
Marks, P. A., 475
Marmor, J., 273
Martin, P. A., 463
Martin, W. R., 86
Marzagao, L. R., 404
Mascia, G. V., 402
Masnik, R., 505
Mason, A. S., 503
Massimo, J. L., 435
Masters, W., 366
Mathews, A. M., 245, 247
Mawson, D., 252, 261
May, P. R. A., 143–83
Mayfield, D. G., 52
Mayou, R., 287, 295
McConaghy, N., 344, 354, 357
McCord, J., 52, 431
McCord, W., 52, 431
McCrady, B. S., 225, 463
McDonald, R., 244
McDonald, R. L., 441
McEvoy, J. P., 3–43
McKenna, G. J., 72
McKinney, W. T., 184–233
McNair, D. M., 441
McPherson, F. M., 243
Meichenbaum, D., 292, 298, 406, 407, 409
Meliek, M., 106, 107, 109–11
Meltzoff, J., 153
Mendel, J. B., 391
Mendelson, J. H., 51
Menninger, K. A., 215, 218
Merry, J., 54
Merskey, H. A., 288
Meyer, H. J., 435
Meyer, J. K., 324
Meyer, R. E., 115–17, 136
Meyer, R. F., 135
Meyer, V., 404
Michaux, W. W., 511
Miller, A. I., 46
Miller, D. H., 162
Miller, M., 398

Miller, P. R., 494
Milligan, W. L., 275, 284
Milman, D. H., 444
Mindham, R. S., 210
Minkoff, K., 412
Minter, R. E., 202, 203
Minuchin, S., 269
Mirin, S. M., 135, 136
Mitchell-Heggs, N., 449
Moan, C. E., 357
Modlin, C., 175
Molling, P. A., 443
Money, J., 321
Monkenmoeller, X., 407
Monroe, L. J., 476
Monroe, R. R., 411, 413
Montgomery, I., 481
Moodie, J. L., 365–86
Moore, D. M., 470
Moore, D. P., 11
Moran, E., 399
Morgenstern, F. S., 354
Morrison, J. R., 412
Mullaney, J. A., 254
Mullen, E. J., 431
Mumford, P. R., 274
Munby, M., 243
Munro, A., 300
Murillo, L. G., 162
Myers, E. D., 509

Nadelson, T., 391–94
Naples, M., 457
Neil, J. F., 133
Nelson, A. A., 504
Nelson, C., 203
Neufeld, H., 354
Neville, J., 310–14
Nichols, M. A., 288, 295
Nicklin, G., 164
Novaco, R. W., 409, 413
Nunes, J., 246

O'Brian, C. P., 168
O'Reilly, R. A., 392
O'Donnell, J. M., 298
Ochitill, H., 266–86, 387–97
Ogata, M., 51
Okasha, H., 284
Okuma, T., 199

Oppendahl, M. C., 99, 100, 101
Oswald, I., 478, 482

Palmer, T. B., 437
Paolino, T. J., 225, 463
Pardes, H., 148
Parfitt, D. N., 312, 314, 315
Parkes, C. M., 459, 461
Parry, H. J., 64
Pasamanick, B., 152
Pathy, M. S., 7
Pattison, E. M., 57
Paul, G. L., 149, 169
Pauly, I., 324
Paykel, E. S., 215
Pelser, H. E., 297
Perley, M. J., 267, 270
Person, E., 163
Persons, R. W., 433, 434
Pesikoff, R., 491
Peters, J., 270
Petersen, R. C., 94, 96, 99, 100–2
Peterson, P., 40
Piercy, M., 216
Pilowsky, I., 288, 295
Pinsky, J. J., 278, 281
Pittel, S. M., 99–102
Platman, S., 188
Polack, R. P., 460, 461
Post, F., 174, 199
Pouissaint, A. F., 494
Powers, E., 431
Powers, G., 288
Prien, R., 189, 191, 198, 211, 212
Prince, V., 332

Quitkin, F. M., 148, 202, 210, 212

Rabavilas, A. D., 243
Rachlin, H. L., 161
Rachman, S., 354
Rada, R. T., 440
Radley, J. J., 285
Raphael, B., 261, 299
Rappaport, J. A., 246
Raskind, M., 174
Rechtschaffen, A., 484–87
Rees, L., 187, 190
Rees, W. D., 461
Rehm, L. P., 219, 220
Reich, T. C., 9

Rekers, G., 328, 330
Resnick, R. B., 136
Reter, D. J., 324
Retterstol, M., 174, 175
Revelle, W., 290
Rickels, K., 300, 441
Riddell, S. A., 160–62
Riding, J., 300
Rieger, W., 388
Ries, R. K., 391
Rifkin, A., 447
Rimm, D. C., 408, 413
Risch, S. C., 22
Rizzo, A. E., 411
Roberts, R. K., 21
Robertson, J. R., 246, 404
Robins, E., 331
Robinson, A. M., 505
Robinson, D. S., 206, 227
Roman, P. M., 58
Rooth, F. G., 354
Rosen, I., 340
Rosenberg, S., 291
Ross, M. W., 341
Roth, B., 486, 487
Roth, M., 174
Rubenfeld, S., 437
Rubin, B., 148
Ruesch, J., 290
Rumans, L. W., 390
Rush, A. J., 221
Russ, D., 493
Russell, M. A. H., 125, 126

Sacher, E. J., 36
Sackett, D. I., 501
Saenger, G., 54, 58
Saghir, M., 331
Sainsbury, P., 152, 287
Salzman, C., 161, 481
Sands, D. E., 275, 284
Sarason, I. G., 436
Sargent, W., 310, 311
Sarno, J. E., 291, 295
Satterfield, S., 324
Scallet, A., 270
Scarf, M., 215
Schachter, S., 292
Schapira, K., 297
Schatzberg, A. F., 447
Schilder, P., 310, 314

Schuckit, M., 52
Schulz, S. C., 164
Schuyler, D., 221
Schwartz, M. S., 148
Schwitzgebl, R., 436
Seager, C. P., 398
Segal, D. S., 484
Sells, S. B., 136, 137
Seltzer, B., 3, 12
Serber, M., 352, 357
Shader, R. I., 11, 21, 63–65, 73, 84, 88, 89, 109, 117, 118, 478, 505
Shafer, D., 494
Shaffer, J. W., 410
Shahar, A., 341
Shakir, S. A., 510
Shapiro, A. K., 295
Sharp, C. W., 102–5
Sheard, M. H., 444, 445
Sheehan, D. V., 251
Sheffield, B. F., 287, 288, 294, 295, 503
Shelley, E. L. V., 432
Sherwin, D., 284
Sherwin, I., 3, 12
Shiomi, K., 288
Shoor, M., 161
Shopsin, B., 188–91
Shore, M. F., 435
Showstack, N., 431
Shuey, I., 35
Shull, H. J., 11, 21
Siegel, P. V., 489
Sifneos, P., 218
Sigell, L. T., 104
Sim, M., 389
Simmel, E., 148
Simpson, G. M., 143–83, 227
Singer, J. C., 292
Skoichet, R. P., 457
Skoloda, T. E., 58
Slater, E. T., 272, 310, 311
Slavson, S. R., 268
Slipp, S., 223
Smith, A. B., 431
Smith, D. I., 71
Smith, J. A., 148
Smith, K., 161
Snyder, S. H., 95
Soldatos, C. R., 473–500
Solomon, K., 442
Sours, J. A., 486

Spadoni, A. J., 148
Spear, F. G., 288, 295
Spellman, M. S., 292
Sperling, M., 328
Spiro, H. R., 391
Squire, L. R., 208
Stalstrom, O. W., 341
Stampfl, T. C., 247
Stanton, A. H., 148
Starfield, B., 494
Stein, A., 222
Stein, L. I., 152
Stein, N., 431
Stephens, J. H., 410
Stern, R. S., 242, 243
Stern, T. A., 391
Stevenson, I., 356, 357
Stevenson, T. I., 291
Stillman, R. C., 94, 96, 99, 100–2
Stillner, V., 132
Stoller, R., 333, 335
Stone, A. R., 267, 291
Stone, M. H., 391, 393
Stone, W. N., 511
Strachan, R. W., 29
Stravynski, A., 341
Strohl, K. P., 488
Strupp, H. H., 260
Stumphauzer, J. S., 404
Suedfeld, P., 431
Sullivan, C., 437
Sullivan, H. S., 148
Summers, W. K., 9

Taber, J. I., 399, 401, 402
Tan, E., 260
Tanner, B. A., 349
Taub, A., 284
Tec, L., 491
Tennant, F. S., 73
Tennent, T. G., 407
Tepperman, J. H., 398
Test, M. A., 152
Thomas, K. B., 295
Thoren, P., 251, 252
Thornton, B. P., 29
Thornton, W. E., 29
Thorpe, F. T., 161
Tilkian, A. G., 488
Tinklenberg, J. R., 79, 82–84, 86–92, 95–98, 107, 109, 110, 114–20, 134, 135

'OUR

VE **Date Due**

Tinling, D. C., 280
Tourney, G., 160
Treffert, D. A., 150
Trice, H. M., 58
Trippett, C. J., 254
Troupin, A. S., 40
Truax, C. B., 293, 405, 434, 435
Truelove, S. C., 287
Tsoi, W. F., 389
Tuma, A. H., 155, 162
Tupin, J. P., 445
Turek, I., 208
Turkington, R. W., 284
Tyndel, M., 389

Uhlenhuth, E. H., 294

Vachon, M. L. S., 460
Valko, R. J., 269
Van Putten, T., 146, 148, 275, 504, 505, 510
Vaughn, C., 167, 169
Vaughn, C. E., 503
Victor, M., 47, 48–50
Victor, R. G., 398
Vilkin, M. I., 447
Voegtlin, W. L., 53
Vosti, K. L., 390

Wagemaker, H., 164
Walberg, L. R., 457
Walinder, J., 324
Walter, C. J., 275
Walters, A., 280
Ward, N. G., 340
Wargo, D. G., 293, 435
Warren, M. Q., 437
Watson, J. P., 243
Weber, J. J., 273
Weeks, H. A., 433
Weil, A., 78

We...
Wei....,......
Weiss, G., 439, 444
Weissman, M. M., 215, 218, 225
Weitzman, E., 489
Wells, C. E., 3–43
Werner, W., 510
Wesson, D. R., 71
Wheeler, E. O., 290
Whitlock, F. A., 387, 388, 389
Wikler, A., 70, 135
Wilkinson, J. C. M., 298
Williams, L. W., 246
Wilmer, H. A., 148
Wilson, W. P., 213
Wing, J. K., 152
Winstead, D. K., 133, 511
Wise, S. P., 411
Wisocki, P. A., 357
Witmer, H. L., 431
Wolpe, J., 356, 357, 383, 406
Wood, D. R., 444
Wooley, S. C., 299
Wulff, M. H., 73
Wyckoff, M., 284
Wynne, L. C., 421

Yalom, I., 222, 268
Yarnell, H., 405
Yassa, R., 391
Yerevanian, B. I., 226
Yorkston, N., 163
Yoss, R. F., 483, 484, 485

Zarcone, V., 484, 486
Zavitzianos, G., 404
Zeifert, M., 161
Zetzel, E. R., 273
Ziegler, V. E., 22, 280
Zitrin, C. M., 251, 252, 383

DRAKE MEMORIAL LIBRARY
WITHDRAWN
THE COLLEGE AT BROCKPORT